Evidence-based Implant Treatment Planning and Clinical Protocols

Dedication

To my wife, Francine, who has modeled enduring love, patience, and an indefatigable positive attitude, and to my children, Elon and Tess, who have inspired me by their commitment to make a difference in the lives of others, and to my granddaughter, Ella, whose curiosity and laughter are without bounds.

Evidence-based Implant Treatment Planning and Clinical Protocols

Edited by

Steven J. Sadowsky, DDS

Professor
University of the Pacific Arthur A. Dugoni School of Dentistry
San Francisco, California, USA

WILEY Blackwell

Editorial Offices
1606 Golden Aspen Drive, Suites 103 and 104, Ames, Iowa 50010, USA
The Atrium, Southern Gate, Chichester, West Sussex, PO19 8SQ, UK
9600 Garsington Road, Oxford, OX4 2DQ, UK

For details of our global editorial offices, for customer services and for information about how to apply for permission to reuse the copyright material in this book please see our website at www.wiley.com/wiley-blackwell.

Library of Congress Cataloging-in-Publication data are available

ISBN: 9781119080039

A catalogue record for this book is available from the British Library.

Wiley also publishes its books in a variety of electronic formats. Some content that appears in print may not be available in electronic books.

Cover images courtesy of Steven J. Sadowsky.

Set in 9.5/12pt Minion by SPi Global, Pondicherry, India

Printed and bound in Singapore by Markono Print Media Pte Ltd

2 2018

Contents

Contributors

Sandra Al-Tarawneh DDS, MS
Assistant Professor
University of Jordan
Amman, Jordan

Sun-Yung Bak DDS
Clinical Assistant Professor
University of North Carolina
Chapel Hill School of Dentistry
Chapel Hill, North Carolina, USA

John Beumer III DDS, MS
Distinguished Professor Emeritus
University of California
Los Angeles School of Dentistry
Los Angeles, California, USA

Avinash S. Bidra BDS, MS
Associate Professor
University of Connecticut School of Dental Medicine
Farmington, Connecticut, USA

S. Andrew Chapokas DMD, MS
San Diego, California, USA

Donald A. Curtis DMD
Professor
University of California
San Francisco, California, USA

Gary R. Goldstein DDS
Professor
New York University College of Dentistry
New York, New York, USA

David G. Gratton DDS, MS
Associate Professor
University of Iowa College of Dentistry
Iowa City, Iowa, USA

Paul B. Greenawalt DDS
Private Practice in Oral and Maxillofacial Surgery
Poulsbo, Washington, USA

W. Peter Hansen DDS
Associate Professor
University of the Pacific Arthur A. Dugoni School of Dentistry
San Francisco, California, USA

Elena Hernandez-Kucey RDH, DDS
Private Practice in General Dentistry
Edmonton, Alberta, Canada

Jay Jayanetti DDS
Assistant Clinical Professor
University of California
Los Angeles School of Dentistry
Los Angeles, California, USA

Parag R. Kachalia DDS
Associate Professor
University of the Pacific Arthur A. Dugoni School of Dentistry
San Francisco, California, USA

Joseph Y.K. Kan DDS, MS
Professor
Loma Linda University School of Dentistry
Loma Linda, California, USA

Mathew T. Kattadiyil BDS, MDS, MS
Professor
Loma Linda University School of Dentistry
Loma Linda, California, USA

James A. Kelly DDS, MS, MBA
Assistant Clinical Professor
Mayo Clinic College of Medicine
Rochester, Minnesota, USA

Sreenivas Koka DDS, MS, PhD, MBA
Professor
Loma Linda University School of Dentistry
Loma Linda, California, USA

Brian Kucey DDS, MSEd
Private Practice in Prosthodontics
Edmonton, Alberta, Canada

Howard M. Landesman DDS, MEd
Professor Emeritus
University of Colorado School of Dental Medicine
and Herman Ostrow School of Dentistry
University of Southern California
Encino, California, USA

Hamilton Le DMD
Private Practice in Prosthodontics
Torrance, California, USA

Jaime L. Lozada DMD
Professor
Loma Linda University School of Dentistry
Loma Linda, California, USA

Karl Lyons MDS, PhD
Professor
Faculty of Dentistry
University of Otago
Dunedin, New Zealand

Glenn E. Minsley DMD
Associate Professor
University of North Carolina
Chapel Hill School of Dentistry
Chapel Hill, North Carolina, USA

Anders Nattestad DDS, PhD
Professor
University of the Pacific Arthur A. Dugoni School of Dentistry
San Francisco, California, USA

Harold Preiskel MDS, MSc
Emeritus Professor
King's College London Dental Institute
London, UK

Kitichai Rungcharassaeng DDS, MS
Professor
Loma Linda University School of Dentistry
Loma Linda, California, USA

Steven J. Sadowsky DDS
Professor
University of the Pacific Arthur A. Dugoni School of Dentistry
San Francisco, California, USA

Thomas J. Salinas DDS
Professor
Mayo Clinic College of Medicine
Rochester, Minnesota, USA

Kumar C. Shah BDS, MS
Associate Clinical Professor
University of California Los Angeles
School of Dentistry
Los Angeles, California, USA

Clark M. Stanford DDS, PhD
Professor
University of Illinois at Chicago
College of Dentistry
Chicago, Illinois, USA

Eric C. Sung DDS
Professor
University of California Los Angeles School of Dentistry
Los Angeles, California, USA

Thomas D. Taylor DDS, MSD
Professor
University of Connecticut School of Dental Medicine
Farmington, Connecticut, USA

Ghadeer Thalji DDS, PhD
Assistant Professor
University of Illinois at Chicago
College of Dentistry
Chicago, Illinois, USA

Istvan Urban DMD, MS, PhD
Associate Professor
University of Szeged
Hungary

Chandur P.K. Wadhwani BDS, MSD
Adjunct Assistant Professor
Loma Linda University School of Dentistry
Loma Linda, California, USA

Robert Ferguson Wright DDS
Professor
University of North Carolina
Chapel Hill School of Dentistry
Chapel Hill, North Carolina, USA

Roy T. Yanase DDS
Clinical Professor
Herman Ostrow School of Dentistry
University of Southern California
Los Angeles, California, USA

George Zarb DDS, MS
Professor Emeritus
University of Toronto Faculty of Dentistry
Toronto, Ontario, Canada

Nicola U. Zitzmann DDS, PhD
Professor
Clinic for Periodontology, Endodontology and Cariology
School of Dental Medicine
University of Basel
Switzerland

Foreword

The 1982 North American introduction of the Osseointegration technique raised expectations for dental treatment outcome standards. It was catalyzed by the ingenious surgical implant protocol described by PI Branemark that readily synergized with available prosthodontic ones. It also virtually coincided with the late David Sackett's introduction of the "clinical science of evidence-based medicine", contributing to exciting times to be engaged in clinical education. In fact, this significant text's editor and contributor selection presided over – indeed contributed to – an unparalleled period of clinical scholarly initiatives to merge the two ideas. An accompanying explosion of continuing education programs in applied osseointegration quickly adopted the new Branemark/Sackett information package into teaching/learning initiatives that sought to reconcile efficacy and effectiveness considerations in orofacial rehabilitation. However, new concerns regarding stewardship for patient-mediated responsibilities quickly surfaced, as the continuing education landscape was rapidly swamped by commercially driven programs and implant-treatment packages that were only pale reflections of traditional clinical scholarship.

A tradition of scrupulous book learning and chairside dialogue has now been virtually usurped by a visual one. The former's primacy in shaping and nurturing clinical education is threatened by an increased reliance on the convenience of electronic learning, so-called personalized courses, and hyper-visual meetings – all promising virtual treatment and formulaic panaceas. It is tempting to assign this approach to a failure to appreciate that the newer treatment options still need to be reconciled with the quality of long-term outcome results that engaged the profession in 1982 when the osseointegration genie first came out of the bottle. And, while the appeal and merits of universally styled educational approaches cannot be underestimated, they risk undermining our discipline's ethos of patient-mediated priorities. Moreover, concerns regarding shifts in societal pyramids are increasingly accompanied by multimorbidity and treatment uncertainties in the elderly cohort. This makes their current and future prosthodontic management more demanding, irrespective of whether these patients wear removable prostheses or implant-supported alternatives. The risk of an unavoidable and unnecessary burden for an aging prosthodontically treated population suggests an insurmountable challenge for our discipline; and the need for easy and repeat access to prudent and balanced information to enrich scope for debate that informs scrupulous decision making, is still best provided via books of this calibre.

A text of this quality and ambition is a welcome, if belated, gift for the profession; and the author has shown admirable judgment in his selection of his book's title and objectives. He also recruited contributions from a roster of gifted and experienced dentists – all beneficiaries of the two seminal ideas that changed the direction of dental clinical schoalrship. Dr Sadowsky's scholarly thrust in identifying and discussing determinants for best treatment decisions for patients' oral rehabilitataive needs, reflects his profound commitment to prosthodontic stewardship in patient management. The text's overall context provides a continuum of implant management needs, together with incisive cognizance of patient-mediated concerns. Above all, Dr Sadowsky ensures that the brilliance of an applied osseointegration technique does not succumb to a formulaic approach, whereby the notion of implant therapy suggests a panacea. This book is an exceptional contribution to the discipline's canon and deserves the widest readership possible. It is also a very reasssuring reminder that written clinical scholarship remains a compelling way to underscore professional education.

George Zarb

Prologue

Per-Ingvar Branemark was the first scientist to report that a commercially pure titanium cylinder appeared to fuse to animal bone in his laboratory research; and it catalyzed his concept of osseointegration. His subsequent studies led to the 1982 Toronto Conference on Osseointegration in Clinical Dentistry, where compelling evidence of its efficacy and effectiveness introduced a new treatment landscape of prosthodontic patient care. The technique of osseointegration introduced a safe and predictable system of dental implant therapy whose positive, evidence-based assessments and outcomes are undeniable. Thirty years later, dentists may be quick to extract natural teeth and replace them with implants in situations where the natural teeth's state is questionable. That said, no technology is a panacea. It's worth tempering the optimism surrounding implants with an investigation of their shortcomings, that allows us to understand the circumstances where they are best used and most likely to offer the greatest benefit. Let's examine the evidence.

Dental implants may not last longer than natural teeth.

Levin and Halperiin-Sternfeld have shown that implant survival rates do not exceed those of compromised, but adequately treated and maintained teeth.[1] We conclude, therefore, that the decision to extract a tooth and place a dental implant requires careful consideration, and that this does not always occur when it should.

Teeth that could be saved and used as support are being extracted and replaced with implants, sometimes on doubtful indications. The natural tooth should not be considered an obstacle, but a possibility, regardless of whether the treatment is to include implant placement.[2] Oral implants – when evaluated after 10 years of service – do not surpass the longevity of natural teeth, "even those that are compromised for periodontal or endodontic reason."[3] Relying on natural teeth in lieu of implants has gained broad support. The European Conference on Evidence-based Reconstructive Dentistry argues, "Implants do not have a better prognosis than teeth with reduced marginal bone support. There is no evidence available to support an aggressive approach of early extraction of teeth to preserve bone for later implant placement."[4]

When implants are used, the cementation of implant restorations increases risks for circum-implant disease – popularly described as peri-mucositis, or else so-called peri-implantitis, when different amounts of marginal bone loss are present.

Dentists must closely monitor patients with cement-retained implant fixed dental prostheses for a range of issues. In spite of dentists' comfort in using designs that are akin to conventional dentistry, differences in the implant/tooth gingival complex favor a screw-retained design. Peri-implant disease includes color changes, bleeding on probing, and suppuration, and is most likely caused by impaction of cement in the gingival sulcus.[5] While the lesion of peri-implant mucositis resides in the soft tissues, so-called peri-implantitis also affects the supporting bone. Peri-implant mucositis occurs in about 50% of sites restored with implants, and peri-implantitis is reported to occur in 12–40% of sites. Although nonsurgical treatment of peri-implantitis remains unpredictable, limited evidence suggests that surgery, coupled with the adjunctive use of systemic antibiotics, may help resolve some peri-implantitis lesions. There was no evidence that so-called regenerative procedures had additional beneficial effects on treatment outcome.[6] Understanding which patients are at greatest risk for peri-implantitis can help dentists make better decisions about who is an appropriate candidate for implants. Peri-implantitis (loss of at least 2 mm of marginal bone) at one or more implant sites has been found to occur in 16–28% of implant patients after 5–10 years and with higher prevalence among patients with multiple implants.[2] Additionally, poor oral hygiene, a history of periodontitis, and cigarette smoking, are risk indicators for peri-implant disease.[7]

Implants are generally not affordable for the average patient seeking dental care.

When a patient is missing a natural tooth, a single implant is as cost effective as placing a three-unit fixed partial denture. However, only the affluent can afford full-mouth rehabilitation with implants. How can the millions of edentulous and partially edentulous patients gain access to dental care and be offered this twenty-first century treatment modality? Should third-party providers change their criteria for reimbursement? Can dental professionals surgically place and restore implants at an affordable price for most consumers? For the totally edentulous patient, should the gold standard be maxillary and mandibular prostheses supported by implants? We need to address the relevant social issues before we can say we have succeeded in our quest to provide the ultimate care for our patients.

Education is a step in the right direction.

With new technology that changes practice, education of practitioners must change, too. All schools of dentistry in the USA now devote significant time in the curriculum to teaching principles of implants. Most offer hands-on experience in restoring an implant. More than one half of schools are teaching DDS students how to place an implant surgically. In 2015, the Commission on Dental Accreditation (CODA) of the American Dental Association (ADA) adopted and approved a new 2016 standard for prosthodontic education, indicating that all dental practitioners who pursue specialty training in prosthodontics will be competent in the surgical placement of dental implants. One hopes that – along with an understanding of how to conduct the procedure – students also learn when and for whom the implants are likely to be successful.

George Zarb, author of this text's Foreword, was responsible for the seminal 1982 Toronto Conference. He enhanced our ability to understand the fundamentals of evidence-based dentistry with his critical thinking, teaching skills, and research. He advocates a more analytical approach to evaluating patient needs; and in an International Journal of Prosthodontics editorial entitled "Inconvenient Truths" reminds us to be cautious when evaluating the efficacy of implants.[8] "Partnerships with commercial enterprise now dominate continuing education," he writes. "New lecture circuit celebrities keep being recruited to promote osseointegration's newer and expanded promises;" and goes on to warn that their work "falls significantly outside the technique's initial oral ecology context." Wary from this admonition, the dental community must arm itself with data that helps us make informed assessments about which situations and patients merit dental implant therapy. This useful bio-technical advance in the profession is not the one tool that will solve all problems.

Howard M. Landesman, DDS, MEd

References

1. Levin L, Halperin-Sternfield M. Tooth preservation or implant placement: a systematic review of long-term tooth and implant survival rates. *J Am Dent Assoc* 2013; **144**(10): 1119–1133.
2. Lundgren D, Rylander H, Laurell L. To save or to extract, that is the question. Natural teeth or dental implants in periodontitis-susceptible patients: clinical decision-making and treatment strategies exemplified with case presentations. *Periodontol 2000* 2008; **47**: 27–50.
3. Holm-Pedersen P, Lang N, Muller F. What are the longevities of teeth and implants? *Clin Oral Implants Res* 2007; **18**(Suppl 3): 15–19.
4. Godfredsen K, Carlsson GE, Jokstad A, *et al.* Implants and/or teeth: consensus statements and recommendations. *J Oral Rehab* 2008; **35**(Suppl 1): 2–8.
5. Wilson TG Jr. The positive relationship between excess cement and peri-implant disease: a prospective clinical endoscopic study. *J Periodontol* 2009; **80**(9): 1388–1392.
6. Lindhe J, Meyle J, Group D of European Workshop on Periodontology. Peri-implant diseases: Consensus Report of the Sixth European Workshop on Periodontology. *J Clin Periodontol* 2008; **35**(8 Suppl): 282–285.
7. Heitz-Mayfield LJ. Peri-implant diseases: diagnosis and risk indicators. *J Clin Periodontol* 2008; **35**(8 Suppl): 292–304.
8. Zarb GA. On inconvenient truths. *J Prosthodont* 2008; **17**(5): 345.

Acknowledgments

I am indebted to the chapter contributors for their tireless efforts in delivering expert content to the book. It has been a privilege to collaborate with illustrious colleagues for the aim of enhancing patient care. I was fortunate to engage the services of Ms Chris Gralapp and Dr Jeff Miles who produced detailed and beautiful illustrations. Mr Justin Nichols and Ms Noori Harchandani were invaluable in reconciling the references. I also would like to thank Dr Marc Geissberger, the chair of my department at University of the Pacific Arthur A. Dugoni School of Dentistry, for liberating time for me to complete this project.

About the Companion Website

This book is accompanied by a companion website:

www.wiley.com/go/sadowsky/implant

The website includes:

- All the figures from the book.
- Five videos:
  1. Surgical template protocol.
  2. Final custom tray fabrication and open tray/closed impression on bench.
  3. Clinical implant final impression.
  4. Clinical implant restoration delivery.
  5. Beam torque wrench protocol.

How to access the website:

- Go to www.wiley.com/go/sadowsky/implant and enter the password.
- The password is the first word of Figure caption 10.1a.

CHAPTER 1
The State of the Evidence in Implant Prosthodontics

Gary R. Goldstein
New York University College of Dentistry, New York, New York, USA

Introduction

Okay, you have been placing and/or restoring implants for numerous years and are pleased with your clinical outcomes and your patient acceptance of this exciting treatment modality. You attend a lecture or read an article about a new product or technique that claims to have a higher insertion torque, less bone loss, etc.; so, how do you decide if you should switch? The rubrics are very simple, so, whether you read a paper in a peer-reviewed journal, a non-peer-reviewed journal, or hear it in a lecture, the rules are the same for all three.

There is a multitude of information available to the clinician, some evidence-based, some theory-based, some compelling and, unfortunately, some useless. Evidence-based dentistry (EBD) gives one the tools to evaluate the literature and scientific presentations. It constructs a hierarchy of evidence which allows the reader to put what they are reading, or hearing, into perspective. As we proceed on this short trail together, I want to state that there is no substitute for your own clinical experience and common sense, and hope that when you are done with this chapter you will understand why. I am not here to trash the literature, rather to propose that not all published works are equal.

Hierarchy of evidence

EBD is a relatively new phenomenon that was introduced in the 1990s. It evolved slowly due to misunderstandings and misrepresentations of what it is and what it means, and, despite a slow start, has picked up traction and is now an ADA Commission on Dental Accreditation (CODA) requirement, mandatory in dental education and the backbone of clinical research and practice. Journal editors and reviewers are well versed in the process and less likely to approve the methodologically flawed project for publication, putting more pressure on the researcher to pay heed to research design.

I could say, "Here is the hierarchy of evidence (Figure 1.1)," and save us, you the reader and me the author, a lot of time, but unfortunately things are not quite that simple. Routinely, if one is asked what the best evidence is, the response would be a meta-analysis or systematic review and, not having that, a randomized controlled trial (RCT). What is also obvious from the figure is the categorization of animal and laboratory studies. While these present critical contributions to our basic knowledge and the background information needed to design clinical studies, they cannot and should not be utilized to make clinical decisions.

According to the Cochrane Collaboration,[1] a Systematic Review (SR) "summarises the results of available carefully designed healthcare studies (controlled trials) and provides a high level of evidence on the effectiveness of healthcare interventions"; and a meta-analysis (MA) is a SR where the authors pool numerical data. I want to bring your attention to the fact that nowhere in the definition does it mention, or limit itself to, RCTs. SRs and MAs are different from the more typical narrative review where an investigator evaluates all, or much, of the available literature and tenders an "expert opinion" of the results. They usually have loose or no inclusion and exclusion criteria and no "ranking" of the articles being reviewed. For those interested in how one categorizes articles, the following websites would be helpful:

http://www.ncbi.nlm.nih.gov/pmc/articles/PMC1891443/

http://www.nature.com/ebd/journal/v10/n1/fig_tab/6400636f1.html#figure-title

http://www.ebnp.co.uk/The%20Hierarchy%20of%20Evidence.htm

We can break down studies into analytic or comparative, those that have a comparative group (randomized controlled trials, concurrent cohort studies, and case control studies) and descriptive, those that do not have a comparative group (cross-sectional surveys, case series, and case reports). Descriptive studies give us useful information about a material, treatment,

Evidence-based Implant Treatment Planning and Clinical Protocols, First Edition. Edited by Steven J. Sadowsky.

Companion website: www.wiley.com/go/sadowsky/implant

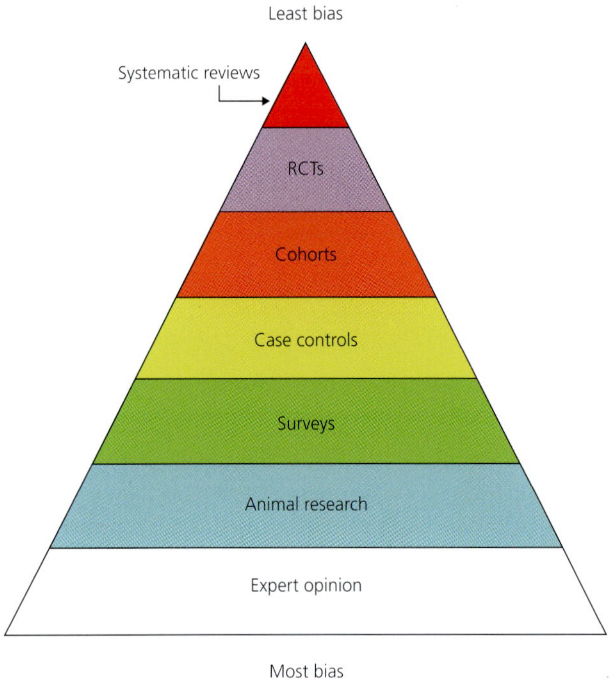

Figure 1.1 Hierarchy of evidence. *Source:* Adapted from http://consumers.cochrane.org.

etc., however, to determine if one material, treatment, etc. is better than another, requires a comparative study.

In addition, studies may be prospective or retrospective. In a prospective study the investigator selects one or more groups (cohorts) and follows them forward in time. In a retrospective study the investigator selects one or more cohorts and looks backwards in time. Prospective studies are considered superior since they can ensure that the cohorts were similar for possible confounding variables at the beginning of the study, that all participants were treated equally, and that dropouts are known and accounted for. Prospective studies allow for randomization or prognostic stratification of the cohorts. Retrospective studies can be very valuable and should not be minimalized, especially in uncovering adverse outcomes that have a low prevalence or take many years to become evident. The adverse effects from smoking have mostly been uncovered by retrospective investigation.

A randomized controlled trial (RCT) is a prospective, comparative study in which the assignment to the treatment or control group is done using a process analogous to flipping a coin. In reality, most projects are randomized utilizing a computer-generated random assignment protocol. The sole advantage of randomization is that it eliminates allocation bias. Feinstein[2] and Brunette[3] feel that the universal dependence on RCTs to achieve this is overestimated and prefer prognostic stratification of the matched cohorts for major confounding variables prior to allocation. What soon becomes obvious, however, is that prognostic stratification is not possible for every potential confounding variable, so only "major" ones are usually accounted for.

Doing an RCT is ideal, but has the constraints of time (can we afford to wait the numerous years necessary to design, implement and publish?) and cost (where can you get the funding?). Furthermore, RCTs are only ideal for certain questions, for example one that involves therapy. If our question is one of harm, it would be unethical to randomize a patient to something with a known harmful effect. To my knowledge, there has never been a RCT that proved smoking was harmful. Could you get an Internal Review Board (IRB) or Ethics Committee approval to assign participants to a group that had to smoke two packs of cigarettes a day for 25 years? Yet, does anyone doubt, given the mass of clinical evidence, that it is better to not smoke? Ultimately, the design is determined by the question.

Sackett,[4] considered by many to be the father of evidence-based medicine, in response to the heated dialogue over which design was the best, and in an effort to refocus the time, intellect, energy, and effort being wasted, proposed that "the question being asked determines the appropriate research architecture, strategy, and tactics to be used – not tradition, authority, experts, paradigms, or schools of thought."

Causation is one of the most difficult things to prove. It is like approaching a single set of railroad tracks. One can feel the warmth of the track and know that a train passed, but in which direction? It is why many studies conclude a "correlation." In the EBM series authored by the McMaster faculty, the Causation section published in the Canadian Medical Journal had David Sackett using the pseudonym Prof. Kilgore Trout as the corresponding author.[5] One can only wonder what motivated him to use the pseudonym rather than his own name to write on this critical topic. Sackett's love of the works of Kurt Vonnegut is well known and one might wonder if, in fact, his Canadian home named the Trout Research & Education Centre, is based on Kilgore or the fish?

While the design is critical, one must also determine the validity of the methodology. According to Jacob and Carr,[6] internal validity is a reflection of how the study was planned and carried out and is threatened by bias and random variation; while external validity defines if the results of the study will be applicable in other clinical settings.

Bias

There are many types of biases and a full explanation of the multitude reported is beyond the scope of this chapter. Still, there are a few that are meaningful to us as clinicians. We can divide bias into the following groups: the reader, the author, and the journal.

The reader

Taleb[7] used the following quote to accent that past experience is not always the best method to judge what we are doing at the present time.

> But in all my experience, I have never been in an accident…of any sort worth speaking about. I have seen but one vessel in distress in all my years at sea. I never saw a wreck and have never been wrecked nor was I ever in any predicament that threatened to end in disaster of any sort.
>
> *E.J. Smith, 1907, Captain RMS Titanic.*

The reader is almost always subject to confirmation bias, which is to believe whatever confirms one's beliefs. It was best stated by Sir Francis Bacon[8]: "The human understanding, once it has adopted an opinion, collects any instances that confirm it, and though the contrary instances may be more numerous and more weighty, it either does not notice them or rejects them, in order that this opinion will remain unshaken." People seek out research in a manner that supports their beliefs. We have all invested time, energy, and money getting a dental education. We have successfully treated patients and are loath to admit that something we have been doing is not as useful, successful, good, etc., as another product, technique, or procedure. This is a form of cognitive dissonance and a common human reaction. It is difficult for a clinician, and especially an educator, to admit that what they have been doing and/or teaching is not currently the best for our patients. Remember, we performed the procedure with "older" information and materials and are evaluating our outcomes or planning new treatment with "newer" evidence. The best recourse is self-reflection. Keeping up to date with clinically proven advances is our obligation as health providers.

The author

Allocation bias, a type of selection bias, is present when the two or more groups being compared are not similar, especially for confounding variables that could affect the outcome of the study. Familiar examples could be smoking, diabetes, osteoporosis, etc. Theoretically, randomization will account for this and is its major advantage, but only in the presence of a compelling number of participants (N).

The problem of allocation bias was demonstrated in a recent study.[9] The investigators were attempting to compare a one-stage protocol with a two-stage protocol with respect to marginal bone loss after 5 years; unfortunately the patients in the two-stage cohort were those who did not have a predetermined insertion torque at placement. As such, the two cohorts were not similar (one-stage = high insertion torque, two-stage = low insertion torque) for a major confounding variable and the internal validity of the study is in question.

Chronology bias refers to how long a clinical study ran and whether you, the reader, feel the time span was sufficient to justify the results and/or reveal expected or unexpected untoward responses. For example, company A has introduced a new implant surface that supposedly allows for faster osseointegration. How long would you expect the trial to run in order to accept the results as meaningful? What was their outcome assessment for success? Let's assume that there was a matched control with an adequate N. Since this is a human study, sacrificing the subjects to get histology would not sit well with your local IRB, but you have confidence that the selected outcome assessment is reliable. They have compelling evidence that a range of 3–6 months proved verifiable in their control group. They run a 6-month study with all subjects completing the full 6-month protocol. Do you feel the time is sufficient? Some will say yes and some would feel more comfortable allowing the study to run for 1 year to be certain of the external validity. Some might question whether the new surface will function under occlusal load and the biologic burden of the oral cavity and feel a multiyear protocol is needed.

In a study examining bone loss around implants, what time sequence would you require, 1 year, 2–3 years, 4–5 years, 5+ years? If a study examined the periodontal response to varying emergence profiles on implant-retained restorations, would you accept a shorter clinical trial than with the previous example? If the study was looking at monolithic zirconia that had surface custom staining and you were concerned about the outer glaze/stain wearing off, how many years would you expect the study to run? If you polled a group of experienced clinicians, you would get different answers to each, so who is correct? Unfortunately, EBD does not give you a definitive answer to this problem. It all comes back to your comfort with the premise and methodology, clinical experience, and need to alter your clinical regimen.

Referral filter bias is a type of selection bias and refers to where the patient is to be treated. For example, tertiary care cancer hospitals like M.D. Anderson or Memorial Slone Kettering have a different patient pool than you would expect to see in your private office. People who get on a plane and travel to the Mayo Clinic are not similar to the ones who are in your office because you practice close to where they work or live. Will the dental school patient be similar to yours? Will the patients in the office of a clinician who does external marketing be similar to yours, or vice versa?

Ideally, clinical projects should be triple blinded in that the person administering the therapy, drug, etc., the patient, and the person doing the outcome assessment are not familiar with what is being tested. The rationale is obvious. I am looking at my work and it all looks great, but you might not be so kind. It is one of the reasons that a case series performed and evaluated by the same group has a lower external and internal validity. In implant therapy studies, blinding often becomes quite difficult. If you are testing a zirconia abutment vs. a titanium abutment, there is a distinct visual difference that is hard to hide. Comparing a locator attachment with a ball attachment is another example that would be impossible to blind, as is one-stage vs. two-stage surgery. But, because the study is not blinded does not mean it is not well done and useful. Here we rely on the integrity of the researcher.

Conflict of interest (COI) is easily understood and it is now mandatory to disclose this in most journals. In a 2013 article in JADA,[10] the authors examined RCTs in 10 journals, three of which did not have mandatory reporting of COI, and found that "RCTs in which authors have some type of COI are more likely to have results that support the intervention being assessed." Here we have a major issue that needs to be addressed. Much of the implant clinical research we see is funded by commercial companies. In the US, it is apparent that the National Institute of Dental and Craniofacial Facial Research's (NIDCR) policy is to fund basic science research and allow companies to fund clinical trials. While this seems counter-intuitive, it is a fact of life. So we as clinicians, and the patients that we treat, are starting with a decided bias in the research being presented. Often SRs have eliminated RCTs for high risk of bias in other parameters but accept those with industry support. Burying our heads in the sand is not appropriate either. We must be realistic in how we evaluate all forms of bias. As with a lack of blinding, the internal validity suffers, but with both, one must assume the integrity of the researcher is intact. While there is a bad egg in every field, for the most part our colleagues are honest and sincere in their desire to do a study that will answer a needed question, undergo peer review, and stand the test of time. In today's digital world, once it is written it is there for all to see for all time.

I wouldn't have seen it if I didn't believe it. Sherlock Holmes, in the novel *A Scandal in Bohemia*,[11] said, "It is a capital mistake to theorize before one has data. Insensibly one begins to twist facts to suit theories, instead of theories to suit facts." This is an unfortunate but sometimes unavoidable consequence for the researcher who has invested time, effort, and money in a project and perhaps is unable to clearly see what was happening. Sometimes it is innocuous, like framing the data in a positive manner. An example of this is the researcher who states they had a 70% success rate instead of a 30% failure rate, or justifying the lower success rate by saying that we save the patient time, money etc. But other times it takes on a more disconcerting approach, which could be a type of apophenia, which, according to the Merriam-Webster Online Dictionary is "the tendency to perceive a connection or meaningful pattern between unrelated or random things (such as objects or ideas)." One of the best examples was given by Cotton[12] in a 1988 editorial in the Journal of Dental Research, in which he described an experiment where a frog was trained to jump when told "jump". After one leg was amputated the frog was still able to jump when told. After two legs were amputated the frog was still able to jump when told. The same occurred after three legs were amputated. After the fourth amputation the frog could not jump so the researchers concluded that quadruple amputation in frogs created deafness. His example explains it all.

The journal

Publication bias is often defined as a preference to publish studies that have a positive finding, and it is true that most studies have historically been positive or neutral. In fact, a recent Cochrane Review[13] found that trials with positive findings were "published more often, and more quickly, than trials with negative findings." There are numerous potential reasons for this finding. Many researchers are reluctant to admit that their premise was incorrect, but these studies have just as much clinical value as positive ones. The negative result always creates a conundrum when the study was funded by a company who now wants to squash the publication and the researcher does not want to risk the loss of future grants. We, as clinicians, should be accepting and thankful to our research colleagues who publish despite these concerns.

There is another form of publication bias which may be imposed by the editor and/or journal board. There have been numerous articles that were rejected by one journal and, when published by another, have gone on to be highly quoted and generated a respectable citation index. Our history is riddled with unfortunate examples of work that had difficulty getting published: gastric ulcers are caused by bacteria; lactic acid buildup in muscles being exercised is good; lobotomies on patients suffering from chronic pain are unacceptable; carotid ligation in people who have suffered a stroke is not indicated; and all teeth that have had root canal therapy, regardless of the remaining tooth structure, should not be decoronated and a post placed 3 mm from the apex to support a core that replaces the removed tooth structure.

Some editors are extremely rigid, in that they require adherence to editorial demands, and others are more accepting, feeling that they have performed their duty in helping to upgrade the quality of the publication and if the authors refuse they would allow reader opinion and history to resolve the conflict. Either way, the journal is not giving a "stamp of approval" to each article published and, again, it is up to the reader to decide if the results are applicable to their patients.

Statistics

Pundits have been famous for analyzing data and coming up with fallacious conclusions. The most famous example is the Chicago Tribune's headline in 1948 predicting that Dewey won the presidential election over Truman. Issues like the mortgage crisis of 2008–2009 and the current debate over the US student loan crisis, show the constant problems with data analysis.

Statisticians are a testy and argumentative group and are almost as bad as prosthodontists. Much of the early work on statistics was derived by intellectuals trying to improve their gambling odds.[14] Many of their theories are based on non-medical protocols which do not translate into the clinical milieu. Statisticians are like bad relatives; we may not want them but we have no choice. They are a critical part of our lives. They help us to determine the N and power of a project and to clarify data collection methodology. They analyze the data to help us interpret and understand the results, but statisticians do not make clinical decisions. Clinicians make the decisions by utilizing the best available evidence to treat the patient. The statistics section should be the shortest and least obtrusive part of the publication, unless some new statistical method is being presented.

Not all statisticians agree on which tests to run on specific issues and many of us have had a journal ask us to rerun data because "their" statistician did not agree with "our" statistician. Some tests are considered more robust than others and sometimes a more rigorous test might show something different. Sometimes the wrong statistics were performed. But sometimes the request is unwarranted or even unreasonable.

There is a difference between statistical significance and clinical significance. Feinstein[15] opined that "statistical significance has become a malignant mental pathogen" as it does not take into consideration the methodology, the clinical implications, or the cause of the difference. Say you now possessed an extremely accurate instrument that could measure bone loss in the nanometer range and were able to show that the mean bone loss after 5 years was 10 nanometers more with implant B when compared to A and the difference was statistically significant, is that clinically significant? In this case no, but in many projects clinicians will have different opinions as to the clinical relevance of the data presented. If we now had a 0.5 mm difference, how would you respond? Or a 1 mm difference?

What does the mean mean? To paraphrase an example given by Wheelan,[16] after reading the latest contract for the sanitation workers in New York City, nine senior dental faculty members went to happy hour at a local bar to share their angst over the current data. When adding up their clinical supervision time, lecture, and/or seminar time, preparation time, research, and personal development time, and comparing it with the hours worked by the sanitation people, it was obvious that the mean salaries of those at the bar were less than the sanitation workers and required another round of drinks. Unbeknownst to them, Warren Buffett walked in and ordered a drink; suddenly the mean salary of the 10 people sitting at the bar skyrocketed to an obscene number. Ok, so you say eliminate Warren as he is the outlier, definitely an accepted technique for statisticians and it indeed makes sense. But what if we are doing a medical or dental clinical trial?

Biostatistics should have different rules than other forms of statistics. Should the data be manipulated? Homogenizing the data by log transforming it or eliminating outliers is acceptable in large survey studies to conform to the Gaussian curve, but is not appropriate in medical and dental clinical studies, especially those with small Ns.

Let's say I'm doing a measurement of pocket depth around implants after 1 year of clinical loading and I decide to take three readings with a periodontal probe and average the three for each patient that I am analyzing. I have 10 patients on whom I am going to take the measurements. If my data set is running between 5 and 6 mm for all of the patients, then using the average of three readings (5.5 mm) would probably suffice. But picture the scenario where I'm getting readings of 0 mm, 5 mm, and 10 mm. It is obvious that by using the mean (5 mm) I've eliminated a major variation (was it the probe, me, or variations in the depth manifested by not being able to be in the same exact location?) which could potentially affect the statistical validity of my sample. What should be done is to enter all three measurements as a subset of the patient. The mean will still be the same but the standard deviation will be much larger in the 0, 5, 10 group which could affect the statistical significance. The statistical programs easily handle this, but many research projects are not designed in this manner.

The over-reliance on statistics that cannot truly assume the effect of chance is also questionable. Derek Richards[17] stated that "when testing a new treatment in a clinical trial, there are three possible explanations for why it did or did not work as expected – chance, bias or the truth."

Chance and the N have a way of intertwining. If I asked you to flip a coin, you would say you have a 50-50 chance of getting a head or tail. If I told you that I flipped the coin and got five heads in a row you might not be surprised. Would you still bet 50-50 on the next flip? If I told you that I had flipped nine heads in a row, some of you might say *okay it's possible* and some of you might say *no way*. But, if I told you that we were going to flip the coin 1000 times everybody would pretty much agree that we would get 500 heads and 500 tails. Would you put a wager on that? John Kerrich, a mathematician who had the bad luck to be spending time in a German prison during World War II, had the time to do 10 000 coin tosses. He had 44% heads after 100 throws and 50.67% at 10 000.[18] So how does chance come into play in a clinical trial with an N of 10 or 20?

The N is determined *a priori* by the clinician who helps determine the expected clinical difference with input from the statistician who helps determine the estimated number. It can also be verified *post hoc* by a power analysis. But does the N make sense to the clinician? One of the biggest problems we see, especially in implant literature, is the inadequate N despite the fact that large numbers of patients are in the clinical trial. Let's look at a clinical trial to determine if implant A will integrate faster using bone grafting material X or Y in the maxillary premolar area, utilizing a split-mouth design, where the patient is their own control, with an N of 40. In this situation the age, sex, medical and dental history, medications etc. are the same for the test group and the control group. Since the confounding variables are equally distributed, the split mouth has the advantage of requiring a smaller N and you may agree that 40 patients are adequate.

In another clinical example, with an N of 100 patients, implants were placed in the maxilla, in the mandible, some were premolars, some were molars, and some were anteriors. In addition, some implants were 8 mm, some were 10, and some were 12. Some implants were wide body, some regular body, and some narrow body. And then, to make matters worse, different brands of implants were also used. So if I am looking for data to determine whether or not I can use a regular body, 10 mm, brand X implant in a maxillary premolar on a 40-year-old female nonsmoker, there may only be an N of one or two whose results are applicable to my patient. This shotgun technique of patient allotment violates basic EBD principles in that a well-defined question was not established or that too many questions (Is brand A better than brand B? Does implant width make a difference? Does implant length make a difference? Does the arch or tooth position matter and what about smoking, age or sex?) were trying to be answered. Each time you add another variable you have to double the N needed, so here 100 patients is not an adequate number.

How do you handle dropouts? One of the key questions in evaluating the validity of a research project is "Were all patients who entered the trial properly accounted for and attributed at its conclusion?"[19] Patients pass away (hopefully not from our dental treatment), move to other areas, or become too sick to return for follow-up. But patients can also drop out because they are unhappy with the treatment, the clinician, or the environment in which the treatment occurred. Patients can also be noncompliant with the protocols such as taking medication or using a prescribed home-care regimen to which they were randomized.

The classical manner of handling dropouts is the "intention to treat" method in which all subjects are followed regardless of adherence. Sackett[20] espoused it and Montori and Guyatt,[21] in a more recent commentary, lambasted alternative strategies. On the other hand, Gerard Dallal[22] in his *Handbook of Statistical Practice* called the "intention to treat" a fraud, and gives many examples where it is severely flawed. But he also questioned the per protocol, in which only data from adherent subjects are analyzed, as well as some other varied attempts to deal with the problem.

For our purposes, say you are doing a study to determine which postoperative antibiotic "regimen", in patients getting immediate placement of an implant, is more efficacious. You have three groups: test group regimen A; test group regimen A and regimen B; and placebo group C. Mr. Smith, who was randomized to group A, never took his medication. "Intention to treat" demands he be included in the data for group A. Are you comfortable with that? This argument will endure for many years before there is any hope of a settlement. It is the researcher's obligation to decide how dropouts will be handled in the protocol stage and however they choose to do this, the number and reason for the dropouts needs to be clearly reported. At the end of the day, dropouts are a problem that affects the internal and external validity of a study. Sackett[23] has said that "it would be unusual for a trial to withstand a worst-case scenario if it lost more than 20% of its patients." It is you the clinician who must decide if you are comfortable with the number of dropouts and how they were handled.

How long should you run a clinical trial to avoid "follow-up not complete"? Some patients will start in the first year of the study, some in the second, etc. The reality is that not every patient starts on day 1, as this is a clinical trial and not a horse or a car race where everyone starts at the same time. If you do a 5-year study and only a small percentage of the patients were treated for 5 years, should you still call that a 5-year study? Statisticians will say okay and that there are formulae that they could use to predict what will actually happen, but how do you feel? In the typical dental studies with small Ns, where chance and outliers wreak havoc, why not just wait until everyone completes the study? It creates numerous problems, not the least of which is time and money, for the research staff, but if everyone does not complete the study, once again we risk putting the decision-making process in the hands of the statistician rather than the clinician.

A major concern in evaluating the outcome of a study, especially on implants, is what was the outcome assessment? Was it the implant, or was it the patient? It all depends on the question. If your question is *Will this new implant integrate?*, then the implant should be the outcome measure. As an example, you are reading a study on implant survival in 30 patients who have six fixture prostheses in the maxilla. At the end of 5 years, seven patients lost two implants, seven patients lost one implant, and one patient lost five implants. Only one patient had the prosthesis compromised sufficiently to require a redo, the patient with five lost implants. The other patients had the failed implants removed from the mouth and the existing prosthesis was deemed usable. If you use the patient as the outcome assessment then only one failure occurred. But, if you use the implant as the outcome assessment, then 26 out of 180 implants failed. The result is two totally different data sets; two totally different conclusions.

In a recent article in the Journal of Dental Research,[24] a retrospective cohort study was conducted to determine the effect of selective serotonin reuptake inhibitors (SSRIs) on implant survival. In this study the question really is *Will SSRIs inhibit osseointegration?*, so the patient should be the outcome measure since the medication affects the patient. The study showed a failure rate in the SSRI group of 10.6% (10/94 failed) and 4.6% (38/822) in the nonuser group, utilizing implants as the outcome assessment. The researchers, to their credit, understanding that SSRIs would affect the patient, ran a separate statistical analysis "to account for cluster effects of multiple implants when placed and evaluated in a single patient." Here you get to see the data both ways and, regardless of your opinion on the outcome assessment, the ability to apply the conclusions.

We seem to have an immense fascination with the Gaussian bell-shaped curve which has lately come under a great deal of criticism. Carl Friedrich Gauss, the German mathematician for whom the bell-shaped curve is named, placed his "proof" inconspicuously in a section at the end of his book *The Theory of the Motion of Heavenly Bodies Moving about the Sun in Conic Sections*. Interestingly, he later considered that proof invalid.[25] Both Feinstein[26] (*On Exorcizing the Ghost of Gauss and the Curse of Kelvin*) and Taleb[27] (The *Bell Curve, That Great Intellectual Fraud*), devoted entire chapters to this.

While data dredging has always been a concern, the user friendly statistical programs currently available have enabled the dredger to easily run a multitude of tests until they finally find one that proves a premise. This has become a more prevalent issue and unfortunately, it may also involve culling or manipulating data and is commonly referred to as p-hacking. While most of the time it is used to try and prove a difference, it can also be used to do the opposite.

Understanding that the P value is a probability of the likelihood that what is seen occurred by chance, it does seem counter-intuitive to say that a $P=.05$ is statistically significance but a $P=.51$ is not. Today it is recommended to look at confidence intervals and see if, and how much, they overlap. While there are formulae to help derive this, it should not be the reader's obligation to do math when analyzing an article. If not provided by the author, the confidence interval (CI) can be simply viewed as two standard errors. For example, let's take a data set where we have a mean of 10 in group A and a mean of 20 in group B. If the standard error (SE) around group A and B are plus or minus 2, then the confidence interval around group A would go from 6 to 14 (2× the SE) and the confidence interval around B would go from 16 to 24. Since the confidence intervals are not overlapping, one can be assured that the groups are different. But let's create a sample where the standard error is plus or minus 5 for both groups. Now the confidence intervals stretch from 0 to 20 in group A and 10 to 30 in group B. Since the confidence intervals are overlapping, in this case severely to demonstrate the point, even if the data were statistically significant (which I doubt, given the exaggerated standard errors in this scenario), one would be tempted to be concerned about the data sets. If there is a large overlap there is a large concern, if there is a small overlap there is much less concern, and, again, if there is no overlap there is no concern.

Classical statistics usually follows the Neyman–Pearson approach, but there is much controversy in that and many people are looking to the Bayesian approach which was first proposed by the Reverand Thomas Bayes in 1763.[28] It states that the probability that A will occur if B occurs is often different than the probability that B will occur if A occurs. The Bayesian theory contradicts standard statistical analysis by bringing prior probability into the equation. Simplistically, it means that if you just look at the data set in and of itself without having background information upon which to apply or how to apply that data set, you will come to a potentially incorrect conclusion. An example is given by Mlodinow.[29] He applied for life insurance and took a routine blood test which came back HIV positive. His doctor told him that he had 1 in 1000 chances of being healthy, since HIV tests will give a false positive in only 1 out of 1000 samples. But, the confusion is that his doctor assumed he would test positive if he was not HIV positive with the chances that he would not be HIV positive if he tested positive. Hence, he was looking at the chance he was not infected out of all negative and positive tests, rather than the chance that he was not infected just out of all positive tests. In order to understand the example, it is important to note that he is a white American, heterosexual male, non-IV drug user and according to the Center for Disease Control (CDC) data, only 1 in 10 000 people in that data set was infected with HIV. Therefore, given that the false-negative rate is almost zero, we can deduce that in the 10 000 men in the proposed sample, 9989 will be testing negative. If we look at the people who tested positive, 10 will be false-positives (1 in 1000 false-positive rate) and one will be a true positive (1 in 10 000 prevalence); so rather than a 1 in 1000 chance that he is HIV positive, his chances are 10 out of 11 that he is not.

Another example given by Siegfried in Science News[30] had to do with steroid testing of baseball players. Using an assumption that the test is 95% accurate and one of the players on your team tested positive, the probability of guilt should be 95%. But using the Bayesian approach you need to know some additional information. Previous data on this type of testing showed that 5% of professional baseball players use steroids. He proposes on a test of 400 players, 20 would be users (the 5%) and 380 would not be users. So, giving a test to all 400 that is 95% accurate, of the 20 users 19 would be identified and, of the 389 nonusers, 19, or 5%, would be incorrectly identified. So testing 400 players would give you 38 positives, 19 of whom were users and 19 of whom were not users. Your player has a 50% chance of being guilty.

Since the classical versus the Bayesian disagreement transcends my pay grade, those of you with interest in this topic can pursue it with the references stated, and others, which can easily be found on the Internet, and I will allow those with more knowledge than me to continue this debate.

Researchers devise questions and in simplistic terms, "will A be better than B?" or, "will A last longer than B?". The statistical consultant desires a null hypothesis to do their data analysis, but why must the reader have to deal with inverted statistical logic? Which is more intuitive, "A is better than B" or the "null hypothesis was rejected"? Perhaps the null hypothesis, which is confusing jargon forced upon us by statisticians, needs to be "rejected" and be null and void in the manuscript conclusion.

Yogi Berra, the great philosopher and Hall of Fame baseball player and coach said, "It is tough to make predictions, especially about the future."[31] Few of us have the background to truly analyze the statistics being utilized in today's clinical studies. What are needed are meaningful answers to our clinical questions, not fancy data manipulation that could possibly obscure the facts we seek. A memorable quote from an esteemed mentor and friend, Dr. Louis Blatterfein, was "if you have nothing to say dazzle them with your footwork." Statistical analyses have to make sense. If you are concerned that the methodology is questionable then don't worry about the statistics; you are not accepting the premise and/or the results. A flawed project cannot be salvaged by exotic statistical manipulation. Remember, "garbage in – garbage out". If the methodology is sound, you can assume the statistics are also.

Evaluation

Sackett[32] states, "Evidence-based medicine is not restricted to randomized trials and meta-analyses. It involves tracking down the best external evidence (from systematic reviews when they exist; otherwise from primary studies) with which to answer our clinical questions." In addition, not all SRs are well done and articles have been written on how to evaluate them.[17,33]

If what you are doing has a 95% success rate, unless you had compelling evidence from a well-designed RCT, why would you change? If what you are doing has a 30% failure rate, why are you still doing it? But, suppose you prefer to frame it in a more positive manner and say a 70% success rate, and you have no other treatment options, can you or your patient wait for the RCT? Each one of us might put a different number for the percentage success rate you would accept or not accept. Here we are directed to the best available evidence, which unfortunately in dentistry may be a case series.

The key aspect to having an evidence-based practice is to be able to critically appraise the article you have been reading. When evaluating an article you look at the methodology first. In the study, was the patient population similar to the patient you are treating? Is the operator expertise similar to your own? Is your environment similar to the one in which the study was performed? Are your inclusion and exclusion criteria for treatment the same? You need to look at the design, the biases, the statistical methods, and the conclusions to make a judgment using your EBD tools to evaluate the internal and external validity and determine *are the results applicable to my patient*? Two people can read an article and after critically appraising it come up with different opinions of its clinical usefulness. And there is nothing wrong with this.

Clinicians function in a different environment than researchers. The researcher is looking for statistical significance, while the practitioner demands clinical significance. In an effort to standardize their cohorts, the researcher has stringent inclusion and exclusion criteria and works with mean populations. Clinicians treat the standard deviation, rarely the mean, and have people in their practice who fall outside of the inclusion/exclusion criteria of the study. We treat the diabetic, the smoker, the pregnant women, the neurologically impaired, and the patient on a wide assortment of medications, etc. What if the patient was referred by your best referring doctor or is the relative of an existing patient who has sent many friends, relatives, and business associates to you? Clinicians also have the concerns of litigation, since they are not under a university or hospital umbrella, and the possibility of the everlasting and insidious negative internet review.

When evaluating a new procedure or product we should never be using only one outcome assessment. Let's look at implant placement procedures A and B. Certainly, implant failure or success is a primary outcome, but what other clinical parameters does the clinician need to take into consideration. For our discussion, A equaled B in terms of failure/success. But, how many surgical procedures were involved? What was the morbidity? What was the cost to the patient? Did one procedure require a shorter treatment time than another? While the implants were still in place, was there more bone loss or soft-tissue issues for one procedure? What other patient management issues are important to you?

Many factors come into play when trying to determine treatment for our patients. Fretwurst *et al.*[34] in an October 2014 article, found residual DNA in the allografts tested. So, what is the clinician to do? Is there a critical mass for residual DNA? What do the numbers mean? Is there clinical evidence of any harm? Is that because we never looked for it? How do public perception and legal consequences enter into our clinical decision-making process?

Is a poorly-done RCT of more value than a well-done non-randomized controlled trial? The answer is unequivocally no. But, is it better or worse than a well-done case series? Here we will get into some disagreements. If you have a few case series that have shown a 95% success rate over 10 years, that is compelling evidence that needs to be accounted for. If they present with a 50% failure rate that is also critical evidence that should not be discarded. Sackett tells us that we should use the best available clinical evidence.[4]

A very significant problem in the literature and one that can have unfortunate consequences in the medical–legal and insurance arenas is misstating the conclusions of a MA or SR. In an article published in Evidence Based-Dentistry in 2010, *Indirect or direct restorations for heavily restored posterior adult teeth*, one RCT that compared composites with crowns on root canal treated premolars was rejected because the clinical scenario was a vital tooth. Two prospective studies comparing large amalgams with crowns (a 5-year and a 17-year follow-up) were rejected because they were not randomized. The author concluded, "The clinician can only say that there is no high quality clinical evidence to suggest that placing a crown on a posterior tooth would lead to its longer retention than a composite or amalgam."[35] This is extremely dangerous as insurance companies, and perhaps government agencies and the press, latch onto this information and misuse it, preventing practitioners from providing the care they feel appropriate for their patients. *Sorry Doc, we won't pay for crowns since there is no evidence that they are better than a composite or amalgam.*

Here we must decide what the question was. "Does it work?" only requires a case series. "Is it better?" requires a comparative study. Since, crowns and amalgams have been in use for many years the onus would be to prove that the composite was as good as a crown or an amalgam in the tooth involved. A major variable in determining which restorative material is indicated is the amount of remaining tooth structure and the opposing occlusion. Also, is "longer retention" the needed outcome assessment? What if the restoration or residual tooth structure fractured? What if the tooth devitalized? What if the tooth wore down occlusally and the opposing tooth extruded? What if there was recurrent decay or periodontal issues? Would "there is no high quality evidence that supports or rejects the practice of placing a crown or onlay on a vital posterior tooth rather than a composite or amalgam restoration to ensure longer tooth survival" have been a better conclusion? Or perhaps, *more clinical research, especially RCTs, is needed*. Absence of evidence is not evidence of absence,[36] especially if a good portion of the evidence has been excluded.

A positive example was a review on whether or not occlusal splints should be routinely prescribed for bruxers undergoing implant therapy.[37] The authors concluded, "The absence of evidence-based studies to recommend occlusal splints in bruxers who have received implant-supported rehabilitation emphasizes the need for well-designed randomized controlled clinical trials." So why am I pointing this out? The conclusion seems valid and well founded and I agree. Unfortunately, many authors would say something like "there is no evidence that an occlusal splint should be prescribed in bruxers undergoing implant therapy," which, if someone was just reading the conclusion would lead them to believe that occlusal splints are contraindicated. This occurs quite often where authors conclude that, since there is inadequate evidence to support a premise, that the premise is fallacious.

Another problem is that someone can perform a systematic review with only RCTs as inclusion criteria and, despite a multitude of clinical trials that were not RCTs, draw a conclusion that there is no evidence to support the question asked. This has limited value, especially in the US, as NIDCR has been reluctant to fund RCTs. Yes, we need them, but who will fund them? Should we depend on industry to fund our RCTs? Will they fund the project whose premise is that the product may not be good? Well-done cohort studies or even case series may be the best available evidence and have significant value. If there are no RCTs, or no well-done RCTs, then the author is obligated to follow the trail to the best available evidence. There is no requirement that a SR needs to only look at RCTs! If you have numerous case series that have shown a 95% success rate over 10 years that is compelling evidence that needs to be accounted for. If they present with a 50% failure rate that is also critical evidence that should not be discarded.

When reading a SR or a MA, what were the inclusion and exclusion criteria? Do you agree with them? Are you comfortable with the ones excluded? Should they have been?[33] Some SRs will include discussions with recognized experts, especially ones who may be performing current research on the topic being reviewed, as well as Grey Literature, which are articles not published in peer-reviewed journals. What is your position on that?

We also have the possibility of committee bias. Are evaluators on a committee evaluating their own work? Are they receiving grants, stipends, or other forms of corporate support? They may be esteemed experts, but should they be on the committee? Even if they recuse themselves from the discussion on their particular paper, what is the risk of bias for the committee evaluations?

Evidence-based practice does not mean that you have to wait for a MA to make decisions. In order to do a MA you need data that can be pooled. Because there are no or few randomized controlled trials available, doesn't mean there is no evidence. If evidence cannot be pooled then the SR is more than adequate. If one finds that there are a few or no RCTs available then one can broaden the inclusion criteria. This is where a critically appraised topic (CAT), which is a defined critical summary of research evidence that answers a clinical question, may be more helpful. Evaluating the available evidence is more fruitful than saying we need more RCTs.

Some journals are moving away from the case series and/or case presentations in favor of RCTs and SRs, and, while it is improving the status of the journal, is it really improving dental care? Where does the innovator publish? In order to get funding for RCTs, there needs to be justifiable evidence to support the researcher's premise. A problem facing dentistry is the inability, given demands of EBD, for imaginative thoughts to have a place to be published. Medicine has recognized this problem and created a Journal of Medical Hypothesis which caters to original ideas that can be the basis for future research rather than RCTs, SRs, and MAs. We in dentistry need to follow suit. Historically most of our articles were expert opinion and much of it did not stand the test of time but, if we cut off the essay or the case presentation because there is no place for it to be published, are we losing the innovation necessary for us to grow? Prospective clinical studies are needed. So please do not misunderstand the thought process here. We still are obligated to make clinical decisions on the highest level of research available, but can we risk cutting off the innovative sparks that may lead us in the future?

Conclusion

EBD gives you, the clinician, the tools to run an evidence-based practice. Once you have ascertained that the results are applicable to your patient, you now have to determine if the results are valid and compelling enough to allow you to feel comfortable applying them. You have earned a BS or BA and a DDS or DMD. Many of you have Master's degrees, and perhaps PhDs. You have taken general practice residency programs, specialty programs, and perhaps specialty certification exams. You have a lifelong commitment to continuing education, attend lectures and seminars, and read professional journals. You have spent years honing your clinical and patient-management skills. You are indeed the real clinical scholars and you make the clinical decisions. EBD is a tool; it can never replace your skill, experience or judgment.[38]

References

1. Cochrane Consumer Network. What is a systematic review [internet]. [updated 2012 Jun 25; cited 2015 June 22]. Available from: http://consumers.cochrane.org/what-systematic-review
2. Feinstein AR. An additional basic science for clinical medicine: II. The limitations of randomized trials. *Ann Intern Med* 1983; **99**(4): 544–550.
3. Brunette DM. *Critical Thinking: Understanding and Evaluating Dental Research.* Chicago: Quintessence Publishing Co 1996; 152.
4. Sackett DL, Wennberg JE. Choosing the best research design for each question: it's time to stop squabbling over the "best" methods. *BMJ* 1997; **315**(7123): 1636.
5. Department of Clinical Epidemiology and Biostatistics, McMaster University Health Science Center. How to read clinical journals, IV: to determine etiology or causation. *Can Med Assoc J* 1981; **124**(8): 985–990.
6. Jacob RF, Carr AB. Hierarchy of research design used to categorize the "strength of evidence" in answering clinical dental questions. *J Prosthet Dent* 2000; **83**(2): 137–152.
7. Taleb NN. *The Black Swan.* New York: Random House Trade Paperbacks 2010; 42.
8. Mlodinow L. *The Drunkard's Walk: How Randomness Rules Our Lives.* New York: Pantheon Books 2008; 189.
9. Berberi AN, Tehini GE, Noujeim ZF, *et al.* Influence of surgical and prosthetic techniques on marginal bone loss around titanium implants. Part I: Immediate loading in fresh extraction sockets. *J Prosthodont* 2014; **23**(7): 521–527.
10. Brignardello-Peterson R, Carrasco-Labra A, Yanine N, *et al.* Positive association between conflicts of interest and reporting of positive results in randomized clinical trials in dentistry. *JADA* 2013; **144**(10): 1165–1170.
11. Kameron Kent Searle. Sherlock Holmes Quotes. 2012–2015 [cited 2015 June 22]. Available from: http://sherlockholmesquotes.com/
12. Cotton WR. How far can a frog jump? A current assessment of pulp biology research. *J Dent Res* 1988; **67**(9): 1251.
13. Hopewell S, Loudon K, Clarke MJ, *et al.* Publication bias in clinical trials due to statistical significance or direction of trial results. *Cochrane Database Syst Rev* 2009; **1**: MR000006. doi: 10.1002/14651858.
14. Mlodinow L. *The Drunkard's Walk: How Randomness Rules Our Lives.* New York: Pantheon Books 2008; 48–50.
15. Feinstein A. *Clinical Biostatistics.* St. Louis: The C.V. Mosby Company 1977; 11.
16.. Wheelan C. *Naked Statistics: Stripping the Dread from the Data.* New York: W.W. Norton & Company 2013; 19.
17. Richards D. Critically appraising randomised trials. *Evid Based Dent* 2009; **10**(3): 88–90.
18. Mlodinow L. *The Drunkard's Walk: How Randomness Rules Our Lives.* New York: Pantheon Books 2008; 95.
19. Goldstein GR, Preston JD. How to evaluate an article about therapy. *J Prosthet Dent* 2000; **83**(6): 599–603.
20. Sackett DL, Richardson WS, Rosenberg W, Haynes RB. *Evidence-Based Medicine: How to Practice & Teach EBM.* New York: Churchill Livingstone 1997; 96.
21. Montori VM, Guyatt GH. Intention-to-treat principle. *Can Med Assoc J* 2001; **165**(10): 1339–1341.
22. Dallal G. *The Little Handbook of Statistical Practice.* [Internet]. 2015 [cited 2015 June 22]. Available from: http://www.jerrydallal.com/LHSP/LHSP.HTM.
23. Sackett DL, Richardson WS, Rosenberg W, Haynes RB. *Evidence-Based Medicine: How to Practice & Teach EBM.* New York: Churchill Livingstone 1997; 95.
24. Wu X, Al-Abedalla K, Rastikerdar E, *et al.* Selective serotonin reuptake inhibitors and the risk of osseointegrated implant failure: a cohort study. *J Dent Res* 2014; **93**(11): 1054–1061.
25. Mlodinow L. *The Drunkard's Walk: How Randomness Rules Our Lives.* New York: Pantheon Books 2008; 143.
26. Feinstein A. *Clinical Biostatistics.* St. Louis: The C.V. Mosby Company 1977; 229–242.
27. Taleb NN. *The Black Swan.* New York: Random House Trade Paperbacks 2010; 229–252.
28. Brunette DM. *Critical Thinking: Understanding and Evaluating Dental Research.* Chicago: Quintessence Publishing Co 1996; 172–174.
29. Mlodinow L. *The Drunkard's Walk: How Randomness Rules Our Lives.* New York: Pantheon Books 2008; 114–117.
30. Siegfried T. Odds Are, It's Wrong: Science fails to face the shortcomings of statistics. Science News [internet]. 2010 March 27 [cited 2015 June 22];177(7):26. Available from: https://www.sciencenews.org/article/odds-are-its-wrong.
31. Taleb NN. *The Black Swan.* New York: Random House Trade Paperbacks 2010; 136.
32. Sackett DL, Richardson WS, Rosenberg W, Haynes RB. *Evidence-Based Medicine: How to Practice & Teach EBM.* New York: Churchill Livingstone 1997; 4.
33. Felton DA, Lang BR. The overview: an article that interrogates the literature. *J Prosthet Dent* 2000; **84**(1): 17–21.
34. Fretwurst T, Spanou A, Nelson K, *et al.* Comparison of four different allogeneic bone grafts for alveolar ridge reconstruction: a preliminary histologic and biochemical analysis. *Oral Surg Oral Med Oral Pathol Oral Radiol* 2014; **118**(4): 424–431.
35. Hurst D. Indirect or direct restorations for heavily restored posterior adult teeth? *Evid Based Dent* 2010; **11**(4): 116–117.
36. Sedgwick P. Understanding why "absence of evidence is not evidence of absence". *BMJ* 2014; **349**: g4751.
37. Mesko ME, Almeida RCCR, Porto JAS, *et al.* Should occlusal splints be a routine prescription for diagnosed bruxers undergoing implant therapy? *Int J Prosthodont* 2014; **27**(3): 201–203.
38. Sackett DL, Richardson WS, Rosenberg W, Haynes RB. *Evidence-Based Medicine: How to Practice & Teach EBM.* New York: Churchill Livingstone 1997; 5.

CHAPTER 2
Systemic Factors Influencing Dental Implant Therapy

Steven J. Sadowsky
University of the Pacific Arthur A. Dugoni School of Dentistry, San Francisco, California, USA

Despite the fact that only a small percentage of adult patients are precluded from dental implant therapy because of absolute contraindications, surgical placement in these individuals may have serious sequelae, including possible implant failure, refractory healing, and even life-threatening consequences. The American Society of Anesthesiologists (ASA) has developed a classification system to stratify patients' physical status in order to assess relative risk for surgical procedures (Table 2.1). Maloney *et al.*[1] have recommended that elective treatment (implant placement) should be reserved for classification I–III. While this can serve as a general guide, implant treatment may run the gamut from simple and minimally invasive to most complicated.[2] Moreover, the degree of systemic disease control can be labile and subtle. Finally, the influence of specific disease entities or medications on dental implant survival is unclear in the literature as there are few randomized controlled trials, if any, evaluating health status as a risk factor.[3]

Suggested absolute contraindications to implant placement include profound immunosuppression, uncontrolled diabetes, intravenous bisphosphonates, bleeding disorders, recent myocardial infarction/stroke, active treatment of malignancy, alcohol/drug abuse, and neuropsychiatric illness. Commonly proposed relative contraindications include osteoporosis, smoking, chronic periodontitis, autoimmune disease (nondiabetic conditions), and lack of surgical experience, but there is weak evidence to support recommended absolute or relative contraindiactions.[4] Temporary contraindications include incomplete growth, pregnancy, and acute infection. A discussion of these potential risk factors will be helpful to assess the best strategy in orchestrating implant therapy, considering the benefit/risk calculus.

Immunocompromised patients

Immunocompromise can diminish the patient's ability to battle infection following implant surgery. There is not a robust body of evidence-based literature to determine the influence of immunosuppression on implant survival.

Case reports and a case series have demonstrated implant survival up to and including more than 5 years' follow-up on patients with organ transplants.[5,6] Despite the fact that long-term cyclosporin A usage has been shown to impair initial peri-implant bone healing and osseointegration in animals, patients receiving liver or kidney transplants and concomitant immunosuppressant therapy have had unremarkable implant outcomes.[7] However, given the low-level evidence and small population size, caution should be used when implants are placed in these patients.

The human immunodeficiency virus (HIV+) has a significant impact on a patient's immune function. The use of highly antiretroviral therapy (HAART) has extended the lifespan of these patients and qualified them for implant treatment.

Patients infected with the HIV+ been reported in the short term to have similar outcome measurements to HIV- patients after activation of implants in a mandibular two-implant overdenture opposing a complete denture scenario.[8] These included 20 patients with a CD4 (glycoprotein on surface of T-helper cells) count ranging from 132–948/mL. Another short-term study substantiated that implant treatment in HIV+ patients proved to be a predictable approach in posterior mandibles.[9] Given the absence of published long-term success, it is propitious to place implants in HIV+ patients when CD4 rates are greater than 250/mL, the viral load is below 50/mL, and the patient is on antiretroviral therapy.[10] Optimized oral hygiene regimens, regular recall appointments, and screening for HIV-related oral lesions and xerostomia are recommended to treat the side effects of antiretroviral therapy.

Systemic corticosteroids can cause suppression of the hypothalamus–pituitary–adrenal axis and patients on systemic steroids are therefore at risk of adrenal insufficiency when undergoing implant surgery. Patients who have completed a short course of this therapy (less than 3 weeks) may be at risk

Evidence-based Implant Treatment Planning and Clinical Protocols, First Edition. Edited by Steven J. Sadowsky.

Companion website: www.wiley.com/go/sadowsky/implant

Table 2.1 ASA classification system for assessing relative risk for surgical procedures.

	ASA I Healthy	ASA II Mild systemic disease	ASA III Severe/not incapacitating disease	ASA IV Incapacitating	ASA V Dying
Walk up two flights of stairs	Yes	Rest at completion	Rest before finishing	Unable	Unable
Examples	Healthy	Drug allergy 140–159 systolic 90–94 diastolic Controlled diabetic Controlled asthmatic Controlled epilepsy Controlled asthma	Stable angina pectoris 160–199 systolic 90–114 diastolic Chronic obstructive pulmonary disease Myocardial infarction (MI) >6 months prior Stroke more >6 months prior	Unstable angina MI <6 months ago >200 systolic >115 diastolic Severe heart failure Uncontrolled diabetes	End-stage disease
Treatment modification	None	Stress reduction protocols where needed	Elective care OK Stress reduction recommended	Noninvasive only	Palliative only

and it is recommended that they be given steroid coverage.[3] On the other hand, a history of recent prescribed doses of less than 10 mg prednisone daily can be treated without additional steroid therapy.[11] Aside from the fact that medical advice should be garnered for immunosuppressed patients and infection-control measures must be strictly enforced, systemic corticosteroid treatment is not an absolute contraindication to implant placement.

Uncontrolled diabetes

Diabetes mellitus is a chronic disorder of carbohydrate metabolism affecting all tissues, often resulting in morbidity and possibly mortality. The American Diabetes Association reported in 2013 that nearly 10% of the US population has diabetes, including 25% of seniors, which makes this metabolic disease the most common. Persistent hyperglycemia in diabetic patients inhibits osteoblastic activity and alters the parathyroid hormone response regulating calcium and phosphorus, decreases collagen formation during the initial callus formation, and induces osteoclastic activity due to a chronic inflammatory response.[12] Type 1 diabetes is caused by an autoimmune reaction resulting in destruction of the beta cells of the pancreas leading to underproduction of insulin. Type 2 diabetics (most commonly seen in the adult population seeking dental implants) are characterized by resistance to insulin and the inability to manufacture compensatory endogenous insulin. Glycated hemoglobin (HbA1c – blood glucose levels measured over 8–12 weeks) greater than 6.5% has been considered a reliable metric indicating the diabetic patient is poorly controlled (Table 2.2, Table 2.3).

Oates *et al.*[13] have reported alterations in early (2–6 weeks) implant stability in direct relation to hyperglycemic conditions, which have been corroborated in a systematic review.[14] However, the same authors later reported on a randomized controlled trial on implant overdenture therapy in normal, controlled, and uncontrolled diabetic patients with no correlation to implant survival after 1 year.[15] This may point to the complexities of

Table 2.2 Glycated hemoglobin (HbA1c) targets.

HbA1c targets	mmol/mol	%
Nondiabetics	20–41	4–5.9
Diabetics	48	6.5
Diabetics at higher risk of hyperglycemia	59	7.5

Table 2.3 Conversion of glycated haemoglobin (HbA1c) to blood glucose level.

HbA1c (%)	Average blood glucose (mg/dL)
6	120
7	150
8	180

diabetes mellitus as well as the import of possible comorbidities. Careful evaluation of the patient's medical status/history and consultation with a physician will lead to a personalized medical approach. At this time, it is not advised to place implants in a patient with uncontrolled diabetes until longer-range follow-up studies are conducted. It is prudent to consider the following regimen for patients with hyperglycemia: 1) good glycemic control pre- and postoperatively;[16] 2) at least 4 months of healing time;[17] 3) use of prophylactic antibiotics and 0.12% chlorhexidine;[18] and 4) increased length and width of implants when native bone volume permits.[3] When patients have had a history of controlled diabetes for more than 10 years, they may also benefit from the aforementioned recommendations.[3]

Intravenous bisphosphonates

Epidemiological studies have suggested a compelling, if not circumstantial, association between intravenous (IV) nitrogen-containing bisphosphonates (BPs) and bisphosphonate-related osteonecrosis of the jaw (BRONJ) (Figure 2.1).[19] BRONJ can be

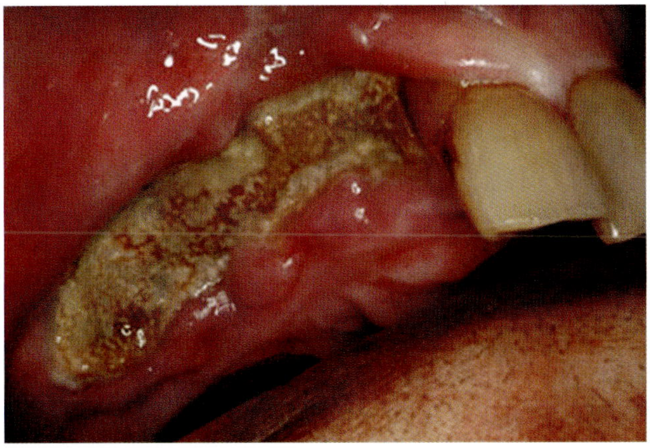

Figure 2.1 Osteonecrosis of the jaw.

Table 2.4 Relative potency of nitrogen-containing bisphosphonates.[21]

Drug name	Generic name	Relative potency*
Fosamax (oral)	Alendronate	1000
Actonel (oral)	Risedronate	5000
Boniva (oral/IV)	Ibandronate	10 000
Aredia (IV)	Pamidronate	100
Zometa (IV)	Zoledronic acid	100 000

*Relative to etidronate (non-nitrogen containing bisphosphonate with relative potency of 1).

a confirmed diagnosis if the patient is on a current or previous treatment with a bisphosphonate, presenting with exposed bone in the maxillofacial region that has persisted for 8 weeks, and no history of radiotherapy to the jaws. BPs are nonmetabolized analogs of pyrophosphate with a half-life in the bone of 11 years and are described as effective inhibitors of osteoclastic function.[20] As BP potency increases, the risk of BRONJ increases. For example, zoledronate is more than 100 times more potent than alendronate (Table 2.4).[22] Frequency estimates for BRONJ risk in patients exposed to IV BPs have ranged from 0.7% to 12%, as opposed to risk with oral BPs ranging from 0.04% (without extractions) to 0.3% (with extractions). The preponderance of cases of BRONJ has been reported in the mandible.

IV BPs are used for the management of hypercalcemia and the treatment of symptomatic bony lesions or prevention of pathologic fracture from multiple myeloma, or metastatic tumors from breast cancer, lung cancer, prostate cancer, and other solid tumors.[23] Hypercalcemia is a common complication of advanced malignancies, impacting 10–20% of patients during their disease state. IV BPs are dosed frequently (e.g. 4 mg of zoledronate monthly) as opposed to the management of osteoporosis which would use zoledronate in a 5 mg annual dose. While current studies suggest no increased risk for patients being managed with IV BPs for osteoporosis,[24,25] the investigations are recent, and the cumulative exposure to IV BPs has been limited. This will further be addressed under the heading of Osteoporosis.

Based on a recent systematic review, implants can be placed successfully in patients with a history of IV BPs, but the studies are of moderate to weak strength of evidence with inherent bias and limitations, and hence results must be interpreted with caution.[26] Until well-controlled trials with higher strength of evidence on larger populations (with homogeneity in terms of BP dosage, frequency, and duration) are conducted, the use of IV BPs should be considered an absolute contraindication to implant placement.

Bleeding disorders

There is no reliable evidence that bleeding disorders should be considered in a class of absolute contraindications for implant placement. Even patients with congenital bleeding abnormalities (hemophiliacs) may be treated successfully with dental implants.[27] However, if there is a history of bleeding problems in the patient/familial line or if medications are linked to clotting problems, laboratory tests, such as platelet count, bleeding time, prothrombin time (PT), and partial thromboplastin time (PTT), are recommended. The platelet count is ascertained in the complete blood count (CBC) and normal values are 200 000–300 000/mL. Values one tenth of normal represent a spontaneous bleeding risk. Bleeding time assesses both platelet function and capillary activity. Extrinsic (outside vessels) and intrinsic pathways (factors VII through XII) of coagulation are evaluated with the PT and PTT, respectively.

Anemia is the most common hematological disorder, resulting in a decreased production of erythrocytes or increased rate of their destruction, possibly from a deficiency in iron. Bone maturation can be impaired in the chronic anemic patient. Decreased density of bone has been found to influence time of integration. Hematocrit levels (volume of blood made up of erythrocytes) should be no lower than 40%. A hemoglobin test (assessment of oxygen-containing protein in blood) is also needed to proceed with surgery (minimum 10 mg/dL).

There is a group of medications that inhibits the production of prothrombin. Patients on anticoagulants (e.g. warfarin) may proceed with implant placement without modifying their prescribed regimen, provided that the International Normalized Ratio (INR) is less than or equal to 2.5 (2.5 times normal to clot) and the surgery does not involve autogenous bone grafts or extensive flaps.[28] If heparin has been prescribed for anticoagulation, a patient should have a PTT scheduled the day of surgery and if it is 1.5 times the normal value, surgery should be postponed. Long-term antibiotic coverage interferes with intestinal bacteria necessary to produce vitamin K, affecting the prothrombin levels in the liver and a PT should be evaluated. Aspirin inhibits platelet function because it interferes with the hepatic production of prothrombin by blocking vitamin K. If four or more tablets (325 mg) are prescribed for more than 1 week, bleeding time and PTT can be affected, signaling a possibility of a bleeding complication. In rare cases, implant placement can

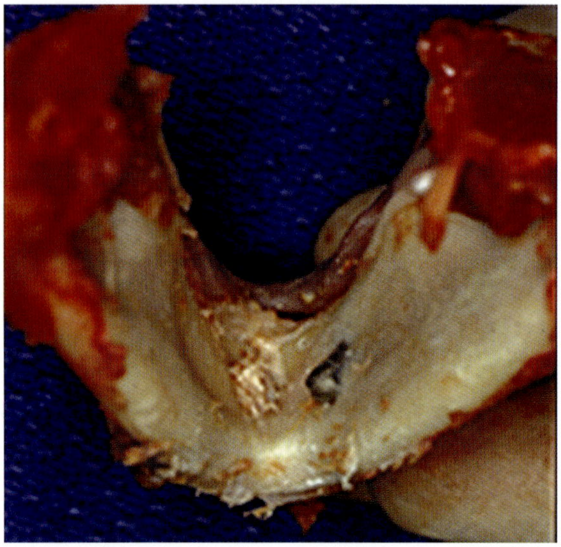

Figure 2.2 Implant perforation of lingual plate.

cause arterial impingement (e.g. perforation of the lingual plate, Figure 2.2) and in patients with bleeding disorders, hemorrhage may be prolonged, raising the risk of a serious complication.[28] However, with patients on antiplatelet therapy (aspirin, nonsteroidal anti-inflammatory drugs) the risks of thromboembolism may outweigh the risk of bleeding after invasive dental procedures and therefore their medication usually is not altered.[29]

Despite the lack of evidence to suggest that bleeding disorders are an absolute contraindication to implant placement, medical advice should obtained before surgery, especially for patients with congenital bleeding maladies. With this cohort of patients, as with others that are medically compromised, a premium is placed on surgical expertise.

Recent myocardial infarction/stroke

It has been purported that some cardiovascular events, such as myocardial infarction, stroke, and cardiovascular surgery, may be classified in the category of absolute contraindications.[30] A number of retrospective studies, however, have failed to link coronary artery disease or hypertension to a significant increase in either early or late implant failures.[31–34] Despite the weight of this evidence, it is propitious to obtain medical advice before any surgical procedure is planned for these patients, as the sequela of bleeding or an ischemic event during placement of implants is possible. To this point, approximately 20% of patients with a recent history of MI will have complications of a recurrent episode with a mortality rate as high as 70%. The risk of recurrence with a surgical procedure decreases with time from 30%, if within 3 months of the MI, to 5% after 1 year post-MI.[35] It is of note when treating patients with unstable hemodynamics, that the efficacy of intravenous sedation using midazolam and propofol synergistically during implant surgery has been well demonstrated in a comparative study.[36]

Active treatment of malignancy

Due to the variability of disease conditions and combinations of treatment regimens, the oncological patient is difficult to categorize regarding implant placement risk. Radiotherapy is commonly used to treat head and neck tumors and has been found to significantly impact dental implant outcomes during the healing period as well as predisposing to osteonecrosis of the jaw because of the induction of endarteritis obliterans.[37] For example, an 8-year follow-up demonstrated 75% implant survival rate of implants in the irradiated mandible.[38] However, implant success rates in irradiated patients have been reported to be linked to the source, dose, and fractionation of irradiation, concomitant therapies, jaw site, and timing of the adjuvant therapies.[39,40] The following guidelines have been proposed to improve implant therapy outcome:[2,41,42]

- the source should avoid implant portals, if possible;
- when the dose is less than 66 Gy, this reduces the risk of osteonecrosis of the jaw (more common in the mandible), and when less than 50 Gy reduces implant failure;
- daily fractions of 1/25 the total target irradiated dose is recommended;
- while controversy persists regarding the concomitant use of hyperbaric oxygen,[40] hyperbaric treatment has been recommended when the therapeutic dose has been greater than 50 Gy.

When implants are inserted after radiotherapy, the implant failure rate can be expected to be lower on the mandible than maxilla (4.4% vs. 17.5%).[42] Implant surgery is optimally carried out either more than 21 days before irradiation therapy or 9 months after. Implant placement is not indicated during radiotherapy or in the presence of mucositis. Immediate loading is not recommended on post-radiation patients.

In regard to implant therapy following chemotherapy, two studies compared data to healthy controls and found no significant difference in implant failure rates when radiotherapy did not accompany treatment.[34,44] On the other hand, a history of therapeutic radiation is considered a relative contraindication to implant treatment, especially on the maxilla. In summary, active radiotherapy is an absolute contraindication to implant placement, but implant placement is not contraindicated in the patient after completing only chemotherapy,[44] although comorbidities must be analyzed carefully. Consultation with the oncologist is recommended in all cases when surgical and prosthodontic treatment is planned for the cancer patient. Dental implants are not necessarily contraindicated in patients with terminal illness as their quality of life may be immensely improved during their time remaining.

Alcohol/drug abuse

While animal studies[45] have found a negative impact of alcohol intake on bone density and osseointegration (bone-to-implant contact), human studies have only established an increased risk of complications such as peri-implantitis in this subset of patients.[46,47] Attendant to more occult conditions, alcoholism has also been shown to be implicated in a myriad of problems from bleeding disorders due to a decrease in platelet production, to impairing nutrition (e.g. vitamin B) and the immune response (elevated levels of cortisol and interleukin [IL]-10).[2] Chronic alcoholism increases infection risk postoperatively due to the T-helper cell ratio of T1 to T2 being depressed.[48] Preoperative alcohol cessation prior to implant therapy was evaluated with two randomized controlled studies using pharmacological strategies for alcohol withdrawal and relapse.[49] The findings demonstrate reduction of postoperative complication rate, including decreased frequency of delirium tremors and postoperative seizures while reducing the need for potent sedatives. Timing, duration, and intensity of intervention, however, need further study. In summary, alcoholism (10% of US population is dependent[50]) is often linked to comorbidities which can magnify the incidence of untoward postsurgical consequences.

In 2010, it was estimated that approximately 8.9% of persons older than 12 years old were illicit drug users, which has increased from 6.3% in 2000.[51,52] Over the last 15 years there has been a 10-fold increase in the use of opioid painkillers. Surgical problems related to the parental drug misuse may have global medical implications which include increase in blood-borne infections, thrombosed veins, and neuropraxia. However, there is a paucity of studies that correlate implant failure to drug abuse. One multicentered retrospective study completed a multivariate analysis of risk for implant failure and noted that addiction to narcotics was a significant factor.[53] Notwithstanding the fact that neither alcoholism nor drug addiction has been demonstrated to be an absolute contraindication to implant therapy, there is little rationale to proceed with an elective surgical procedure until there is substance abuse cessation.

Neuropsychiatric/neuromuscular illness

A limited number of case reports and case series predominate in the literature addressing the influence of psychiatric and neuromuscular conditions on implant integration.[54–56] Mental, psychiatric, and physical disabilities have not been analyzed with granularity to assess which patients would be poor candidates for osseointegrated rehabilitation. The fact that patients with cerebral palsy,[57] severe epilepsy,[58] and Parkinson's disease[59] have been treated successfully over a medium- to long-term period is promising, but patient selection remains paramount in considering prognosis and prosthetic strategy. For example, lower implant survival rates have been reported in Parkinson's disease patients compared to healthy patients.[59] However, implant and prosthetic success are not well documented due to heterogeneity. For example, design considerations for patients with poor compliance in home care or parafunctional habits may favor a removable implant prosthesis and also facilitate maintenance care. On the other hand, retention security with a locking mechanism may be essential to counteract the effects of seizures or dislodging behavior habits common to neuropsychiatric patients. In summary, while the presentation of unrealistic expectations is considered an absolute contraindication to dental implant placement, neuropsychiatric or neuromuscular illness may not be. However, it is important to analyze the constellation of specific ailments in this classification that may contribute to the severity of the risk. This supports the admonition to seek a psychiatric/medical consult for collaboration in implant and prosthetic treatment planning.

Osteoporosis

Osteoporosis has been defined as a condition that is present if the patient's bone mineral density level is 2.5 standard deviations below that of a mean young population, using dual energy X-ray absorptiometry.[60] After the age of 60, almost 33% of the population has this disorder with twice the occurrence in women vs. men.[61] As of 2010, more than 10 million Americans have osteoporosis and 44% of the population has low bone mass.[62] Currently osteoporosis is responsible for 1.5 million fractures annually, which have as high as a 20% mortality rate after 1 year.[63] This has prompted the ubiquitous use (27 million prescriptions written in 2008) of oral bisphosphonates (BPs) to prevent osteoporotic fractures.[64] Dental implant therapy has been found to be successful in osteoporosis/osteopenia patients when compared to healthy controls.[65] No association has been revealed between bone mineral density status, mandibular bone mineral status, bone quality, and implant loss in a systematic review.[66]

Regarding the risk of bisphosphonate-related osteonecrosis of the jaw (BRONJ) with osteoporotic patients taking oral BPs (e.g. alendronate), the estimated prevalence rate has been reported to be 0.01–0.04% or one case per 2260–8470 prescriptions.[67] The incidence of BRONJ after an average of 3.3 years of oral BP therapy following implant insertion with or without tooth extraction is also minimal, comparable to rates found in nonbisphosphonate users.[68] Concern regarding longer-term use of oral BPs[69] have prompted the recommendation of a drug holiday in preventing the risk of BRONJ associated with implant placement, but has not been validated.[64] Urinary C-telopeptide (CTX, measure of type 1 collagen in urine possibly indicating increased activity of osteoclasts) may eventually show value in assessing the effects of BPs in the bone of patients.[70] However, current evidence consists of only a case series and variability in the test and lack of replication has resulted in uncertainty in its prognostic reliability.[71] In 2009, a systematic review tracking patients with chronic intake of oral BPs during dental implant treatment concluded that dental implants might be considered a safe procedure in patients taking oral BPs for less than 5 years.[72] While there is no convincing data that implant placement in patients taking oral BPs is contraindicated, patients should understand the small risk of compromised bone healing.[73]

Annual IV administration of zoledronate 5 mg has been recommended for osteoporosis patients to address esophageal irritation from oral BPs and poor compliance. This regimen has proved to be effective in reducing spinal fractures by 71% and hip fractures by 41%.[74] The incidence of osteonecrosis in patients taking an annual IV dose has been documented at less than 1 in 14 200 patient treatment years.[75] It is of note that low levels of CTX were not associated in this study with increased risk of developing BRONJ.

Smoking

It has been estimated in 2012 that 18.1% of all adults or approximately 42 million people are cigarette smokers.[76] The relative risk (RR) of lung cancer and oral cancer is 23 times and 3.43 times higher respectively in smokers compared to nonsmokers.[77] Data on the link between smoking and epigenetic mechanisms have emerged, with recent studies showing that hypermethylation in the promotor region of tumor suppressor genes prompted a repression of these genes in head and neck cancer.[78] Additionally, cigarette bioactive chemicals, such as nicotine, nitrosamines, aldehydes, carbon monoxide, and benzene, have been shown to have a deleterious effect on bone healing.[79,80] For example, nicotine reduces osteoblastic activity impacting the amount of collagen available to form the extracellular matrix, decreases the blood flow and nutrients in healing zone, and decreases the proliferation of macrophages that participate in the immune response.[81–83]

A meta-analysis with multivariable-adjusted relative risk in 33 studies, including over 35 000 implants, demonstrated that smoking was associated with almost twice the risk of dental implant failure (RR = 1.92) than that in nonsmokers.[84] A case-control investigation compared turned and oxidized implants and concluded that oxidized implants have similar failure rates with nonsmokers.[85] However, a recent 2-year prospective study using textured implants has addressed the outcome of immediately loaded single implants placed in the anterior maxilla in nonsmokers and smokers, with a focus on papilla regrowth and midfacial recession. Nonsmokers showed significantly more papillae regrowth and midfacial overgrowth compared to inactive soft tissue heights in smokers.[86] Smoking more than 15 cigarettes a day has also been linked to complications with sinus and onlay grafting.[87–89]

Given that smoking behavior has been found to have a debilitating effect on both wound healing and bone healing, it is important to address cessation with patients. Smoking cessation for 4 weeks prior to surgery has been shown to reflect a similar complication rate as that of nonsmokers.[90,91] It may be important as well to consider comorbidities for smokers when assessing risk. For example, both higher alcohol consumption and a greater prevalence of aggressive periodontitis have been found in smokers.[92–95] Heavy smokers may also be linked to a positive IL-1 genotype which has been shown to be correlated to higher implant complications.[96] In summary, a smoking habit should be considered a relative contraindication to implant placement, but in motivated patients can be terminated or at the very least suspended, leading to substantive improvement in healing potential.

Chronic periodontitis

Patients with a history of chronic periodontitis have been shown to have as high as a 25-fold increase in the probability of incidence of peri-implant disease.[43] Authors have shown common pathways in etiology of peri-implant and periodontal disease.[97–99] The microbiota associated with both disease entities are rich in Gram-negative bacteria, although other Gram-positive pathogens, such as *Staphylococcus aureus*, may also facilitate peri-implantitis. It is of note that persistent biofilm accumulation may prompt a more pronounced inflammatory reaction in the peri-implant gingival tissues than in the dentogingival unit. This has been explained by the natural tooth's gingival complex superiority in vascularity, fibroblast to collagen ratios, and the functional matrix of perpendicular or oblique Sharpey's fibers (terminal ends of the periodontal ligament) which insert in the cementum, acting as a barrier to the epithelial migration of pathogens.[97] On the other hand, connective tissue fibers run a parallel course to the implant surface and their adhesion to implants has a poor mechanical resistance compared to that of the natural dentition.[100]

Single implants have been documented at higher failure rates in patients with periodontitis, but there was no observed effect with time of placement.[101] While implant survival has been shown to be compromised in patients with a history of periodontitis, those undergoing strict periodontal maintenance care achieved an implant survival rate of 96.2%, after 5 years.[102] Mechanical and chemical antimicrobial intervention with the application of diligent home oral hygiene regimens are recommended and can be assessed after a series of strict 3-month recalls before implant therapy is initiated.[103]

Autoimmune disease

According to the Autoimmune Related Diseases Association, autoimmune disease affects up to 50 million Americans.[104] Seventy-five percent of those affected are women.[105] There are as many as 80 types of autoimmune disease, including rheumatoid arthritis, scleroderma, Sjogrens syndrome, and systemic lupus erythematosus. All share a common pathogenesis of an immune system misinterpreting healthy cells as foreign, initiating a concerted defense against them. Diagnosis intends to test the level of antibodies and inflammation in the body. These tests include antinuclear antibody tests, autoantibody tests, complete blood count, C-reactive protein, and erythrocyte sedimentation rate.

Rheumatoid arthritis (RA) affects the joints with pain, swelling, and stiffness, and has a varied course and duration. Retrospective studies evaluating implant prosthodontic rehabilitation of patients with RA, either isolated RA or with concomitant connective tissue disease (CCTD), revealed a high implant survival rate, albeit with small samples.[106,107] However, patients with CCTD may demonstrate pronounced marginal bone resorption and bleeding on probing. Scrupulous oral hygiene and a recall program appear to be essential in maintaining vulnerable soft tissue conditions.

Scleroderma is characterized by inflammatory and sclerotic changes in the skin and organs with a highly variable clinical presentation that may include taut skin and thinning of the lips (possibly hindering implant insertion) as well as indurations of the tongue.[108,109] There is a paucity of literature on dental implants in scleroderma patients represented by case reports on only a few patients with up to a 3-year follow-up.[110–112]

Sjogren's syndrome is a chronic autoimmune disease of the exocrine glands involving the salivary and lacrimal glands. Its principle presentation is xerostomia and dry eyes as well as malaise. Difficulty with caries control, swallowing, and use of removable prostheses have all been documented.[113] The use of dental implants in patients with Sjogren's syndrome has only been reported in case reports. One study placed 54 implants in eight patients with 87.1% implant survival at abutment connection and 83.3% survival after 1 year.[114] While the prospect of providing a fixed implant restoration is appealing to patients with desiccated soft tissues, only one case report has been published.[115]

Systemic lupus erythematosus (SLE) may present with a facial rash that resembles a butterfly and it can affect joints, skin, kidneys, blood cells, heart, and lungs. Implants in patients with SLE have been documented in only one case report providing an implant fixed complete denture to address severe xerostomia.[116]

Dental implant placement in patients with autoimmune disease (other than diabetes) has been investigated mainly with case reports and therefore should remain a relative contraindication. Comparative studies evaluating larger populations observed over a longer period of follow-up are needed. Documentation of implant success outcomes, not only survival, will facilitate prognostic acumen and appropriate patient selection.

Lack of surgical experience

Relative contraindications generally do not include surgical experience. However, three of four studies have demonstrated a significantly higher level of failures when implants were placed by less experienced surgeons.[117–120] Specifically, Lambert *et al.*[120] noted that surgeons with less than 50 implants placed had twice the failure rate (3.5% vs. 1.8%); notably with the first nine cases showing the greatest difference. Careful site selection and preoperative planning in collaboration with experienced surgeons could flatten out the learning curve.

Temporary contraindications

Incomplete growth

Routinely, implants have been reserved for patients after craniofacial/skeletal growth is completed. When the epiphysis of the radius fuses and forms a bony union with the diaphysis as seen in a hand–wrist radiograph, the adult level of skeletal growth has been attained.[121] Superimposing tracings of serial cephalometric radiographs taken at least 6 months apart also is a reliable index, but requires greater irradiation and time.[122] Implants placed after the age of 15 in girls and 18 in boys have been reported to have the most predictable prognosis.[123]

In the presence of natural teeth, early implant insertion can result in an apically submerged implant (similar to ankylosed primary tooth), progressive infraocclusion, and possible harm to adjacent teeth.[124] Transverse palatal growth along the suture line can create esthetic and functional problems when implants are placed in the posterior maxillae of a prepubertal child.[125] Although the mandibular symphyseal suture closes within months of birth and early placement of anterior implants may have a reasonable prognosis, flexibility in prosthetic design must be planned to accommodate 5–6 mm of dental height caused by mandibular growth.[124] With these caveats in mind, Sharma *et al.*[126] have identified two groups of young patients which would benefit from early implant placement: children who are missing more than a few teeth, but have permanent teeth present adjacent to edentulous sites, and children who are virtually or completely edentulous (e.g. ectodermal dysplasia). In these cases, subsequent surgical and/or restorative interventions will be planned as the child matures.[127] An in-depth review of the indications, treatment phases, and outcomes in the implant treatment of the growing patient will be addressed in Chapter 13.

Pregnancy

Dental implant placement is contraindicated until after term for the gravid patient. Radiographs, medication, increased stress, and possible surgical complications related to the procedure are best postponed. Only emergency dental procedures and caries control should be considered, and preferably during the second or third trimesters. In the middle to late third trimester, caution is advised when treating the expectant mother in the supine position as hypotension may result from the pressure of the fetus on the inferior vena cava.[2] Meticulous home care and regular prophylaxis are recommended as periodontitis is often magnified during pregnancy, especially in those 30 years or older.[128]

Summary

In conclusion, there has been a dearth of prospective studies to clearly establish absolute or relative contraindications for implant placement. However, a number of systemic conditions has been shown to elevate the risk for implant failure or complications in specific subsets of the population. A careful assessment of the patient's disease state with medical consultation when necessary, will allow for a customized informed consent of the risk factors, given the best available evidence. The clinician should not minimize the potential to motivate the patient to improve their health status by cessation of destructive habits and commitment to long-term health and dental maintenance care.

References

1. Maloney WJ, Weinberg MA. Implementation of the American Society of Anesthesiologists physical status classification in periodontal practice. *J Periodontol* 2008; **79**(7): 1124–1126.
2. Misch CE. *Contemporary Implant Dentistry*, 2nd edn. St. Louis: Mosby 1999.
3. Bornstein MM, Cionca N, Mombelli A. Systemic conditions and treatments as risks for implant therapy. *Int J Oral Maxillofac Implants* 2009; **24**(Suppl): 12–27.
4. Diz P, Sully C, Sanz M. Dental implants in the medically compromised patient. *J Dent* 2013; **41**(3): 195–206.
5. Heckmann SM, Heckmenn JG, Linke JJ, *et al.* Implant therapy following liver transplantation: clinical and microbiological results after 10 years. *J Periodontol* 2004; **75**(6): 909–913.
6. Gu L, Yu YC. Clinical outcome of dental implants placed in liver transplant recipients after 3 years: a case series. *Transplant Proc* 2011; **43**(7): 2678–2682.
7. Sakakura CE, Marcantonio Jr E, Wenzel A, *et al.* Influence of cyclosporine A on quality of bone around integrated dental implants: a radiographic study in rabbits. *Clin Oral Implants Res* 2007; **18**(1): 34–39.
8. Stevenson GC, Riano PC, Moretti AJ, *et al.* Short-term success of osseointegrated dental implants in HIV-positive individuals: a prospective study. *J Contemp Dent Pract* 2007; **8**(1): 1–10.
9. Oliveira MA, Gallottini M, Pallos D, *et al.* The success of endosseous implants in human immunodeficiency virus-positive patients receiving antiretroviral therapy: a pilot study. *J Am Dent Assoc* 2011; **142**(9): 1010–1016.
10. Streizel FP, Rothe S, Reichart PA, *et al.* Implant-prosthetic treatment in HIV-infected patients receiving highly active antiretroviral therapy: Report of cases. *Int J Oral Maxillofac Implants* 2006; **21**(6): 951–956.
11. Nicholson C, Burrin JM, Hall GM. Peri-operative steroid supplementation. *Anesthesia* 1998; **53**(11): 1091–1104.
12. Dubey RK, Gupta DK, Singh AK. Dental implant survival in diabetic patients: review and recommendations. *Natl J Maxillofac Surg* 2013; **4**(2): 142–150.
13. Oates TW, Dowell S, Robinson M, *et al.* Glycemic control and implant stabilization in type 2 diabetes mellitus. *J Dent Res* 2009; **88**(4): 367–371.
14. Oates TW, Huynh-Ba G, Vargas A, *et al.* A critical review of diabetes, glycemic control, and dental implant therapy. *Clin Oral Implants Res* 2013; **24**(2): 117–127.
15. Oates TW, Galloway P, Alexander P, *et al.* The effects of elevated hemoglobulin A1c in patients with type 2 diabetes mellitus on dental implants. Survival and stability at one year. *JADA* 2014; **145**(12): 1218–1226.
16. Ciancio SG, Lauciello F, Shibly O, *et al.* The effect of an antiseptic mouthrinse on implant maintenance: plaque and peri-implant gingival tissues. *J Periodontol* 1995; **66**(11): 962–965.
17. Morris HF, Ochi S, Winkler S. Implant survival in patients with type 2 diabetes: placement to 36 months. *Ann Periodontol* 2000; **5**(1): 157–163.
18. Balshi TJ, Wolfinger GJ. Dental implants in the diabetic patient: a retrospective study. *Implant Dent* 1999; **8**(4): 355–359.
19. Dodson TB. Intravenous bisphosphonate therapy and bisphosphonate-related osteonecrosis of the jaws. *J Oral Maxillofac Surg* 2009; **67**(5Suppl): 44–52.
20. Marx RE. Oral and intravenous bisphosphonate-induced osteonecrosis of the jaws: history, etiology, prevention, and treatment. Chicago: Quintessence 2007; 12.
21. Marx RE. A decade of bisphosphonate bone complications: what it has taught us about bone physiology. *Int J Oral Maxillofac Implants* 2014; **29**(2): 247–258.
22. Fantasia JE. Bisphosphonates: practical considerations. *J Oral Maxillofac Surg* 2009; **67**(5 Suppl): 53–60.
23. Mehrotra B. Bisphosphonates – role in cancer therapies. *J Oral Maxillofac Surg* 2009; **67**(5 Suppl): 19–26.
24. Black DM, Delmas PD, Eastell R, *et al.* Once-yearly zoledronic acid for treatment of postmenopausal osteoporosis. *N Engl J Med* 2007; **356**(18): 1809–1822.
25. Lyles KW, Colon-Emeric CS, Magaziner JS, *et al.* Zoledronic acid in reducing clinical fracture and mortality after hip fracture. *N Engl J Med* 2007; **357**: 1799.
26. Chadha GK, Amadieh A, Kumar S, *et al.* Osseointegration of dental implants and osteonecrosis of the jaw in patients treated with bisphosphonate therapy: a systematic review. *J Oral Implantol* 2013; **39**(4): 510–520.
27. Gornitsky M, Hammouda W, Rosen H. Rehabilitation of a hemophiliac with implants: a medical perspective and case report. *J Oral Maxillofac Surg* 2005; **63**(5): 592–597.
28. Scully C. *Medical Problems in Dentistry*, 6th edn. London: Elsevier 2010.
29. Napenas JJ, Hong CH, Brennan MT, *et al.* Frequency of bleeding following invasive dental treatment in patients receiving single and dual antiplatelet therapy. *J Am Dent Assoc* 2009; **140**(6): 690–695.
30. Hwang D, Wang HL. Medical contraindications to implant therapy. Part I. Absolute contraindications. *Implant Dent* 2006; **15**(4): 353–360.
31. Khadivi V, Anderson J, Zarb GA. Cardiovascular disease and treatment outcomes with osseointegration surgery. *J Prosthet Dent* 1999; **81**(5): 533–536.
32. Alsaadi G, Quirynen M, Komarek A, *et al.* Impact of local and systemic factors on the incidence of late implant loss. *Clin Oral Implants Res* 2008; **19**(7): 670–676.
33. Moy PK, Medina D, Shetty V, *et al.* Dental implant failure rates and associated risk factors. *Int J Oral Maxillofac Implants* 2005; **20**(4): 560–577.
34. Alsaadi G, Quirynen M, Komarek A, *et al.* Impact of local and systemic factors on incidence of oral implant failures, up to abutment connection. *J Clin Periodontol* 2007; **34**(7): 610–617.

35. Pell S, D'Alonzo CA. Immediate mortality and 5-year survival of employed men with a first myocardial infarction. *N Eng J Med* 1964; **270**: 915.
36. Taguchi T, Fukuda K, Sekeine H, *et al.* Intravenous sedation and hemodynamic changes during dental implant surgery. *Int J Oral Maxillofac Implants* 2011; **26**(6): 1301–1308.
37. Linsen SS, Martini M, Stark H. Long-term results of endosteal implants following radical oral cancer surgery with and without adjuvant radiation therapy. *Clin Implant Dent Rel Res* 2012; **14**(2): 250–258.
38. Yerit KC, Posch M, Seemann M, *et al.* Implant survival in mandibles of irradiated oral cancer patients. *Clin Oral Implants Res* 2006; **17**(3): 337–344.
39. Chiapasco M. Implants for patients with maxillofacial defects and following irradiation. In: Lang NP, Karring T, Lindhe J (eds). *Proceedings of the 3rd European Workshop on Periodontology*. Berlin: Quintessence Int 1999: 557–607.
40. Granstrom G. Osseointegration in irradiated cancer patients: an analysis with respect to implant failures. *J Oral Maxillofac Surg* 2005; **63**(5): 579–585.
41. Granstrom G. Radiotherapy, osseointegration and hyperbaric oxygen therapy. *Periodontol 2000* 2003; **33**: 145–162.
42. Collela G, Cannavale R, Pentenero M, *et al.* Oral implants in radiated patients: a systematic review. *Int J Oral Maxillofac Implants* 2007; **22**(4): 616–622.
43. Kovacs AF. Influence of chemotherapy on endosteal implant survival and success in oral cancer patients. *Int J Oral Maxillofac Surg* 2001; **30**(2): 144–147.
44. De Araujo Nobre M, Malo P, Antune E. Influence of systemic conditions on the incidence of peri-implant pathology: a case-control study. *Implant Dent* 2014; **23**(3): 305–310.
45. De Deco CP, Marchini AM, Marchini L, *et al.* Extended periods of alcohol intake negatively affects osseointegration in rats. *J Oral Implantol* 2015; **41**(3): e44–49.
46. Heitz-Mayfield LJ. Peri-implant diseases: diagnosis and risk indicators. *J Clin Periodontol* 2008; **35**(8 Suppl): 292–304.
47. Galindo-Moreno, Cabrera-Leon A. Sanchez-Fernandez E. Influence of alcohol and tobacco habits on peri-implant marginal bone loss: a prospective study. *Clin Oral Implants Res* 2005; **16**(5): 579–586.
48. Lau A, von Dossow V, Sander M, *et al.* Alcohol use disorder and perioperative immune dysfunction. *Anesth Analg* 2009; **108**(3): 916–920.
49. Oppedal K, Moller AM, Pedersen B, *et al.* Preoperative alcohol cessation prior to elective surgery. *Cochrane Database Syst Rev* 2012; **7**: CD008343.
50. Hurst GB. Alcohol and surgery: don't miss the risk. *OR Nurse* 2008; **2**: 30–35.
51. DrugFacts: Nationwide trends (2012). Retrieved Sept. 8, 2012 from http://www.drugabuse.gov/publications/drugfacts/nationwide-trends
52. Calder KK, Severyn FA. Surgical emergencies in the intravenous drug user. *Emerg Med Clin N Am* 2003; **21**(4): 1089–1116.
53. Ekfeldt A, Christiansson U, Eriksson T, *et al.* A retrospective analysis of factors associated with multiple implant failures in maxillae. *Clin Oral Implants Res* 2001; **12**(5): 462–467.
54. Addy L, Korszun A, Jagger RG. Dental implant treatment for patients with psychiatric disorders. *Eur J Prosthodont Restor Dent* 2006; **14**(2): 90–92.
55. Feijoo JF, Limeres J, Dinis M, *et al.* Osseointegrated dental implants in patients with intellectual disability: a pilot study. *Disabil Rehabil* 2012; **34**(23): 2025–2030.
56. Oczakir C, Bahmer S, Mericske-Stern R. Implant-prosthodontic treatment for special care patients: a case series study. *Int J Prosthodont* 2005: **18**(5): 383–389.
57. Rogers JO. Implant stabilized complete mandibular denture for a patient with cerebral palsy. *Dent Update* 1995; **22**(1): 23–26.
58. Cune MS, Strooker H, van der Reijden WA, *et al.* Dental implants in persons with severe epilepsy and multiple disabilities: a long-term retrospective study. *Int J Oral Maxillofac Implants* 2009; **24**(3): 534–540.
59. Packer M, Nikitin V, Coward T, Fiske J. The potential benefits of dental implants on oral health quality of life of people with Parkinson's disease. *Gerontology* 2009; **26**(1): 11–18.
60. Glazer DL, Kaplan FS. Osteoporosis: definition and clinical presentation. *Spine* 1997; **22**(24 suppl): 125–165.
61. Sones S, Fazio R, Fang L (eds). *Principles and Practice of Oral Medicine*. Philadelphia: WB Saunders 1984.
62. Wright NC, Looker AC, Saag KC, *et al.* The recent prevalence of osteoporosis and low bone mass in the United States based on the bone mineral density at the femoral neck or lumbar spine. *J Bone Miner Res* 2014; **29**(11): 2520–2526.
63. Becker DJ, Kilgore ML, Morrisey MA. The societal burden of osteoporosis. *Curr Rheumatol Rep* 2010; **12**(3): 186–191.
64. Assael L. Oral bisphosphonates as a cause of bisphosphonate-related osteonecrosis of the jaws: clinical findings, assessment of risks, and preventive strategies. *J Oral Maxillofac Surg* 2009; **67**(5 Suppl): 35–43.
65. Famili P, Zavoral JM. Low skeletal bone mineral density does not affect dental implants. *J Oral Implantol* 2015; **41**(5): 550–553.
66. Slagter KW, Raghoebar GM, Vissink A. Osteoporosis and edentulous jaws. *Int J Prosthodont* 2008; **21**(1): 19–21.
67. Mavrokokki T, Cheng A, Stein B, *et al.* Nature and frequency of bisphosphonate-associated osteonecrosis of the jaws in Australia. *J Oral Maxillofac Surg* 2007; **65**(3): 415–423.
68. Fugazzotto PA, Lightfoot WS, Jaffin R, *et al.* Implant placement with or without simultaneous tooth extraction in patients taking oral bisphosphonates: postoperative healing, early follow-up, and incidence of complications in two private practices. *J Periodontol* 2007; **78**(9): 1664–1669.
69. Wang HL, Weber D, McCauley LK. Effect of long-term oral bisphosphonates on implant wound healing: literature review and case report. *J Periodontol* 2007; **78**(3): 584–594.
70. Rosen HN, Moses AC, Garber J. Serum CTX: a new marker of bone resorption that shows treatment effects more often than other markers because of low coefficient of variability and large changes with bisphosphonate therapy. *Calcif Tissue Int* 2000; **66**(2): 100.
71. Marx R, Cillo J, Ulloa J. Oral bisphosphonate-induced osteonecrosis: risk factors, prediction of risk using serum CTX testing, prevention and treatment. *J Oral Maxillofac Surg* 2007; **65**(12): 2397–2410.
72. Madrid C, Sanz M. What impact do systemically administered bisphosphonates have on oral implant therapy? A systematic review. *Clin Oral Implants Res* 2009; **20**(Suppl 4): 87–95.
73. Otomo-Corgel J. Osteoporosis and osteopenia: implications for periodontal and implant therapy. *Periodontol 2000* 2012; **59**(1): 111–139.
74. Black DM, Delmas PD, Eastell R, *et al.* Once-yearly zolendronic acid for treatment of postmenopausal osteoporosis. *N Eng J Med* 2007; **356**(18): 1809–1822.
75. Grbic JT, Black DM, Lyles KW, *et al.* The incidence of osteonecrosis of the jaw in patients receiving 5 mg of zoledronic acid: data from

health outcomes and reduced incidence with zoledronic acis once yearly clinical trials program. *J Am Dent Assoc* 2010; **141**(11): 1365–1370.
76. Jamal A, Agaku IT, O'Connor E, *et al.* Current cigarette smoking among adults – United States, 2005-2013. *MMWR Morb Mortal Wkly Rep* 2014; **63**(47): 1108–1112.
77. Levin L, Kessler-Baruch O. Cigarette smoking and alveolar bone around teeth and dental implants. *NY State Dent J* 2013; **79**(5): 53–59.
78. Chang HW, Ling GS, Wei WI, *et al.* Smoking and drinking can induce p15 methylation in the upper aerodigestive tract of healthy individuals and patients with head and neck squamous cell carcinoma. *Cancer* 2004; **101**(1): 125–132.
79. Supervia A, Nogues X, Enjuanes A, *et al.* Effect of smoking and smoking cessation on bone mass, bone remodeling, vitamin D, PTH and sex hormones. *J Musculoskelet Neuronal Interact* 2006; **6**(3): 234–241.
80. Pereira ML, Carvalho JC, Peres F, *et al.* Simultaneous effects of nicotine, acrolein and acetaldehyde on osteogenic-induced bone marrow cells cultured on plasma-sprayed titanium implants. *Int J Oral Maxillofac Implants* 2010; **25**(1): 112–122.
81. Garg A. Pathophysiology of tobacco use and wound healing. *Dent Implantol Update* 2010; **21**(1): 1–4.
82. Shibli JA, Piatteli A, Iezzi G, *et al.* Effect of smoking on early bone healing around oxidized surfaces: a prospective, controlled study in human jaws. *J Periodontol* 2010; **81**(4): 575–583.
83. Balatsouka D, Gotfredsen K, Lindh CH, *et al.* The impact of nicotine on bone healing and osseointegration. *Clin Oral Implants Res* 2005; **16**(3): 268–276.
84. Chen H, Liu N, Xu X, *et al.* Smoking, radiotherapy, diabetes and osteoporosis as risk factors for dental implant failure: a meta-analysis. *PloS One* 2013; **8**(8): e71955.
85. Sayardoust S, Grondahl K, Johansson E, *et al.* Implant survival and marginal bone loss at turned and oxidized implants in periodontitis-susceptible smokers and never-smokers: a retrospective, clinical, case control study. *J Periodontol* 2013; **84**(12): 1775–1782.
86. Raes S, Rocci A, Raes F, *et al.* A prospective cohort study on the impact of smoking on soft tissue alterations around single implants. *Clin Oral Implants Res* 2015; **26**(9): 1086–1090.
87. Testori T, Weinstein RL, Taschieri S, *et al.* Risk factor analysis following maxillary sinus augmentation: a retrospective multicenter study. *Int J Oral Maxillofac Implants* 2012; **27**(5): 1170–1176.
88. Zinser MJ, Randelzhofer P, Kuiper L, *et al.* The predictors of implant failure after maxillary sinus floor augmentation and reonstruction: a retrospective study of 1045 consecutive implants. *Oral Surg Oral Med Oral Pathol Oral Radiol* 2013; **115**(5): 571–582.
89. Nystrom E, Nilson H, Gunne J, *et al.* A 9–14 year follow-up of onlay bone grafting in the atrophic maxilla. *Int J Oral Maxillofac Surg* 2009; **38**(2): 111–116.
90. Truntzer J, Vopal B, Feldstein M, *et al.* Smoking cessation and bone healing: optimal cessation timing. *Eur J Orthop Surg Traumatol* 2015; **25**(2): 211–215.
91. Wong J, Lam DP, Abrishami A, *et al.* Short-term preoperative smoking cessation and postoperative complications: a systemic review and meta-analysis. *Can J Anesth* 2012; **59**(3): 268–279.
92. Dani JA, Harris RA. Nicotine addiction and comorbidity with alcohol abuse and mental illness. *Nat Neurosci* 2005; **8**(11): 1465–1470.
93. Grant BF. Age at smoking onset and its association with alcohol consumption and DSMIV alcohol abuse and dependence: results from National Longitudinal Alcohol Epidemiologic Survey. *J Subst Abuse* 1997; **9**: 103–110.
94. Genco RJ, Bornnakke WS. Risk factors for periodontal disease. *Periodontol 2000* 2013; **62**(1): 59–94.
95. Jansson H. Studies on periodontitis and analyses of individuals at risk for periodontal diseases. *Swed Dent J Suppl* 2006; **180**: 5–49.
96. Gruica B, Wang HY, Lang NP, *et al.* Impact of IL-1 genotype and smoking status on the prognosis of osseointegrated implants. *Clin Oral Implants Res* 2004; **15**(4): 393–400.
97. Heitz-Mayfield LJ, Lang NP. Comparative biology of chronic and aggressive periodontitis vs. peri-implantitis. *Periodontol 2000* 2010; **53**: 167–181.
98. Heydenrijk K, Meier HJ, van der Reijden WA, *et al.* Microbiota around root-form endosseous implants: a review of the literature. *Int J Oral Maxillofac Implants* 2002; **17**(6): 829–838.
99. Silverstein LH, Kurtzman D, Garnick JJ, *et al.* The microbiota of the peri-implant region in health and disease. *Implant Dent* 1994; **3**(3): 170–174.
100. Dhir S, Mahesh L, Kurtzman GM, *et al.* Peri-implant and periodontal tissues: a review of differences and similarities. *Compend Contin Educ Dent* 2013; **34**(7): e69–75.
101. Evian CI, Emling R, Rosenberg ES, *et al.* Retrospective analysis of implant survival and the influence of periodontal disease and immediate placement on long-term results. *Int J Oral Maxillofac Implants* 2004; **19**(3): 393–398.
102. Garcia-Bellosta S, Bravom, Subira C, *et al.* Retrospective study of the long-term survival of 980 implants placed in a periodontal practice. *Int J Oral Maxillofac Implants* 2010; **25**(3): 613–619.
103. Slots J, Jorgensen MG. Efficient antimicrobial treatment in periodontal maintenance care. *J Am Dent Assoc* 2000; **131**(9): 1293–1304.
104. Autoimmune Disease Fact Sheet. Womenshealth.gov. July 2012, http://womenshealth.gov/publications/our-publications/factsheet/autoimmune-diseases.cfm
105. Autoimmune Disease in Women. American Autoimmune Related Diseases Association. July 2012, http://www.aarda.org/women_and_autoimmunity.php
106. Weinlander M, Krennmair G, Piehslinger E. Implant prosthodontic rehabilitation of patients with rheumatic disorders: a case series report. *Int J Prosthodont* 2010; **23**(1): 22–28.
107. Krennmair G, Seemann R, Piehslinger E. Dental implants in patients with rheumatoid arthritis: clinical outcome and peri-implant findings. *J Clin Periodontol* 2010; **37**(10): 928–936.
108. Arnett FC, Cho M, Chatterjee S, *et al.* Familial occurrence frequencies and relative risks for systemic sclerosis (scleroderma) in three United States cohorts. *Arthritis Rheum* 2001; **44**(6): 1139–1162.
109. Clements PJ, Furst DE. *Systemic Sclerosis*, 2nd edn. Philadelphia: Lippincott, Williams & Wilkins 2004.
110. Zigdon H, Gutmacher Z, Teich S, *et al.* Full-mouth rehabilitation using dental implants in a patient with scleroderma. *Quintessence Int* 2011; **42**(9): 781–785.
111. Patel K, Welfare R, Coonar HS. The provision of dental implants and a fixed prosthesis in the treatment of a patient with scleroderma: a clinical report. *J Prosthet Dent* 1998; **79**(6): 611–612.
112. Nam J, Janakievski J, Raigrodski AJ. Complete transition from failing restorations to implant-supported fixed prostheses in a patient with scleroderma. *Comp Contin Educ Dent* 2012; **33**(10): 746–756.
113. Mathews SA, Kuien BT, Scofield RH. Oral manifestations of Sjogrens syndrome. *J Dent Res* 2008; **87**(4): 308–318.

114. Isador F, Brondum K, Hansen HJ, *et al.* Outcome of treatment with implant-retained dental prostheses in patients with Sjogren syndrome. *Int J Oral Maxillofac Implants* 1999; **14**(5): 736–743.
115. Binon PP. Thirteen-year follow-up of a mandibular implant supported fixed complete denture in a patient with Sjogren's syndrome: a clinical report. *J Prosthet Dent* 2005; **94**(5): 409–413.
116. Ergun S, Katz J, Ciffer ED, *et al.* Implant-supported oral rehabilitation of a patient with systemic lupus erythematosus: case report and review of the literature. *Quintessence Int* 2010; **41**(10): 863–867.
117. Adell R, Eriksson B, Lekholm U, *et al.* Long-term follow-up study of osseointegrated implants in the treatment of totally edentulous jaws. *Int J Oral Maxillofac Implants* 1990; **5**(4): 347–359.
118. Block MS, Kent JN. Long-term follow-up on hydroxyapatite-coated cylindrical dental implants: a comparison between developmental and recent periods. *J Oral Maxillofac Surg* 1994; **52**(9): 937–943.
119. Minsk L, Polson AM, Weisgold A, *et al.* Outcome failures of endosseous implants from a clinical training center. *Compend Contin Educ Dent* 1996; **17**(9): 848–856.
120. Lambert P, Morris H, Ochi S. Positive effect of surgical experience with implants on second-stage implant survival. *J Oral Maxillofac Surg* 1997; **55**(12 Suppl 5): 12–18.
121. Shah RA, Mitra DK, Rodrigues SV, *et al.* Implants in adolescents. *J Indian Soc Periodontol* 2013; **17**(4): 546–548.
122. Op Heij DG, Opdebeek H, van Steenberghe D, *et al.* Age as compromising factor for implant insertion. *Periodontol 2000* 2003; **33**: 172–184.
123. Westwood RM, Duncan JM. Implants in adolescents: a literature review and case reports. *Int J Oral Maxillofac Implants* 1996; **11**(6): 750–755.
124. Cronin RJ, Oesterle LJ, Ranly DM. Mandibular implants and the growing patient. *Int J Oral Maxillofac Implants* 1994; **9**(1): 55–62.
125. Oesterle LJ, Cronin RJ, Jr, Ranly DM. Maxillary implants and the growing patient. *Int J Oral Maxillofac Implants* 1993; **8**(4): 377–387.
126. Sharma AB, Vargervik K. Using implants for the growing child. *J Calif Dent Assoc* 2006; **34**(9): 719–724.
127. Heuberer S, Dvorak G, Mayer C, *et al.* Dental implants are a viable alternative to compensating oligodontia in adolescents. *Clin Oral Implants Res* 2015; **26**(4): e22–27.
128. Usin MM, Tabares SM, Parodi RJ, *et al.* Periodontal conditions during pregnancy associated with periodontal pathogens. *J Investig Clin Dent* 2013; **4**(1): 54–59.

CHAPTER 3

Maintenance Considerations in Treatment Planning Implant Restorations

Donald A. Curtis[1], Hamilton Le[2], and Roy T. Yanase[3]

[1] University of California, San Francisco, California, USA
[2] Private Practice in Prosthodontics, Torrance, California, USA
[3] Herman Ostrow School of Dentistry, University of Southern California, Los Angeles, California, USA

The concept of maintenance is simple. As clinicians, we have a choice: either we accept the short-term encumbrance of developing a meaningful in-office and at-home maintenance plan, or we face the long-term prospect of providing an uncomfortable justification for re-treatment.

Maintenance programs are not sexy. They are not esthetic. There is no wow factor in the dialogue necessary to craft a meaningful maintenance program. However, evidence clearly supports the need for a patient-specific maintenance program that takes into account patient risk factors. Most importantly, it is the right thing to do.

General considerations

There are few comparative studies to support how clinicians should best maintain dental implants or the tissues supporting implants.[1,2] This is not because maintenance is not important, but because few studies have compared protocols specific to the maintenance of dental implants. As a result, the default approach by clinicians has often been to use existing recall and maintenance protocols established for patients with natural dentition. This has worked adequately because debridement benefits the tissues proximal to both dentition and implants. Ideally, maintenance protocols for dental implants would account for the unique biologic processes of tissues around implants as well as the differing prosthetic designs seen in implant-supported restorations. The focus of this chapter will be clinician-based considerations and patient-based responsibilities in the maintenance of dental implants.

Maintenance programs for patients with dental implants are often not considered until restorative care is complete or until the patient has a maintenance issue. This is a mistake. It is important we consider maintenance programs during diagnosis and treatment planning of implant restorations, especially when extensive treatment is planned or when patients present with significant risk factors for peri-implant disease. Information gathered during diagnosis and treatment planning becomes important when considering the patient's ability to maintain and clean a planned prosthesis or how the clinician should manage expected functional forces. For example, if the patient was diagnosed as a bruxer, then the developed treatment plan, informed consent, and maintenance protocol would all need to account for controlling, monitoring, and/or dissipating forces. Similarly, if the patient has a history of active or ongoing periodontal disease, maintenance programs and recall patterns should be oriented towards microbial and biofilm management. It is also important that we consider the patient's compliance and dexterity at the time of treatment, and project 5 years out from the time of treatment on their anticipated dexterity and visual acuity, competence for manipulating cleaning brushes and devices, motivation to maintain healthy tissues, and mobility for office visits.

Maintenance is often seen as the patient's responsibility, and restorative failures are similarly seen as a result of the patient's noncompliance. This is an unfortunate perspective. Incentives for the clinician are often prioritized towards satisfying the patient's immediate esthetic goals and the patient is often fatigued and oriented to completing the lengthy and often involved treatment. Patients are frequently unaware of maintenance needs of their new implant restorations, and may consider their expensive dental implant investment as permanent and "bullet-proof". It is easy for both the clinician and patient to be dismissive of maintenance needs. However, maintenance should be considered as a shared responsibility and discussed early during treatment planning. More successful restorative outcomes occur with regular in-office recalls and follow-up with reinforcement of at-home maintenance.[1,3] Likewise, evidence shows that when maintenance programs are not followed, biologic and mechanical complications can occur rapidly, asymptomatically, and without obvious early warning signs.[1–4] The importance of maintenance programs is well illustrated in a study by Costa *et al.* in which 80 partially edentulous patients restored with implants and diagnosed with peri-implant mucositis were monitored to

Evidence-based Implant Treatment Planning and Clinical Protocols, First Edition. Edited by Steven J. Sadowsky.

Companion website: www.wiley.com/go/sadowsky/implant

determine how often they progressed to peri-implantitis over a 5-year period.[3] Patients participating in a maintenance program progressed to peri-implantitis much less frequently (18%) compared to those not participating in a maintenance program (43.9%).[3] Another recent article showed that the incidence of dental implant failure was 90% less in subjects who were enrolled in a maintenance program as opposed to subjects who were not enrolled.[5] Recently, numerous articles have pointed to the importance of patient-specific maintenance programs.[4–10] Clearly, certain groups seem more vulnerable to maintenance problems, and maintenance programs are important to improving outcomes. Identifying vulnerable individuals during diagnosis, and developing an appropriate treatment and maintenance plan is important (Figures 3.1 and 3.2).

A limitation to establishing meaningful protocols for maintenance of implants is that the etiology of marginal bone loss around dental implants is not completely understood.[2] Peri-implant mucositis around implants is most often thought to be plaque-related microbial-based inflammation.[13,14] The microbial-based model and progression of mucositis to peri-implantitis has been adapted from natural dentition where gingivitis can progress to periodontitis.[11] This model makes sense, in that the microbiota in health and disease are similar with teeth and implants; healthy implants are predominately associated with Gram-positive cocci and rods, and peri-implantitis is associated with more Gram-negative anerobic biofilm and a *Porphyromonas gingivalis* and *Fusobacterium nucleatus* complex.[15] However, there are important differences between implants and teeth in how they react to microbial insults; implants have less of a permucosal seal than teeth, allowing a deeper penetration of bacterial products with more inflammatory cytokines that is more difficult to reverse.[2,15,16]

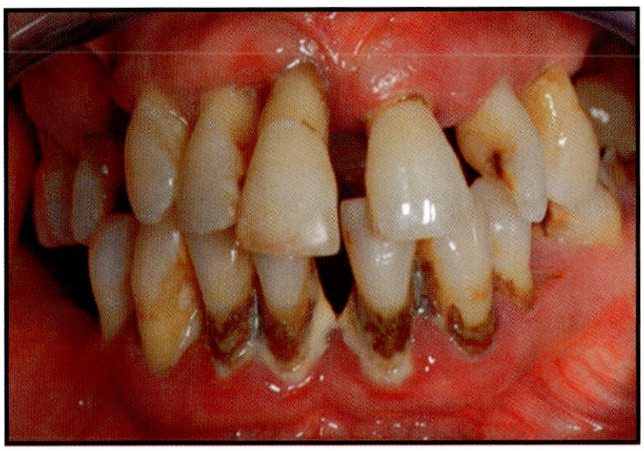

Figure 3.1 In the patient who presents with periodontal disease and poor compliance, the increased risks of implant loss need to be reviewed, and a maintenance program agreed to.[1,4,11]

It is interesting that comparison studies attempting to reverse mucositis around implants have not been as successful as studies attempting to reverse induced gingivitis around teeth.[1] This has led some to question whether peri-implantitis is entirely explained by a primary infectious process or if the bacteria are opportunistic after the tissue has broken down from nonmicrobial processes.[17,18] Bone loss has also been considered to be mediated by strain, with loading causing susceptible bone to microfracture, resulting in a secondary inflammatory process.[18] A second contribution to marginal bone loss could also be an aseptic foreign-body reaction to the implant.[18] Because of our incomplete understanding of marginal bone loss, our ability to develop predictable maintenance protocols that target all the known etiologies of marginal bone loss is limited. Yet, even without a complete understanding of the etiologies of marginal bone loss, strong evidence exists that a maintenance program is important, especially with high-risk groups such as those with a history of periodontal disease.[3,4,19]

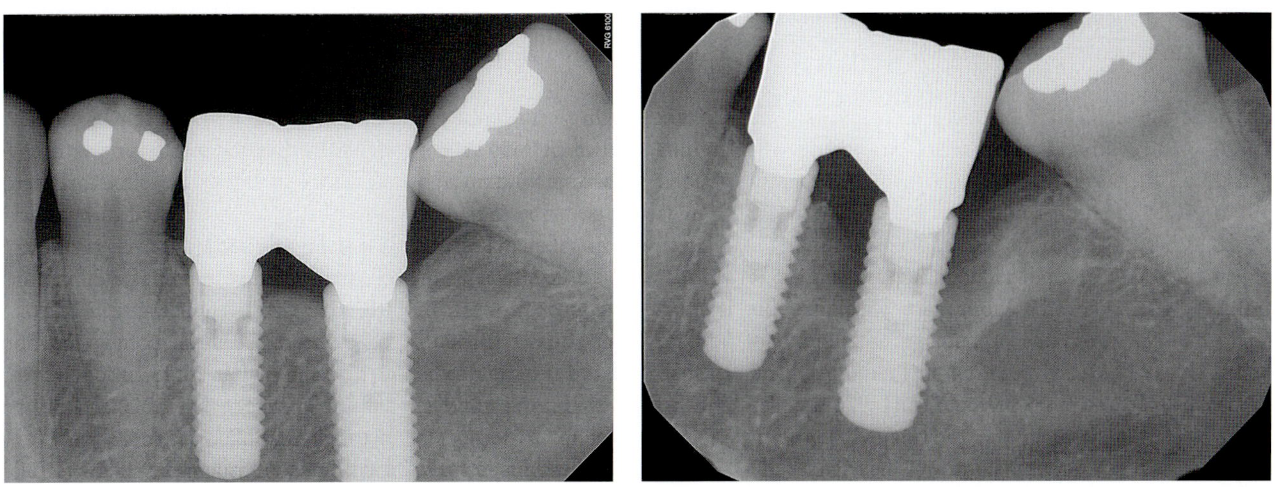

Figure 3.2 At the treatment planning appointment, especially in patients with poor compliance, it is often helpful to show clinical examples of how bone can be lost quickly and asymptomatically around a dental implant. Guiding the patient to articulate a desire for compliance early in treatment can improve outcomes. This is called motivational interviewing and has resulted in improved outcomes in medicine by improving compliance.[12]

Five-year implant success rates of dental implants exceed 95%,[20] and this has allowed dentists to predictably improve function and comfort for many patients. While this is encouraging, it has also been estimated that over 67 000 dental implants failed in Europe alone in 2008.[21] In 2007, replacement costs for implant failures in the US were estimated at over $338 million.[21] Our goals are no longer just osseointegration but also for an enduring functional, stable, and esthetic restorative result. This requires a renewed commitment by the profession to promote and reinforce the need for maintenance programs. Maintenance programs can decrease implant failures. It is important that patients are educated to realize the value of maintenance programs and that clinicians use forethought in planning a patient-specific maintenance program based on patient characteristics and needs, prosthesis design and material, patient compliance, how the patient does in the provisional restoration, and how marginal bone levels respond to the initially developed recall and maintenance program.

Purpose, outline, and definition of terms

The purpose of this chapter is to outline clinician- and patient-based considerations to improve maintenance programs for patients with dental implants. Clinician-based considerations include: identifying risk factors during diagnosis that impact maintenance, reducing modifiable risk factors, appropriate application of medicaments considered to improve maintenance following delivery, and recommended recall patterns during the maintenance phase. The patient-based considerations include: recommended at-home protocols, and suggestions for motivation and reinforcement of at-home maintenance programs. We will also outline specific recommended maintenance protocols with varied prosthesis designs by using a number of clinical examples. This chapter will include the personal opinions of the authors and a review of the literature relevant to maintenance of implant restorations. An emphasis of the chapter will be a series of publications sponsored by the American College of Prosthodontists, which includes a systematic review on maintenance regimens for patients with implant restorations and a clinical practice guideline (CPG).[11,22–24] The CPG includes input from representatives of the American Dental Association, the Academy of General Dentistry, and the American Dental Hygienists Association. Our definition of maintenance includes clinician-based planning and recommended at-home interventions designed to decrease mechanical and biologic aftercare needs.

Clinician decisions influencing maintenance programs

Identifying risk factors during diagnosis and treatment planning to develop an appropriate patient-specific maintenance program

There are many risk factors that can be identified during the history and diagnosis stage of treatment that are relevant to developing a maintenance program. Identifying patients with a history of bruxism, periodontal disease or refractory periodontitis, smoking, diabetes, use of bisphosphonates, or radiation treatment are all relevant to the risk of biologic and/or mechanical complications.[25–68] An early dialogue with the patient regarding anticipated maintenance needs and recall recommendations will likely result in improved patient compliance once treatment is completed.

During the diagnosis and treatment-planning phase, it is important to assess potential occlusal and parafunctional forces developed by the patient. This information can be learned through patient history, but also by carefully evaluating the patient's existing dentition. In a 10-year retrospective study of 397 patients being evaluated for mechanical and biologic complications, Wittneben *et al.*[20] showed a strong association between attrition in the pre-treatment evaluation of dentition and incidence of later mechanical complications of implant restorations. Specifically, with no, localized, or generalized signs of attrition, the incidence of porcelain fracture increased from 10.9%, to 21.9%, and 26.9%, respectively. This means that the pre-treatment evaluation of attrition may be a valuable indicator in informed consent, material selection, number of implants used, and in developing a patient-specific maintenance protocol. In bruxers, the use of a nightguard and more frequent recalls to monitor screw loosening should be considered. Wittneben *et al.*[20] also showed that multiple-unit splinted crowns had a higher risk of porcelain chipping than single units. Individuals with higher force should have a treatment plan with more implants, more detailed informed consent, and more regular recall patterns to monitor potential mechanical complications. In a retrospective study of 152 patients, Kinsel and Lin showed that patients with bruxism had seven times the incidence of porcelain fracture as compared to non-bruxers.[25] The authors also showed that patients had fewer complications when a nightguard was used or when the patient had canine-protected occlusion in their restorations. Clearly, there is evidence for the need to complete a thorough history of potential bruxing habits, to evaluate the dentition carefully for attrition, and to appropriately plan the use of materials, occlusion, and potential use of a nightguard to help maintain the designed implant prosthesis (Figure 3.3).

The relationship between overloading and bone loss is not completely understood. A review of clinical and animal studies was recently completed by Naert *et al.*[36] who concluded that, in the absence of peri-implant inflammation, overload did not significantly contribute to peri-implant bone loss. They did find out, however, that with high loads and poor oral hygiene in susceptible patients, bone loss may occur.

Patients with a history of periodontal disease are particularly vulnerable to peri-implant disease, making a maintenance program especially important to consider.[1,6,7] Unfortunately, the criteria to establish a diagnosis of peri-implant disease remain controversial and are inconsistently applied by investigators, so it is not surprising that there is a wide variation in reported incidence of peri-implant disease.[18] The incidence of peri-implant

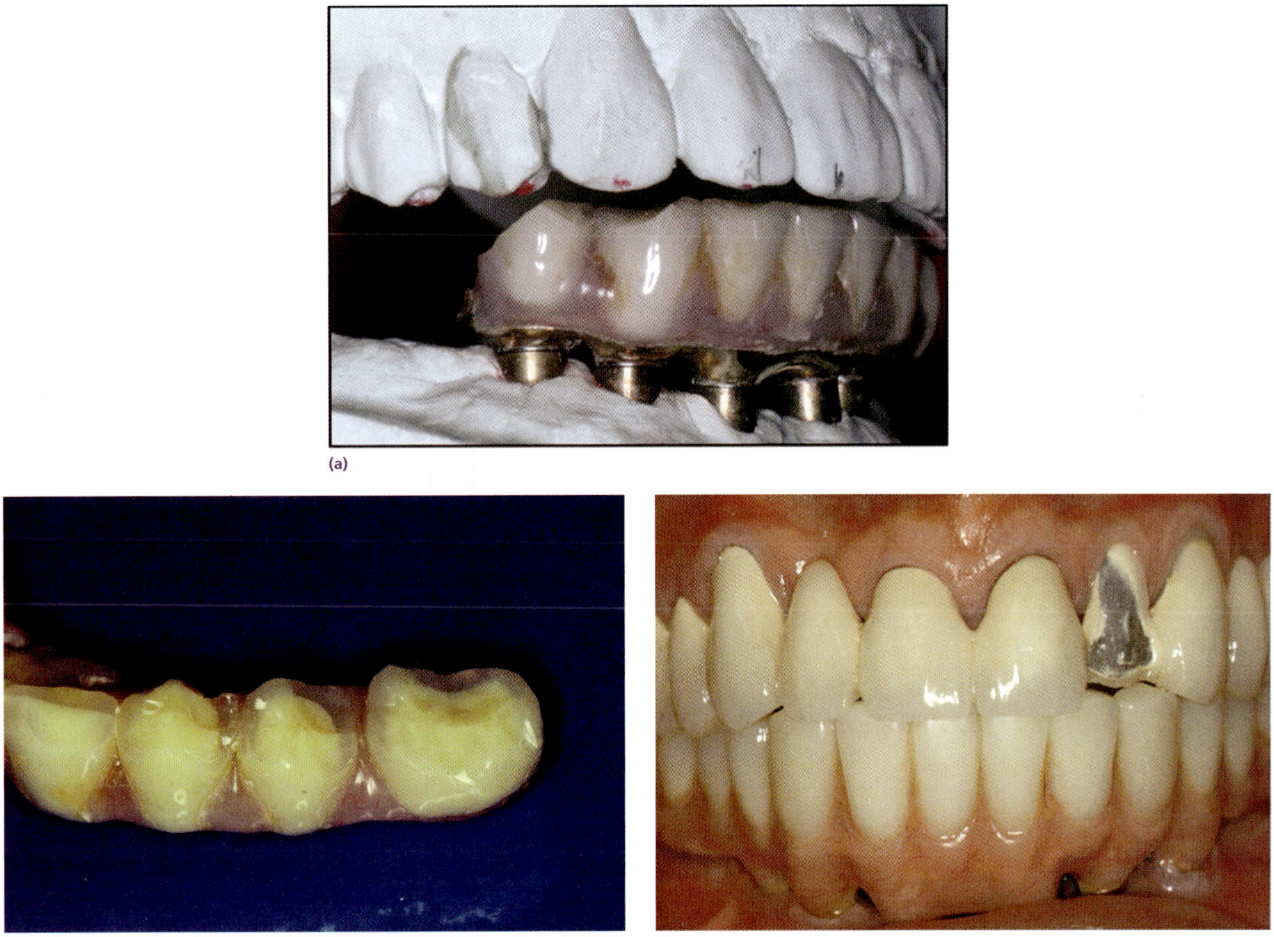

(a)

(b) (c)

Figure 3.3 (a–c) Maintenance needs are expected with implant restorations. In a recent systematic review of technical and biologic complications over a 10-year period, only 8.6% of prostheses did not have complications.[52] Both the patient and clinician need to prepare for this potential.[52] The most common biologic complications were hypertrophy or hyperplasia of tissue and inflammation under the prosthesis. The most common technical complications included chipping/fracture of veneering material, screw loosening, screw fracture, fabrication of new opposing prostheses, replacement resin teeth, wear of resin teeth, framework fracture, and patient dissatisfaction.[52]

disease varies depending on the group studied and the disease criteria, but it has been conservatively estimated to occur in 10% of implants and 20% of patients during a 5–10-year period.[18] Other estimates from a recent systematic review estimate that peri-implant mucositis occurs in 43% of patients, and peri-implantitis in 22% of patients.[1] In contrast, Abrektsson *et al.*[18] suggest, in a review of three modern implant brands with 10-year or longer follow-up data, that the diagnostic value of bleeding on probing may be less valuable than originally thought. His review showed that the incidence of peri-implantitis was less than 3% during a 7–16-year period.[18] Interestingly, and in contrast to Albrektsson *et al.*, a recent systematic review and expert consensus statement found that bleeding on probing was considered the most consistent way to diagnose peri-implant disease, but that changes in probing depth also should also be considered.[1] It has also been suggested that using a light probing force (0.25 N) will minimize damage to the supporting tissues.[1,51]

The literature on maintenance programs and monitoring of peri-implant disease is often based on convenience samples that are usually of limited size, often from university clinics, variable in follow-up time, and predominantly retrospective.[6,13,26] Therefore, the patient populations studied are often heterogeneous and not representative, which makes it difficult to identify trends. The clinical measures used to establish a diagnosis of peri-implant mucositis or peri-implantitis have not been consistent among studies, which makes combining data in systematic reviews or meta-analyses difficult.[1,13] Furthermore, comparative clinical studies of definitive maintenance protocols are lacking.[28] Therefore, the progression of peri-implant disease and the impact of specific homecare and recall regimens are not well understood,[13] which makes establishing the efficacy of maintenance protocols and recommendations problematic.

Several studies, including a recent systematic review, have shown no difference in implant survival rate in patients with periodontitis and those without periodontitis if the patient is enrolled in a maintenance program.[28,29] However, patients with a history of periodontitis did have more marginal bone loss around their implants, and peri-implantitis was more prevalent in patients with periodontitis, which would have implications in long-term follow-up.[27] In a retrospective study of 97 patients, Hardt *et al.* evaluated bone loss and implant loss in patients with or without periodontal disease in their natural dentition.[4] The investigators determined that 64% of patients with periodontal disease on natural dentition had peri-implant bone loss of more than 2 mm compared to 24% of the nonperiodontal patients. In a prospective 5-year randomized trial of 51 patients with a total of 149 implants, Wennstrom *et al.* concluded that, while in a maintenance program, patient's bone loss was minimal, even for those with a background of periodontal disease.[19] Conversely, Monje *et al.* showed the risk ratio for implant failure in patients with generalized aggressive periodontitis to be 4.0, when compared to healthy patients.[17] In a systematic review of patient history of periodontitis on implant success, Ramanauskaite *et al.* concluded that survival rates among those with a history of periodontitis are comparable with nonperiodontitis patients, but that there is a trend for more marginal bone loss in periodontitis patients.[27] It appears from the literature that those patients with a history of periodontal disease are at a significant short-term potential for increased bone loss and a long-term potential for increased implant loss when compared to those without a history of periodontal disease. Maintenance plans have been shown to partially mitigate this trend.[29]

Diabetes is a risk factor for biologic complications that can potentially adversely impact outcomes, especially if coupled with other risk factors such as periodontitis, poor oral hygiene or smoking.[34,35,39] Significant factors include the amount of time the patient has been diabetic and if the HbA1C level is above 7%.[35] The mechanism behind the increased incidence of peri-implantitis and marginal bone loss in diabetics is related to the disruption of collagen.[35,39] Smoking may also potentiate implant failure in diabetics.[38] Although a recent systematic review did not find an association between type 2 diabetes and implant failure, it did find a difference between marginal bone loss and a diabetes diagnosis.[35] The mechanism of bone loss is not entirely understood, but in susceptible diabetic patients, it includes the disruption of collagen formation and integrity.[39]

Decreasing modifiable risk factors to improve maintenance of implant restorations

The most obvious modifiable risk factor for implant success is minimizing or eliminating smoking habits. Tobacco products contribute significantly to periodontal disease and smoking is an avoidable risk factor for biologic complications with dental implants.[38–40] Patients who are heavy smokers, defined by smoking more than 30 cigarettes a day, have increased odds of implant loss compared to those who smoke fewer cigarettes.[39] Smoking also increases the risk of postoperative infections, and may result in epigenetic changes that increase risk for implant failure by downregulating of osteopontin and type II collagen.[38,39] In patients under a regular maintenance program, the impact of smoking appears to be lessened.[29] However, poor oral hygiene has been shown to result in more bone loss in smokers than in nonsmokers.[40]

Cemented restorations can be a risk for peri-implant disease, both because of residual cement and because of retained plaque at the subgingival margins. Cemented restorations should be supragingival if possible, and specific techniques should be used to limit cement into the sulcus. In a double-blind prospective study of 29 patients, Heitz-Mayfield *et al.*[37] evaluated the baseline soft-tissue measures in patients with mucositis by measuring bleeding on probing, pocket depth, suppuration, and plaque. Debridement was then completed on all 29 patients and follow-up provided after 1 month and 3 months. The authors showed that patients with cemented restoration margins that were subgingival demonstrated less improvement in probing depth measurements than in patients with supragingival restorations. Planning adequately for a screw-retained prosthesis should be a goal in treatment planning, and when cementing is necessary, having margins supragingival should be used to improve soft-tissue responses. Clinicians can also consider pre-cementation procedures to decrease extrusion of cement.

There are modifiable risk factors in material selection as well. If there are planned posterior opposing implant restorations, it is advisable to be especially careful in material selection. The use of metal occlusals, the use of a nightguard, and the goal of anterior disclusion are favorable in order to decrease mechanical complications.[25] As the esthetics of monolithic zirconia restorations improves, more of these restorations are likely to be utilized as long as wear of titanium fixtures from the zirconia can be minimized.

Many of the long-term maintenance problems can be evaluated in the provisional. This is especially important for full-arch implant-supported fixed restorations. If the patient has higher occlusal forces than anticipated and starts fracturing the provisional, a more suitable material for the definitive restoration can be considered, and at times more implants or a segmented prosthesis can be recommended. If the patient has speech or spitting issues, as sometimes happens with a maxillary prosthesis, the position and adaptation of the prosthesis can be modified in the provisional. If the patient is having difficulty accessing tissues, then the provisional can be recontoured to allow suitable oral hygiene (Figure 3.4). If the peri-implant tissues are easily irritated and patient is not able to comfortably brush the tissues, then grafting attached tissue should be considered during the time the provisional is being used (Figure 3.5). The authors strongly recommend the use of a provisional to evaluate functional and esthetic issues in order to decrease maintenance needs and complications in the definitive restoration (Figure 3.6). Once recontoured, the provisional can be used for copy milling to the definitive restoration.

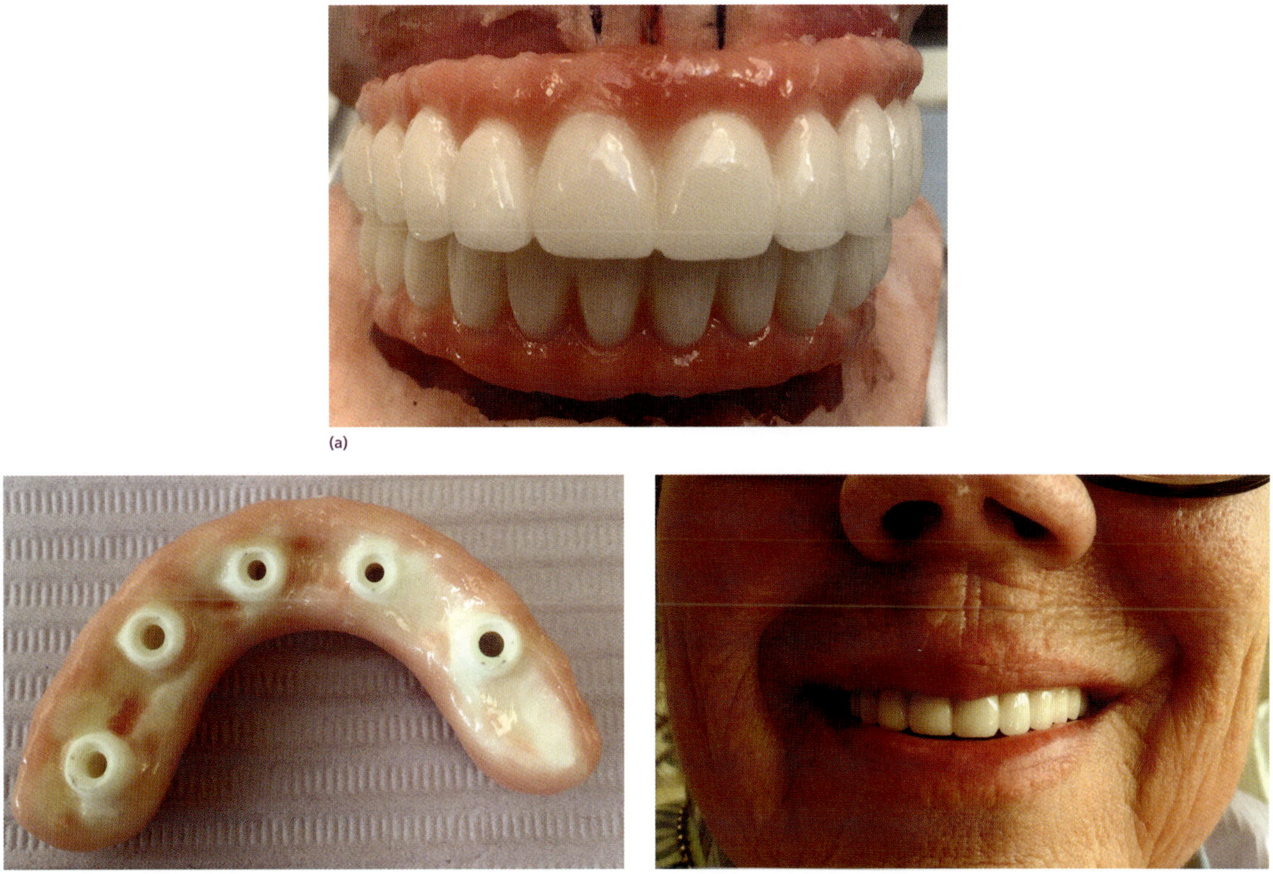

(a)

(b)

(c)

Figure 3.4 (a–c) For this patient ready to receive a maxillary and mandibular implant-supported fixed prostheses fabricated from zirconia, access for cleaning was established early with re-contouring of the provisional until the patient could maintain tissue health. Since the most common biologic complications are gingival hypertrophy and inflammation under the prosthesis, it is important the patient be able to maintain peri-implant tissue health before delivery of the definitive restoration.[52]

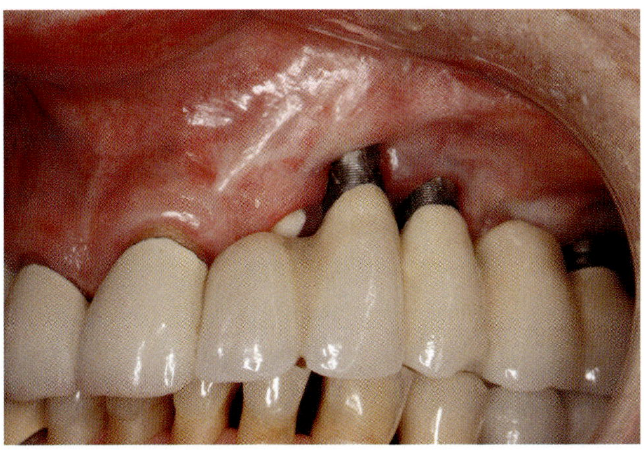

Figure 3.5 Lack of attached tissue is a risk factor around implants and encourages food impaction.[1] Note the high muscle attachment proximal to the cuspid, which creates moving tissue not just movable tissue, potentiating patient discomfort. In such a situation, a connective tissue graft is recommended, ideally during the time the patient is wearing a provisional restoration, before the definitive restoration.[63]

Medicaments to improve health of tissues around dental implants

The use of chlorhexidine has been advocated in management protocols for patients with mucositis but with limited benefit and for a limited period of time.[42–44] It appears that mechanical debridement is more impactful than trying to control the biofilm with the use of chlorhexidine. In a double-blind prospective study of 29 patients, Heitz-Mayfield *et al.*[37] evaluated the baseline soft-tissue measures in patients with mucositis by measuring bleeding on probing, pocket depth, suppuration, and plaque. Debridement was then completed on all 29 patients and follow-up was provided after 1 month and 3 months. Clorhexidine gel (0.5%) was used on 15 patients and a placebo gel was used on 14 patients. Overall, the nonsurgical debridement resulted in significant improvement of soft-tissue measures, although the supplemental use of chlorhexidine did not improve soft-tissue measures compared to debridement without chlorhexidine.[37] The authors did find that patients with cemented restoration margins that were subgingival showed less

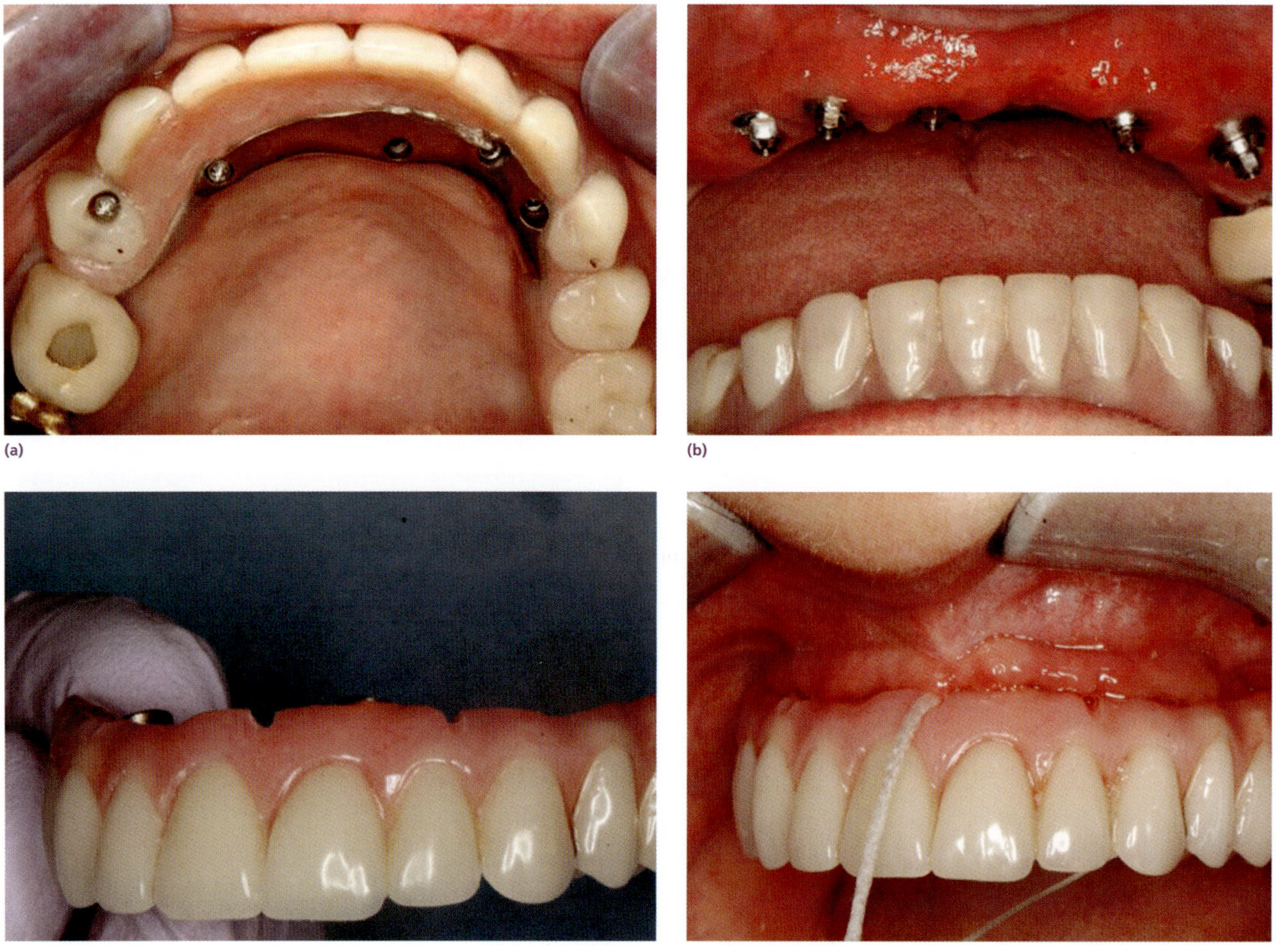

(a) (b) (c) (d)

Figure 3.6 (a) Example of extensive prosthesis coverage of gingiva and marginal tissues of implants. (b) The resulting marginal irritation should be avoided if possible. The patient's ability to maintain the tissue should be evaluated in the provisional. If the restoration contours cannot be modified, frequent recalls, use of a water flosser, floss threaders, and triclosan-containing toothpaste should be considered. (c, d) One modification that facilitates hygiene access is the contouring of gingival grooves in the prosthetic flange. *Source*: Courtesy of Dr. Steve Parel.[45–48]

improvement in probing depth than in patients with supragingival restorations.[37] It is also noteworthy that although the number of implant sites with mucositis diminished, complete resolution of bleeding on probing was only seen in 38% of the patients. This is important because mucositis does not appear to be as reversible as gingivitis, which means a rigorous maintenance program to avoid mucositis is desirable.[1]

In a study of 30 patients who received debridement and used a 1% chlorhexidine gel or 0.2% mouthwash, De Siena *et al.*[43] found a decrease in bleeding on probing, but there was no observable difference between patients who used the rinse and gel, although patients preferred the gel. For compliance, use of the gel may make sense. In a group of 13 partially edentulous patients who received a full-mouth scaling, patients using chlorhexidine did not have improved bleeding on probing scores when compared to patients not using chlorhexidine when patients were evaluated at 1, 2, 4, and 8 months.[42] In a very interesting use of chlorhexidine, Paolatonio *et al.* evaluated microbial penetration in the peri-implant tissue in 30 subjects over an 8-month period. When a 1% chlorhexidine gel was used in the internal part of the fixture prior to abutment placement, a decrease in internal bacterial colonization was observed when compared to no gel being used.[42] The authors of this chapter feel that the application of chlorhexidine into the internal part of the fixture is appropriate in patients with a higher risk of developing peri-implant disease. In conclusion, chlorhexidine may have beneficial effects post-surgically and in selected uses such as outlined by Paolatonio *et al.*, but the effect size, as a stand-alone treatment for patients with peri-implant disease, is limited.

The use of triclosan-containing toothpastes has resulted in improvement of soft-tissue measures in patients with both implants and teeth, and in an edentulous population restored with implants and diagnosed with peri-implant mucositis.[45,46] In a 6-month study of the effects of a 0.3% triclosan/copolymer toothpaste on oral biofilms and gingival inflammation, Sreenivasan *et al.*[45] evaluated 120 subjects divided into groups of patients who used or did not use triclosan. This double-blind, two-treatment parallel study included baseline measures of dental plaque, gingival inflammation, bleeding on probing, and microbiological analysis. Results after 3 and 6 months indicated that the groups using triclosan/copolymer

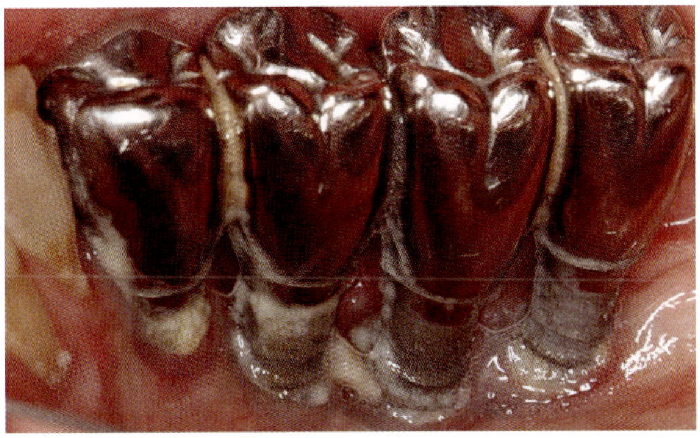

(a)

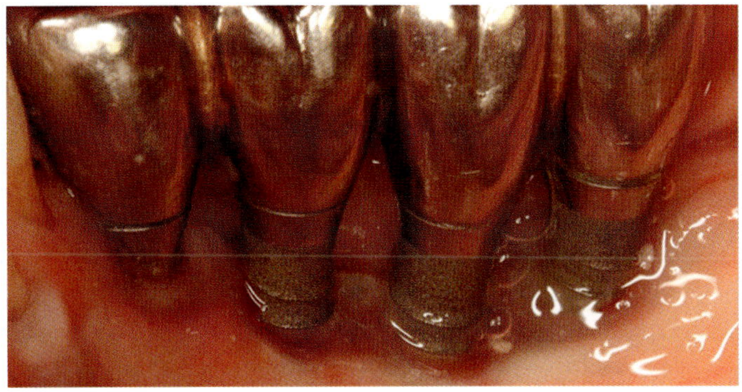

(b)

Figure 3.7 (a) In a patient with poor oral hygiene, the patient needs to understand that without appropriate maintenance they are much more likely to have maintenance complications that can create esthetic concerns and result in the loss of implants. (b) This patient responded to 2-month recalls with reinforcement, triclosan-containing gum, and use of brushes.[47,48]

toothpaste group had significantly lower levels of dental plaque, gingivitis, and bleeding on probing compared to the group not using the triclosan.[45] In a related study of 60 edentulous patients restored with at least two implants and later diagnosed with mucositis, the impact of triclosan on pocket depth, bleeding on probing, and plaque was evaluated at baseline, 3 and 6 months.[46] Patients using triclosan had reduced bleeding on probing scores from 53.8% to 29.1%, while the control group had an increase in bleeding on probing from 52.3% to 58.8%. Because triclosan has been shown to have some hormonal effects, the authors recommend using triclosan in those with higher risk for peri-implant disease. Triclosan-containing toothpastes appear to offer the potential for improved soft tissues around implants and should be considered for patients diagnosed as being at risk for peri-implant disease, in patients with difficult to access marginal tissues, or in those with diagnosed peri-implant disease (Figures 3.6 and 3.7).

Recommended recall patterns and at-home maintenance for patients with implants

Recall patterns should fit the risk profile of the patient and be discussed with the patient at the time of diagnosis and treatment planning. Although there are short-term disadvantages of time and expense for the patient to actively engage in an in-office recall program, the long-term benefits are substantial.[11,58] Patients with existing natural dentition that has been extensively restored should be counseled on diet and oral hygiene to prevent future secondary decay.[23] Having 3-month recall schedules planned for smokers, especially heavy smokers, is highly recommended. In patients with long-standing diabetes or with HbA1C levels above 7%, the 3-month recall schedule is also advised, although the authors are not aware of studies directly evaluating recall at 3-month intervals versus other intervals in patients with risk factors. However, debridement and reinforcement are both evidence-based approaches to improving maintenance outcomes.[1,6,7] The 3-month recall interval can be modified to sequentially longer recall periods after the first year, if at-home maintenance results in healthy tissues. We also recommend the use of triclosan-containing toothpastes in high-risk groups, such as those with a history of periodontal disease, poorly controlled diabetes, or in those wearing prostheses that limit access to the marginal tissues. The use of water flossers is also recommended for patients who have dexterity or visual limitations, or in patients who have a prosthesis that makes access to the marginal tissue of implants difficult.[47,48] Many of the full-arch fixed zirconia prostheses being designed have significant tissue coverage and access to marginal implant tissues is often limited. It is important that the patient demonstrate the ability to maintain the provisional restoration before moving to the definitive restoration.

It is the authors' opinion that maintenance programs should start aggressively with more interventions and slowly decrease the maintenance once compliance and a favorable biologic response have been established. Starting a maintenance program only after a biologic complication has occurred is a mistake. This is an important point and we should be mindful that gingivitis is reversible around teeth but mucositis is less reversible,[18] making early aggressive maintenance and reinforcement a must.

In the future, maintenance will likely include at-home monitoring of cytokine levels in the crevicular fluid, perhaps as frequently as once a week for patients at high risk for peri-implant disease. The use of proinflammatory cytokines (IL-1β) as markers of inflammation around implants has historically been primarily a research tool.[65,66] The future prospects for monitoring proinflammatory cytokine levels, tumor necrosis factor, or osteoclastogenesis-related cytokines (RANKL) look promising.[67]

In-office procedures for maintenance for the patient with implant restorations

The recall appointment should include a review of the medical and dental history, an evaluation of the occlusion and potential changes in occlusal contacts, as well as the stability of proximal contacts. There is a natural mesial drift of dentition and contacts with natural teeth open more often on the mesial side of implants than on the distal.[53] Some authors have suggested mesial migration and resulting proximal instability increases in patients with higher biting forces.[53] Continuing craniofacial growth can also result in open contacts.[54] Using a screw-retained restoration with a porcelain proximal contact, especially on the mesial, can allow easier correction of an open contact. The authors recommend a broader contact area between an implant crown and a natural tooth, which is often easier to accomplish by lightly disking the adjacent tooth prior to impressions. Some investigators have reported stable contacts opening as soon as 3 months following delivery, although the authors have not observed contacts opening so soon after delivery. If an open contact does occur, it is usually not until 2 years after delivery of the restoration.[53] The use of a nightguard to help hold tooth position may be a benefit, but has not been studied. The consequences of open contacts can include proximal decay, peri-implant disease, or periodontal disease on the adjacent natural tooth.

The authors recommend appropriate diagnostic orthogonal radiographs at prosthesis delivery and 6 months following delivery, and then as needed to monitor crestal bone levels (Figure 3.8). Depending on the type of material used and if the prosthesis is screw-retained, it can be an advantage to remove the prosthesis to more accurately evaluate peri-implant health, instruct the patient on areas needing improved oral hygiene, and, if appropriate, recontour and polish the tissue surface of the prosthesis to improve patient access. Reshaping the prosthesis for access is ideally worked out in the provisional restoration. The patient's ability to access and clean all areas of the prosthesis should be determined, and the use of suitable brushes and floss techniques should be reviewed. The use of floss threaders can also be helpful in selected individuals. At the recall appointment, the soft tissue examination should include probing depth (PD) and changes in probing depth over time. Bleeding on probing (BOP) should also be noted, as BOP is an important marker for inflammation and peri-implant disease (Figure 3.9).[1] The clinician and patient should be mindful that healing of the sulcus around an implant requires 4–5 days after probing, but that probing should be completed, even around healthy implants.[1] Minimizing damage to peri-implant tissues when probing can be accomplished by using a calibrated probe with the goal of 0.25 N probing force.[51] Suppuration should also be recorded, and can be determined by using the gloved thumb and forefinger on the buccal and lingual of the tissue at the implant apex and applying mild pressure coronally to visualize suppuration from the sulcus. Cleaning should be done with plastic or graphite scalers for plaque removal and should be completed at appropriate intervals. See also Figure 3.10.

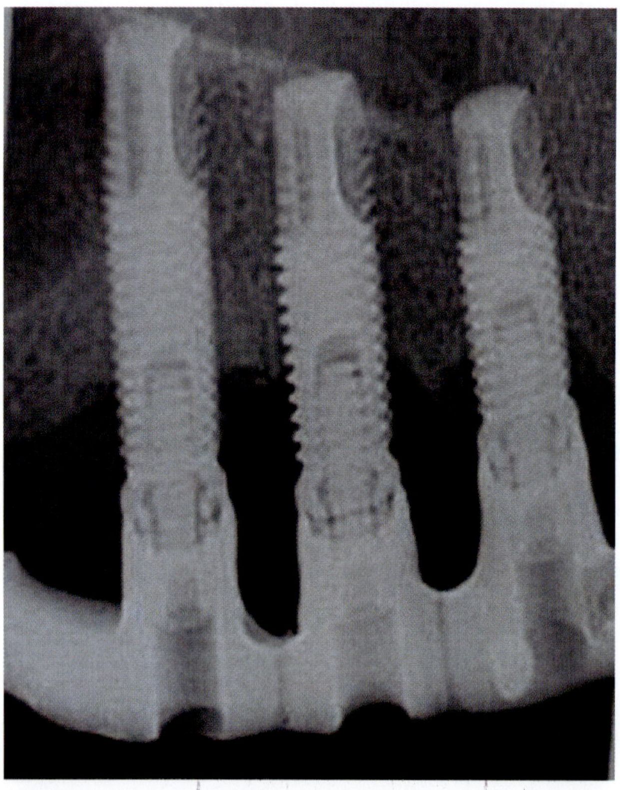

Figure 3.8 Ideally a maintenance plan will be developed while treatment planning. When a patient is referred who has existing implants with bone loss, a more aggressive maintenance program should be considered.

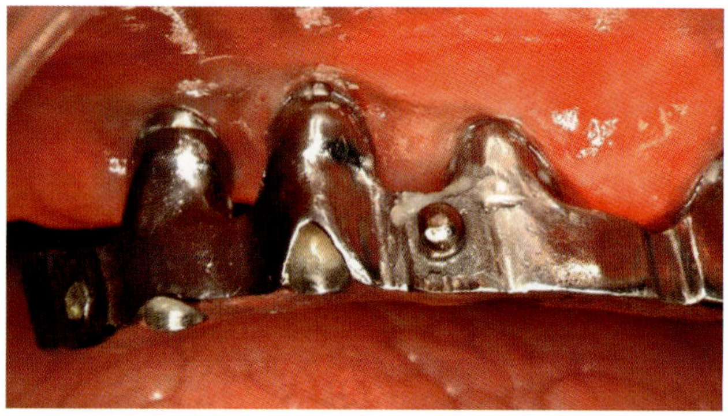

Figure 3.9 This patient has mucositis defined as bleeding on light probing. The abutment connections were open leaving a nidus for plaque accumulation. Additionally, the patient wore their prosthesis at night and had difficulty cleaning. Placing the patient on frequent recalls helped improve tissue health.

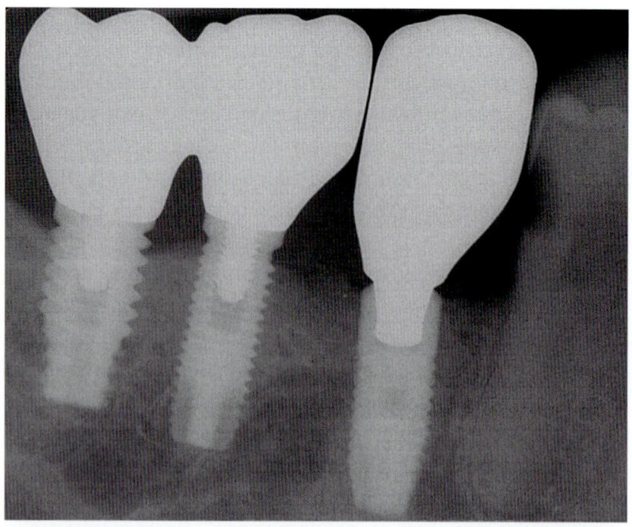

Figure 3.10 There is an increased potential for caries on teeth adjacent to implant restorations. The maintenance plan needs to account for this. Often teeth adjacent to implant restorations have recession and are susceptible to root caries. A high-fluoride toothpaste for at-home maintenance and fluoride varnish for in-office recall appointments should be considered.[60]

Recall intervals for those with high occlusal forces should be very specific to the potential for material fracture, compliance in use of a nightguard, risk and need for monitoring screw loosening, and at-home maintenance. Patients with high occlusal forces may be at higher risk for developing open contacts. It is important to remember that high forces are a maintenance issue due to material complications and high forces and can, with inflammation, accelerate biologic changes such as marginal bone loss.[36]

Development of a patient-specific maintenance program based on the risk factor checklist

The first step in developing a patient-specific maintenance program is to complete the checklist representing cumulative risk for biologic and mechanical complications (Table 3.1). The higher the checklist point total, the greater the risk for complications and the greater the need for proactive in-office

Table 3.1 Risk factors for biologic and mechanical complications (CAMBRA, caries management by risk assessment; CHX, chlorhexidine; OHI, oral hygiene instruction; SSRIs, selective serotonin reuptake inhibitors).

Risk factors	Points	Intervention
Risk factors based on history		
Smokes 10 but <30 cigarettes/day[62]	1	Counseling, medical referral, motivational interviewing[12]
Smokes >30 cigarettes/day[62]	2	Counseling, medical referral, motivational interviewing[12]
Controlled diabetic	0	
HbA1C levels above 7%[35,61]	0.5	Counseling, medical referral for control before surgery, increased long-term risk for peri-implantitis, motivational interviewing[12]
HbA1C levels above 7% for >5 years[61]	1	Counseling, medical referral for control before surgery, increased long-term risk for peri-implantitis, motivational interviewing[12]
HbA1C levels above 7% for >5 years with periodontal disease, and <30 cigarettes smoking[61]	1.5	Counseling, medical referral, OHI, control before surgery, increased risk for peri-implant disease when coupled with other risk factors; marginal bone loss, motivational interviewing[12]
History of previous implant loss[55]	1	Patient education, more frequent recalls
Low motivation for at-home maintenance[11,12,39]	2	Identify from history and initial examination, monitoring and reinforcement
Low motivation for in-office recalls[3,5,11,12]	2	Identify from history, motivational interviewing, additional recall attempts
Body dysmorphic disorder, thin tissue biotype, high lip line, anterior restorations[57]	1	Additional informed consent, screw-retained more important
Medications altering bone capacity such as IV bisphosphonates,[56] SSRIs, heavy drinking of alcohol, other medications	1	Additional consent, options to medications
Risk based on clinical findings		
Generalized aggressive periodontal disease, not in maintenance program[17]	2.5	Periodontal treatment prior to implant placement
Periodontal disease, not in maintenance program[3,17,42]	2	Referral for periodontal treatment, pocket reduction, triclosan, CHX during treatment[42]
Periodontal disease but in maintenance program[29,42]	0.5	Continue in maintenance program, more frequent recalls, triclosan, CHX during treatment[42]
Thin tissue biotype, lack of attached tissue, and/or subgingival margins[1,58]	1	Patient education, screw-retained design rather than cementation, subgingival, connective tissue grafting before definitive prosthesis if brushing irritates tissue
Occlusal disharmony, parafunction[18,20,53]	1	Equilibration, establish occlusal plane, material and prosthesis selection, recall for screw loosening, nightguard, increased potential for open contacts
Parafunction with poor oral hygiene[18,36,53]	1.5	Patient education of the impact of overload and inflammation, material selection, nightguard, increase potential for open contacts, CAMBRA if natural dentition[60]
High plaque levels at presentation[12]	1	Patient education, OHI, more frequent recalls
Limited dexterity, vision, or cognition	1	Treatment plan to accommodate, electric toothbrush with timer, more frequent recalls[47,48]
Risk based on clinician/implant factors		
Inexperienced clinicians in surgical or restorative phase of treatment,[58] not using postoperative antibiotics	1	More likely to make mistakes in implant selection, placement, position and restoration; outcomes not as favorable overall[58]
Treatment plan includes prostheses that limit access for cleaning	1	Consider alternate prosthesis if patient has numerous other risk factors; evaluate in provisional restoration, water flosser[47,48]
Subgingival cemented restoration in patient with thin tissue biotype,[1] lack of 2 mm of attached tissue[63]	1	Treatment plan screw-retained design if practical, clean residual cement, good adaptation of components, access for cleaning
Placing implants <2 mm from each other or having multiple implants[58,68]	1	Provide brushes to allow cleaning; some authors have shown multiple implants are a risk factor for peri-implantitis[58,68]
Placing implants too facial, especially in patient with high smile line	1	Esthetic concerns; color, recession
Risk of implant type[58]	1	Some implants systems appear to be more susceptible to peri-implant disease and may require additional maintenance to avoid peri-implant disease[58]

and at-home maintenance interventions. The categories of risk can be broken down into risk factors determined from patient history, clinical exam, and clinician factors. The checklist should be completed during treatment planning.

The checklist may serve as a tool to motivate patients and guide the clinician, and may also be used following treatment to monitor changes in the risk profile of the patient. We have often found using the checklist influences prosthesis selection. For example, in a patient with poor oral hygiene and active periodontal disease, a planned prosthesis with extensive tissue coverage would not be planned (see Figure 3.4). In using the checklist with patients, the true value has been in establishing a dialogue during treatment planning so that the prosthesis selection and design are consistent with the patient-specific needs and motivational risk factors. Improved patient understanding has resulted in an improved willingness of the patient to engage in reducing risk. We find patients are more willing to be actively engaged to decrease their risk point total, and by doing so are more likely to decrease or stop smoking, understand the cost of using a provisional restoration, and be more compliant in recalls.

Developing a patient-specific maintenance program using the risk factor checklist

1 Gather history to identify risk factors that could create maintenance issues.
2 Discuss findings with patient.
3 Establish a dialogue with the patient to decrease modifiable risk factors such as smoking, high HbA1C levels, poor oral hygiene, and those at increased risk for proximal contact instability, materials failure, and adherence. Motivational interviewing is often helpful.
4 Select treatment after dialogue with patient regarding the checklist.
5 The authors recommend a signed agreement with the patient regarding the recommended recall schedule and patient responsibilities. We feel this will enlist support and recognition of the importance of maintenance. The signed agreement should also include a provision that the definitive prosthesis might be changed based on how the patient does with the provisional restoration.

Maintenance schedules based on point totals

- **Low risk**: <3 points. Regular 6-month recalls, routine cleaning patterns, and routine toothpaste. Recall and management program as you would for healthy natural dentition.
- **Intermediate risk**: 3–6 points. Patient educated about risk factors and counseled to decrease avoidable risk factors. Medical referral to reduce HbA1C and decrease or eliminate smoking, if appropriate. Discuss 4-month in-office recalls with patient prior to treatment, use of water flosser if access is an issue, and use of timer on electric toothbrush if there is a compliance/cognitive issue. Application of 1% chlorhexidine in implant prior to abutment connection if abutment(s) are removed and/or if screws are replaced.[42] During provisionalization, especially if an implant-supported fixed prosthesis, evaluate the patient's ability to access and clean prosthesis and modify accordingly (Figures 3.4, 3.6, 3.11). If that patient is a thin tissue biotype or if there is no attached tissue, careful evaluation during the provisional stage and consideration of a connective tissue graft if they are unable to comfortably maintain peri-implant tissues is recommended.[63]
- **High risk**: >6 points. Patient should be educated about risk factors and counseled to decrease avoidable risk factors. Motivational interviewing can be helpful. Discuss 2–3-month in-office recalls in the first year following delivery of the prosthesis and 3-month recalls thereafter until tissues and prosthesis appear stable. We recommend the use of triclosan-containing toothpaste twice a day. Medical referral to reduce HbA1C and decreasing or eliminating smoking should be recommended, if appropriate. Suggest the use of a water flosser if access is an issue, and the use of a timer on an electric toothbrush if lack of compliance is an issue. Application of 1% chlorhexidine in implant prior to abutment connection if abutment(s) are removed and/or if screws replaced.[42] Use of a screw-retained prosthesis becomes more important, especially if the patient develops high occlusal forces. During provisionalization it is important to evaluate the patient's ability to access and clean the prosthesis. If patient is a thin tissue biotype or if there is no attached tissue, a connective tissue graft may be recommended to improve the ability of the patient to brush without discomfort.[63] It is the authors' opinion that in patients identified as high risk, screw-retained restorations should be strongly considered and crown restorations should be kept 2 mm away from marginal bone.[58]

When a patient presents with existing implants, it is still prudent to use the same checklist but use the supplemental risk factor categories given in Table 3.2.

Conclusions

There are many risk factors that can adversely impact implant restorations and the tissues around dental implants. The use of the risk factor checklist is one way to gather relevant information by which to plan restorative care and a maintenance program. The maintenance program needs to reflect risk, and risk is established by diagnosis. It is the responsibility of the clinician to identify the risk factors, educate the patient, and to use established techniques, such as motivational interviewing, to reinforce the need for patient compliance. Developing a patient-specific maintenance program needs to be considered as important as patient-specific restorative care. We don't fabricate all implant restorations the same way; rather, restorations are unique to the functional and esthetic needs of the patient. In the same way, maintenance programs need to be specific, based on risk, and developed during the diagnosis and treatment planning. Use of the risk factor checklist can help identify risk factors and lead to a dialogue with the patient about maintenance. Patient involvement and understanding drive motivation and compliance.

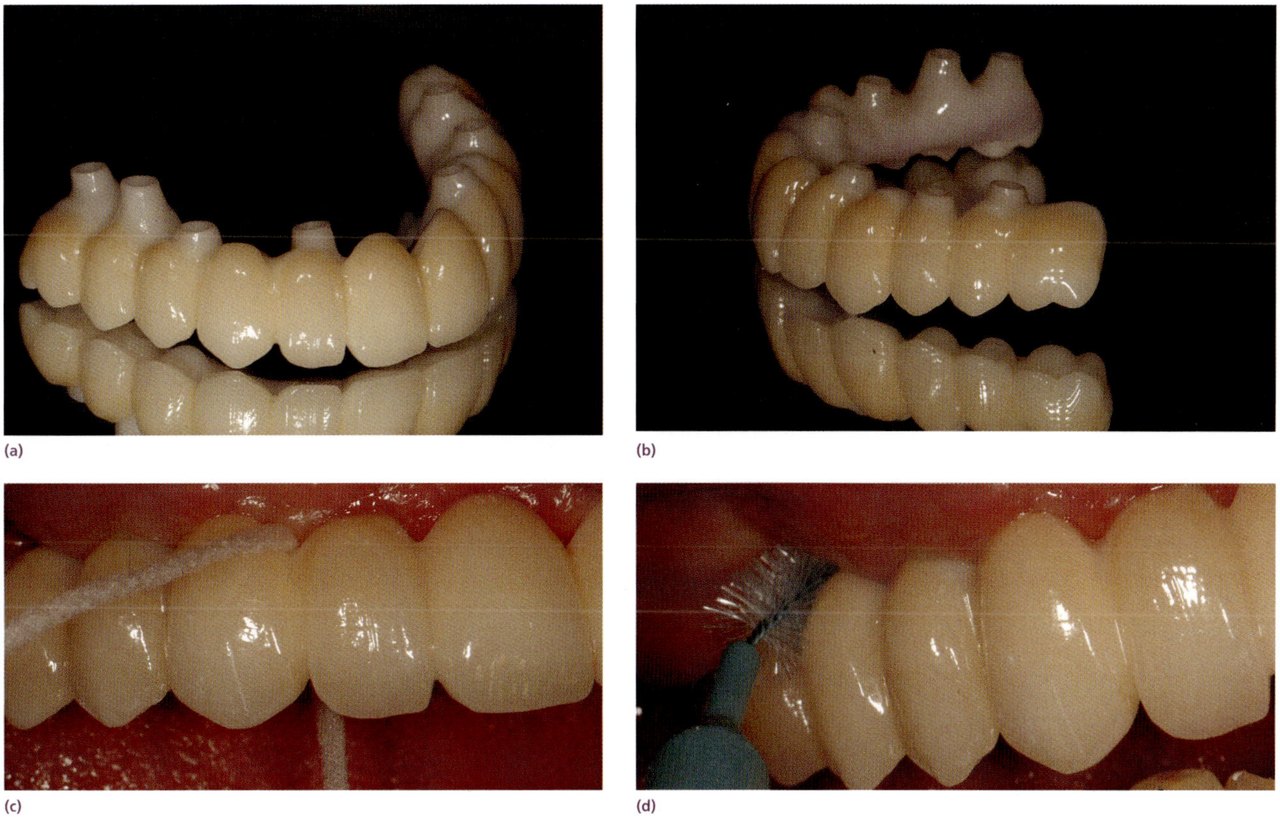

(a) (b) (c) (d)

Figure 3.11 (a–d) This implant-supported fixed prosthesis was completed in zirconia. The prosthesis has minimal tissue coverage and was evaluated in the provisional for patient access for cleaning, speech, and comfort. Extensive tissue coverage can be avoided through careful patient selection. *Source:* Reproduced with permission from Mike Singer, DDS, and Arun Sharma, BDS.

Table 3.2 Clinical risk factors determined after patient has implants (CHX, chlorhexidine).

Risk factors	Points	Intervention
Bleeding with light (0.25 N) probing indicates mucositis[42,45,46]	2	3–4-month recall until inflammation resolves, triclosan-containing toothpaste, use CHX as remove, replace restoration[42]
Increasing pocket depth on successive appointments[42,45,46]	2	3–4-month recall until inflammation resolves, triclosan-containing toothpaste, use CHX as remove, replace restoration[42]
Suppuration[58]	1	3–4-month recall until stable bone levels established, triclosan-containing toothpaste, use CHX as remove, replace restoration[42]

References

1. Jepsen S, Berglundh T, Genco R, *et al.* Primary prevention of peri-implantitits: managing peri-implant mucositis. *J Clin Periodontol* 2015; **42**: S152–157.
2. Qian J, Wennerberg A, Albrektsson T. Reasons for marginal bone loss around oral implants. *Clin Implant Dent Rel Res* 2012; **14**(6): 792–807.
3. Costa FO, Takenaka-Martinez S, Cota LO, *et al.* Peri-implant disease in subjects with and without preventive maintenance: a 5-year follow-up. *J Clin Periodontol* 2012; **39**(2): 173–181.
4. Hardt CR, Grondahl K, Lekholm U, *et al.* Outcome of implant therapy in relation to experienced loss of periodontal bone support: a retrospective 5-year study. *Clin Oral Implant Res* 2002; **13**(5): 488–494.
5. Gay IC, Tran DT, Weltman R, *et al.* Role of supportive maintenance therapy on implant survival: a university-based 17 years retrospective analysis. *Int J Dent Hygiene* 2015. doi:10.1111/idh.12188.
6. Monje A, Aramda L, Diaz KT, *et al.* Impact of maintenance therapy for the prevention of peri-implant diseases: a systematic review and meta-analysis. *J Dent Res* 2015; 1–8. [Epub ahead of print]
7. Schwarz F, Becker K, Sanger M. Efficacy of professionally-administered plaque removal with or without adjunctive measures for the treatment of peri-implant mucositis. A systematic review and meta-analysis. *J Clin Periodontol* 2015; **42**: S201–212.
8. Renvert S, Polyzois I. Risk indicators for peri-implant mucositis. A systematic literature review. *J Clin Periodontol* 2015; **42**: S172–186.
9. Zitzmann NU, Berglundh T. Definition and prevalence of peri-implant diseases. *J Clin Periodontol* 2008; **35**(8 Suppl): 286–291.
10. Carcuac O, Berglundh T. Composition of human peri-implantitis and periodontitis lesions. *J Dent Res* 2014; **93**(11): 1083–1088.
11. Bidra AS, Daubert DM, Garcia LT, *et al.* A systematic review of recall regimen and maintenance regimen of patients with dental restorations. Part 2: Implant-borne restorations. *J Prosthodont* 2016; **25**(S1): S16–31.

12. Gao X, LoEC, Kot SC, *et al.* Motivational interviewing in improving oral health: a systematic review of randomized controlled trials. *J Periodontol* 2014; **85**(3): 426–437.
13. Mombelli A, Marxer M, Gaberthuel T, *et al.* The microbiota of osseointegrated implants in patients with a history of periodontal disease. *J Clin Periodontol* 1995; **22**(2): 124–130.
14. Renvert, S, Polyzois I. Risk indicators for peri-implant mucositis. A systematic literature review. *J Clin Periodontol* 2015; **42**(Suppl.16): S172–**186**.
15. Lee A, Wang HL. Biofilm related to dental implants. *Implant Dent* 2010; **19**(5): 387–391.
16. Zitzmann NU, Berglundh T, Ericsson I, *et al.* Spontaneous progression of experimentally induced peri-implantitis. *J Clin Periodontol* 2004; **31**(10): 845–859.
17. Monje A, Alcoforado G, Padial-Molina M, *et al.* Generalized aggressive periodontitis as a risk factor for dental implant failure: a systematic review and meta-analysis. *J Periodontol* 2014; **85**(10): 1398–1407.
18. Albrektsson T, Buser D, Sennerby L. Crestal bone loss and oral implants. *Clin Implant Dent Rel Res* 2012; **14**(6): 783–791.
19. Wennstrom Jl, Ekestubbe A, Grondahl Karlsson S, *et al.* Oral rehabilitation with implant-supported fixed partial dentures in periodontitis-susceptible subjects. A 5-year prospective study. *J Clin Periodontol* 2004; **31**(9): 713–724.
20. Wittneben J, Buser D, Salvi GE, *et al.* Complication and failure rates with implant-supported fixed dental prostheses single crowns: a 10-year retrospective study. *Clin Implant Dent Rel Res* 2014; **16**(3): 356–364.
21. Nevins M, Kim D. Comprehensive treatment planning for the patient with oral or systemic inflammation. In: Jokstad, A (ed). *Osseointegration and Dental Implants.* Oxford: Wiley Blackwell 2009.
22. Masri R. Dental recall and maintenance regimens: toward an evidence-based philosophy for care of the prosthodontic patient. *J Prosthodont* 2016; **25**(S1): S1.
23. Bidra AS, Daubert DM, Garcia LT, *et al.* A systematic review of recall regimen and maintenance regimen of patients with dental restorations. Part 1: Tooth-borne restorations. *J Prosthodont* 2016; **25**(S1): S2–15.
24. Bidra AS, Daubert DM, Garcia LT, *et al.* Clinical practice guidelines for recall and maintenance of patients with tooth-borne and implant-borne dental restorations. *J Prosthodont* 2016; **25**(S1): S32–40.
25. Kinsel, RP, Lin D. Retrospective analysis of porcelain failures of metal ceramic crowns and fixed partial dentures supported by 729 implants in 152 patients: patient-specific and implant-specific predictors of ceramic failure. *J Prosthet Dent* 2009; **101**(6): 388–394.
26. Derks J, Tomasi C. Peri-implant health and disease. A systematic review of current epidemiology. *J Clin Periodontol* 2015; **42**(Suppl 16): S158–171.
27. Ramanauskaite A, Baseviciene N, Wang HL, *et al.* Effect of history of periodontitis on implant success: meta-analysis and systematic review. *Implant Dent* 2014; **23**(6): 687–696.
28. Romanos GE, Weitz D. Therapy of peri-implant diseases. Where is the evidence? *J Evid Based Dent Pract* 2012; **12**(3 Suppl): 204–208.
29. Garcia-Bellosta S, Bravo M, Subira C, *et al.* Retrospective study of the long-term survival of 980 implants placed in a periodontal practice. *Int J Oral Maxillofac Implants* 2010; **25**(3): 613–619.
30. Alsaadi G, Quirynen M, Komarek A, *et al.* Impact of local and systemic factors on the incidence of oral implant failures, up to abutment connection. *J Clin Periodontol* 2007; **34**(7): 610–617.
31. Bain CA, Weng D, Meltzer A, *et al.* A meta-analysis evaluating the risk for implant failure in patients who smoke. *Compend Contin Educ Dent* 2002; **23**(8): 695–699.
32. Clementini M, Rossetti PHO, Penarrocha D, *et al.* Systemic risk factors for peri-implant bone loss: a systematic review and meta-analysis. *Int J Oral Maxillofac Surg* 2014; **43**(3): 323–334.
33. Chrcanovic BR, Albrektsson T, Wenneberg A. Diabetes and oral implant failure: a systematic review. *J Dent Res* 2014; **93**(9): 859–867.
34. Klokkevold, PR, Han TJ. How do smoking, diabetes, and periodontitis affect outcomes of implant treatment? *Int J Oral Maxillofac Implants* 2007; **22** Suppl: 173–202.
35. Tawil G, Younan R, Azar P, *et al.* Conventional and advanced implant treatment in the type II diabetic patient: surgical protocol and long-term clinical results. *Int J Oral Maxillofac Implants* 2008; **23**(4): 744–752.
36. Naert I, Duyck J, Vandamme K. Occlusal overload and bone/implant loss. *Clin Oral Implants Res* 2012; **23**(Suppl 6): 95–107.
37. Heitz-Mayfield LJ, Salvi GE, Botticelli D, *et al.* Implant complication research group. Anti-infective treatment of peri-implant mucositis: a randomised controlled clinical trial. *Clin Oral Implants Res* 2011; **22**(3): 237–241.
38. Chrcanovic BR, Albrektsson T, Wennerberg A. Smoking and dental implants: a meta-analysis. *J Dent* 2015; **43**(5): 487–498.
39. Razzouk S, Sarkis R. Smoking and diabetes. Epigenetics involvement in osseointegration. *N Y State Dent J* 2013; **79**(2): 27–30.
40. Lindquist L, Carlsson G, Jemt T. Association between marginal bone loss around osseointegrated mandibular implants and smoking habits: a 10-year follow-up study. *J Dent Res* 1997; **76**(10): 1667–1674.
41. Levin L, Kessler-Baruch O. Cigarette smoking and the alveolar bone around teeth and dental implants. *N Y State Dent J* 2013; **79**(5): 53–58.
42. Paolantonio M, Perinetti G, D'Ercole S, *et al.* Internal decontamination of dental implants: an in vivo randomized microbiologic 6-month trial on the effects of a chlorhexidine gel. *J Periodontol* 2008; **79**(8): 1419–1425.
43. Thöne-Mühling M, Swierkot K, Nonnenmacher C, *et al.* Comparison of two full-mouth approaches in the treatment of peri-implant mucositis: a pilot study. *Clin Oral Implants Res* 2010; **21**(5): 504–512.
44. De Siena F, Francetti L, Corbella S, *et al.* Topical application of 1% chlorhexidine gel versus 0.2% mouthwash in the treatment of peri-implant mucositis. An observational study. *Int J Dent Hyg* 2013; **11**(1): 41–47.
45. Sreenivasan PK, Vered Y, Zini A, *et al.* A 6-month study of the effects of 0.3% triclosan/copolymer dentifrice on dental implants. *J Clin Periodontol* 2011; **38**(1): 33–42.
46. Ramberg P, Lindhe J, Botticelli D, *et al.* The effect of a triclosan dentifrice on mucositis in subjects with dental implants: a six-month clinical study. *J Clin Dent* 2009; **20**(3): 103–107.
47. Swierkot K, Brusius M, Leismann D, *et al.* Manual versus sonic-powered toothbrushing for plaque reduction in patients with dental implants: an explanatory randomised controlled trial. *Eur J Oral Implantol* 2013; **6**(2): 133–144.
48. Magnuson B, Harsono M, Stark PC, *et al.* Comparison of the effect of two interdental cleaning devices around implants on the

reduction of bleeding: a 30-day randomized clinical trial. *Compend Contin Educ Dent* 2013; **34**(8): 2–7.

49. Heitz-Mayfield LJ. Peri-implant diseases: diagnosis and risk indicators. *J Clin Periodontol* 2008; **35**(8 Suppl): 292–304.
50. Etter TH, Hakansom I, Lang NP, *et al.* Healing after standardized clinical probing of the perlimplant soft tissue seal: a histomorphometric study in dogs. *Clin Oral Implants Res* 2002; **13**(6): 571–580.
51. Todescan S, Lavigne S, Kelekis-Cholakis A. Guidance for the maintenance care of dental implants: clinical review. *J Can Dent Assoc* 2012; **78**: 1–8.
52. Papaspyridakos P, Chen CJ, Chuang SK, *et al.* A systematic review of biologic and technical complications with fixed implant rehabilitations for edentulous patients. *Int J Oral Maxillofac Implants* 2012; **27**(1): 102–110.
53. Greenstein G, Carpentieri J, Cavallaro J. Open contacts adjacent to dental implant restorations: etiology, incidence, consequences, and correction. *J Am Dent Assoc* 2016: **147**(1): 28–34.
54. Daftary F, Mahallati R, Bahat O, *et al.* Lifelong craniofacial growth and the implications for osseointegrated implants. *Int J Oral Maxillofac Implants* 2013; **28**(1): 163–169
55. Weyant RJ, Burt BA. An assessment of survival rates and within-patient clustering of failures for endosseous oral implants. *J Dent Res* 1993; **72**(1): 2–8.
56. Liddelow G, Klineberg I. Patient-related risk factors for implant therapy. A critique of pertinent literature. *Austr Dent J* 2011; **56**: 417–426.
57. Sarwer DB, Crerand CE, Magee L. Body dysmorphic disorder in patients who seek appearance-enhancing medical treatments. *Oral Maxillofac Surg Clin North Am* 2010; **22**(4): 445–453.
58. Derks J, Schaller D, Hakansson J, *et al.* Effectiveness of implant therapy analyzed in a Swedish population: prevalence of peri-implantitis. *J Dent Res* 2016; **95**(1): 43–49.
59. Tarnow DP. Increasing prevalence of peri-implantitis: how will we manage? *J Dent Res* 2016; **95**(1): 7–8.
60. Featherstone JDB, Singh S, Curtis DA. Caries risk assessment and management for the prosthodontics patient. *J Prosthodont* 2011; **20**: 2–9.
61. Marchand F, Raskin A, Dionnes-Hornes A, *et al.* Dental implants and diabetes: conditions for success. *Diabetes Metab* 2012; **38**: 14–19.
62. Jacob V, Vellappally S, Smejkalova J. The influence of cigarette smoking on various aspects of periodontal health. *Acta Medica* 2007; **50**(1): 3–5.
63. Ferreira CF, Buttendorf AR, deSouza JG, *et al.* Prevalence of peri-implant diseases: analyses of associated factors. *Eur J Prosthodont Restor Dent* 2015; **23**(4): 199–206.
64. Wu X, Al-Abedalia K, Rastikerdar E, *et al.* Selective serotonin reuptake inhibitors and the risk of osseointegrated implant failure: a cohort study. *J Dent Res* 2014; **93**(11): 1054–1061.
65. Kao RT, Curtis DA, Richards DW, *et al.* Increased interleukin-1β in the crevicular fluid of diseased implants. *Intl J Oral Maxillofac Implants* 1995; **10**(6): 696–701.
66. Curtis DA, Kao R, Plesh O, *et al.* Crevicular fluid analysis around two failing implants: a case report. *J Prosthodont* 1997; **6**(3): 210–214.
67. Duarte PM, Serrao CR, Miranda TS, *et al.* Could cytokine levels in the peri-implant crevicular fluid be used to distinguish between healthy implants and implants with peri-implantitis? A systematic review. *J Periodont Res* 2016; Jan 16. doi: 10.1111/jre.12354: 1–10. [Epub ahead of print]
68. Passoni BB, Dalago HR, Filho GS, *et al.* Does the number of implants have any relation with peri-implant disease? *J Appl Oral Sci* 2014; **22**(5): 403–408.

CHAPTER 4

Three-Dimensional Radiographic Imaging for Implant Positioning

Anders Nattestad
University of the Pacific Arthur A. Dugoni School of Dentistry, San Francisco, California, USA

Introduction

Dental implants are one of the most significant developments in dentistry in the last four decades. The treatment modality has quickly emerged as the most advanced approach to replacing missing teeth. The treatment is, however, relatively costly and can be quite complex from both a surgical and restorative perspective. The surgical challenges frequently evolve around loss of tissue support (bone and soft tissue) for the implants that does not always allow for the implants to be placed in the ideal position for the prosthetic superstructure. Also, as these treatments have become increasingly complex, the need for knowledge sharing and collaboration between the surgeon and the restorative doctor becomes increasingly important. The inherent challenge is often that the ideal position and angle of the implants may not be possible or predictable, which can leave the restorative doctor with the need to compromise the esthetic and/or functional aims. Prior to the availability of three-dimensional (3-D) imaging, the restorative doctor would typically manually fabricate a surgical guide based on the ideal position of the implant without always knowing if there was bone to support the implants in that position. During surgery, if it became apparent that the ideal implant position could not be achieved, it was most often not possible to discuss the alternative options with the restorative doctor, and the surgeon would make the unilateral decision how to compromise. With the entry of 3-D imaging, it is more realistic to analyze the availability of bone in greater detail and to simulate the possible outcomes of different treatment options. Ultimately the technology could allow for greater accuracy of the placement of the implants by using 3-D guided surgery. This chapter will describe the technology and evaluate the current evidence behind this treatment option.

Three-dimensional radiographic imaging

The use of 3-D radiographic imaging was initially confined to large hospitals using either computed tomography (CT) or magnetic resonance imaging (MRI). The latter does not show hard tissue well and is used little for dental applications. CT was at first very expensive, difficult to access, and came with a high radiation dose that limited its elective use in dentistry.[1] This changed with the development of cone-beam computed tomography (CBCT), where the radiation was sent out as a beam rather than a full-size slice, dramatically reducing the radiation dose. The CBCT technology also offered availability and affordability to 3-D imaging, and because of these benefits has become an important tool, especially in implant dentistry.[2] There have even been discussions about whether or not CBCT should be considered the standard of care in implant dentistry and thus recommended for all patients. However, although it is widely agreed that CBCT is a very useful tool for most patients, there may be a limited number of cases where this technology offers inconsequential additional information and advantage.[3]

With the addition of 3-D information in implant dentistry, it is now possible to consider not just evaluating the patient in three dimensions, but also to do virtual treatment planning, and ultimately a completely digital workflow from surgical placement through a 3-D image-guided template to an all-digital impression.[2] This technology obviously requires great accuracy to be predictable and this chapter will address this important issue in detail.

The contemporary choice for 3-D radiographic imaging is *de facto* the CBCT. No other 3-D radiographic options should be considered at this time for implant treatment planning.[3] The early generations of CBCT were characterized by low resolution and the only way to increase the resolution was to increase the amount of radiation and the time it took to capture the volume. In later generations, the quality of the sensor was improved and

Evidence-based Implant Treatment Planning and Clinical Protocols, First Edition. Edited by Steven J. Sadowsky.

Companion website: www.wiley.com/go/sadowsky/implant

that allowed for less radiation and shorter volume capture times.[4] The latter also reduced the risks of movement during the scan, improving the quality of the captured volume. In the current generation of CBCT, the quality of the image is adequate for diagnostic needs and the radiation has been minimized to a level that should not limit the use of this technology in dental practices. One important consideration for investing in CBCT technology is medical–legal liability. From a medical–legal standpoint, the practitioner is responsible for identifying pathology – even if it is outside the dental field or outside the experience of the practitioner. The simplest way to reduce that concern is to minimize the field of view to the required area only. This will allow for a reduction in radiation as well. The other option to consider is outsourcing a radiographic interpretation from a board-certified radiologist. This will add to the cost of using the machine, but will reduce the medical–legal concerns.[2,5]

The issue of radiation

The first use of conventional CT scanning in implant dentistry came with a significant amount of radiation, deeming it unfeasible for routine use (Table 4.1). With the emergence of CBCT, the radiation became a much more manageable issue; even so, over the last couple of years concerns over radiation from CBCT machines in dental offices have emerged. Most of those concerns stem from a misunderstanding of how the newest-generation CBCT machines can minimize radiation by reducing the field of view (FOV). This brings a CBCT scan down to about the same as a panoramic x-ray or five times that of the annual naturally occurring background radiation (Table 4.1, Table 4.2). It would appear from Tables 4.1 and 4.2 that concerns over radiation should be minimal when a CBCT scan is taken with a modern

Table 4.1 Effective radiation dosages (in micro-sieverts) from different sources.[1,2,5] *Source:* Data from Bouserhal 2002.[1]

Radiation source	Effective radiation (μsv)
Conventional CT scan	500–3000
Full-mouth series periapical x-rays on film	150
Conebeam CT (see Table 4.2)	10–200
Panoramic x-ray (digital)	14
Flying at 30 000 feet per hour	4
Background radiation per year	<3

Table 4.2 Radiation dosage for different CBCT machines and different field of view (FOV). *Source:* Data from Benavides *et al.* 2012.[5]

Device and FOV	Effective radiation (μsv)
ICAT first-generation 13–22 cm	69
ICAT newest generation at 6 cm	11–15
Kodak 9000 3D	5–38
Accuitomo 4 × 4 cm	13

CBCT machine with the minimal amount of field of view, and when there is diagnostic information in the images that enhances the outcome of implant surgery.[1,2,5] The trend is clearly that the newest-generation machines have the smallest FOV, and the quickest scans with a smaller and smaller amount of radiation, leading to either the same or improved image quality as compared to the earlier version.

Levels of adjunct use of CBCT in implant dentistry

During the past decade, there has been a significant development in the level of sophistication with which CBCT technology is being used to aid implant dentistry.[5] Initially the technology was used mainly to diagnose and visualize the 3-D availability of bone using multiple cross-sectional slices of the potential implant sites (passive or CBCT). Later additional tools became available to allow for simulation or virtual treatment planning, and tools to aid the positioning during surgery (semi-active or CBCT guided), and most recently the use of CBCT combined with a guidance system to facilitate the correct positioning of surgical instrumentation (active or fully CBCT guided).[6] This technology is still in very early stages of development and there has been relatively little development in this technology as compared to the use of guides to facilitate implant accuracy. At this time there is no evidence that this approach can or will become more accurate than guided surgery described in more detail in this chapter. For the remainder of this chapter, the focus will be placed on the first two levels.

Diagnostic use of CBCT (passive or CBCT aided)

The CBCT scan is used primarily to evaluate the anatomy of the implant site in three dimensions. The advantage over conventional radiographs is the added third dimension that can be difficult to evaluate clinically depending on the case. The 3-D representation will help evaluate the cross-sectional width of the bone around the implant site and the proximity to important anatomical landmarks, such as nerves and vessels. In addition, it can serve as a more accurate tool for measuring the vertical amount of bone in the maxilla, where the maxillary sinuses often limit the availability of bone. The diagnostic value depends on the assessment of clinical findings and the conventional radiographs, which may indicate an adequate amount of bone in the implant site both vertically and horizontally, and in those cases CBCT will add little extra diagnostic value.

The CBCT volumetric data can also be used to evaluate the bone density. Soft tissue will similarly be assigned different shades of grey (in the darker spectrum). It is, however, very difficult to see the difference between gingiva, tongue, and lips. Therefore, it has been shown useful to scan patients with cotton rolls or gauze to keep these tissues apart. This will increase the diagnostic quality of the image.[5,7] This gradient in radiodensity is often expressed in Hounsfield units (HU), which is a linear scale based on the difference between the radiodensity of air and water. This scale is very useful with medical or conventional CT scans, which are calibrated to this scale. There is third-party software available on the market that will apply this scale to CBCT imaging, which is not as reliable as medical CT, as the CBCT is not calibrated in the same fashion due to the volumetric data acquisition and reconstruction of CBCT. However, recent studies suggest that there may be a strong correlation between high CBCT Hounsfield units and increased bone density and correlation to good bone quality and higher initial insertion torque of implants.[5] It has been suggested, for example, that implants placed in bone with HU below 500 should not be loaded immediately.[8] Except for this facility of bone density evaluation and Hounsfield units, the diagnostic level of sophistication with CBCT and implants can usually be accomplished without any third-party imaging software or special equipment. Most CBCT scanners come with software to scan and view the images captured and many will allow for a read-only viewer to be delivered with the image, if the machine is not on site.

Implant planning (semi-active or CBCT guided)

The next level of sophistication of the use of CBCT in implant dentistry is to use third-party software that can simulate the brand, width, and length of the implant, and be used to visualize the implant when placed relative to the bony architecture and in proximity to relevant anatomical landmarks, such as the inferior alveolar nerve and the maxillary sinuses. This simulation aids in the determination of appropriate width and length of implants and may result in a decision to graft bone either concurrent with the implant or months before the implant is placed.[6] As such, these 3-D simulations are also very useful in communications between the involved parties, such as referring dentist, surgeon, and/or laboratory. If the CBCT is captured with a radiographic template (Figure 4.1) it will allow for the position of the implants to be correlated to the desired position of the crown and the relative trajectory of the implants can be discussed between the surgeon and the restorative doctor. The preoperative availability of virtual planning can improve the quality of the discussion of the design requirements of screw- vs. cement-retained restorations. It is also possible to drill the desired trajectory of the implant in the radiographic guide. This "access hole" can be visualized with gutta percha or other fiduciary radiopaque material on the CBCT image and, if this fits well with where the bone is, the radiographic guide can be converted into a surgical guide or manual modifications can be made as necessary. At this basic level of sophistication, the surgical guide is not customized accurately to the implant brand, size, or exact position, but rather to be used in a semi-guided approach to placing the implant. It should not be expected at this level that there is a great correlation between the planned and actual position of the implant.[9]

The next level of sophistication is to digitally replicate the initial and/or revised planned brand, size, and position of the implants in a surgical guide that is fabricated more directly, based on the virtual planned position of the implant(s) on the CBCT. There are several different ways to achieve this and they have been shown to not all be equally accurate.[5,10] The first comprehensive systematic review of these systems was done by Jung *et al.*[6] in 2009 using published reports until the end of 2007. They reported on three different approaches to this transfer of the virtual treatment planning to the surgical placement of the implants: a) mechanical positioning devices or the use of drilling machines based on a transfer of a coordinate system from the patient's CBCT scan; b) CAD/CAM stereolithographic (SLA) models; and c) navigation systems, where the position of the implant driver was recorded in three dimensions and compared in the planning. The outcomes in terms of accuracy and

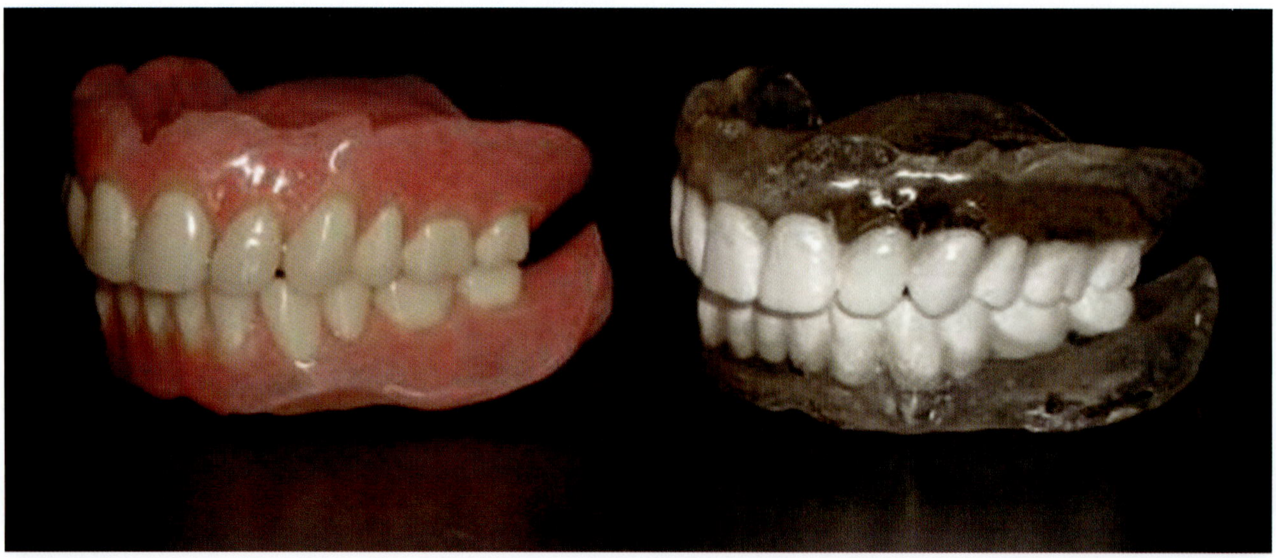

Figure 4.1 Radiographic template used for identifying the desired position of the restored teeth, here marked by barium sulfate. *Source:* Reproduced with permission from Charles Goodacre.

survival of implants were very mixed among different studies and techniques.[6] There has been a significant amount of research done on types a) and b). These are described below, differentiated by manufacturing process and how the guide is fixed to the patient. As for type c), the navigation system, it is still in a very early stage of development and it would appear that additional data and refinement of the technology are necessary before that technology is ready for a more comprehensive deployment.

Generations of guides for CBCT-guided surgery

During the last 10 years, CBCT image-guided implant surgery has gone through several generations of the imaging and fabrication process. During this iteration process, reports of varying outcomes have been plagued with heterogeneity, leading to difficulty in assessing the critical variables for accuracy. The first variable was the quality of the CBCT, including the slice thickness. Some early studies used very large slice thickness and later studies had much finer details, with slice thickness down to about 0.2 mm. A second variable was that guides can be placed on bone, soft tissue, or teeth. A third variable was the fabrication method for the guide. Some studies used printed stereolithographic (SLA) guides and other used a vacuum-formed splint on a printed SLA model. Finally, a fourth variable was the method and amount of guidance. Some of the early generations had a metal sleeve for the pilot drill only, whereas others used a series of handles to center the osteotomy of more/all of the drill diameters. Some guides and drill systems allow for placement of the implant through the guide and some have a vertical stop on the delivery process to indicate when the implant is at the planned vertical position. Due to the complexity of combining simultaneous variations in these four parameters, guided surgery experiences have varied and studies have revealed significant variation in outcomes. In the following paragraphs, it has been attempted to describe the most common combinations of these variables and correlate them to outcomes as evaluated by accuracy and implant survival. It is critically important to evaluate these variations to understand the opportunities and limitations with this technology.

Bone-level and SLA printed guides

The first guides that were described were SLA printed to be placed on bone. An early comprehensive report on this approach was by van Steenberghe *et al.*,[11] which evaluated edentulous patients receiving multiple implants with an immediate loading protocol. This study was predominantly focusing on the protocol and patient satisfaction with the Nobel Biocare "Teeth-in-an-hour" concept, which has since been discontinued in its original form. Another of the early reports on guided surgery was by Lal *et al.*[12,13] in 2006, where the use of SLA templates to plan and place implants was described. This was mostly a proof-of-concept study with a case report. The approach used was a bone level guide made on a SLA printed model of the jaw based on a CT scan with 1 mm slice thickness. The printed SLA model, slice thickness, and use of bone to position the guide have later all proven to be the least accurate approach to guided implant surgery. Later in 2008, Nikzad and Azari[14] published on a methodology very similar to that of Lal *et al.*[12] with a printed SLA model and one case report. The guide was also a bone level guide. No data on accuracy or survival were presented. By nature of the positioning the guides on bone, extensive flaps to position and secure the guide are required. At the time it was speculated that in the future, perhaps soft-tissue-based guides could be less invasive.[12,13] At that time, using teeth for positioning and fixation was not possible as these were not accurately enough captured by the CBCT and reproduced in the SLA printing, partly due to the slice thickness of the CBCT and the scatter from metal objects in the teeth.

Soft-tissue-level guides and flapless surgery

Conventional implant surgery has almost always included exposing the implant site with an incision and flap. With the additional 3-D information about the architecture of the underlying bone, it has been one of the alluring aspects of guided surgery to avoid an incision and a flap. This would imply that the guide is placed and held on soft tissue and that osteotomies be done and implants be placed with a guide based on the CBCT plan. One of the first studies to review such an approach was by Merli *et al.*[15] in 2008, where they planned no flap and bone exposure by a computer-guided flapless approach in the edentulous maxilla, in a pilot prospective case series on 13 consecutive patients receiving a total of 89 implants. They used Procera software and a NobelGuide® approach to place the implants in atrophic fully edentulous patients with a flapless approach. Merli *et al.* reported 5.6% failure rate of implants, which, for the atrophic edentulous maxilla, is similar to non-guided approaches. They reported no data on accuracy, but commented that a learning curve was evident from their experience in that many of the failures occurred in the early cases. However, later studies found similar and higher failure rates with the same approach.[16,17]

Another study looked at accuracy of guided implants in a flapless approach on edentulous patients.[18] They found a mean deviation of the entry point of the implants of 2.17 mm in the maxilla and 1.42 mm in the mandible. The angle deviation was similar in the upper and lower jaw at around 1.9°. A similar flapless approach with NobelGuide® was published by Komiyama *et al.*[19] in 2008, where 29 edentulous patients received 176 implants in an immediately loaded approach. They found 11% failure rate of implants and a higher than normal incidence of surgical and technical complications. They concluded that this methodology should be regarded to be in the exploratory phase of development. Another long-term survival study was published by Orentlicher *et al.*[16] They reported on a 7-year retrospective analysis of cumulative survival rate of implants placed "fully guided". They analyzed 796 implants placed in 177 patients using CBCT-guided surgery. The cumulative survival rate was 96.98% and they found no reduction in survival when immediately loading implants. Similar survival results were found by

Vasak *et al.*[17] in reviewing 163 implants in 30 patients with a cumulative survival rate of 98.8%.

The limiting factor with flapless surgery is that it is not possible to confirm either the availability of bone or the accurate placement of the implant. Positioning and holding of the guide in the planned position on the soft tissue has been suggested to be done with pins that can be incorporated into the guide.[15,20] This still does not solve the issue of possibly not positioning the guide accurately on soft tissue alone. This issue was addressed by Holst *et al.*[21] in a proof-of-concept study with a case report. The approach included placing at least three positioning screws in the edentulous jaw before taking impressions for a radiographic template. In this template a Lego block was embedded as a fiduciary marker. This served to orient the laboratory model according to the CBCT when transferring the planned position of the implants from the CBCT to a surgical guide that would be positioned according to the screws in the patient's jaw and fixed on these during implant placement. This approach would require an additional surgical procedure to place the positioning screws and subsequent removal. It has not been elaborated on since its original description in 2007.

Other attempts have been made to address the issue of fiduciary markers and transfer of coordinate systems between the CBCT scan of the patient and the laboratory setting for fabrication of a surgical guide that replicates the planned position of the implants. With such an intent being the accurate transfer of the virtual planning to the surgical template, Nickenig *et al.*[22] in 2007, used three fiduciary markers in a scanning template that the patient wore during the CBCT. The planned position of the implants was then determined using a special laboratory appliance and sleeves were inserted into a guide after drilling through the radiographic scanning template, converting it into a surgical guide. This was similar to several other systems on the market at the time, such as the Straumann GonyX system (Straumann USA, Andover, Massachusetts). In this study, a total of 102 patients received 250 implants. About 7% of the patients were edentulous and the guides were soft tissue based and held with pins. The goal was to do flapless surgery, which was done in roughly 60% of the implant sites. The remaining sites needed bone augmentation, ridge splitting, or sinus lift augmentation, and a flap was used. This illustrates an important point when planning guided flapless surgery: the surgeon must be prepared and skilled to raise a flap and do adjunct procedures such as ridge splitting and bone augmentation. This supports the conclusion reached after a comprehensive review by Hammerle *et al.*[23] that guided flapless surgery should be reserved for experienced clinicians and not performed by novices, because of repeated intraoperative complications and frequent need for adjunctive procedures.

Tooth-borne guides

In partially edentulous patients it would make sense to use the remaining teeth for placement and anchorage of the guide, and difficulty in capturing the teeth accurately was overcome through digital scanning technology. In 2008 and 2009, companies began experimenting with 3-D scanning of stone models of the teeth (and later direct intraoral scans using iTero [Align Technology, San Jose, CA] or similar intraoral scanners). These 3-D surface models could then be superimposed on the CBCT plan and allow for much greater accuracy in fabrication of the surgical guide (Figures 4.2 and 4.3). One of the first studies to report on this modification to the planning and production of tooth-borne guides was Abboud *et al.*[24] in 2012. The study compared two different guide systems and found an overall survival of 98.7% and, in contrast to other studies, no intraoperative complications were seen. This is contrary to previous bone-level and soft-tissue-level guides, where intraoperative complications were common. No data on accuracy were provided, but the survival rate is generally higher than what previously had been reported with guided surgery. Another study[25] used principally the same technology and did report some interesting data on accuracy on 132 implants placed with guided surgery in 52 patients. The average deviation at the platform of the implant was 0.27 mm and at the implant apex 0.46 mm average deviation with an angle deviation of 1.84°. These data were more promising than earlier studies, especially when compared to bone- and soft-tissue-borne guides, although the maximum deviation at the implant platform was 0.97 mm and 1.38 mm at the apex of the implant. The larger discrepancy at the apex of the implant than the platform has been verified in other studies and is attributed to simple geometry of the greater distance from the guidance of the sleeve in the guide to the apex of the implant. Further studies are needed to increase our knowledge base with teeth-borne guides, but at this time it appears to be the most promising approach to guided surgery, both when looking at overall survival and accuracy of the implants.

Comparative accuracy of guided surgery with different approaches

The overall key challenge with guided surgery is the many steps in the process, where error can be introduced. Many studies have tried to investigate each of the steps in order to glean improvements to that part of the process. Some of the earlier studies focused on implant survival as the only measure of outcome, whereas later studies started looking at the discrepancy between the planned and actual position of the implants. It is important to differentiate outcomes based on the fabrication process and the seating method of the guide. In 2009, Ozan *et al.*[26] reported on accuracy of the guides and compared outcomes based on the type of seating of the guide comparing tooth-, bone-, and soft-tissue-supported guides in the same study. This was one of the first studies that compared the accuracy between the planned and actual position of the implant using these three different approaches to the surgical guide. The result of the study showed a clear advantage of the tooth-supported guide compared to the other two when it came to accuracy of the implant relative to the planned position. The increased accuracy of guides placed on teeth was confirmed by Arisan *et al.*[27] in a study of SLA printed guides based on either teeth, soft tissue or bone. They found the

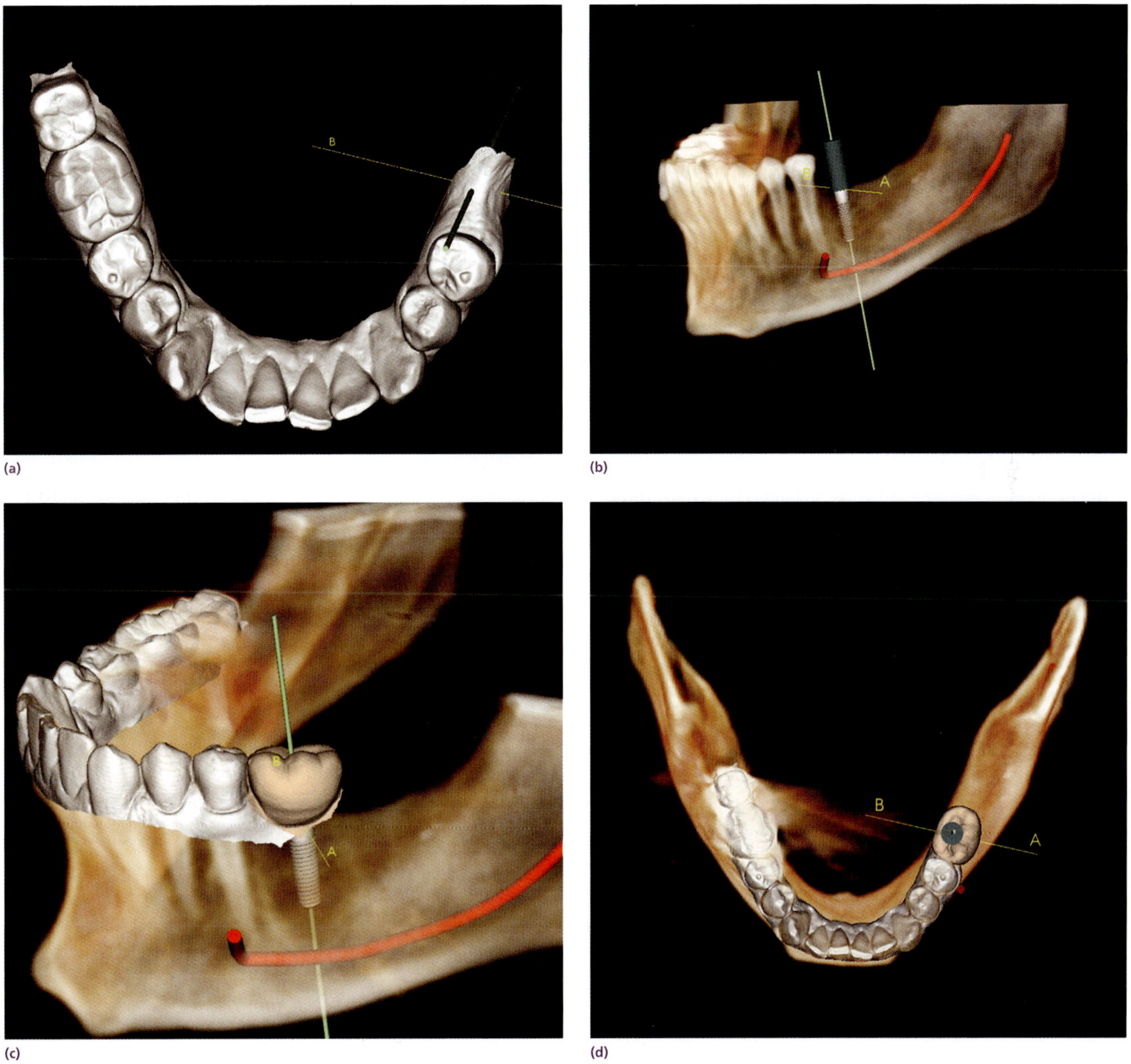

Figure 4.2 CBCT virtual 3D planning tool for implant positioning. **(a)** Mandibular arch generated from intraoral scan. **(b)** Sagittal position of implant in #19 site. **(c)** Sagittal view of implant in #19 site with superimposition of radiographic template. **(d)** Occlusal view of implant in #19 site with superimposition of radiographic template.

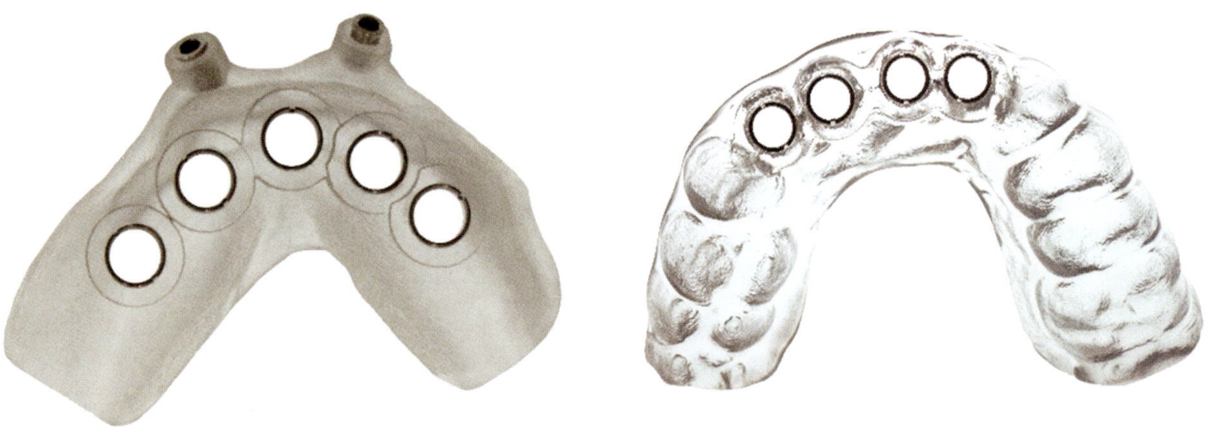

Figure 4.3 Different approaches to guide fabrication showing soft-tissue-supported guide on the left with fixation pins, and tooth-supported guide on the right. *Source:* Reproduced with permission from Anatomage Inc.

tooth-borne guides to be significantly more accurate than both soft-tissue- and bone-borne guides. They also recommended that if soft-tissue-borne guides are used, that the accuracy of those can be improved by fixating them with screws. This has subsequently become even clearer. Similar levels of accuracy were seen in a smaller study by Van Assche *et al.*[28]

Despite the relative superior accuracy of tooth-borne guides versus other designs, deviations may be of concern. Valente *et al.*[29] reviewed the accuracy by contrasting the planned versus actual position of the implants. Their data, however, were collected between 2004 and 2006 and studied both partially edentulous and fully edentulous patients using bone-supported, soft-tissue-supported, and tooth-supported guides in a flapped or flapless approach. The guides were printed (SLA) based on the CBCT. The surgeries were done at two different locations and two different implant systems were used. The guides were only used to drill the osteotomy and the implants were inserted without guidance. They evaluated 89 implants, but, due to the different locations, different implants, and different guide support, each group was relatively small. The overall mean deviation between planned and actual position of the implant was 1.4 mm at the coronal aspect, 1.6 mm at the apical aspect, 1.1 mm depth deviation and 7.9° average angle deviation of the implants. In reviewing the variation, it was seen that 28% of the implants were more than 2 mm deviated from the planned position. The data seemed to suggest that the soft-tissue-based guides were more accurate that the tooth-supported guides, which is contrary to later findings in many other studies. The cumulative survival was 96%. They concluded that, although the survival was similar to nonguided cases, the accuracy was not clinically acceptable in a fourth of the implants and therefore that guided surgery with this methodology should be pursued with caution. Similar results were reported by Schneider *et al.*[30] in a systematic review of the literature on CBCT-guided surgery outcomes in terms of accuracy and survival. The authors found eight studies (some of which have been mentioned earlier) and found survival to vary between 91 and 100%. They also reported that guided surgery came with a fair number of technical perioperative complications and that the accuracy was reasonable, but with relatively high maximum deviations. The authors reported average deviations around 1.1–1.6 mm and concluded that it may not be reliable enough to justify a "blind" implantation, which would be the case with flapless surgery.

The most recent systematic review on computer technology applications in surgical implant dentistry was done by Tahmaseb *et al.*[31] in 2014. They found 14 survival and 24 accuracy studies that met the criteria for inclusion in the review. The survival rates and accuracies reported were similar to earlier studies. Behneke *et al.*[32] studied factors that affected the transfer accuracy and found that flapped or flapless surgery did not significantly influence accuracy. They did, however, find that improved accuracy was seen when the implants were placed fully guided (all drill steps and implant placement occur through the guide) as compared to freehand placement of the implant with all drilling done guided and when the final drill sequence was freehand and only the first drill(s) guided. These studies illustrate another variable that, as of yet, is not well reported on, which is whether the guide was used for the initial drill (pilot) or subsequent drills as well. Also, if the implant was placed through the guide with a vertical stop or by freehand. Further studies are needed to fully understand the importance of these variables.

Complications

Most of the studies that have been published focusing on survival of implants placed traditionally and guided have not found great differences in the ultimate complication: implant failure.[15,16,24,30] The majority of these studies were retrospective in design. This was, however, not the case in a prospective mono-center study,[33] where data were published on 114 implants placed with guided surgery in 26 patients. The 1-year survival of the implants was only 88.6%, and when looking at smokers and nonsmokers, the survival rates were 69.2% and 98.7% respectively. They concluded that smoking might need to be considered a contraindication to guided implant surgery. Some of the implants were placed in edentulous patients and some in partially edentulous. All implants were placed flapless. Some of the implants in this study were immediately loaded and they showed higher failure rate than those not loaded immediately. Other studies[16,17] before and after the above study have not seen similar high failure rates, neither with immediate loading nor in heavy smokers. Further studies are needed to explain these variations.

There are also several advantages with guided implant surgery such as the ability to place implants without raising a mucoperiosteal flap, which reduces the overall time and morbidity of the surgery. These advantages should, however, be carefully evaluated against the possible disadvantages. The most important disadvantage of the fully guided flapless approach is that the bone is poorly visualized and if poor planning or lack of precision of the technique guides the implant outside the bone, it is difficult to appreciate and correct the error. The advantages and disadvantages have been summarized in Table 4.3.

Table 4.3 Advantages and disadvantages of computer image guided surgery in implant dentistry.

Advantages	Disadvantages
Flapless surgery[34,35]	Radiation from CBCT[2]
Patient satisfaction and improved recovery,[36] tolerance[14,15,19,34,37]	Lack of accuracy[38]
Saves time[39]	Increase risk of failure in some studies[33,40]
Improved soft tissue response[28]	Ongoing bone loss with immediate loading[41]
More accurate than freehand surgery[9,27,42]	Not easier than conventional approach due to many intraoperative complications[35]
	Difficult to fit instrumentation in the posterior mandible or with limited opening[22]
	Making flapless surgery appear deceptively easy[23]
	Challenge to cool bone through guide while drilling[38]

Operator sensitivity/learning curve influence

In 2008 a group at the Fourth ITI consensus conference was tasked to review the status and make recommendations for computer-assisted clinical procedures in implant dentistry. The outcome of that review was published in 2009.[23] The group expressed concern over the lack of long-term data and the variability of studies on accuracy of this new technology. They found that the technology of CBCT-guided surgery was technique sensitive and that there was a significant learning curve with the technology. They cautioned that flapless surgery may have advantages in terms of less trauma and postoperative discomfort, but that it should be reserved for skilled and experienced surgeons that utilize comprehensive 3-D planning.

As has been mentioned before, there are numerous steps in doing CBCT-guided implant surgery and each step can introduce error. One step is the tolerance of surgical instrumentation through the guide, which may be particularly prone to operator error and thus affected by a learning curve when first employing guided surgery. This tolerance of the drilling was studied by Schneider *et al.*,[43] and they found that, even when using a conventional guide with fitted metal sleeves there was significantly more flexing than compared to a printed guide without metal sleeves. The study was based on an *in vitro* model and has not been confirmed in a clinical study.

More recently, another consensus conference was held by European Academy of Osseointegration (EAO) in 2015 with many of the same authors as previous reports from similar consensus conferences. The main report by Hammerle *et al.*[44] stresses that, although guided implant surgery clearly reduces the inaccuracy as compared to freehand surgery, there is still a risk of introducing cumulative errors in the design, fabrication, and clinical use of guides. They conclude that future research should focus on reducing the number of steps needed in this process to reduce the variation in accuracy currently reported by many. They also mention that further research is necessary to find out which categories of patients may benefit most from guided surgery.

From the same conference, Vercruyssen *et al.*[45] summarized the status of computer-supported implant planning and guided surgery. This report formed part of the background for the report by Hammerle *et al.*,[44] and thus the findings and conclusions overlap. It seems clear that optical scanning and 3-D printing are technologies that will be part of the foundation for the future of guided implant surgery and stressed again the need to improve accuracy by reducing the number of steps in the process of planning, fabrication, and clinical use of guides.

Post-surgical evaluation of implant positions

CBCT has been used to evaluate the outcome of grafting procedures since the technology became available. Today it is also frequently being used to evaluate the position of guided implants after placement relative to the planned position.[18,25,28,29] This was previously a little more controversial due to the radiation involved. However, as the CBCT technology continues to improve and the field of view is kept small, the radiation is relatively low and is significantly less of a hindrance to using the technology for this purpose. Some have suggested alternative approaches to registering the position of the implants, for example from scanning of the master cast and superimposition on the planned position.[42,46] A challenge with both techniques is that the superimposition required to compare the implants before and after has an inherent inaccuracy as well. New digital imaging, such as optical coherence tomography (OCT) and spectrophotometry, can also be used to access outcomes in terms of soft-tissue and bone defects and misfit between the reconstructions and the implants.[47]

Conclusion

This review of the current evidence base in the literature clearly supports the use of CBCT as a diagnostic aid and to facilitate communication about surgical and restorative options and restrictions. The next level of using CBCT to guide the position of implants is more controversial and there are currently conflicting reports in the literature. The use of guides in implant dentistry has evolved quickly and has been promoted by the industry before there are reliable outcome data in terms of survival of implants and accuracy of the placement. The positive reports in the literature outweigh the negative, but the presence of variation in outcomes is a cause of concern at the moment. Future studies are needed to improve this technology and explain the variation currently seen. At this time, until further information is available, guided flapless surgery in edentulous cases should be planned with great care and applied only to cases where there is at least 2 mm bone available in any direction. In contrast, tooth-supported guides have recently shown much greater accuracy, by incorporating direct or indirect intraoral scans (digital impressions) overlaid on the CBCT plan and by using guided systems that have vertical stops on drills, where all drilling is done through the guide and where the implant can be placed through the guide with a vertical stop as well. In general, guided surgery has the potential to make implant surgery more accurate, faster, and with less postoperative discomfort for the patient than the conventional approach to implant surgery. However, it is clear from this review that very limited evidence exists yet to suggest that computer-assisted surgery is superior to conventional procedures in terms of safety, outcomes, morbidity, or efficiency.

What we have learned from the last decade is that tooth-borne guides are superior in accuracy to both soft-tissue-supported and bone-supported guides. We have also learned how to incorporate the superior accuracy of intraoral scanning into the CBCT treatment plan, which has increased the accuracy of the fit of guides, especially the tooth-borne guides. We have also learned some of the limitations of flapless guided surgery, such as when limited bone is available. The currently available outcomes data from different studies show varying outcomes due to different approaches to fabrication and positioning approaches. As the pros and cons of the different variables become more clear, we are likely to see a maturation process, where outcomes of guided surgery become less variable and further refinements can take place based on stronger-pedigree investigations.

When evaluating guided surgery, it is important to understand that, although fully guided surgery (all drilling and implant placement is done through a guide) is possible even with a flapless approach, it does require a significant safety margin in terms of bone availability. If that bone is not available, it may be preferable to do a partially guided flapped procedure, where the initial or first couple of drills are done guided and then the availability of bone is reviewed and the remainder of the osteotomy is drilled nonguided with a flap and the implant is placed manually as well. Thus, adjunctive procedures such as ridge splitting and bone grafting can be employed. In this way, the accuracy of the implant, when comparing the planned versus the actual position of the implant, may not be ideal, but the trajectory of the implant is likely to be appropriate for the planned prosthetic solution, and the implant has a higher chance of being well encased in adequate bone. This underscores the importance of operator expertise to override the guided approach when necessary. Further studies are needed to determine the effectiveness of this partially guided approach and to identify which cases could be done fully guided and flapless.

References

1. Bouserhal C, Jacobs R, Quirynen M, *et al.* Imaging technique selection for the preoperative planning of oral implants: a review of the literature. *Clin Implant Dent Relat Res* 2002; **4**(3): 156–172.
2. Jansen CE. CBCT technology for diagnosis and treatment planning: what general practitioners should consider. *Compend Contin Educ Dent* 2014; **35**(10): 749–753.
3. Bornstein MM, Al-Nawas B, Kuchler U, *et al.* Consensus statements and recommended clinical procedures regarding contemporary surgical and radiographic techniques in implant dentistry. *Int J Oral Maxillofac Implants* 2014; **29**(Suppl): 78–82.
4. Dawood A, Patel S, Brown J. Cone beam CT in dental practice. *BDJ* 2009; **207**(1): 23–28.
5. Benavides E, Rios HF, Ganz SD, *et al.* Use of cone beam computed tomography in implant dentistry: the International Congress of Oral Implantologists consensus report. *Implant Dent* 2012; **21**(2): 78–86.
6. Jung RE, Schneider D, Ganeles J, *et al.* Computer technology applications in surgical implant dentistry: a systematic review. *Int J Oral Maxillofac Implants* 2009; **24**(Suppl): 92–109.
7. Wouters V, Mollemans W, Schutyser F. Calibrated segmentation of CBCT and CT images for digitization of dental prostheses. *Int J Comput Assist Radiol Surg* 2011; **6**(5): 609–616.
8. Block MS, Chandler C. Computed tomography-guided surgery: complications associated with scanning, processing, surgery, and prosthetics. *J Oral Maxillofac Surg* 2009; **67**(11 Suppl): 13–22.
9. Farley NE, Kennedy K, McGlumphy EA, *et al.* Split-mouth comparison of the accuracy of computer-generated and conventional surgical guides. *Int J Oral Maxillofac Implants* 2013; **28**(2): 563–572.
10. Bedrossian E. Laboratory and prosthetic considerations in computer-guided surgery and immediate loading. *J Oral Maxillofac Surg* 2007; **65**(7 Suppl1): 47–52.
11. van Steenberghe D, Glauser R, Blomback U, *et al.* A computed tomographic scan-derived customized surgical template and fixed prosthesis for flapless surgery and immediate loading of implants in fully edentulous maxillae: a prospective multicenter study. *Clin Implant Dent Relat Res* 2005; **7**(Suppl 1):S111–S120.
12. Lal K, White GS, Morea DN, *et al.* Use of stereolithographic templates for surgical and prosthodontic implant planning and placement. Part I. The concept. *J Prosthodont* 2006; **15**(1): 51–58.
13. Lal K, White GS, Morea DN, *et al.* Use of stereolithographic templates for surgical and prosthodontic implant planning and placement. Part II. A clinical report. *J Prosthodont* 2006; **15**(2): 117–122.
14. Nikzad S, Azari A. A novel stereolithographic surgical guide template for planning treatment involving a mandibular dental implant. *J Oral Maxillofac Surg* 2008; **66**(7): 1446–1454.
15. Merli M, Bernardelli F, Esposito M. Computer-guided flapless placement of immediately loaded dental implants in the edentulous maxilla: a pilot prospective case series. *Eur J Oral Implantol* 2008; **1**(1): 61–69.
16. Orentlicher G, Horowitz A, Goldsmith D, *et al.* Cumulative survival rate of implants placed "fully guided" using CT-guided surgery: a 7-year retrospective study. *Compend Contin Educ Dent* 2014; **35**(8): 590–600.
17. Vasak C, Kohal RJ, Lettner S, *et al.* Clinical and radiological evaluation of a template-guided (NobelGuide) treatment concept. *Clin Oral Implants Res* 2014; **25**(1): 116–123.
18. Vieira DM, Sotto-Maior BS, Barros CA, *et al.* Clinical accuracy of flapless computer-guided surgery for implant placement in edentulous arches. *Int J Oral Maxillofac Implants* 2013; **28**(5): 1347–1351.
19. Komiyama A, Klinge B, Hultin M. Treatment outcome of immediately loaded implants installed in edentulous jaws following computer-assisted virtual treatment planning and flapless surgery. *Clin Oral Implants Res* 2008; **19**(7): 677–685.
20. de Almeida EO, Pellizzer EP, Goiatto MC, *et al.* Computer-guided surgery in implantology: review of basic concepts. *J Craniofac Surg* 2010; **21**(6): 1917–1921.
21. Holst S, Blatz MB, Eitner S. Precision for computer-guided implant placement: using 3D planning software and fixed intraoral reference points. *J Oral Maxillofac Surg* 2007; **65**(3): 393–399.
22. Nickenig HJ, Eitner S. Reliability of implant placement after virtual planning of implant positions using cone beam CT data and surgical (guide) templates. *J Craniomaxillofac Surg* 2007; **35**(4–5): 207–211.
23. Hammerle CH, Stone P, Jung RE, *et al.* Consensus statements and recommended clinical procedures regarding computer-assisted implant dentistry. *Int J Oral Maxillofac Implants* 2009; **24**(Suppl): 126–131.
24. Abboud M, Wahl G, Guirado JL, *et al.* Application and success of two stereolithographic surgical guide systems for implant placement with immediate loading. *Int J Oral Maxillofac Implants* 2012; **27**(3): 634–643.
25. Behneke A, Burwinkel M, Knierim K, *et al.* Accuracy assessment of cone beam computed tomography-derived laboratory-based surgical templates on partially edentulous patients. *Clin Oral Implants Res* 2012; **23**(2): 137–143.

26. Ozan O, Turkyilmaz I, Ersoy AE, *et al.* Clinical accuracy of 3 different types of computed tomography-derived stereolithographic surgical guides in implant placement. *J Oral Maxillofac Surg* 2009; **67**(2): 394–401.
27. Arisan V, Karabuda ZC, Ozdemir T. Accuracy of two stereolithographic guide systems for computer-aided implant placement: a computed tomography-based clinical comparative study. *J Periodontol* 2010; **81**(1): 43–51.
28. van Assche N, van Steenberghe D, Quirynen M, *et al.* Accuracy assessment of computer-assisted flapless implant placement in partial edentulism. *J Clin Periodontol* 2010; **37**(4): 398–403.
29. Valente F, Schiroli G, Sbrenna A. Accuracy of computer-aided oral implant surgery: a clinical and radiographic study. *Int J Oral Maxillofac Implants* 2009; **24**(2): 234–242.
30. Schneider D, Marquardt P, Zwahlen M, *et al.* A systematic review on the accuracy and the clinical outcome of computer-guided template-based implant dentistry. *Clin Oral Implants Res* 2009; **20**(Suppl 4): 73–86.
31. Tahmaseb A, Wismeijer D, Coucke W, *et al.* Computer technology applications in surgical implant dentistry: a systematic review. *Int J Oral Maxillofac Implants* 2014; **29**(Suppl): 25–42.
32. Behneke A, Burwinkel M, Behneke N. Factors influencing transfer accuracy of cone beam CT-derived template-based implant placement. *Clin Oral Implants Res* 2012; **23**(4): 416–423.
33. D'Haese J, Vervaeke S, Verbanck N, *et al.* Clinical and radiographic outcome of implants placed using stereolithographic guided surgery: a prospective monocenter study. *Int J Oral Maxillofac Implants* 2013; **28**(1): 205–215.
34. Nikzad S, Azari A. Custom-made radiographic template, computed tomography, and computer-assisted flapless surgery for treatment planning in partial edentulous patients: a prospective 12-month study. *J Oral Maxillofac Surg* 2010; **68**(6): 1353–1359.
35. Hultin M, Svensson KG, Trulsson M. Clinical advantages of computer-guided implant placement: a systematic review. *Clin Oral Implants Res* 2012; **23**(Suppl 6): 124–135.
36. Youk SY, Lee JH, Park JM, *et al.* A survey of the satisfaction of patients who have undergone implant surgery with and without employing a computer-guided implant surgical template. *J Adv Prosthodont* 2014; **6**(5): 395–405.
37. Fortin T, Bosson JL, Isidori M, *et al.* Effect of flapless surgery on pain experienced in implant placement using an image-guided system. *Int J Oral Maxillofac Implants* 2006; **21**(2): 298–304.
38. D'Haese J, Van De Velde T, Komiyama A, *et al.* Accuracy and complications using computer-designed stereolithographic surgical guides for oral rehabilitation by means of dental implants: a review of the literature. *Clin Implant Dent Relat Res* 2012; **14**(3): 321–335.
39. Orentlicher G, Abboud M. Guided surgery for implant therapy. *Oral Maxillofac Surg Clin North Am* 2011; **23**(2): 239–242vi.
40. Chrcanovic BR, Albrektsson T, Wennerberg A. Reasons for failures of oral implants. *J Oral Rehabil* 2014; **41**(6): 443–476.
41. Browaeys H, Dierens M, Ruyffelaert C, *et al.* Ongoing crestal bone loss around implants subjected to computer-guided flapless surgery and immediate loading using the All-on-4® concept. *Clin Implant Dent Relat Res* 2015; **17**(5): 831–843.
42. Nickenig HJ, Wichmann M, Hamel J, *et al.* Evaluation of the difference in accuracy between implant placement by virtual planning data and surgical guide templates versus the conventional free-hand method – a combined in vivo–in vitro technique using cone-beam CT (Part II). *J Craniomaxillofac Surg* 2010; **38**(7): 488–493.
43. Schneider D, Schober F, Grohmann P, *et al.* In-vitro evaluation of the tolerance of surgical instruments in templates for computer-assisted guided implantology produced by 3-D printing. *Clin Oral Implants Res* 2015; **26**(3): 320–325.
44. Hammerle CH, Cordaro L, van Assche N, *et al.* Digital technologies to support planning, treatment, and fabrication processes and outcome assessments in implant dentistry. Summary and consensus statements. The 4th EAO Consensus Conference 2015. *Clin Oral Implants Res* 2015; **26**(Suppl 11): 97–101.
45. Vercruyssen M, Laleman I, Jacobs R, *et al.* Computer-supported implant planning and guided surgery: a narrative review. *Clin Oral Implants Res* 2015; **26**(Suppl 11): 69–76.
46. Giordano M, Ausiello P, Martorelli M, *et al.* Reliability of computer designed surgical guides in six implant rehabilitations with two years follow-up. *Dent Mater* 2012; **28**(9): e168–e77.
47. Benic GI, Elmasry M, Hammerle CH. Novel digital imaging techniques to assess the outcome in oral rehabilitation with dental implants: a narrative review. *Clin Oral Implants Res* 2015; **26**(Suppl 11): 86–96.

CHAPTER 5

Decision Making in Bone Augmentation to Optimize Dental Implant Therapy

Jaime L. Lozada[1], Istvan Urban[2], and Joseph Y.K. Kan[1]
[1] Loma Linda University School of Dentistry, Loma Linda, California, USA
[2] University of Szeged, Hungary

In order to provide bone support for osseointegrated dental implants, a variety of bone augmentation techniques has been used to treat simple and complex defects. Some of the defects that may interfere with implant placement are horizontal defects, vertical defects, combination defects, alveolar ridge defects, and maxillary sinus pneumatization. There are different indications, numerous alternative techniques, and various biologically active agents and biomaterials currently used to augment bone.

The materials can be itemized as follows: autografts, allografts, xenografts, and alloplastic materials; the surgical techniques include: onlay grafting, inlay grafting, ridge expansion, guided bone regeneration (GBR), and distraction osteogenesis. The techniques can use each of the materials listed or a combination of them. The treatment options have many permutations with surgical proponents claiming that a particular material or technique results in improved dental implant success.

This chapter will focus exclusively on techniques aimed at the decision making and the implementation of procedures to augment the bone in a horizontal and vertical direction, utilizing GBR techniques, and maxillary sinus grafting procedures.

GBR techniques for horizontal and vertical augmentation

Horizontal bone augmentation procedures are any techniques aimed at making the recipient bone wider or thicker in order to receive dental implants of adequate diameter (usually of a 3.5 mm diameter or wider) (Figure 5.1). Vertical bone augmentation procedures are any techniques aimed at making the recipient bone higher in a vertical dimension in order to receive dental implants of adequate length (usually 8 mm or longer) (Figure 5.2).

The application of GBR procedures for horizontal augmentation is well documented, with high rates of implant success and low complication rates for the augmentation procedure.[1–4] Complications reported with vertical augmentation have involved membrane exposure and/or subsequent infection, with rates ranging between 12.5% and 17%.[5–7]

Horizontal augmentations

The so called knife-edge ridge, or Cawood and Howell Class IV edentulous jaw, presents a unique problem for horizontal augmentation. The necessary height of the ridge is adequate on the lingual/palatal aspect, but the width is insufficient, thereby making implant placement often impossible without prior treatment.[8]

One of the factors that may lead a grafting procedure to failure is movement, pressure, or instability of the graft during the initial healing phase. There is a good prognosis for this treatment if the residual ridge can be used to stabilize the bone graft. GBR for the treatment of bucally resorbed ridges utilizes both resorbable and nonresorbable membranes.[9–11] Resorbable membranes have shown better soft tissue compatibility compared with nonresorbable membranes.[12] Hammerle *et al.*[11] used anorganic bovine bone-derived mineral (ABBM) in combination with a more rapidly resorbing natural collagen membrane and concluded that this was an effective treatment for horizontal ridge augmentation. A recent prospective case series reported on the use of a more slowly resorbing, synthetic membrane in combination with autogenous bone mixed with ABBM. In this case series the amount of horizontal bone gain was more than in previously reported studies.

Urban *et al.*[10] investigated prospectively the use of a more rapidly resorbing natural collagen membrane and a 1:1 mixture of autogenous particulated bone/ABBM as grafting material for horizontal augmentation. On the basis of a case series, the authors evaluated clinically and histologically the use of a more rapidly resorbing membrane with the mixture of the bone graft previously described in horizontal augmentation of knife-edge ridges. The case series consisted of patients with an indication

Evidence-based Implant Treatment Planning and Clinical Protocols, First Edition. Edited by Steven J. Sadowsky.

Companion website: www.wiley.com/go/sadowsky/implant

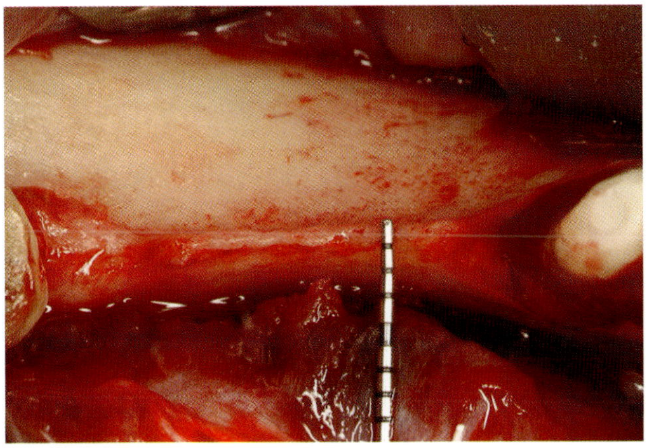

Figure 5.1 Preoperative view of a "knife-edge" ridge depicting a horizontal bone defect.

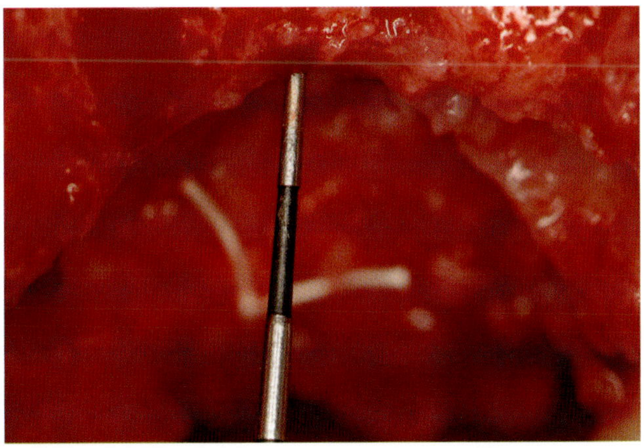

Figure 5.2 Typical vertical ridge defect in an interdental situation.

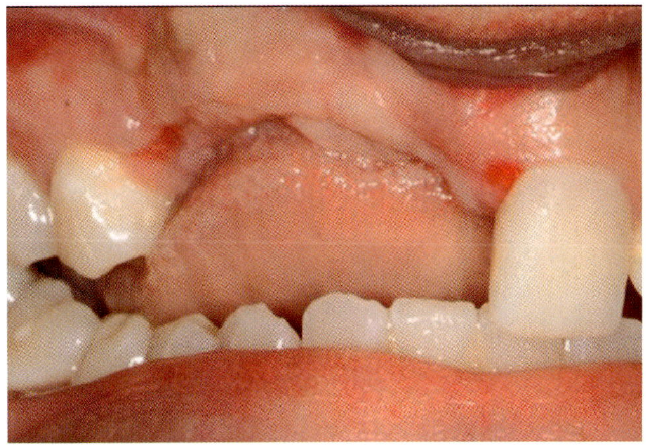

Figure 5.3 Preoperative view of a patient presenting with a horizontal and vertical defect.

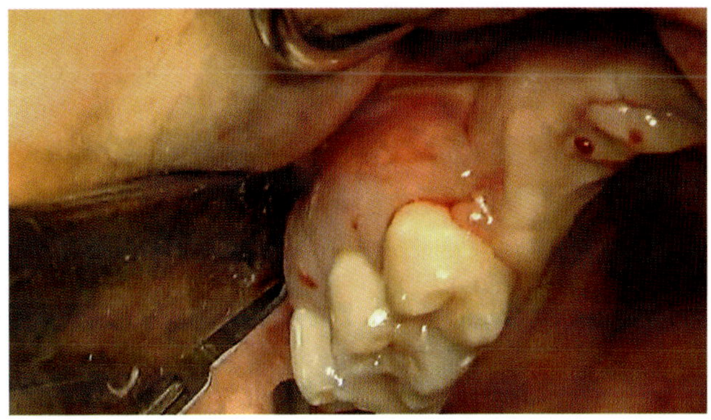

Figure 5.4 The divergent vertical releasing incision is made three teeth away from the defect in order to help mobilize the flap.

for horizontal ridge augmentation generally resulting from the lack of horizontal bone width in the posterior maxilla and mandible. All patients presented with a horizontal width of 4 mm or less and in need of horizontal ridge augmentation prior to dental implant placement. The presurgical protocol required that all patients be free of periodontal disease, maintain good oral hygiene, and were willing to comply with a list of requirements for postoperative care after the surgery. Based on these authors' experience, patients that were current smokers, engaged in excessive alcohol consumption, or had uncontrolled systemic conditions or periodontal disease, presented a significant number of complications, and thus should not be eligible for this type of treatment. Urban *et al.*[10] reported the medications, flap design, sutures, and bone harvesting procedures recommended for these types of procedures. The protocol initiates with the premedication of patients with amoxicillin (2 g) 1 hour before surgery and 500 mg three times a day for 1 week following surgery. In the event of penicillin allergy, clindamycin (600 mg) can be used for premedication and following surgery (300 mg four times a day for 1 week). Prior to surgery, the patients are also instructed to rinse with 0.2% chlorhexidine solution for 1 minute to disinfect the surgical site. For such procedures, sterile surgical drapes are also used to minimize the potential contamination from extraoral sources. For local anesthesia, xylocaine with epinephrine, 1/100 000 was used. The flap design is one of the most important aspects of these surgical procedures to ensure successful outcomes after surgery. The design must confirm primary tension-free closure after the bone grafting procedure, despite the increased dimension of the ridge. For such situations, remote flaps that include crestal and vertical releasing incisions can be used. In the area of the crest of the ridge, a midcrestal incision into the keratinized gingiva needs to be made. The divergent vertical incisions can be made at least one tooth away from the surgical site. In edentulous areas, the vertical incisions can be placed 5 mm away from the augmentation site (Figures 5.3 and 5.4).

After the primary incisions have been made, periosteal elevators can be used to reflect a full-thickness flap beyond the mucogingival junction and at least 5 mm beyond the bone defect. In the posterior mandible, the lingual flap can be elevated beyond the mylohyoid line. Sensitive anatomical locations, such as the mental and infraorbital nerves, always need to be protected.

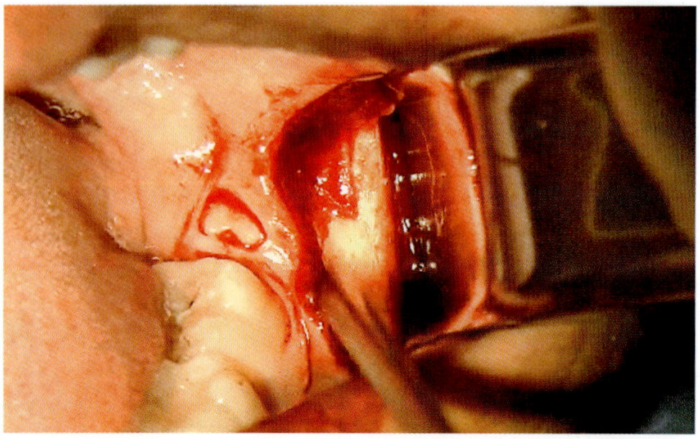

Figure 5.5 Incision made lateral to the retromolar area to obtain access to the donor autogenous bone site.

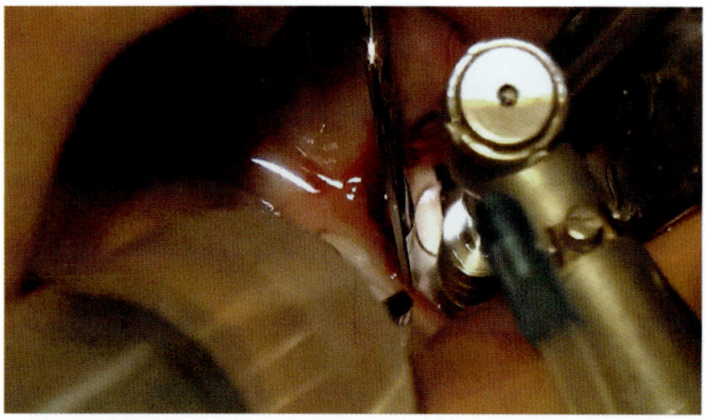

Figure 5.6 Trephine burs used to harvest autogenous bone cores.

Several techniques have been described for harvesting autogenous bone from an intraoral source. These authors' preference is to use the retromolar area and the ascending ramus in the mandible as the donor site, utilizing trephine burs. Harvested bone graft material can be particulated using a bone mill (R. Quetin Bone-Mill, Roswitha Quetin Dental Products, Leimen, Germany) and combined with the ABBM in a 1:1 ratio (Figures 5.5 and 5.6).

The recipient bony site requires preparation before graft placement. First, the exposed augmentation site needs to be cleaned of all soft tissue remnants. During clinical studies and case reports, ridge measurements can be made to evaluate the augmentation results after several months. The recipient bony bed also needs to be prepared with multiple decortication holes using a small round bur (Figure 5.7).

Proper flap reflection must be performed at this point to evaluate the size of the defect for precise trimming of the membrane. A previously sterilized foil sheet can be used as a template to determine the size of the membrane. The membrane needs to be trimmed to cover the entire volume of the graft. Once properly sized, the membrane needs to be fixated in at least two points on the lingual/palatal side with titanium tacks. The composite graft is prepared and reconstituted in a sufficient amount of saline solution to allow for easy handling of the graft and placement into the defect. The membrane can be folded over the graft and fixed into place with additional titanium tacks on the vestibular side. Special care must be taken to ensure that the membrane completely encloses the graft and that no openings are visible between the membrane and the recipient bone where soft tissue can invaginate into the area and affect graft maturation (Figures 5.8, 5.9, and 5.10).

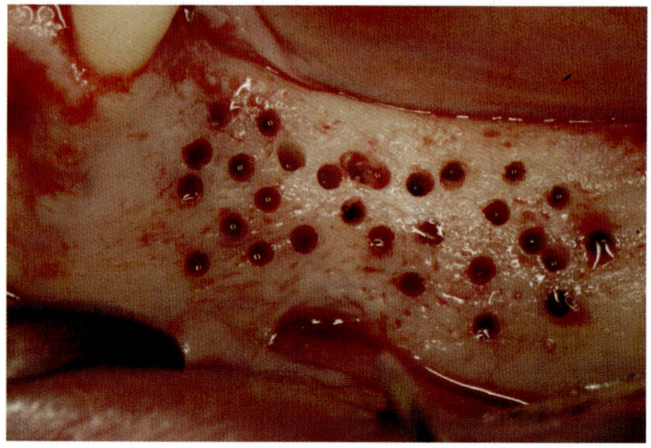

Figure 5.7 Example of multiple decortication holes to help vascularize the bone graft.

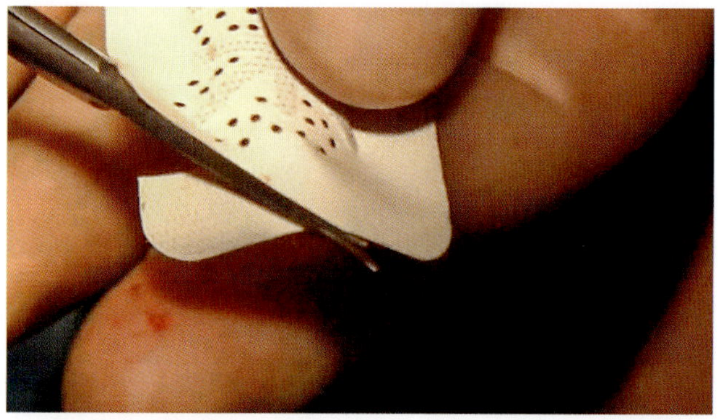

Figure 5.8 Trimming the nonresorbable membrane to adequately contain the graft.

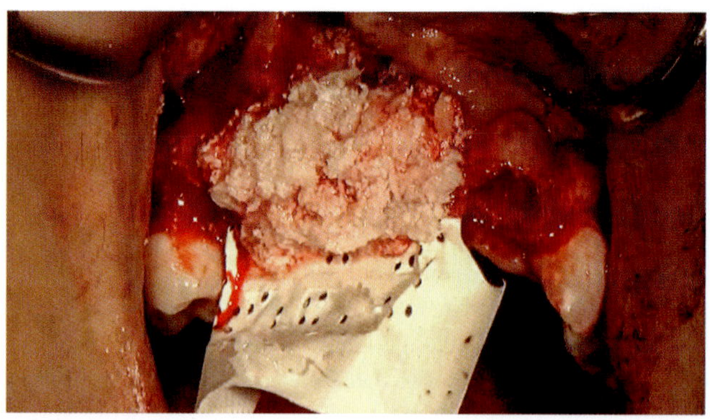

Figure 5.9 The nonresorbable membrane is attached to the palatal bone and the graft material is incorporated into the area.

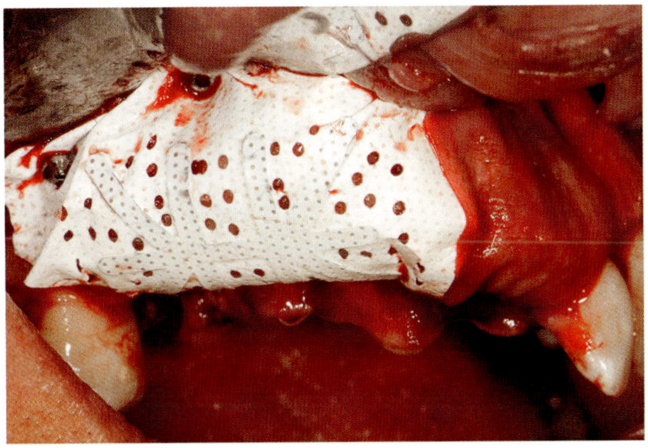

Figure 5.10 Notice the multiple titanium tacks fixing the nonresorbable membrane.

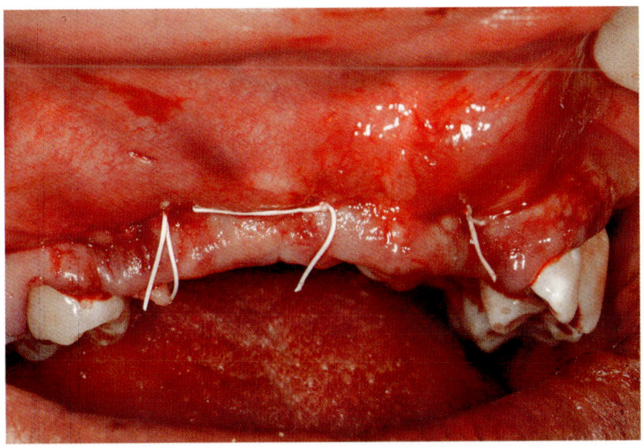

Figure 5.11 Horizontal mattress sutures approximating the flaps for the first suture layer.

After the membrane is completely secured, periosteal incisions connecting or approximating the vertical incisions can be performed to achieve elasticity and mobility of the flap to permit tension-free primary closure. The flap should be sutured in two layers. First, horizontal mattress sutures (GORE-TEX CV-5 Suture, Gore & Associates) need to be placed 4 mm from the incision line; then, single interrupted sutures with the same suturing material are used to close the edges of the flap. This suturing technique allows for a 4 mm thick connective tissue barrier between the membrane and the oral epithelium. This intimate contact of the everted connective tissue flaps can help prevent exposure of the membrane. The vertical incisions can be closed with single interrupted suture (Figures 5.11 and 5.12). These sutures can be removed between 10 and 14 days after surgery, and the mattress sutures after 2–3 weeks (Figures 5.13 and 5.14).[10] The average healing time for this type of grafting procedure and graft material is 8 months. In some publications the authors have reported harvesting of biopsy specimens at the time of implant placement. Cylindrical biopsy specimens from selected healed and augmented surgical sites using a trephine bur have been obtained. The specimen preparation has been previously reported according to the technique described by Richardson *et al.*[13]

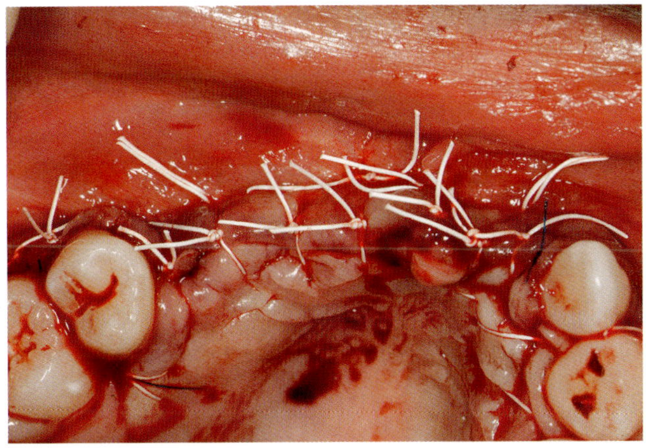

Figure 5.12 Multiple single interrupted sutures for complete closure of the entire area.

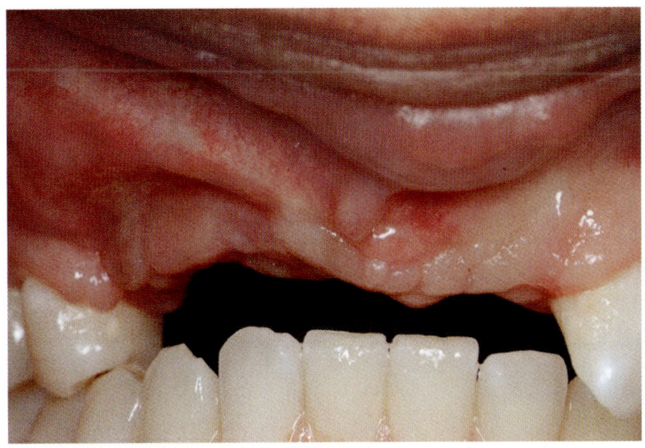

Figure 5.13 Postoperative view of the grafted area 2 months after surgery.

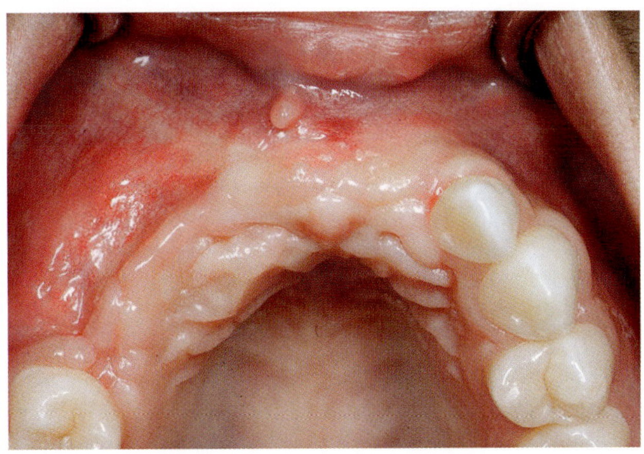

Figure 5.14 Occlusal view depicting the healthy appearance of the augmented site after 2 months.

The case series presented by Urban *et al.*[10] demonstrates that the combination of particulated autogenous bone and ABBM

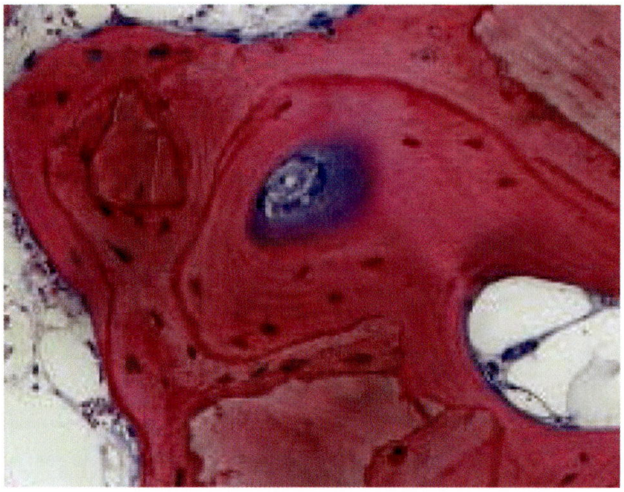

Figure 5.15 Histology of the mixture of autogenous bone and ABBM, demonstrating that the ABBM is connected by a dense network of newly formed bone.

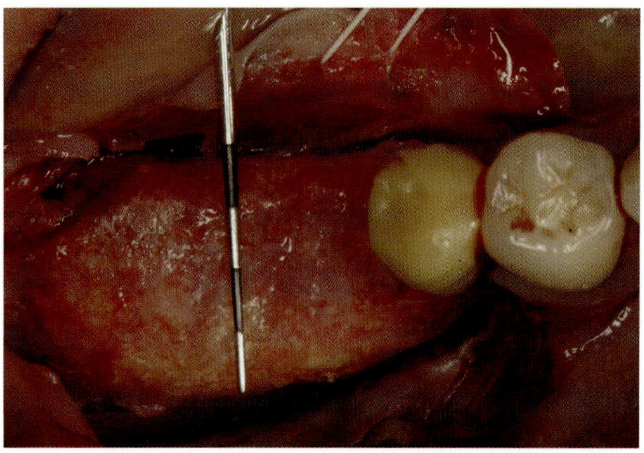

Figure 5.16 A clinical example of an horizontally augmented ridge before implant placement.

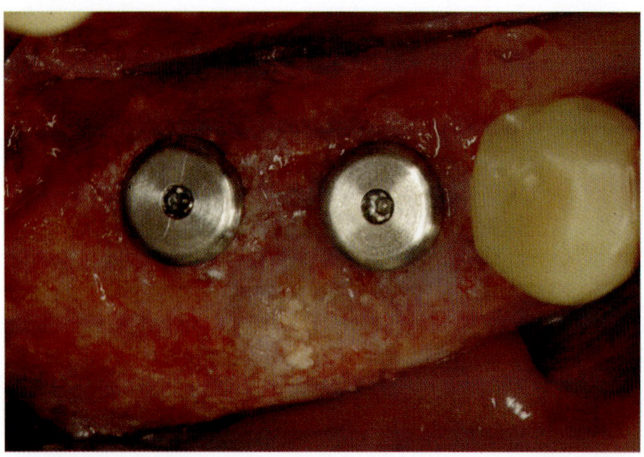

Figure 5.17 Implants placed during the second stage of treatment of the horizontally regenerated ridge.

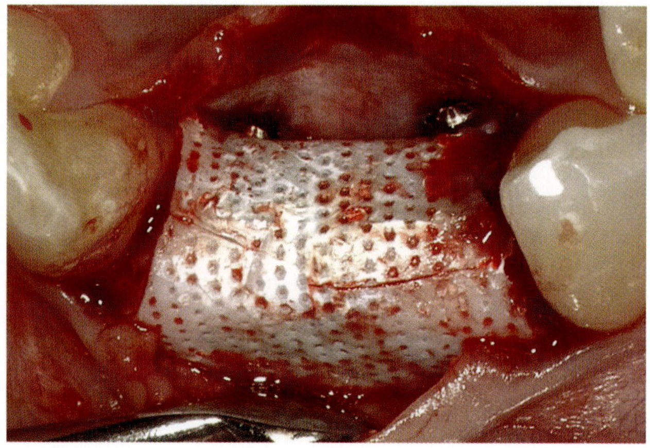

Figure 5.18 A clinical example depicting the presence of a nonresorbable membrane before its removal after 6 months of healing.

with a resorbable membrane can be used safely and effectively for horizontal augmentation of knife-edged ridges in the posterior maxilla and mandible. The report also indicates a 100% survival rate of the implants placed in the grafted bone for more than 32 months.[14]

Other publications have reported the gain of 4.6 mm of horizontal bone when autogenous bone blocks covered with ABBM particles and resorbable membranes have been used.[9] Less favorable results have reported 3.6 mm of horizontal bone gain when using ABBM particles alone as grafting material with collagen membranes.[11]

The histological evidence of the mixture of autogenous bone and ABBM demonstrates that the ABBM is connected by a dense network of newly formed bone (Figure 5.15). Other published reports, in which autogenous bone blocks were covered with ABBM particles and collagen membranes, showed that the particles of ABBM were encapsulated by fibrous tissue and with no evidence of osseous integration.[9] The use of bone grafting materials and resorbable membranes to treat knife-edged defects with horizontal augmentation may lead to less morbidity in the treatment of patients with these defects. In addition, the use of ABBM in these procedures may lessen the need for harvested autogenous bone and generally lead to decreased morbidity and, therefore, increased patient comfort and satisfaction associated with these regenerative procedures (Figures 5.16, 5.17, 5.18, and 5.19).

Vertical augmentations

The application of GBR for supracrestal augmentation was introduced and the surgical technique described in 1998.[5] A recent systematic review of the literature by Esposito *et al.*[15] analyzed the outcomes of vertical augmentations among other interventions for replacing missing teeth. This review shows that various augmentation techniques are able to augment bone in a vertical direction, however, there is insufficient evidence to indicate which is the preferred technique. Bone substitutes, such as ABBM, may be a valid, and less expensive, alternative to autogenous bone, particularly when bone is harvested from extraoral locations,

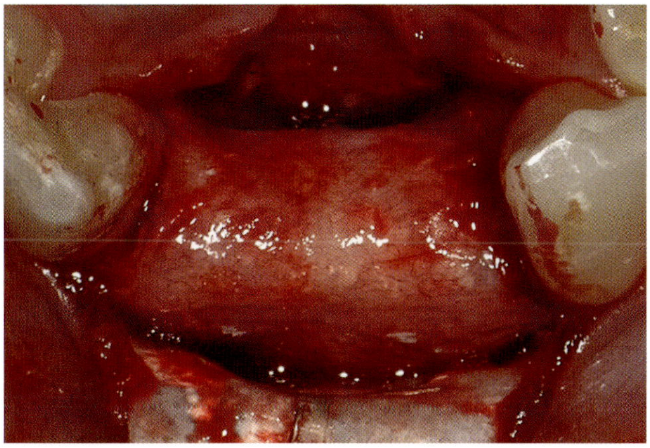

Figure 5.19 Notice the regenerated bone after removal of the e PTFE membrane.

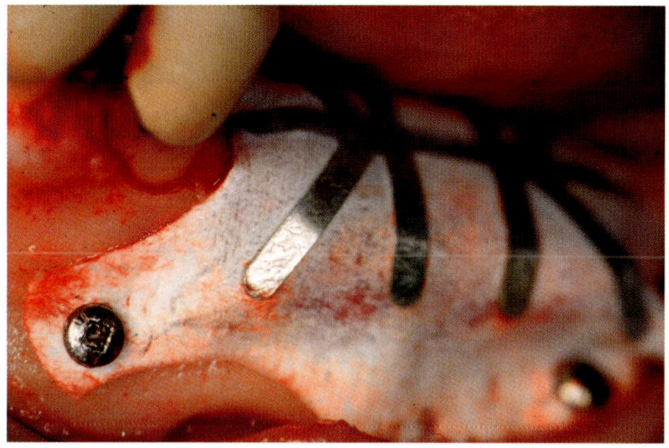

Figure 5.20 The clinical picture demonstrates the required distance between the edges of the membrane and adjacent teeth and mental nerve.

since bone substitutes are associated with less postoperative morbidity. Osteodistraction allows for more vertical augmentation but it is of little use in the presence of thin ridges. All the vertical augmentation techniques evaluated were associated with high complication rates ranging from 60% to 20%.[15–17] The complications involved membrane exposure and/or subsequent infection. The review by Esposito *et al.*[15] also concluded that clinicians and patients should carefully evaluate the benefits and risks in relation to the desired outcome when deciding whether to use vertical ridge augmentation techniques.

Urban *et al.*[14] stated that fewer publications had reported long-term results on vertical ridge augmentation following GBR. In their publication, the authors reported the results of vertical GBR with particulated autogenous bone grafts, the clinical and radiographic success and survival rates of implants placed in surgical sites after prosthetic loading, and the success rates of implants placed in defects treated simultaneously with sinus augmentation and vertical GBR.[18] This retrospective study evaluated patients that were consecutively treated who required vertical bone regeneration to achieve the necessary bone volume to place dental implants and to improve the crown/implant ratio and esthetics. The preoperative and surgical protocol was performed as previously described in the horizontal augmentation section of this chapter. The primary difference for this particular procedure is the type of membrane used for the augmentation. All patients in the study were treated with a titanium-reinforced, nonresorbable, expanded polytetrafluoroethylene (e-PTFE) membranes (Gore & Associates, Flagstaff, AZ).

For this particular technique, a remote full-thickness flap must be elevated in the edentulous area and the residual ridge prepared carefully to receive an e-PTFE membrane properly trimmed to the volume of the graft. Special care must be taken to avoid contact of the edges of the membrane with the adjacent teeth (Figure 5.20). In the same study, the authors described the surgical approach for those cases with both severe vertical crestal bone atrophy and enlarged maxillary sinus cavities, where a combined procedure of vertical GBR and maxillary sinus grafting was used. The description of the maxillary sinus graft procedure will be outlined in more detail in a later section of this chapter.

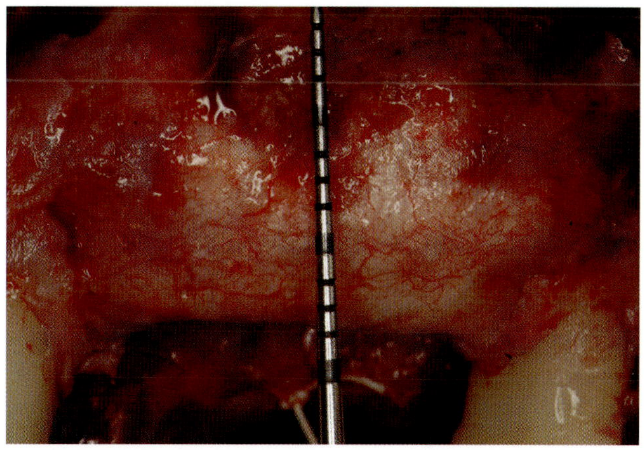

Figure 5.21 Typical appearance of a successful vertically regenerated ridge.

As previously described in the horizontal augmentation section of this chapter, the graft material needs to be immobilized and covered with a nonresorbable membrane, which is stabilized with titanium tacks. The surgical site is allowed to heal for 6–9 months. The membrane is then removed and implants are placed (Figure 5.21). In the experience of these authors, during implant placement, a resorbable collagen membrane should be placed over the newly formed bone to protect the graft from early resorption. Additional healing time of 4–6 months is also recommended for implants in grafted bone.

When evaluating the results of other studies with the published experience of these authors, there is a marked difference when comparing the outcomes. In a study that combined maxillary sinus augmentation and vertical GBR, the implant survival and implant success rates was reported to be 92% and 76% respectively,[19] whereas 100% implant success was achieved in a similar population in the published study by Urban *et al.* (Figures 5.22, 5.23, 5.24, and 5.25).[18]

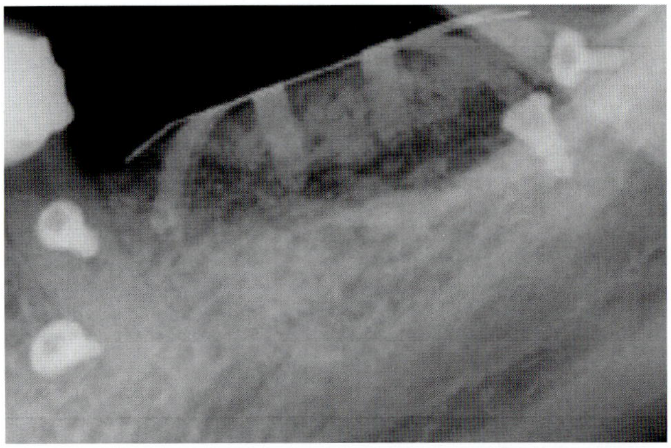

Figure 5.22 Postoperative radiograph of a vertical augmentation procedure clearly showing the titanium strips embedded in the nonresorbable membrane.

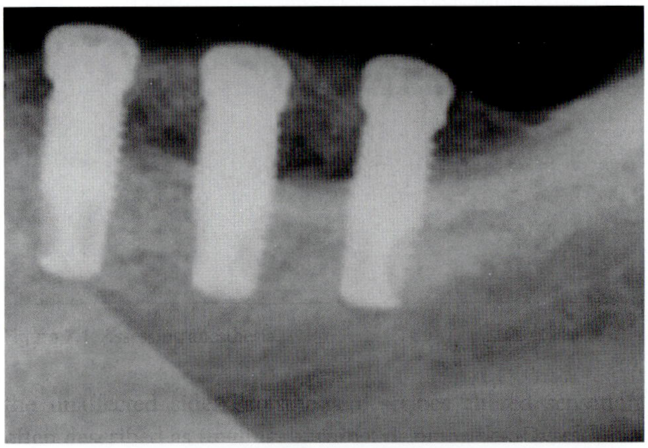

Figure 5.23 Postoperative radiograph of the placement of three implants in the grafted site. Notice that the membrane has been removed.

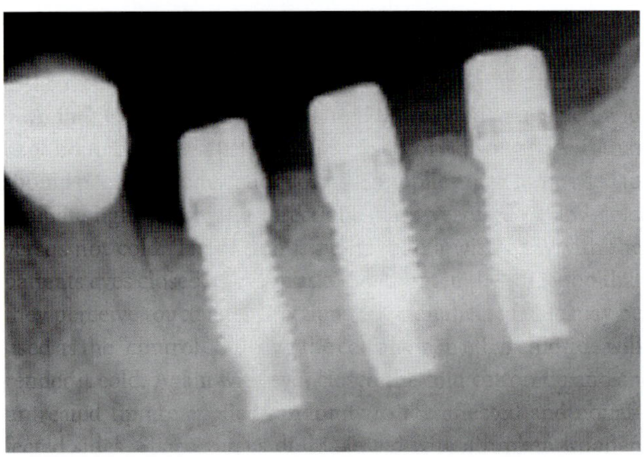

Figure 5.24 Postoperative radiographic view of the three endosseous implants recently uncovered after 4 months of healing.

In examining the differences in results, we can recognize that previous studies have used nonsurface-treated implants and they were also placed simultaneous with the graft, whereas a staged technique and surface-enhanced implants may be a more beneficial treatment, as shown in the published data by these authors.

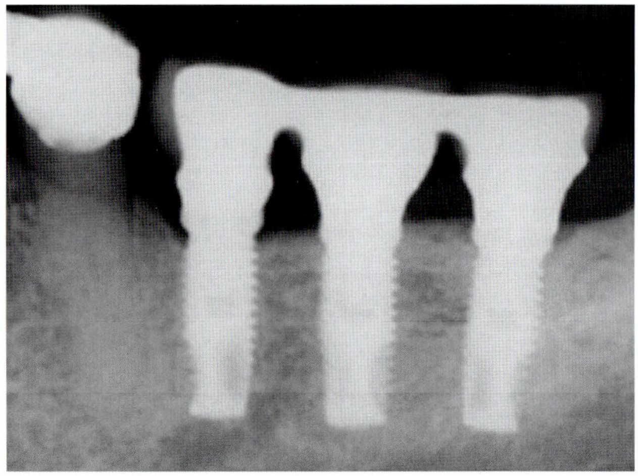

Figure 5.25 Radiograph taken 7 years post loading, depicting adequate marginal bone levels.

As previously described, high complication rates have been reported associated with this technique.[15] The study referenced here reported a complication rate of 2.78%. It should be noted that the reported techniques could be considered similar, however the described technical differences and the fact that there is no initial learning curve with the procedure, are some of the reasons that these authors report more encouraging results with this and more current published data.[20] The studies should be analyzed in a meta-analytic fashion to coalesce the data into a more meaningful assessment of the current state of the science on vertical augmentation.

Maxillary sinus grafts

Maxillary sinus graft procedures are presently routine surgical techniques for the treatment of posterior edentulism, after being first proposed by Tatum in 1977 and then first published by Boyne and James in 1980.[21,22]

Access into the maxillary sinus can be made either through the crest or the lateral wall of the maxillary sinus. In this section, only the lateral approach technique will be described. Boyne and James[22] reported the use of a large round carbide bur to obliterate the wall of the sinus to make a window access for the placement of an autogenous bone graft. Multiple modifications to this technique have been published over the years. The original rotary techniques, with either surgical handpieces or high-speed handpieces were first described by Smiler and Holmes in 1987,[23] and then Smiler *et al.*[24] reviewed multiple technique variations in 1992. In 2001, Vercellotti *et al.*[25] introduced the piezoelectric technique, and in 2011 the Dentium Advanced Sinus Kit (DASK) technique was first published by Lozada *et al.*[26]

Wallace *et al.*[27] stated that the introduction of new techniques for lateral approach to the sinus are surgical modifications designed to increase the predictability of the procedure while reducing the occurrence of the two main intraoperative complications: profuse bleeding and sinus membrane perforation.

Starting with the presurgical evaluation of the patient, the surgeon must obtain sufficient diagnostic information before proceeding with the surgical technique, including the prosthodontic treatment plan and the presurgical CT scan or cone-bean scan, assessing the current condition of the maxillary sinus area (Figure 5.26). After proper flap design and execution, an osteotomy can be made in the lateral sinus wall to gain access to the Schneiderian membrane for the purpose of elevating it. Depending on the amount of available bone below the pneumatized maxillary sinus, the surgical technique can be a two-stage or a one-stage treatment.

The two-stage treatment via a lateral approach is recommended for patients with complete pneumatization of the maxillary sinus. During the first stage the placed bone graft material is allowed to heal for several months after surgery. The second stage consists of implant placement. The one-stage treatment is recommended for patients with partial pneumatization of the maxillary sinus, where the bone graft and implants can be placed simultaneously. In such instances, the remaining bone, ideally between 3 and 7 mm, can be used to stabilize the implants (Figure 5.27).

The most commonly used techniques to access the maxillary sinus cavity are rotary, piezoelectric, and DASK techniques. The rotary technique utilizes a high-speed handpiece or surgical straight handpiece motor with external irrigation to create a "window" in the lateral sinus wall. The lateral window, with the sinus membrane still attached, is then debilitated enough to be pushed inward and elevated to create the space for the graft material in the floor of the maxillary sinus cavity (Figure 5.28). The piezoelectric technique consists of a surgical technique invented by Tomaso Vercellotti,[25] and first published in the US in 2001. It utilizes low-frequency ultrasonic vibration to create the lateral window and elevate the sinus membrane. This technique eliminates the "drag" created by rotary instrumentation and is therefore less likely to damage blood vessels or the Schneiderian membrane. Elevation and displacement of the membrane can then be continued with either angled piezoelectric elevator inserts or the more commonly used hand elevators and maxillary sinus curettes (Figure 5.29).

The DASK lateral window approach has been described by Lozada *et al.* as a lateral bone-planing or obliteration antrostomy

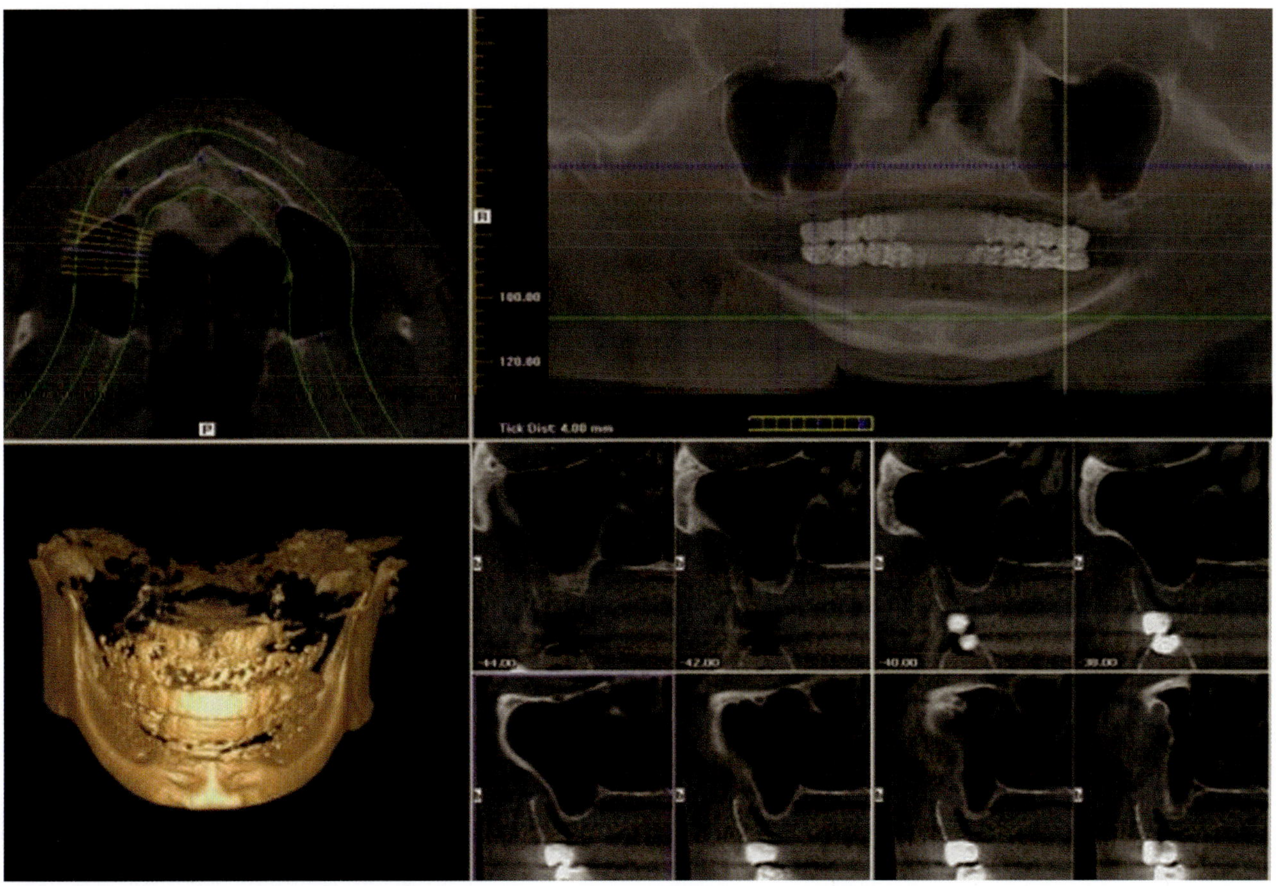

Figure 5.26 Cone beam CT preoperative image depicting a pneumatized maxillary sinus.

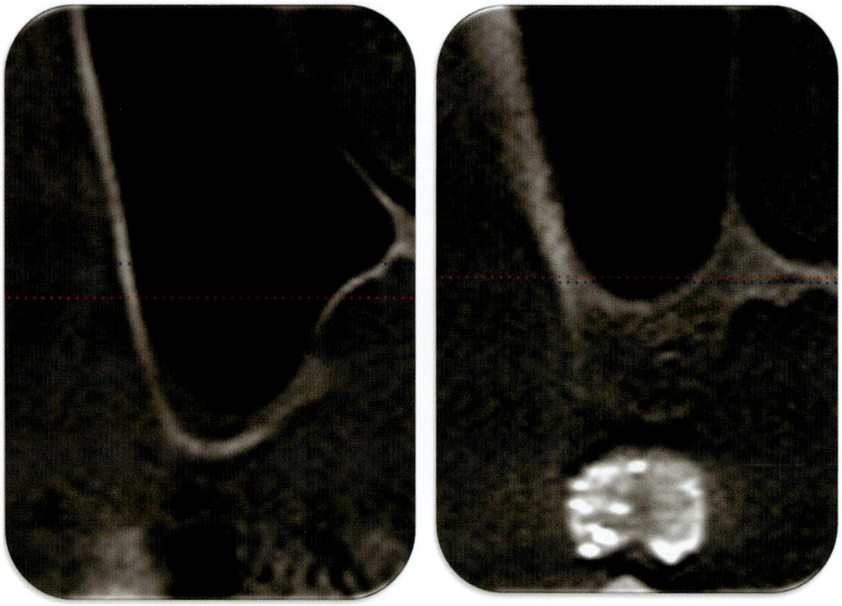

Figure 5.27 CBCT images of a completely (left) pneumatized sinus and a partially (right) pneumatized sinus.

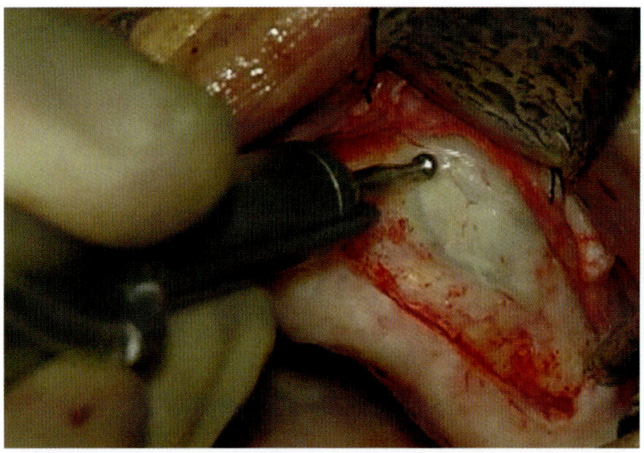

Figure 5.28 Rotary osteotomy instrumentation for the lateral approach to the maxillary sinus cavity.

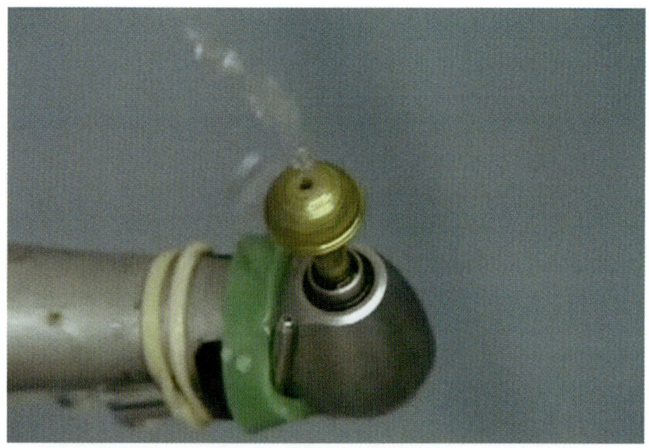

Figure 5.30 Notice the internal irrigation capability of a DASK drill for the lateral approach to the maxillary sinus cavity.

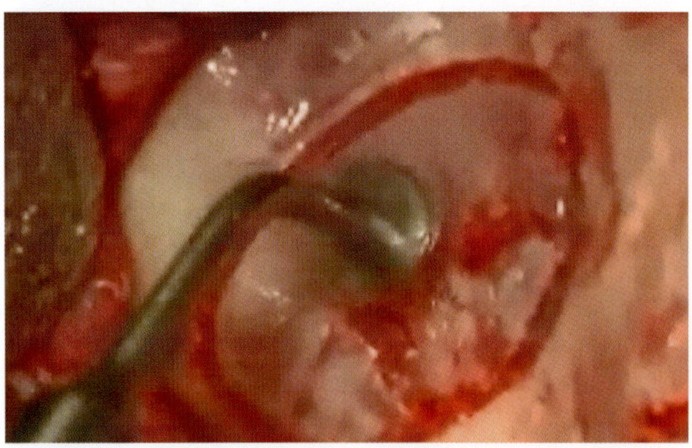

Figure 5.29 Piezosurgery instrumentation depicting the initial separation of the membrane before the use of sinus curettes.

technique. The DASK technique makes use of either a 6 or 8 mm diameter × 4 mm high dome-shaped drill with a nonaggressive diamond grit and both internal and external irrigation (Figure 5.30). The drills are operated at 800–1200 rpm and produce little or no "drag" when compared with traditional rotary instrumentation. The drill is used with light pressure to plane or thin the bone of the lateral wall. As the bone is thinned, the blue shadow of the sinus membrane becomes more apparent. With proper technique, a very thin, movable layer of bone remains attached to the sinus membrane. It is often possible to see the microvasculature of the lateral wall intact within this layer. The thin bony layer and membrane can be elevated as a unit or the bone fragments can be gently removed with a curette, creating a complete osteotomy, allowing for ideal access and visibility to elevate the sinus membrane. Just as with the other techniques,

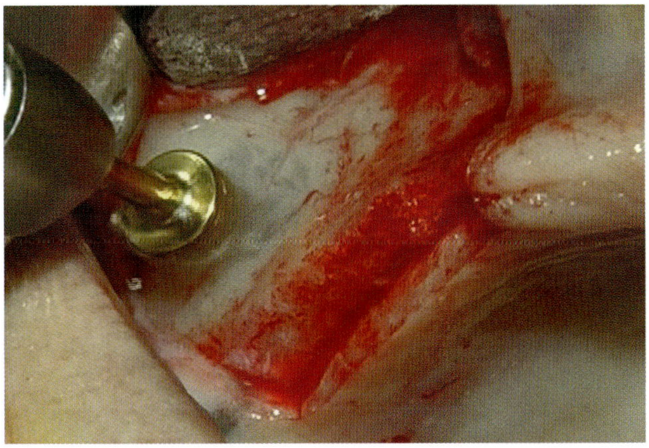

Figure 5.31 Clinical photograph of the DASK osteotomy instrumentation technique thinning the lateral bony aspect of the maxillary sinus cavity. Notice the blueish appearance of the bone as the drilling action approximates the maxillary sinus membrane.

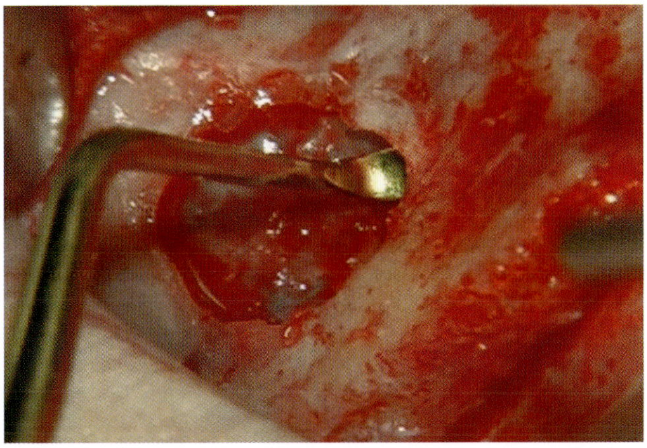

Figure 5.32 Maxillary sinus curettes in the initial stages of the maxillary sinus elevation.

the elevation and displacement of the membrane can then be completed with hand elevators and maxillary sinus curettes (Figures 5.31 and 5.32).

From 2003 until the present day, there have been at least nine evidence-based reviews reporting on the efficacy of all forms of graft materials.[28–36] The reviews conclude that more favorable results have been achieved with bone replacement grafts than with autogenous bone. The same reviews substantiate, however, the finding that implant survival with bone replacement grafts, such as xenografts, is equal to or better than that achieved with autogenous bone. These data, along with the reduction in patient morbidity by eliminating the need for a secondary surgical donor site, appear to position bone replacement as the graft material of choice today (Figure 5.33).

The maxillary sinus graft procedure is today considered to be one of the most predictable pre-prosthetic surgical techniques. Success rates and implant survival in the grafted maxillary sinus have been reported to be between 90 and 96% when utilizing the proven evidence-based decisions to use rough-surfaced implants and xenogeneic bone replacement grafts. With such high success rates, the developing technologies of bone graft enhancement factors (BMPs, growth factors, and stem cell products) are unlikely to result in any dramatic change. Piezoelectric surgery, and recently the DASK technique, have demonstrated the capability to dramatically reduce the perforation rate.[27]

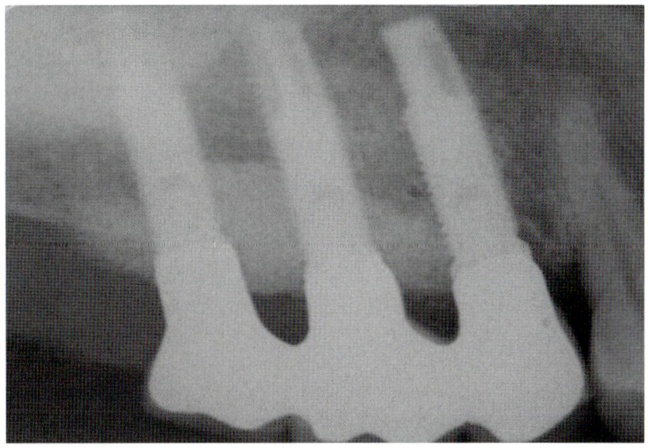

Figure 5.33 Radiograph taken 8 years after a simultaneous maxillary sinus graft procedure and vertical ridge augmentation. Notice the relatively radiopaque crest of the ridge and maxillary sinus cavity.

Summary

Currently, and within the limitation of the published data, the treatment of horizontal and vertical deficient ridges with the GBR techniques, using autogenous bone mixed with ABBM and membranes, can be regarded as successful treatment and may lead to a significant improvement in implant survival. The possibility of predictably grafting the maxillary sinus cavity and simultaneously augmenting vertically deficient ridges it is also a significant benefit to our patients. It is our experience that the newer surgical techniques to access the maxillary sinus cavity have resulted in a significant reduction in membrane perforations, thus permitting the possibility of performing simultaneous procedures that otherwise need to be staged. Further documentation using controlled long-term, randomized clinical trials are necessary to prove that these techniques and materials are applicable in the regular practice of surgical implant dentistry.

References

1. Buser D, Bragger U, Lang NP, *et al.* Regeneration and enlargement of jaw bone using guided tissue regeneration. *Clin Oral Implant Res* 1990; **1**: 22–32.
2. Jovanovic SA, Spikermann H, Richter EJ. Bone regeneration around titanium dental implants in dehisced defects sites: a clinical study. *Int J Oral Maxillofac Implants* 1992; **7**: 233–245.

3. Buser D, Dula K, Hirt HP, *et al.* Lateral ridge augmentation using autogenous grafts and barrier membranes: a clinical study with 40 partially edentulous patients. *J Oral Maxillofac Surg* 1996; **54**: 420–432.
4. Buser D, Ingimarsson S, Dula K, *et al.* Long term stability of osseointegrated implants in augmented bone: a 5-year prospective study in partially edentulous patients. *Int J Periodontics Restorative Dent* 2002; **22**: 109–117.
5. Tinti C, Parma-Benfenati S. Vertical ridge augmentation: surgical protocol and retrospective evaluation of 48 consecutively inserted implants. *Int J Periodontics Restorative Dent* 1998; **18**: 434–443.
6. Simion M, Tristi P, Piattelli A. Vertical ridge augmentation using a membrane technique associated with osseointegrated implants. *Int J Periodontics Restorative Dent* 1994; **14**: 496–511.
7. Simion M, Jovanovic SA, Tristi P, *et al.* Vertical ridge augmentation around dental implants using a membrane technique and autogenous bone or allografts in humans. *Int J Periodontics Restorative Dent* 1998; **18**: 18–23.
8. Cawood JI, Howell RA. A classification of edentulous jaws. *Int J Oral Maxillofac Implants* 1988; **17**: 232–236.
9. Proussaefs P, Lozada J. The use of resorbable collagen membrane in conjunction with autogenous bone graft and inorganic bovine mineral for buccal/labial alveolar ridge augmentation: a pilot study. *J Prosthetic Dent* 2003; **90**: 530–538.
10. Urban IA, Nagursky H, Lozada J. Horizontal ridge augmentation with a resorbable membrane and particulated autogenous bone with or without anorganic bovine bone mineral: a prospective case series in 22 patients. *Int J Oral Maxillofac Implants* 2011; **26**: 404–414.
11. Hammerle CHF, Jung RE, Yaman D, *et al.* Ridge augmentation by applying bioresorbable membranes and deproteinized bovine bone mineral: a report on twelve consecutive cases. *Clin Oral Implants Res* 2008; **19**: 19–25.
12. Zitzmann NU, Naef R, Scharer P. Resorbable versus nonresorbable membranes in combination with Bio-Oss for guided bone regeneration. *Int j Oral Maxillofac Implants* 1997; **12**: 844–852.
13. Richardson KG, Jarett L, Finke EH. Embedding in epoxy resins for ultrathin sectioning in electron microscopy. *Stain Technol* 1960; **35**: 313–325.
14. Urban IA, Nagursky H, Lozada J, *et al.* Horizontal ridge augmentation with a collagen membrane and a combination of particulated autogenous bone and anorganic bovine bone-derived mineral: a prospective case series in 25 patients. *J Periodontics Restorative Dent* 2013; **33**: 299–307.
15. Esposito M, Grusovin MG, Felice P, *et al.* Interventions for replacing missing teeth: horizontal and vertical bone augmentation techniques for dental implant treatment. *Cochrane Database Syst Rev* 2008 **16**; 3: pub3.
16. Bianchi A, Felice P, Lizio G, *et al.* Alveolar distraction osteogenesis versus inlay bone grafting in posterior mandibular atrophy: a prospective study. *Oral Surg Oral Med Oral Path Oral Radiol Endodont* 2008; **105**(3): 282–292.
17. Felice P, Marchetti C, Lezzi G, *et al.* Vertical augmentation of the posterior mandible with inlay grafts: bone from the iliac crest versus bovine bone. Results up to 1 year after loading from a randomized controlled clinical trial. *Eur J Oral Implantol* 2008; **1**: 183–187.
18. Urban IA, Jovanovic SA, Lozada JL. Vertical ridge augmentation using guided bone regeneration (GBR) in three clinical scenarios prior to implant placement: a retrospective study of 35 patients 12 to 72 months after loading. *Int J Oral Maxillofac Implants* 2009; **24**(3): 502–510.
19. Simion M, Fontana F, Rasperini G, *et al.* Long-term evaluation of osseointegrated implants placed in sites augmented with sinus floor elevation associated with vertical ridge augmentation: a retrospective study of 38 consecutive implants with 1- to 7-year follow-up. *Int J Periodontics Restorative Dent* 2004; **24**(3): 208–221.
20. Urban IA, Lozada JL, Jovanovic SA, *et al.* Vertical ridge augmentation with titanium-reinforced, dense-PTFE membranes and a combination of particulated autogenous bone and anorganic bovine bone-derived mineral: a prospective case series in 19 patients. *Int J Oral Maxillofac Implants* 2014; **29**(1): 185–193.
21. Tatum H Jr. Maxillary and sinus implant reconstruction. *Dent Clin North Am* 1986; **30**: 207–229.
22. Boyne PJ, James RA. Grafting of the maxillary sinus floor with autogenous marrow and bone. *J Oral Surg* 1980; **38**: 613–616.
23. Smiler DG, Holmes RE. Sinus lift procedure using porous hydroxyapatite: a preliminary clinical report. *J Oral Implantol* 1987; **13**(2): 239–253.
24. Smiler DG (1), Johnson PW, Lozada JL, *et al.* Sinus lift grafts and endosseous implants. Treatment of the atrophic posterior maxilla. *Dent Clin North Am* 1992; **36**(1): 151–186.
25. Vercellotti T, De Paoli S, Nevins M. The piezoelectric bony window osteotomy and sinus membrane elevation: introduction of a new technique for simplification of the sinus augmentation procedure. *Int J Periodontics Restorative Dent* 2001; **21**: 561–567.
26. Lozada JL, Goodacre C, Al-Ardah A, *et al.* Lateral and crestal bone planing antrostomy: a simplified surgical procedure to reduce the incidence of membrane perforation during maxillary sinus augmentation procedures. *J Prosthet Dent* 2011; **105**: 147–153.
27. Wallace SS, Tarnow DP, Froum SJ, *et al.* Maxillary sinus elevation by lateral window approach: evolution of technology and technique. *J Evid Based Dent Pract* 2012; **12**(3 Suppl): 161–171.
28. Wallace SS, Froum SJ. Effect of maxillary sinus augmentation on the survival of endosseous dental implants. A systematic review. *Ann Periodontol* 2003; **8**: 328–343.
29. Del Fabbro M, Testori T, Francetti L, *et al.* Systematic review of survival rates for implants placed in the grafted maxillary sinus. *Int J Periodontics Restorative Dent* 2004; **24**: 565.
30. Aghaloo T, Moy PK. Which hard tissue augmentation techniques are the most successful in furnishing bony support for implant placement? *Int J Oral Maxillofac Implants* 2007; **22**(Suppl): 49–70.
31. Pjetursson BE, Tan WC, Zwahlen M, *et al.* A systematic review of the success of sinus floor elevation and survival of implants inserted in combination with sinus floor elevation. Part I: lateral approach. *J Clin Periodontol* 2008; **35**(Suppl 8): 216–224.
32. Del Fabbro M, Rosano G, Taschieri S. Implant survival rates after maxillary sinus augmentation. *Eur J Oral Sci* 2008; **116**: 497–506.
33. Nkenke E, Stelzle F. Clinical outcomes of sinus floor augmentation for implant placement using autogenous bone or bone substitutes: a systematic review. *Clin Oral Implants Res* 2009; **20**(Suppl 4): 124–133.
34. Jensen SS, Terheyden H. Bone augmentation procedures in localized defects in the alveolar ridge: clinical results with different bone grafts and bone-substitute materials. *Int J Oral Maxillofac Implants* 2009; **24**(suppl): 218–238.
35. Esposito M, Grusovin MG, Rees J, *et al.* Interventions for replacing missing teeth: augmentation procedures of the maxillary sinus. *Cochrane Database Syst Rev* 2010; **3**:CD008397.
36. Del Fabbro M, Bortolin M, Taschieri S, *et al.* Implant survival in maxillary sinus augmentation. An updated systematic review. *J Osteol Biomat* 2010; **1**: 69–79. Erratum in: *J Osteol Biomat* 2010; **1**: 186.

CHAPTER 6

Immediate Implant Placement and Provisionalization of Maxillary Anterior Single Implants

Joseph Y.K. Kan, Kitichai Rungcharassaeng, and Jaime L. Lozada
Loma Linda University School of Dentistry, Loma Linda, California, USA

Introduction

Achieving optimal gingival esthetics around anterior single implants is a challenging procedure,[1,2] and maintaining it over time can be an equally demanding task. Despite the high success rates achieved with osseointegrated implants,[3] the peri-implant mucosal response is not clearly understood. For anterior single implants, up to 16% of gingival recession has been reported.[3] On the other hand, spontaneous rebound of the receded gingiva has also been observed following a few years of function.[4–6] The peri-implant mucosa changes had been postulated to be an attempt to establish a stable biological dimension.[7] An understanding of the dentogingival complex and its implant counterpart (peri-implant mucosa) allows clinicians to predictably balance the biologic/physiologic requirement and esthetic demand of single implant restorations in the esthetic zone.

The impending loss of a single tooth in the esthetic zone in a patient with an otherwise healthy periodontium can be a distressing experience.[1,8–10] An inevitable loss of soft and hard tissue after tooth extraction can be expected in a compromised site for anterior implant esthetics. Various augmentation techniques have been advocated as corrective procedures, but they are time consuming and not always predictable.[4,11–13] Therefore, the fundamental concept of site development for an anterior single implant is to preserve the existing gingival and osseous tissue of the failing tooth, if possible.[1] Since 1998, when Wohlre[14] first demonstrated success with immediate implant placement and provisionalization (IIPP) of single anterior maxillary implants, numerous studies have substantiated the viability of such treatment.[9,15–26] One of the most desirable features of IIPP is its efficacy in optimizing esthetic success by preserving the existing osseous and gingival architecture.[8,9,14,27]

The esthetic success of IIPP procedures is influenced by a number of factors that can be identified as intrinsic or extrinsic.[28] Intrinsic factors are patient dependent, and include the relationship between hard and soft tissues, gingival biotype, and sagittal root position in the alveolar bone.[29,30] Extrinsic factors, on the other hand, are clinician dependent and include three-dimensional (3-D) implant position and angulation, as well as contour of the abutment and provisional restoration.[8,29]

Diagnosis and treatment planning

Proper diagnosis of the patient's condition allows clinicians to devise a suitable treatment plan that can be predictably executed. By recognizing unfavorable conditions, adjunctive procedures can be incorporated to avert compromised situations. The following parameters must be evaluated for an IIPP procedure.

1 *Gingival level* of the failing tooth should be: 1) the same as (or more coronal than) that of the contralateral tooth and 2) harmonious with adjacent dentition, as some gingival recession can be expected after the procedure (Figure 6.1).[1] Furthermore, it is more challenging to coronally reposition an existing recession for IIPP procedures. Therefore, when the gingival level of the failing tooth is more apical than that of the contralateral tooth, orthodontic forced eruption, if possible, should be implemented prior to IIPP.[31]
2 *Osseous–gingival tissue relationship* can be evaluated by bone sounding and should measure 3 mm on the facial aspect of the failing tooth and 4.5 mm on the proximal aspect of adjacent teeth (Figure 6.2). There is a propensity for tissue recession after extraction with or without immediate implant placement in low crest situations, in which bone sounding measurements are greater (more than 3 mm mid-facial pocketing) than those indicative of an optimal relationship.[29] Depending on the gingival level, orthodontic and/or periodontal treatment can be used to improve the osseous–gingival tissue relationship.
3 *Gingival biotype* can be assessed during bone sounding and categorized according to the visibility of the underlying periodontal probe (SE Probe SD12 Yellow, American Eagle Instruments Inc., Missoula, MT) through the gingival tissue (visible = thin, and not visible = thick) (Figure 6.2).[32,33] Higher

Evidence-based Implant Treatment Planning and Clinical Protocols, First Edition. Edited by Steven J. Sadowsky.

Companion website: www.wiley.com/go/sadowsky/implant

visibility corresponds to lower levels of thickness. Thin gingival biotype, which has been shown to sustain more tissue recession after surgical insults than thick biotype, can be enhanced by using a bilaminar subepithelial connective tissue graft (SCTG) at the time of IIPP.[28]

4 *Sagittal root position (SRP)*[30] of the failing tooth in the alveolar bone can be identified via cone-beam computed tomography (CBCT) and can be categorized as one of four different classes (Figure 6.3):
   - class I: the root is positioned against the labial cortical plate;
   - class II: the root is centered in the middle of the alveolar housing without engaging either labial or palatal cortical plates at the apical one-third of the root;
   - class III: the root is positioned against the palatal cortical plate;
   - class IV: at least two-thirds of the root is engaging both labial and palatal cortical plates.

5 It is important for clinicians to recognize cases that are favorable for IIPP (class I SRP), cases that are more technique sensitive and entail additional attention (class II and class III SRP), and cases that are contraindicated for IIPP, requiring hard and/or soft tissue augmentation prior to implant placement (class IV SRP).[30] *Buccolingual width and interradicular mesiodistal widths* of the failing tooth determine the diameter of the implant to be used and can be evaluated using CBCT and periapical radiographs (Figure 6.4).

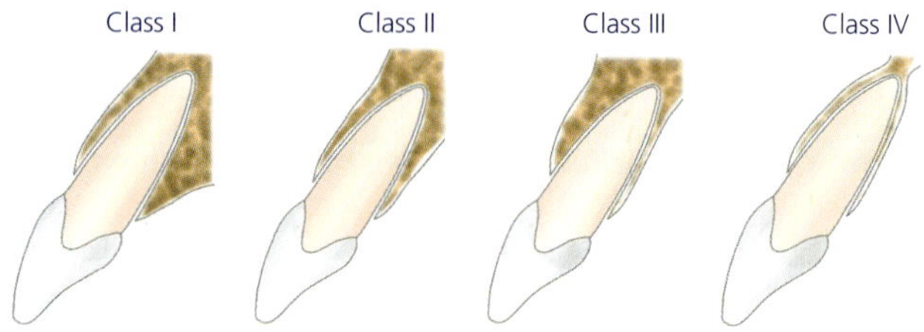

Figure 6.3 Sagittal root position classification. Class I: the root is positioned against the labial cortical plate. Class II: the root is centered in the middle of the alveolar housing without engaging either labial or palatal cortical plates at the apical one-third of the root. Class III: the root is positioned against the palatal cortical plate. Class IV: at least two-thirds of the root is engaging both labial and palatal cortical plates. *Source:* Courtesy of Jeff Miles.

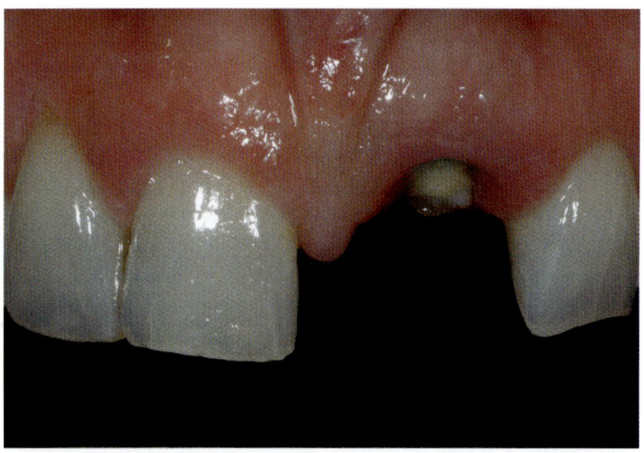

Figure 6.1 Gingival level of the failing tooth (#9) should be (1) the same as (or more coronal than) that of the contralateral tooth and (2) harmonious with the adjacent dentition, as some gingival recession can be expected after the procedure.

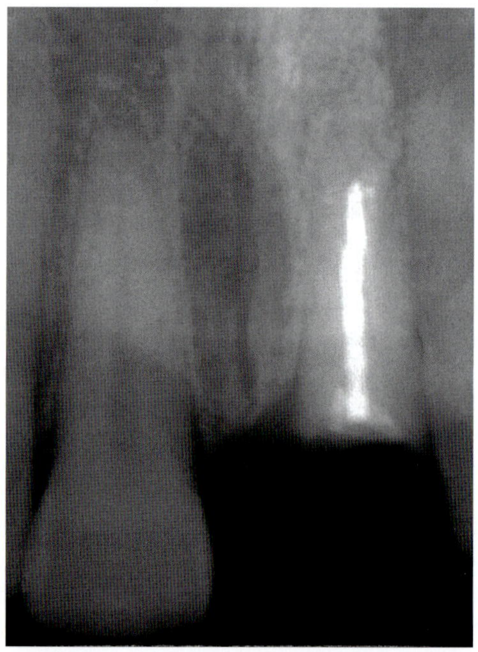

Figure 6.4 Periapical radiograph of the failing tooth.

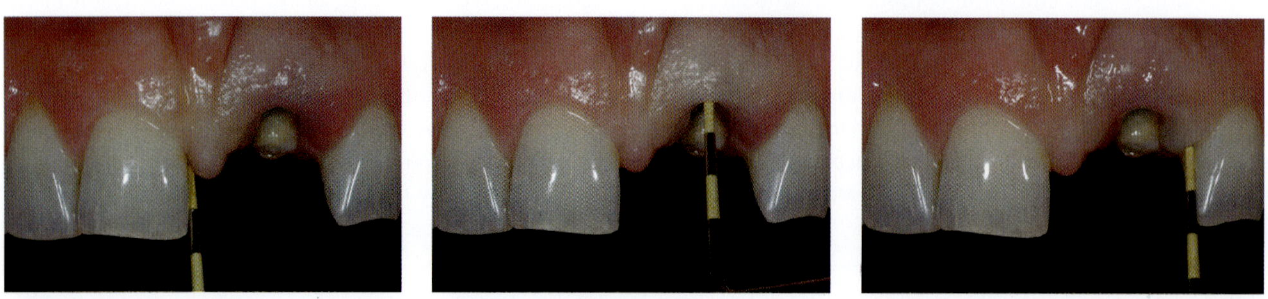

Figure 6.2 Osseous–gingival tissue relationship can be evaluated by bone sounding and should measure 3 mm on the facial aspect of the failing tooth and 4.5 mm on the proximal aspect of adjacent teeth.

Clinical procedure

Diagnostic waxing

A diagnostic waxing of the failing tooth on the study cast should: 1) represent, as closely as possible, the definitive restoration; 2) match the contralateral tooth; and 3) be harmonious with the adjacent dentition. Proper diagnostic waxing provides information necessary for treatment planning, especially when adjunctive procedures (orthodontic and/or periodontal intervention) are required. A provisional restoration, as well as implant and soft tissue surgical templates, can be accurately fabricated from a well-executed diagnostic waxing. It may be possible, before the provisional crown is fabricated, for the patient to preview the intended morphology of the definitive restoration with a smile design using a composite resin replica inside a vacuum-formed template generated from a cast of the wax-up. On the other hand, where the crown portion of the failing tooth is intact and esthetically acceptable, it can be modified after extraction to be used as a natural-looking provisional restoration.

Surgical procedure

Immediate implant placement entails extraction of the failing tooth followed by placement of an osseointegrated implant. The extraction must be minimally traumatic with controlled expansion of the bony socket to avoid soft and/or hard tissue damage. This can be accomplished by first using a periotome (Nobel Biocare, subsidiary of Danaher, Washington DC) to make a sulcular incision with transeptal fiberectomy that extends apically beyond the marginal bone. This incision separates the tooth from the periodontal tissue, facilitating extraction with zero or minimal damage to the usually thin labial bony plate. After the extraction, the integrity of the labial plate must be verified using a periodontal probe. Fenestrations located at least 5 mm apical to the intact facial marginal bone are generally inconsequential to the IIPP procedure, as these defects can be addressed predictably with grafting.

When a facial osseous dehiscence/defect is detected, the predictability of the IIPP in conjunction with guided bone regeneration (GBR) procedures is determined by the shape/size of the defect.[34] A V-shaped defect, which is isolated only to the mid-facial portion of the facial bony plate, responds favorably to IIPP with GBR (Figure 6.5). It should be noted, however, that significant facial gingival recession after 1 year of function has been reported when IIPP with GBR was attempted on failing teeth with U-shaped (extends to mesial and/or distal aspect of the failing tooth) or UU-shaped (extends to the mesial and distal aspect of the immediately adjacent teeth) defects (Figure 6.5).[34] Therefore, a failing tooth with a U-shaped or UU-shaped defect is contraindicated for IIPP.

Primary implant stability is the prerequisite for IIPP and is usually achieved by engaging the palatal wall and the bone 4–5 mm beyond the apex of the extraction socket. Therefore, class I SRP, with a considerable amount of bone present on the palatal aspect for implant engagement to attain primary stability, is optimal for IIPP. Class IV SRP, with a limited amount of bone for implant engagement, is a contraindication.[30] Class II and III SRP present compromised and/or challenging conditions for IIPP.[30] In class III SRP, implant stability must rely on its engagement with the available bone on the labial aspect, which can potentially lead to facial fenestration or perforation.[30] In class II SRP, as available bone on both the palatal and labial aspects is inadequate, the implant stability relies primarily on the amount of available bone beyond the apex of the extraction socket.[30]

The final implant diameter should be within the confines of the tooth socket, but should not engage the usually thin coronal portion of the labial plate. This will help to prevent perforation. Furthermore, a minimal distance of 2 mm between the implant and adjacent teeth is recommended to minimize marginal bone loss due to encroachment.[35] The final implant position and angulation are in accordance with the following guidelines (Figure 6.6).

- Mesiodistally: the implant should be placed at the center of the predetermined mesiodistal width of the final restoration with a minimal distance of 2 mm from the adjacent tooth.
- Labiopalatally: the implant should be placed along the palatal wall of the extraction socket for primary stability. At the cervical level, the implant should emerge slightly lingual to the predetermined buccolingual width of the

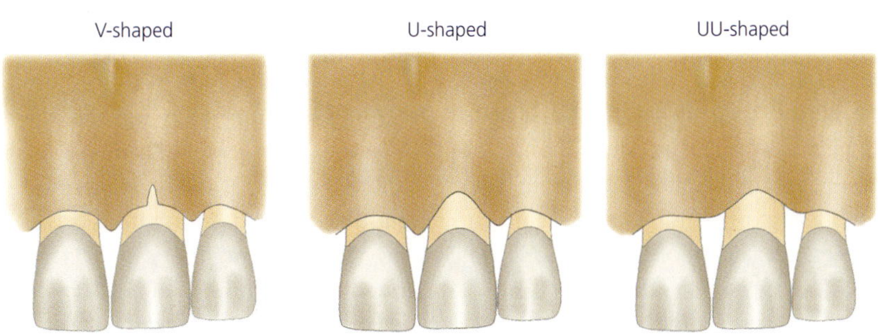

Figure 6.5 Facial bone defect classification. V-shaped defect: isolated only to the mid-facial portion of the facial bony plate. U-shaped defect: extends to the mesial and/or distal aspect of the failing tooth. UU-shaped defect: extends to the mesial and distal aspects of the immediately adjacent teeth. *Source:* Courtesy of Jeff Miles.

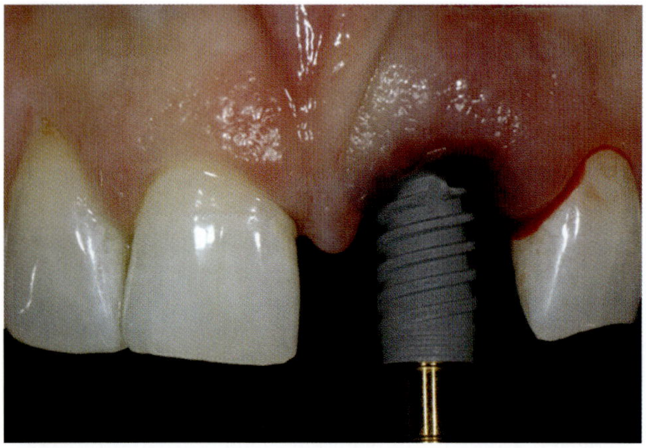

Figure 6.6 The implant should be placed at the center of the predetermined mesiodistal width of the final restoration with a minimal distance of 2 mm from the adjacent tooth.

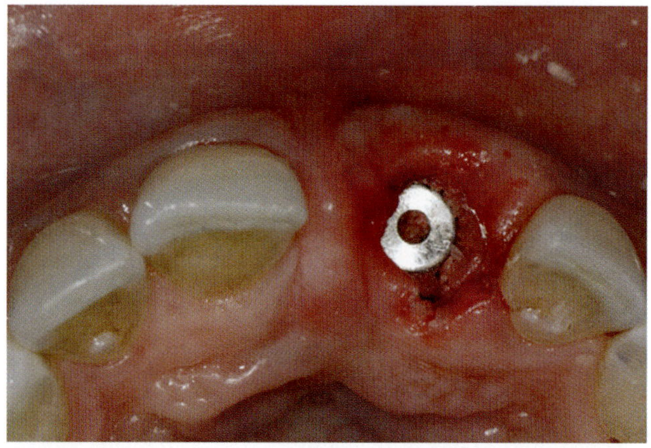

Figure 6.7 Bone graft material is placed into the gaps between the implant and the bony socket to maintain facial osseous contour.

final restoration. At the incisal level, the implant should emerge at the incisal edge of the final restoration, if cement-retained design is elected. With this labiopalatal position/placement, a gap of at least 1.5 mm between the implant and the buccal bone is maintained and the integrity of the labial bone ensured.

- Apicocoronally: the neck of the implant is placed approximately 3 mm apical to the predetermined facial free gingival margin of the final restoration.

Immediate provisionalization

For immediate provisionalization, a prefabricated zirconium abutment (Nobel Biocare) or metal temporary abutment is manually prepared extraorally and then hand-tightened onto the implant. The provisional shell is then relined with light polymerized acrylic resin (Ultradent Products, Inc., South Jordan, UT) to capture the cervical gingival emergence of the extracted tooth, and adjusted to clear all centric and eccentric functional contacts. The provisional restoration can be screw-retained or cement-retained. A cement-retained provisional restoration is usually more esthetic, especially when the implant access opening is at or facial to the incisal edge. However, it also is at higher risk of gingival inflammation at the abutment–cement–restoration interface as well as cement debonding.

It has recently been demonstrated that following immediate implant placement in an anterior tooth socket, the facial bony plate undergoes remodeling, characterized by bone fill from the inside of the socket and resorption of the labial bony plate from the outside.[26] Without a bone graft, this usually results in significant horizontal and vertical facial bone loss and, subsequently, facial gingival tissue loss.[36–40]

To maintain the facial osseous contour, bone graft material (Bio-Oss, Osteohealth, Shirley, NY and Puros, Zimmer Dental, Carlsbad, CA) is placed into the gaps between the implant and the bony socket (Figure 6.7). If thin gingival biotype is present, a subepithelial connective tissue graft (SCTG) can be placed subgingivally between the labial free gingival margin and the labial bone to improve the gingival condition (Figure 6.8).[28] Cementation of the provisional restoration with provisional cement (Temp-bond, Kerr USA, Romulus, MI) should be performed simultaneously with the SCTG placement (Figure 6.8).

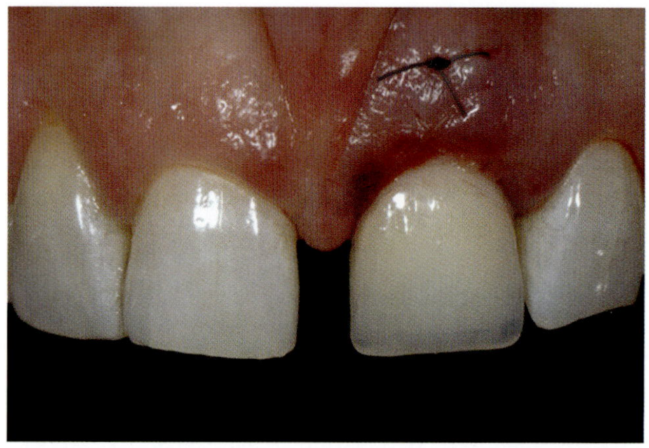

Figure 6.8 Subepithelial connective tissue graft (SCTG) can be placed simultaneously with cementation of the provisional restoration.

The amount of cement used should be minimal and mostly isolated at the intaglio incisal and lingual area of the provisional for ease of later cement removal. Light finger pressure must be applied over the grafted site with moist gauze for 5 minutes to minimize blood clot formation between the graft and its underlying and overlying tissues. A thick blood clot can potentially hinder the anastomosis of new capillary buds from the recipient bed, thus jeopardizing graft survival.[41] The fit of the prosthesis with a radiopaque abutment can be ascertained with a periapical radiograph (Figure 6.9).

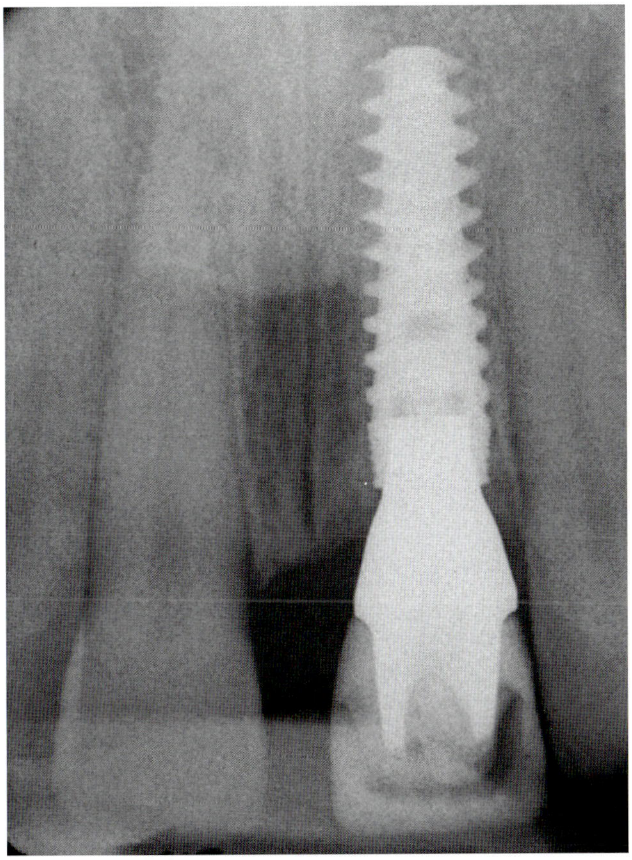

Figure 6.9 Periapical radiograph of IIPP of #9.

Postoperative instruction

Appropriate antibiotics and analgesics are prescribed for postoperative use. The patient is instructed not to brush the surgical site, but instead rinse gently with 0.12% chlorhexidine gluconate (Peridex, Procter & Gamble, Cincinnati, OH). A liquid diet is required for 2 weeks after the operation, and a soft diet is recommended for the remaining duration of the implant healing phase, which typically lasts 4 months (Figure 6.10). The patient is also advised against any activity that could irritate the surgical site.

Definitive restoration

The final implant impression is usually made 6 months after the surgery. A customized zirconia/gold alloy abutment (Procera, Nobel Biocare) is fabricated, duplicating the gingival emergence profile of the provisional restoration (Figure 6.11). The abutment should be tightened onto the implant with the manufacturer's recommended amount of torque, and the fit should be verified with a periapical radiograph. Subsequently, definitive cement (Ceramir, Doxa Dental Inc., Newport Beach, CA) should be used for the definitive restoration (Figures 6.12 and 6.13a). Follow-up appointments with the patient should occur at 1 month, 3 months, 6 months, 12 months, and annually thereafter in order to ascertain the functional and esthetic outcome (Figure 6.13).

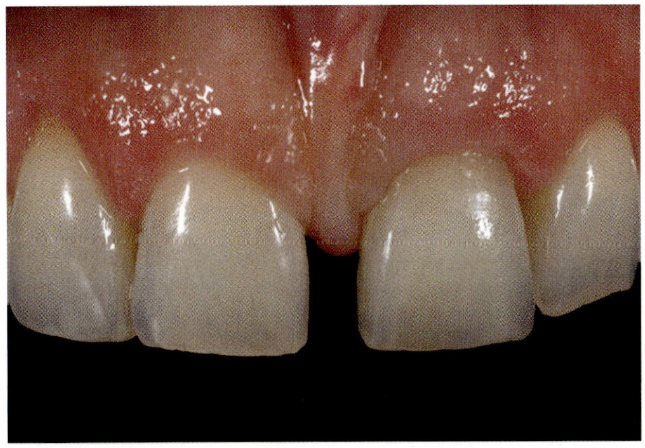

Figure 6.10 Clinical image of provisional restoration after 4 months of healing.

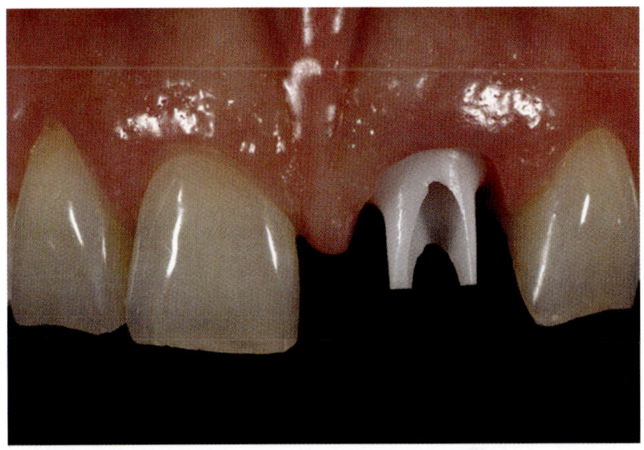

Figure 6.11 Customized zirconium abutment.

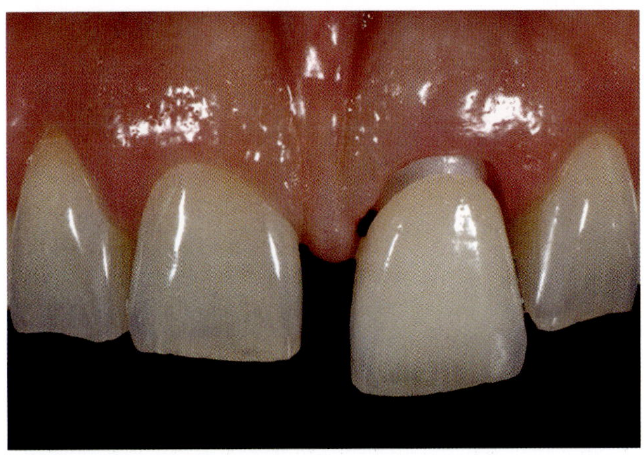

Figure 6.12 Cementation of an all-ceramic definitive restoration.

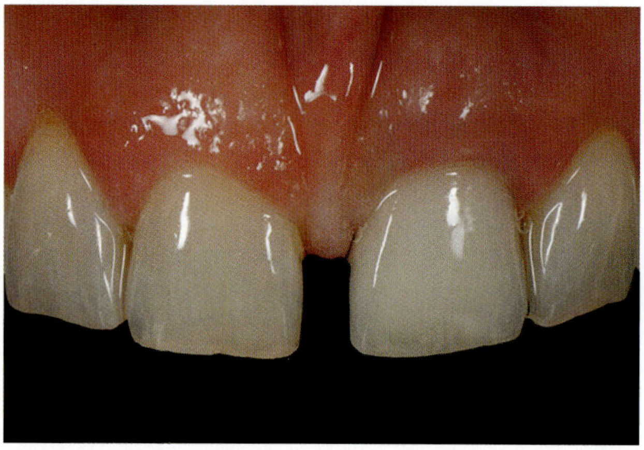

(a)

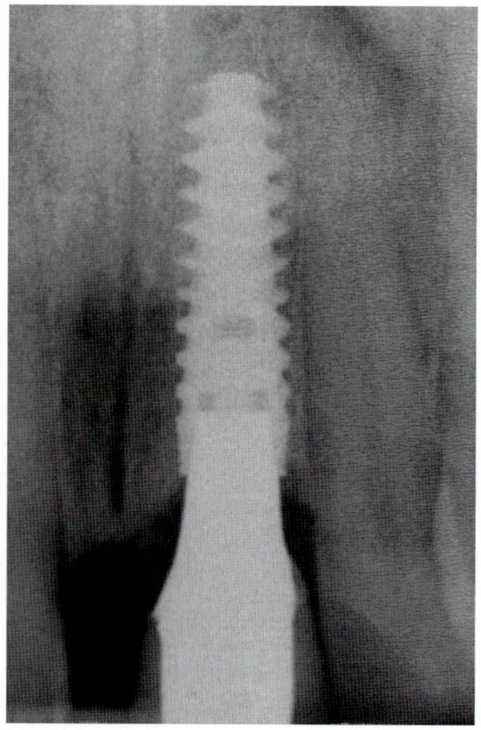

(b)

Figure 6.13 (a) Clinical and (b) radiographic images of the definitive restoration 4 years after surgery.

The challenge and potential solution of maintaining the inter-implant papilla when replacing a tooth adjacent to an implant

To develop an implant restoration that mimics the contralateral tooth in the esthetic zone is daunting enough. However, when the immediately placed and restored implant is adjacent to an implant restoration, the papilla is often compromised as the tooth to be extracted is the sole preserver of the interproximal bone on that side. An innovative approach to this scenario has been reported in the literature.

Papilla loss is common when replacing multiple adjacent failing teeth with implants in the anterior maxillary esthetic zone.[42] This is due to the fact that the implant platform is positioned based on the facial bone level, and since most available dental implants are uniplanar (flat), the implant platform will be positioned apical to the proximal bone level. In addition, long-term maintenance of the proximal bone coronal to the implant platform has been shown to be more of an exception than the rule,[43] even with the use of implants with a scalloped[44] or unmatched (platform switch) platform.[45] As a result, the proximal implant marginal bone level is often more apical than that of the adjacent natural teeth, ultimately leading to diminished papillary soft tissue, despite stable marginal bone levels of both the implant and adjacent tooth. Methods, such as alternate immediate implant placement and provisionalization (IIPP) on one failing tooth after the integration of another, proper spacing (at least 3 mm of inter-implant/radicular distance), immediate prosthetic support of the papilla, as well as flapless surgery, have been advocated with some degree of success of minimizing, but not preventing, papilla loss.[42] Recently, the proximal socket-shield technique, utilizing the retained proximal portion of the root in an attempt to preserve the interproximal bone after IIPP, has been described, and promising clinical results have been reported.[46] The next section describes the technique of maintaining the inter-implant papilla when replacing a failing tooth adjacent to an implant restoration using the proximal socket-shield (PSS) procedure in conjunction with IIPP.

A typical scenario would be a patient with a high smile line presenting with a failing left maxillary lateral incisor (#10) due to root resorption, 2 years after implant placement at the left maxillary central incisor (#9) (Figure 6.14). The following novel procedure elucidates the use of a residual root to maintain the papillary tissue. After administration of local anesthesia, the maxillary left lateral incisor (#10) was sectioned (#557 L, Brasseler, Savannah, GA) buccolingually (Figure 6.15) and the distal half of the root was removed atraumatically without flap reflection. The crown portion of the remaining distal tooth structure was then sectioned horizontally leaving the root with a cervical extension ~1 mm coronal to the mesial marginal bone. The distal root fragment was removed, creating a 1.5–2 mm uniformly thick C-shaped root fragment spanning from the mesiobuccal to the mesiolingual line angles. After the mesial portion of the tooth socket was debrided and

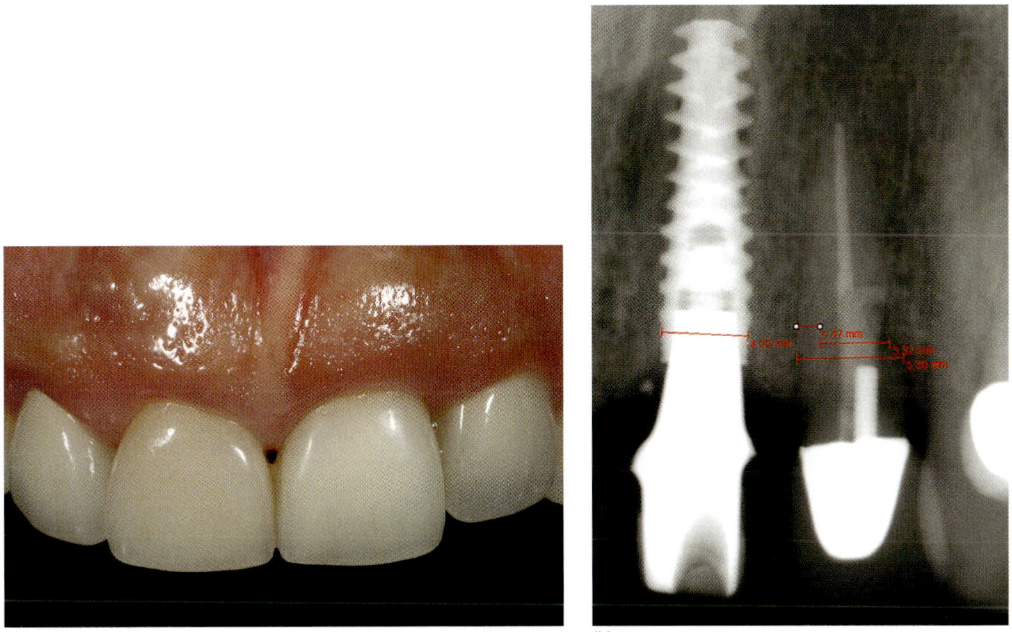

(a) (b)

Figure 6.14 (a) Pretreatment frontal view of failing maxillary left lateral incisor (#10). (b) Pretreatment periapical radiograph of #10.

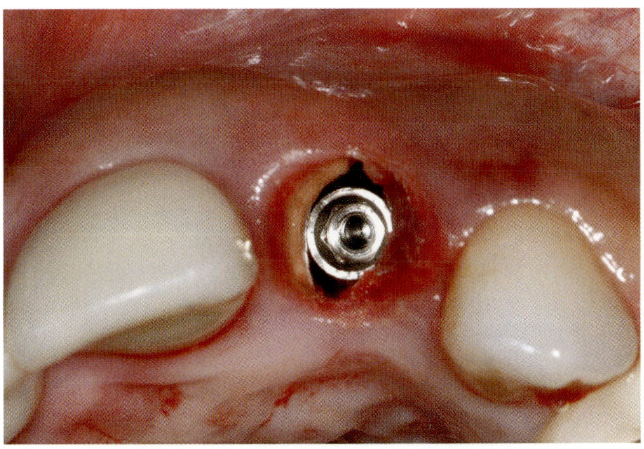

Figure 6.15 Immediate implant placement after preparation of a 1.5–2 mm uniformly thick C-shaped mesial root fragment.

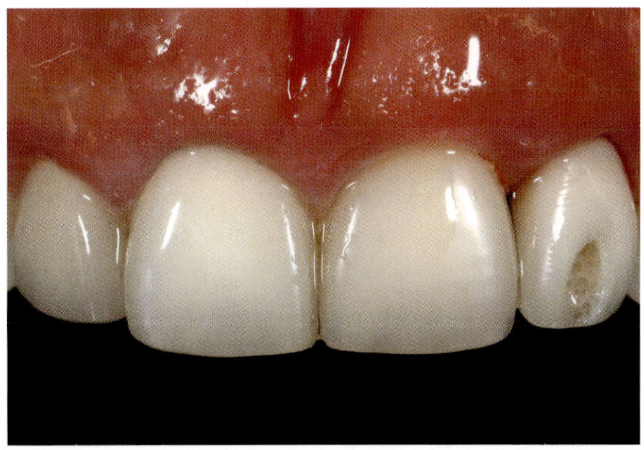

Figure 6.17 The screw-retained provisional restoration was hand tightened onto the implant.

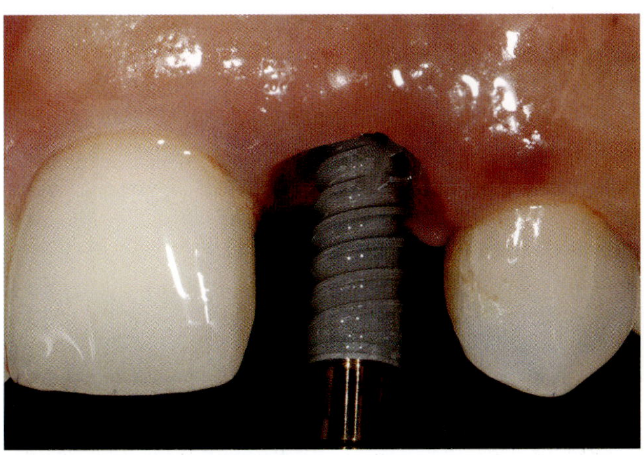

Figure 6.16 Immediate implant placement at the maxillary left lateral incisor position.

detoxified, sequential implant osteotomy was performed to achieve the desired three-dimensional implant (NobelActive, Nobel Biocare) position in relationship to the distal root fragment (Figures 6.16, 6.17, and 6.18). Bone graft materials (Bio-Oss, Osteohealth, Shirley, NY and Puros, Zimmer Dental, Carlsbad, CA) were placed into the gaps between the implant and the bony socket as well as the mesial root fragment. A provisional shell was then relined onto a zirconia abutment and adjusted to clear all centric and eccentric functional contacts.

Appropriate antibiotics and analgesics were prescribed. The patient was instructed not to brush the surgical site, but to rinse gently with 0.12% chlorhexidine gluconate (Peridex, Procter & Gamble) and be on a soft diet for 2 weeks. The patient was advised against functioning activities to

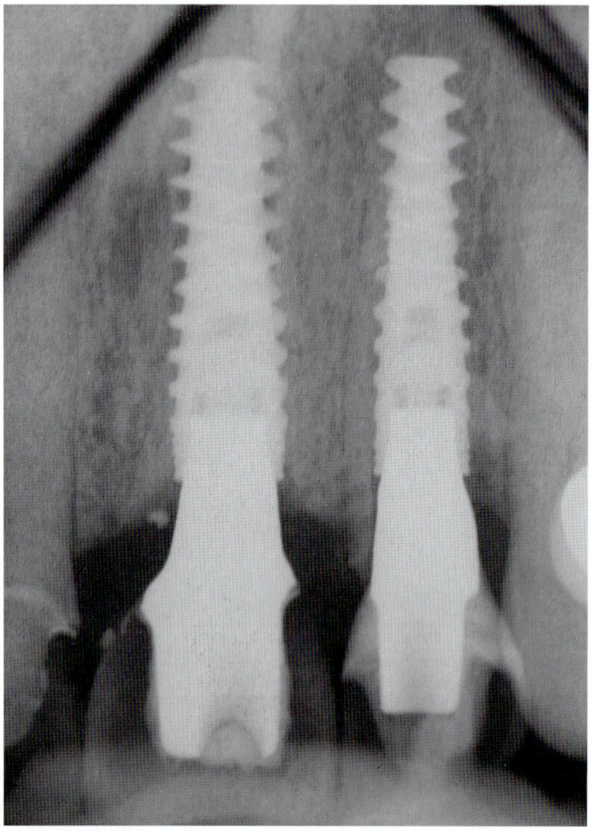

Figure 6.18 Periapical radiograph of proximal socket-shield with immediate implant placement and provisionalization.

the implant site for the duration of the implant healing phase (6 months).

The final implant impression was made 6 months after the surgery. The definitive all-ceramic crown (Procera, Nobel Biocare) with a customized zirconia abutment (Procera, Nobel Biocare) was fabricated and cemented. Clinical and radiographic images at 4 years showed satisfactory esthetic results with a well-maintained inter-implant papilla between #7 and #8 (Figure 6.19).

The benefits of the proximal socket-shield (PSS) procedure with IIPP in maintaining both the bone level and the dentogingival supercrestal fibers have been reported in the literature.[47] Nevertheless, this is a technique-sensitive procedure with limited long-term evidence. Therefore, proper case selection and execution as well as close monitoring in larger-scale studies are needed to substantiate the validity of the procedure.

Conclusions

While a well-executed IIPP of anterior maxillary single implants has been shown to be a predictable treatment modality, its success depends primarily on careful patient selection, accurate diagnosis, and proper planning. Nonetheless, operator-sensitive procedures are required to deliver a harmonious and functional restoration in the esthetic zone.

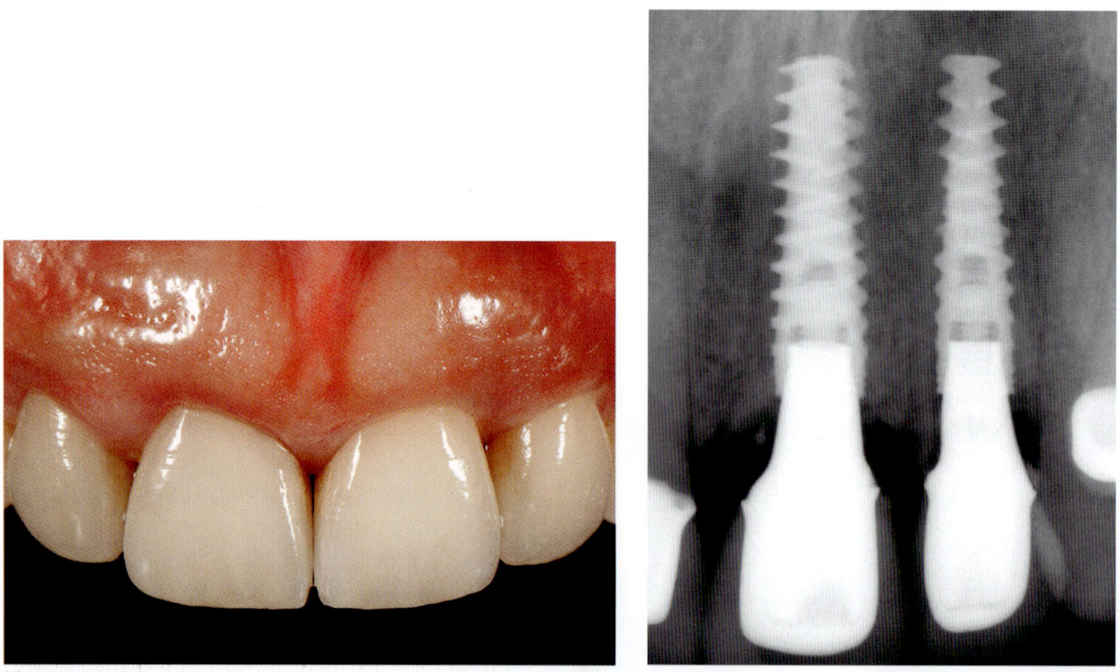

(a) (b)

Figure 6.19 (a) Definitive restoration of #10 at 4-year follow-up. Note the maintenance of the interproximal peri-implant papilla. (b) Periapical radiograph of definitive restoration of #10 at 4 years.

References

1. Kan JYK, Rungcharassaeng K. Site development for anterior implant esthetics: the dentulous site. *Compend Contin Educ Dent* 2001; **22**(3): 221–232.
2. Phillips K, Kois JC. Aesthetic peri-implant site development. The restorative connection. *Dent Clin North Am* 1998; **42**(1): 57–70.
3. Goodacre CJ, Kan JYK, Rungcharassaeng K. Clinical complications of osseointegrated implants. *J Prosthet Dent* 1999; **81**(5): 537–552.
4. Jemt T. Regeneration of gingival papillae after single-implant treatment. *Int J Periodontics Restorative Dent* 1997; **17**(4): 326–333.
5. Jemt T. Restoring the gingival contour by means of provisional resin crowns after single-implant treatment. *Int J Periodontics Restorative Dent* 1999; **19**(1): 20–29.
6. Cooper L, Felton DA, Kugelberg CF, *et al.* A multicenter 12-month evaluation of single-tooth implants restored 3 weeks after 1-stage surgery. *Int J Oral Maxillofac Implants* 2001; **16**(2): 182–192.
7. Bengazi F, Wennstrom JL, Lekholm U. Recession of the soft tissue margin at oral implants. A 2-year longitudinal prospective study. *Clin Oral Implants Res* 1996; 7(4): 303–310.
8. Kan JYK, Rungcharassaeng K. Immediate placement and provisionalization of maxillary anterior single implants: a surgical and prosthodontic rationale. *Pract Periodontics Aesthet Dent* 2000; **12**(9): 817–824.
9. Kan JYK, Rungcharassaeng K, Lozada JL. Immediate placement and provisionalization of maxillary anterior single implants: 1-year prospective study. *Int J Oral Maxillofac Implants* 2003; **18**(1): 31–39.
10. Kan JYK, Rungcharassaeng K. Immediate implant placement and provisionalization of maxillary anterior single implants. In: Torabinejad M, Sabeti MA, Goodacre CJ (eds). *Principles and Practice of Single Implant and Restoration*, 1st edn. Missouri: Elsevier Saunders 2013; 119–131.
11. Beagle JR. Surgical reconstruction of the interdental papilla: case report. *Int J Periodontics Restorative Dent* 1992; **12**(2): 145–151.
12. Nemcovsky CE, Moses O, Artzi Z. Interproximal papillae reconstruction in maxillary implants. *J Periodontol* 2000; **71**(2): 308–314.
13. Palacci P. Peri-implant soft tissue management: Papilla regeneration technique. In: Palacci P, Ericsson I, Engstrand P, Rangert B (eds). *Optimal Implant Positioning and Soft Tissue Management for the Branemark System*. Chicago: Quintessence 1995; 59–70.
14. Wohrle PS. Single-tooth replacement in the aesthetic zone with immediate provisionalization: fourteen consecutive cases reports. *Prac Periodontics Aesthet Dent* 1998; **10**(9): 1107–1114.
15. Hui E, Chow J, Li D, *et al.* Immediate provisional for single-tooth implant replacement with Branemark system: preliminary report. *Clin Implant Dent Relat Res* 2001; **3**(2): 79–86.
16. Kan JYK, Rungcharassaeng K, Liddelow G, *et al.* Periimplant tissue response following immediate provisional restoration of scalloped implants in the esthetic zone: a one-year pilot prospective multicenter study. *J Prosthet Dent* 2007; **97**(6 suppl): S109–118.
17. De Rouck T, Collys K, Cosyn J. Immediate single-tooth implants in the anterior maxilla: a 1-year case cohort study on hard and soft tissue response. *J Clin Periodontol* 2008; **35**(7): 649–657.
18. Kan JYK, Rungcharassaeng K, Sclar A, *et al.* Effects of the facial osseous defect morphology on gingival dynamics after immediate tooth replacement and guided bone regeneration: 1-year results. *J Oral Maxillofac Surg* 2007; **65**(7 Suppl 1): 13–19.
19. Barone A, Rispoli L, Vozza I, *et al.* Immediate restoration of single implants placed immediately after tooth extraction. *J Periodontol* 2006; **77**(11): 1914–1920.
20. Palattella P, Toresllo F, Cordarro L. Two-year prospective clinical comparison of immediate replacement vs. immediate restoration of single tooth in the esthetic zone. *Clin Oral Implants Res* 2008; **19**(11): 1148–1153.
21. Norton MR. A short-term clinical evaluation of immediately restored maxillary TiOblast single-tooth implants. *Int J Oral Maxillofac Implants* 2004; **19**(2): 274–281.
22. Ferrara A, Galli C, Mauro G, *et al.* Immediate provisional restoration of postextraction implants for maxillary single-tooth replacement. *Int J Periodontics Restorative Dent* 2006; **26**(4): 371–377.
23. Tsirlis AT. Clinical evaluation of immediate loaded upper anterior single implants. *Implant Dent* 2005; **14**(1): 94–103.
24. Crespi R, Cappare P, Gherlone E, *et al.* Immediate versus delayed loading of dental implants placed in fresh extraction sockets in the maxillary esthetic zone: a clinical comparative study. *Int J Oral Maxillofac Implants* 2008; **23**(4): 753–758.
25. Canullo L, Rasperini G. Preservation of peri-implant soft and hard tissues using platform switching of implants placed in immediate extraction sockets: a proof-of-concept study with 12- to 36-month follow-up. *Int J Oral Maxillofac Implants* 2007; **22**(6): 995–1000.
26. Groisman M, Frossard WM, Ferreira HM, *et al.* Single-tooth implants in the maxillary incisor region with immediate provisionalization: 2-year prospective study. *Pract Proced Aesthet Dent* 2003; **15**(2): 115–124.
27. Garber DA, Salama MA, Salama H. Immediate total tooth replacement. *Compend Contin Educ Dent* 2001; **22**(3): 210–218.
28. Kan JYK, Rungcharassaeng K, Lozada JL. Bilaminar subepithelial connective tissue grafts for immediate implant placement and provisionalization in the esthetic zone. *J Calif Dent Assoc* 2005; **33**(11): 865–871.
29. Kois JC, Kan JYK. Predictable peri-implant gingival aesthetics: surgical and prosthodontic rationales. *Pract Proced Aesthet Dent* 2001; **13**(9): 691–698.
30. Kan JYK, Roe P, Rungcharassaeng K, *et al.* Classification of sagittal root position in relation to the anterior maxillary osseous housing for immediate implant placement: a cone beam computed tomography study. *Int J Oral Maxillofac Implants* 2011; **26**(4): 873–876.
31. Salama H, Salama MA. The role of orthodontic extrusive remodeling in the enhancement of soft and hard tissue profiles prior to implant placement: a systematic approach to the management of extraction sites defects. *Int J Periodontics Restorative Dent* 1993; **13**(4): 312–333.
32. Kan JYK, Rungcharassaeng K, Umezu K, *et al.* Dimensions of peri-implant mucosa: an evaluation of maxillary anterior single implants in humans. *J Periodontol* 2003; **74**(4): 557–562.
33. Kan JYK, Morimoto T, Rungcharassaeng K, *et al.* Gingival biotype assessment in the esthetic zone: visual versus direct measurement. *Int J Periodontics Restorative Dent* 2010; **30**(3): 237–243.
34. Kan JYK, Rungcharassaeng K, Sclar A, *et al.* Effects of the facial osseous defect morphology on gingival dynamics after immediate tooth replacement and guided bone regeneration: 1-year results. *J Oral Maxillofac Surg* 2007; **65**(7Suppl1): 13–19.
35. Esposito M, Ekestubbe A, Grondahl K. Radiological evaluation of marginal bone loss at tooth surfaces facing single Branemark implants. *Clin Oral Implants Res* 1993; **4**(3): 151–157.

36. Araujo MG, Lindhe J. Dimension ridge alterations following tooth extraction. An experimental study in the dog. *J Clin Periodontol* 2005; **32**(2): 212–218.
37. Araujo MG, Sukekava F, Wennstrom JL, *et al.* Ridge alterations following implant placement in fresh extraction sockets: an experimental study in the dog. *J Clin Periodontol* 2005; **32**(6): 645–652.
38. Botticelli D, Berglundh T, Lindhe J. Hard-tissue alterations following immediate implant placement in extraction sites. *J Clin Periodontol* 2004; **31**(10): 820–828.
39. Chen ST. Immediate implant placement postextraction without flap elevation. *J Periodontol* 2009; **80**(1): 163–172.
40. Covani U, Cornelini R, Barone A. Bucco-lingual bone remodeling around implants placed into immediate extraction sockets: a case series. *J Periodontol* 2003; **74**(2): 268–273.
41. Nabers J. Free gingival grafts. *Periodontics* 1966; **4**(5): 243–245.
42. Kan JY, Rungcharassaeng K. Interimplant papilla preservation in the esthetic zone: a report of six consecutive cases. *Int J Periodontics Restorative Dent* 2003; **23**(3): 249–259.
43. Bateli M, Att W, Strub JR. Implant neck configurations for preservation of marginal bone level: a systematic review. *Int J Oral Maxillofac Implants* 2011; **26**(2): 290–303.
44. Kan JY, Rungcharassaeng K, Liddelow G, *et al.* Peri-implant tissue response following immediate provisional restoration of scalloped implants in the esthetic zone: a one-year pilot prospective multicenter study. *J Prosthet Dent* 2007; **97**(6 Suppl): S109–118.
45. Canullo L, Fedele GR, Iannello G, *et al.* Platform switching and marginal bone-level alterations: the results of a randomized-controlled trial. *Clin Oral Implants Res* 2010; **21**(1): 115–121.
46. Crespi R. Cappare P, Gherlone E. Radiographic evaluation of marginal bone levels around platform-switched and non-platform-switched implants used in an immediate loading protocol. *Int J Oral Maxillofac Implants* 2009; **24**(5): 920–926.
47. Kan JYK, Rungcharassaeng K. Proximal socket shield for interimplant papilla preservation in the esthetic zone. *Int J Periodontics Restorative Dent* 2013; **33**(1): e24–31.

CHAPTER 7
Surgical Complications in Implant Placement

Paul B. Greenawalt
Private Practice in Oral and Maxillofacial Surgery, Poulsbo, Washington, USA

Dental implants have become a widely used component of comprehensive treatment planning to restore partially and completely edentulous patients.[1] In spite of their documented long-term survival rates,[2] there has been a tendency to underappreciate the incidence and complexity of restorative and surgical complications. When planning an implant-borne prosthesis, it is critical to develop a restoratively driven blueprint in order to identify the optimal location, diameter, and angulation of the implant(s). Surgical templates may be constructed from diagnostic wax-ups, generated from three-dimensional (3-D) imaging such as cone-beam computed tomography (CBCT), or from a model fabricated by a CAD/CAM machine. The purpose of this guide is to communicate the pertinent spatial requirements and restrictions for implant placement to support a functional and esthetic restoration. However, precise execution of this task continues to be challenging due to potential mishaps in the light of the many variables that must be taken into account.

Avoidance of surgical complications can be enhanced by a thorough knowledge of local and regional anatomy, pretreatment imaging, and sound surgical principles. Untoward results may be related to host limitations, anatomic constraints, or execution of implant placement. As with any medical implantable device there are associated risks and ensuing problems. This chapter will focus on complications associated with implant surgery as well as their prevention and management.

Complications during execution

Neurologic disturbances

To discuss nerve injuries, and their sequelae, we shall first review classification of injuries. Seddon,[3] in 1942, described injuries as belonging to one of three classifications: neurapraxia, axonotmesis, and neurotmesis. Sunderland,[4] in 1978, then described injuries and classified them from 1 to 5. MacKinnon/Dellon[5] (M/D), in 1988, further described a sixth classification that is a neuroma-in-continuity. The purpose of classifying injuries to nerves is to better prognosticate the likelihood of recovery, and to what degree (Table 7.1).

Neurapraxia (Sunderland 1, M/D 1) is characterized by a temporary loss of sensation that returns in days to weeks. The nerve trunk is continuous, as is the axon, however there is demyelination or loss of the myelin sheath. Axonotmesis (Sunderland 2 or 3, M/D 2 or 3) is also characterized as loss of sensation. With class 2 injuries, sensation typically returns in 3–6 months whereas type 3 injuries have incomplete resolution in 3–6 months. The nerve trunk is continuous, however the axon is not and there is demylelination. There is progressively more axonal damage in class 3 as compared to class 2. Neurotmesis (Sunderland 4 or 5, M/D 4, 5, or 6) is characterized by incomplete resolution of symptoms after 3–6 months to no sensation after 3–6 months. Class 6, or the neuroma-in-continuity, has a mixed response after 3–6 months and slightly better long-term prognosis compared to the class 4 or 5 injury. With class 4, 5, and 6 injuries there is nerve trunk disruption, partial to complete, axons are not continuous, with accompanying demyelination.

Nerve injuries may also be classified in a qualitative fashion. This is somewhat easier to relate to patient symptoms and clinical presentation of the injury but is too broad and subjective to quantify the injury. Nevertheless, it is helpful when discussing a nerve injury with a patient. Anesthesia, or adding the qualifier "total" anesthesia, is a term used to describe a complete loss of sensation. In this scenario, noxious stimuli elicit no response (Figure 7.1). More frequently, patients describe an area of profound numbness and also may have a diminished response to noxious stimuli. For example, when testing for perception of sharp versus dull stimulus, patients with anesthesia will note no difference, while partial anesthesia may allow for a diminished ability to discern. They may be able to identify that there is a difference but they simply are unable to replicate sensations on

Evidence-based Implant Treatment Planning and Clinical Protocols, First Edition. Edited by Steven J. Sadowsky.

Companion website: www.wiley.com/go/sadowsky/implant

Table 7.1 Classifications of nerve injuries.

	Sunderland	Seddon	Description of Injury	Recovery period
Least severe	I	Neurapraxia	Conduction block, no Wallerian degeneration	<3 months
	II	Axonotmesis	Axonal discontinuity, nerve remains intact	25 mm (1 inch)/month
	III		Extensive scarring of the endoneurium hinders axon regeneration	<25 mm (1 inch)/month
	IV		Nerve still in-continuity, scar blocks nerve regeneration	Surgical intervention required to remove scar tissue
Most severe	V	Neurotmesis	Rupture of nerve	Recovery requires surgery

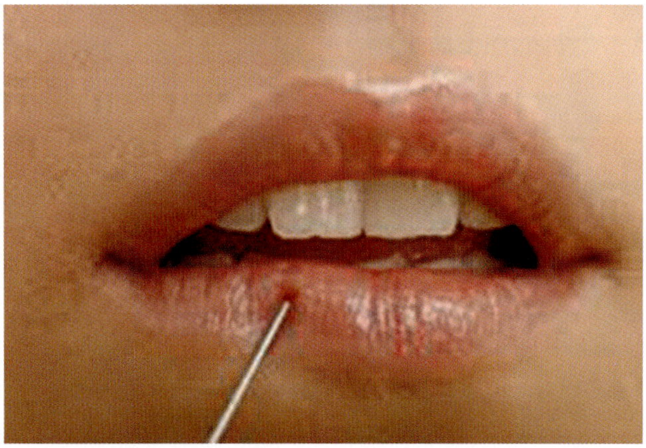

Figure 7.1 Assessing anesthesia.

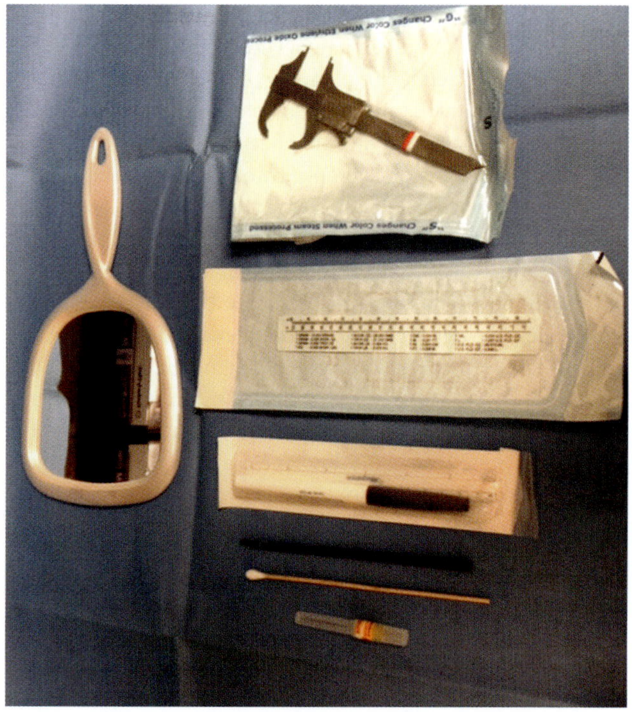

Figure 7.2 Kit for evaluating nerve injuries.

the unaffected side. Paresthesia describes altered sensation, often described as tingling, burning, or pinpricks. Dysesthesia, however, is a condition whereby ordinary stimuli are perceived as noxious and unpleasant. Paresthesia is seen with minor or incomplete injuries, particularly immediately following surgery. Anesthesia typically results from a more severe injury, including transection. Dysesthesia is frequently a late-onset symptom that is the result of scarring, a neuroma, or neuroma-in-continuity.

A simple assessment kit (Figure 7.2) may be assembled and kept on hand to evaluate a patient's sensory disturbance if that should occur. Wooden stick cotton tip applicators can be used to evaluate light touch and direction, sharp versus dull, and cold versus not cold. The cotton is pulled into a wisp and, with the patients eyes closed, they are asked to point in the direction that they perceive touch and direction. The nonaffected side may be used as the "control". Soaking the cotton tip in ethyl chloride will render it cold. Again with eyes closed the cold cotton tip and an untreated tip are applied randomly to the affected and nonaffected sides. Sharp versus dull is tested with a broken wooden stick cotton tip applicator and the cotton tip itself. If desired, two-point discrimination with ordinary calipers can be used to document the sensory disturbance.

In implant dentistry, the nerve most at risk is the inferior alveolar nerve. This can occur with over-instrumentation during osteotomy or overseating the implant, thereby compressing the canal from above. Over-instrumentation can occur in the mandible when firm pressure is required to penetrate the dense cortical plate. When the cortex is breached, the cancellous bone beneath provides little resistance and inadvertent overpenetration can ensue. Drill guards, intraoperative radiographs, and surgical restraint can all help to reduce this risk. Additionally, measuring the twist drill prior to use will confirm the accuracy of the depth markings relative to the actual implant length. Nerve injuries may be avoided with meticulous preparation, imaging, and execution. Treatment planning or mock surgery using the radiographic image with correction for image magnification is very helpful in avoiding this misadventure. A minimum distance of 2 mm must be maintained between the implant and the nerve canal.[6] The mental foramen, the point of exit for the inferior alveolar nerve from its bony canal, poses particular anatomic challenges. The nerve will typically form an anterior loop, or genu, in the body of the mandible before exiting through the mental foramen. The loop is variable but has been reported to be between 1 and at least 5 mm anterior to the foramen. A survey of dried mandibles by Misch and Crawford[7] reported lengths of the loop to be up to 5 mm. To safely place an implant, the implant body needs to be 2 mm from the nerve. Considering the greatest extent of the loop, 5 mm, plus the 2 mm safety margin, the implant should be no closer than 7 mm from the mental foramen. It is with this guideline that Bedrossian[6] creates a path of insertion for an angled posterior implant that avoids the nerve by a minimum of 2 mm. This is achieved by placing the inferior-most point of the implant 7 mm anterior to the mental foramen (Figure 7.3).

Nerve injury can also occur through poor flap design, poor flap development, and excessive retraction. Failing to account for the mental nerve and its branches as they course through soft tissue is but one way of securing a nerve injury. As the inferior alveolar nerve travels through the mandible from the mandibular foramen to the mental foramen it also trends outward from the lingual cortex to the internal aspect of the buccal cortex.[7] Three-dimensional imaging can accurately identify the inferior alveolar canal as it wends its way from proximal to distal. Treatment-planning software can also aid in identifying potential sites for nerve injury during implant placement. A partial-thickness flap rather than a full-thickness flap can directly traumatize a nerve. Meticulous attention to develop a subperiosteal plane for elevation will help to protect the nerve as it courses through soft tissue. The periosteum is tethered to the mental nerve as it exits the mental foramen. If an extensive flap must be elevated in this area, careful dissection of periosteum from the nerve may be necessary to prevent traction on the nerve. Flapless procedures also carry inherent risk due to lack of direct visualization and potentially "losing one's way".

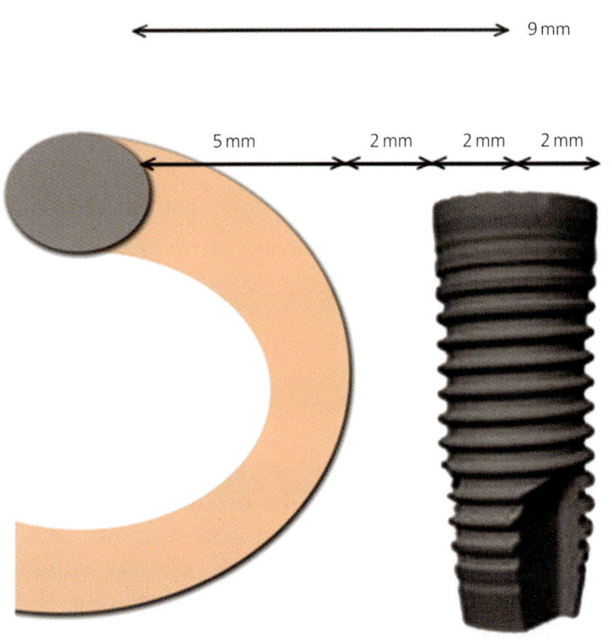

Figure 7.3 Distance from anterior loop of the inferior alveolar nerve, measuring for safe distance from the mental foramen.

A sound understanding of anatomy coupled with 3-D imaging can reduce this risk.

Direct trauma from injection of local anesthesia as well as chemical trauma from the anesthetic agent itself may also play a role in the constellation of causative factors for nerve injuries.[8,9] An increasing percentage of local anesthetic carries with it additional risk for chemical trauma. Hillerup *et al.*[10] in 2011 concluded that local anesthetic in a 4% solution posed a statistically significant greater risk of nerve injury than a lower concentration, such as 2%.

Management of nerve injuries

If, on initial examination of the patient postoperatively, there is altered sensation, a critical examination of radiographs is essential to determine if the implant violated the canal. If the apex of the implant is within the 2 mm "safety" margin, then the surgeon must consider that the implant is compressing the overlying bone and thereby the nerve. If feasible, backing the implant out a few turns may alleviate the compression. This, however, may impact initial stability and/or the position of the head of the implant relative to crestal bone. Inflammation may often be a component of nerve injury in addition to the physical injury. Steroid therapy with or without concurrent nonsteroidal anti-inflammatory drug (NSAID) therapy will mitigate the inflammatory response. Ibuprofen, 800 mg three times per day for a minimum of 14 days, is a typical NSAID regimen. High-dose prednisone in a rapid taper has been shown to greatly suppress the inflammatory response.[11,12] A regimen that has been proffered is 60 mg for 3 days, 40 mg for 3 days, and finally 20 mg for 3 days. Second- and third-generation anticonvulsants such as oxcarbapine (Trileptal), zonisamide (Zonegram), topirimate (Topamax), levetiracetam (Keppra), and lamotrigine (Lamictal), have shown promise, possibly due to their gamma amino butyric acid (GABA) effects as a neuroinhibitor (Figure 7.4).[13] Earlier-generation anticonvulsants, such as carbamazapine (Tegretol), have also been prescribed.

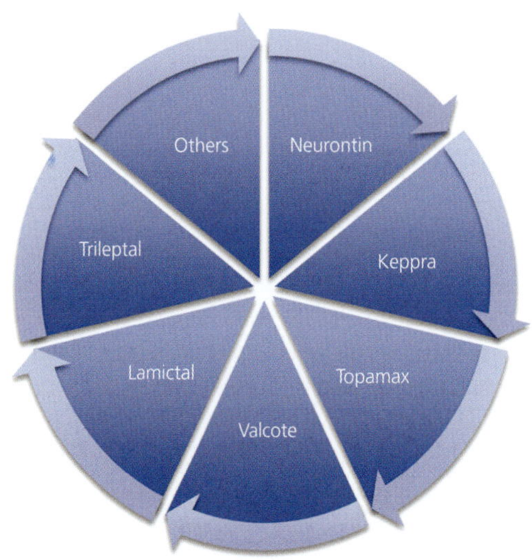

Figure 7.4 Drugs for medical management of nerve injuries.

Antiviral drugs and hyperbaric oxygen (HBO) are also strategies effective in reducing endoneurial edema. Beyond these strategies, B-complex vitamins may also be of benefit. If improvement is noted with medical management, the surgeon may elect to continue the therapy for an additional 3 weeks.

If anesthesia is persistent, or if, after 16 weeks, dysesthesia persists, the patient should be referred to a microneurosurgeon for consultation. It has been suggested that if repair is performed before Wallerian degeneration of the injured nerve takes place, patients report favorable responses.[14] Wallerian degeneration, as described by Augustus Volney Waller,[15] in 1850, is the degeneration of the nerve, particularly the Schwann cells distal to the injury. Typically, the distal nerve trunk has not reached its maximum degeneration for 4–6 months after nerve injury. Sensation may not be restored but subjective improvement is often perceived after degeneration is complete. This degeneration is a slow process, and the reconstructive surgeon may elect to delay the repair or repair the nerve immediately.

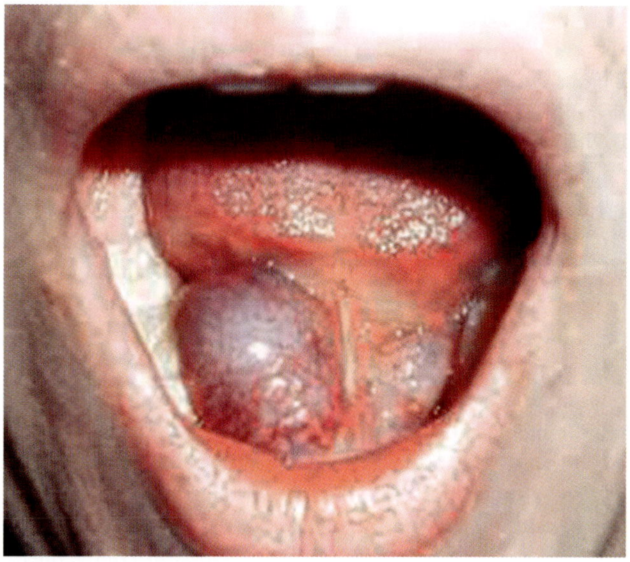

Figure 7.5 Intraoral presentation of ranula.

Floor of mouth injuries

The contents of the floor of the mouth are both numerous and varied. The lingual artery, its branches, and bone perforations will be discussed later in this chapter. Other structures include muscles, salivary glands and their ducts/orifices, as well as nerves.

Muscles in the floor of the mouth not only provide movement but also act as a hammock delineating superficial and deeper spaces. The mylohyoid muscle originates on the lingual aspect of the mandible at the mylohyoid ridge and inserts on the superior aspect of the hyoid bone. Its function is to elevate the contents of the floor of mouth thereby aiding in mastication and swallowing. The ridge is closest to the alveolar crest in the posterior and deepest in the anterior. The mylohyoid muscle serves as an anatomic barrier between the sublingual space and the submandibular space. Violation of it allows for introduction of materials such as bacteria, saliva, and bone into deeper spaces, perhaps raising the risk of a deep space infection. The genioglossus muscles are a paired set that originate on the genial tubercles which arise on the lingual aspect of the mandible, deep to the alveolus. They insert on the deep oropharynx mucosa, lingual fascia, and epiglottis. Their function is to depress and protrude the tongue. In the severely resorbed mandible, the tubercles are often directly below the mucosa. Intrusion into the genioglossus muscle provides the possibility for profound bleeding, introduction of bacteria into deep spaces, and potential airway difficulty.

The tongue itself is also subject to injury, though more likely from a high-speed rotary instrument or disc. Moreover, if a limited alveoplasty is being performed to create adequate width for the implant head then it too can engage the errant tongue, even with an alert surgeon and assistant. Immediate exploration of any injury is vital so as to determine the extent of the injury and initiate a repair if indicated.

The sublingual glands, the smallest of the major salivary glands, are paired and located underneath the plica fimbriata in the floor of the mouth. They are a mixed salivary gland, although they produce more mucinous than serous saliva. There are generally 8–10 ducts for each gland whose orfices are found on the plica. Injury to the sublingual gland may result in formation of a ranula. Ranula in Latin means frog, referring to the typical appearance of the ranula as looking like a frog's belly. Saliva from the damaged gland or duct cannot exit to the oral cavity and a submucosal pseudocyst develops. A further complication of duct or gland injury is a cervical or plunging ranula – a much more serious and involved injury that requires repair. The plunging ranula arises from the same sublingual gland injury or injury to the ducts of Rivini. Rather than being confined to the sublingual space, it follows fascial planes below the mylohyoid muscle into the deep spaces of the neck. Ranulas and plunging ranulas require surgical removal of the offending gland as well as evacuation and debridement of the pseudocyst. Surgical treatment of ranulas and cervical ranulas are beyond the scope of this chapter (Figures 7.5 and 7.6).

Dentoalveolar complex

Implants, when properly positioned, are housed completely within alveolar bone. Lacking adequate residual alveolar height, the surgeon may place the fixtures in the residual alveolar and basilar bone. Structures residing within the maxilla and mandible are therefore susceptible to errant or inaccurate implant placement. Teeth, nerves, the maxillary sinus, and circulatory vessels are all in the path of the errant implant.

Typically, vessels within the maxilla are small nutrient arteries or perforating small branches from the overlying mucosa and soft tissues. However, the greater palatine canal and incisive canal contain relatively sizeable vessels. The incisive canal, located between and palatal to the central incisors, contains the nasopalatine nerve and artery. The greater palatine foramen is located midway between the alveolar crest and palate midline, typically in the area of the second molar. Both arteries are

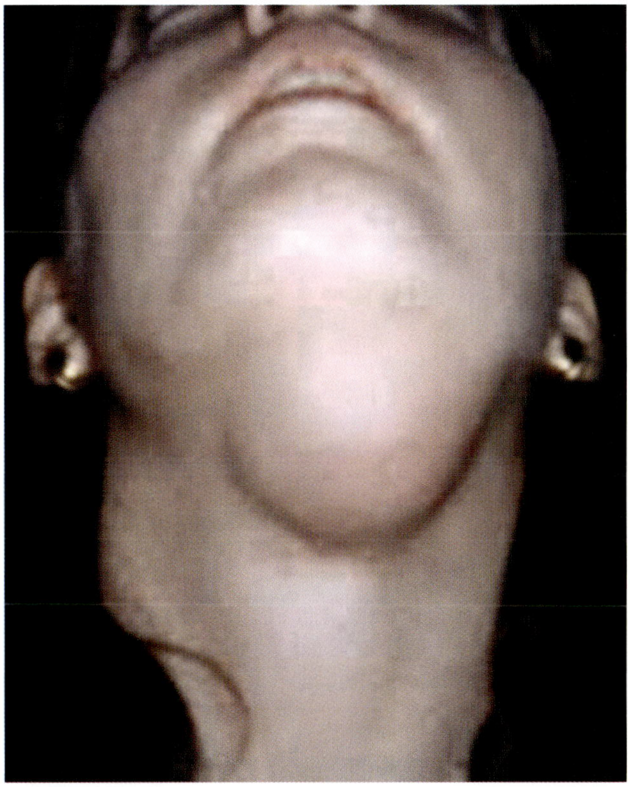

Figure 7.6 Extraoral presentation of plunging ranula.

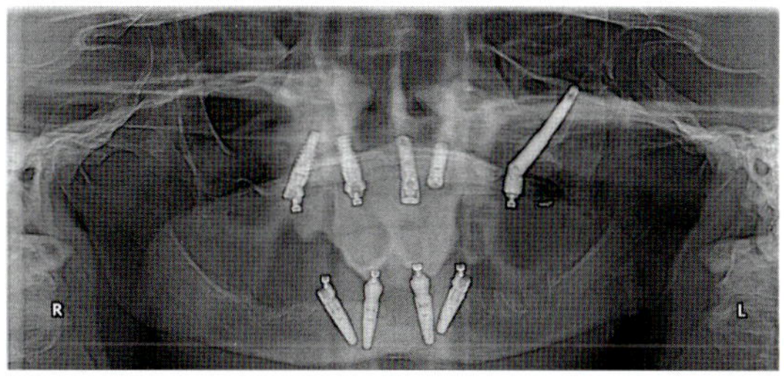

Figure 7.7 Zygomatic implant (left posterior site).

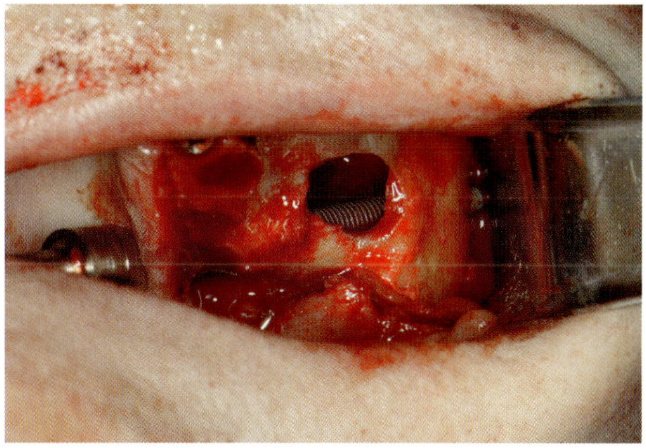

Figure 7.8 Zygoma implant traversing the maxillary sinus and engaging the zygomatic process.

terminal branches of the maxillary artery, a primary branch of the external carotid artery. While unlikely to be injured due to their locations relative to the alveolus, errant surgeons may find themselves venturing into these regions. In situations of severe bone resorption, implants may need to be angled so as to remain within bony confines, thereby potentially bringing these structures into the surgical field.

The maxillary sinus is typically found superior to and adjacent to the root apices of the premolars and molars. Sinus pneumatization occurs as we age and appears to be hastened by tooth loss.[16] This enlargement provides opportunity for the surgeon to violate the sinus floor. Small perforations are typically well handled by the patient but larger perforations may lead to lack of implant stability as well as sinus infections. The sinus is not a sterile environment and the contaminated implant surface may act as a repository for bacteria as well as a nidus for infection. It must also be noted that perforation of the sinus membrane has not been shown to significantly reduce the success rate of bone grafts or implants.[17] The zygomatic implant intentionally traverses the maxillary sinus in order to engage the zygomatic process of the maxilla (Figures 7.7 and 7.8).

Adjacent structures

The nasal floor and piriform aperture have dense cortical plates that may be engaged, when the maxilla is atrophic, for implant stabilization. Potential complications of these techniques are perforation of the nasal floor, and, subsequently, the nasal mucosa. Other structures surrounding the piriform rim subject to injury are the nasal turbinates, particularly the inferior turbinate, and the levator muscles of the upper lip. One can imagine that given the thin tissue overlying the anterior maxilla, perforation of the oral mucosa may also occur. This may develop during instrumentation whilst performing the osteotomy. Repair of injured tissues followed by reorienting the twist drills into bone is appropriate to place the implant within the confines of the maxilla. If implant stability cannot be achieved and the implant is not contained wholly within the bony confines, then removal of the fixture and grafting to re-establish architecture is advisable.

Teeth may be damaged directly by instrumentation, the implant themselves, or by violating the minimum width necessary between implant and tooth. That distance has been reported variably as between 1.5 and 2 mm.[18] Space between adjacent implants must be at least 3 mm to maintain crestal bone height.[18,19] Teeth can tolerate close proximity to adjacent roots and may actually contact an adjacent tooth root. That is not the case when considering implant-to-tooth relationships. Intraoperative radiographs to confirm proper orientation are a critical adjunct to successful implant placement. If, after the initial twist drill is used, the orientation is not ideal, the surgeon may still correct the angulations using the subsequent twist drills. A suggested protocol is to use the initial twist drill, but only to a depth of 5 mm. The guide pin is then inserted and an initial radiograph is taken. Should the angulation need to be changed,

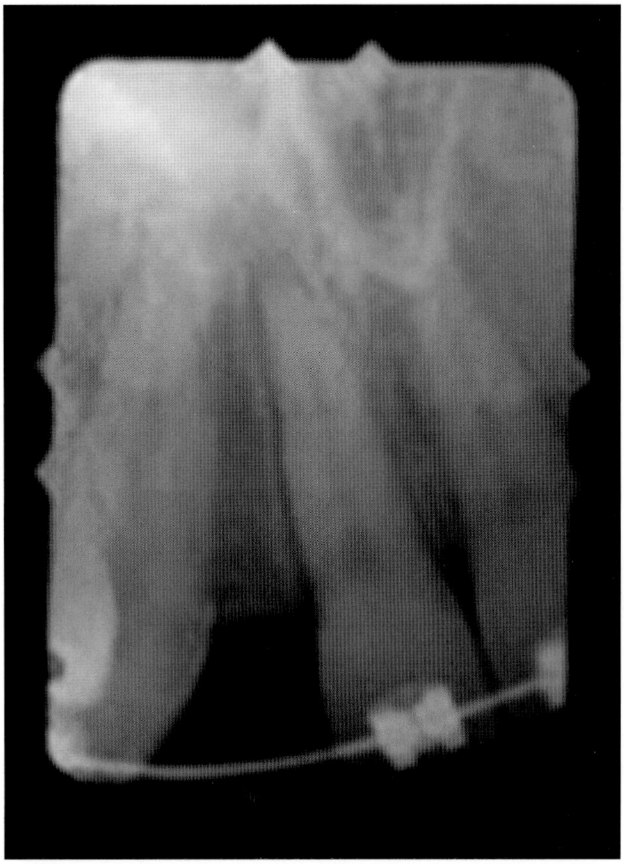

Figure 7.9 Periapical radiograph demonstrating convergent root apices.

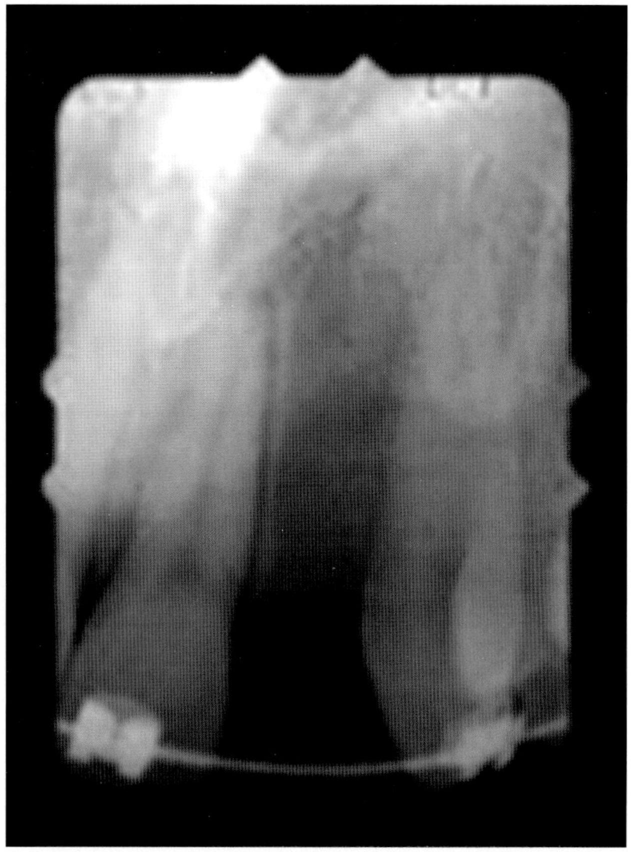

Figure 7.10 Periapical radiograph depicting adequate apical spread.

native bone is available between the 5 mm depth and the osteotomy final depth. All periodontal and endodontal issues in the peri-implant area should be addressed prior to implant placement.[20] If not treated, these issues may arise later in the form of peri-implantitis, loss of bone support, and even loss of the implant. Indolent apical lesions in the adjacent teeth may also become active with close instrumentation for implant placement.

If there is not adequate space between adjacent tooth roots or if excessive tipping of the adjacent teeth is present, then an orthodontic consultation for uprighting, manipulation of root apex position, and idealization of occlusion is warranted. There are few circumstances as frustrating to the patient as, when in the case of congenitally absent teeth, the adjacent root apices are not managed by the orthodontist during treatment. When the patient presents to the surgeon it is not infrequently their unhappy task to show the patient the limitations to implant treatment in that edentulous space. Retreatment with orthodontic appliances is necessary to achieve adequate adjacent root separation. This is disappointing and causes delay in treatment. Establishing good communication between all specialties caring for the patient is critical to timely success. This includes a pretreatment discussion of treatment goals and desired outcomes. Ongoing evaluation during treatment will ensure that those goals are being met (Figures 7.9 and 7.10).

Perioperative complications

A tenet of good surgical technique is to achieve tension-free closure of flaps. Flap design must be undertaken in a considered approach. Attention to adjacent and underlying structures along with the location of attached and unattached mucosa, coupled with direction of muscle pull and frenum attachments, are all critical components to good design. Prominent underlying bone will tend to "thin" the overlying mucosa as well as present a physical impediment to tension-free closure. Muscle attachments and presence of frena often occur at right angles to a planned incision.[21] Reorienting the incision obliquely reduces muscle pull. Release of frenum attachments at the periosteum will temporarily relieve the pull of these structures on the incision. Undermining the flap, as well as releasing the periosteum on the underside of the flap, will also aid in closure. Care must be taken, however, to score the periosteum only and not perforate the mucosa, as vascular compromise of the flap may be a direct consequence of perforation.

Dehiscence of the soft tissue flap will result in exposure of underlying structures. Bone, whether grafted or native, is subject to contamination when exposed to the oral environment. The relatively rough and porous nature of bone makes it a natural recipient bed for bacteria and foreign material, such as food particles, thereby raising the risk of infection or, at least, bone loss. If bone grafting is performed at the time of implant placement, the natural consequence of wound dehiscence is partial to complete loss of the grafted bone. Fixture screws used to gain primary stability of a block graft are easily contaminated with wound dehiscence. Barrier membranes, whether resorbable or nonresorbable, present another nidus for infection, bone loss, and ultimately compromise of the implant. The implant itself, with its highly textured surface, presents an ideal substrate for harboring bacteria. Occasionally, with two-stage surgery, the soft tissue overlying the implant cover screw is too thin to maintain adequate vascularity in spite of tension-free closure. If adequate attached mucosa is present, the patient is compliant, and esthetic constraints allow, converting the implant to a healing abutment from the cover screw is an appropriate management technique of this complication.

Bleeding and hemorrhage

Bleeding, as defined by Webster's Dictionary is, "...to lose blood from the vascular system, either internally or externally through a natural orifice or break in the skin." Hemorrhage is defined as, "...a profuse discharge of blood, as from a ruptured blood vessel, any widespread or uncontrolled loss or diffusion."[22] Bleeding and/or hemorrhage may be related to anatomic factors and variations as well as surgical misadventure. Bleeding may also be exacerbated by medications, supplements, and vitamins taken by the patient.

In today's world of supplement stores, instant nutrition, and the ability to obtain nutrition from sources other than food, many potentiators of bleeding are available and often ingested by the patient without knowledge or concern for unintended side effects. A short, but by no means comprehensive, list includes vitamin E, fish oil, ginko, garlic, ginger, ginseng, saw palmetto, dong quia, and licorice.[23] Patients also will self-medicate with aspirin, having read of its cardioprotective effects, but not disclose it on a health history.[24]

Prescription medications may have a mild to significant effect on postoperative bleeding and normal coagulation. Drugs typically used for anticoagulation or platelet aggregation inhibition are Coumadin (warfarin), aspirin, platelet-aggregation inhibitors such as Plavix (clopidogrel) or Effient (prasugrel), and factor inhibitors such as Xarelto (rivroxaban). Knowing the patient's INR (International Normalized Ratio) when taking Coumadin/warfarin will guide the surgeon as to relative risk of bleeding. Physicians managing anticoagulation and surgeons placing implants must agree on acceptable risk. The physician typically requires an INR between 2.0 and 3.0. Many surgeons are comfortable placing implants when a patient's INR is equal to or below 2.5. Some, however are comfortable with a higher number. This information is best obtained by the surgeon directly from the prescribing physician, thereby not relying on the patient's memory. Short drug holidays may be beneficial in the case of drugs such as Plavix.[25]

Patients with a recent history of cardiac catheterization with stent placement will receive one of two types of stents. The first is nondrug-eluting or bare metal stent. This patient will typically be placed on a platelet-aggregation inhibitor such as Plavix (clopidogrel), with or without aspirin for 1.5 to 12 months. Patients who receive a drug-eluting stent will most often be placed on a dual anti-platelet therapy (DAPT) combination such as Plavix and aspirin for at least 1 year with or without Coumadin.[25] Cardiologists are loath to withdraw antithrombotic therapy in these patients due to the high risk of thrombosis in the stent. Any attempt to adjust or withdraw antithrombotic therapy must only be done with full knowledge, consent, and under the direction of the cardiologist.

Patients may have undiagnosed conditions or disorders of the coagulation system (hemostasis), disorders of platelets, and disorders of blood vessels. Idiopathic thrombocytopenia purpura, coagulation disorders, and factor deficiencies, such as von Willebrand's disease and the hemophilias, must also be considered in the patient experiencing abnormal bleeding. Platelet abnormalitites may be quantitative, such as inadequate production or splenic sequestration, or be drug induced. Inadequate production is seen with undiagnosed leukemias and aplastic anemia. Sequestration may be the result of liver cirrhosis with subsequent congestive splenomegaly.

Thrombocytopenia caused by drugs is well known. Hundreds of drugs have been implicated with their effect being either a disruption of platelet production or platelet destruction.[26] Drugs, such as sulfonamides, quinines, antibiotics, anticonvulsants and gold salts used in treating arthritis, are known to cause destruction of platelets.

There may also be qualitative defects in platelets. Examples of this are medication-induced change in function such as aspirin (ASA), NSAIDs, Plavix, etc.[27] Systemic factors and diseases such as uremia and multiple myeloma may also exert a qualitative effect on platelets. Vascular disorders are seen in patients with amyloidosis, Ehlers–Danlos, osteogenesis imperfecta, Marfan syndrome, and others, resulting in fragility of the vasculature.

Bleeding is a common and expected occurrence during an oral surgical procedure. Mild bleeding, in the absence of the considerations discussed earlier, is generally self-limiting. When faced with brisk or excessive bleeding, an assessment must be quickly made to determine if anatomic boundaries have been violated. When certain that the surgical procedure is proceeding as planned and the bone cortices have not been violated, bleeding is often controlled with local measures. Direct pressure helps by slowing blood flow and allowing the patient's natural clotting ability to begin to work. Pressure in the form of stretched moistened gauze carefully packed into the osteotomy and then held in place with firm finger pressure is usually enough to quell brisk bleeding. Vessel retraction and constriction, coupled with platelet aggregation and the initiation of fibrin formation, slows bleeding. Collagen products absorb many times their weight in blood; via the intrinsic pathway of clotting, they also cause platelet aggregation.[28,29] Aggregated platelets degranulate and release clotting factors such as thromboxane A, all of which aid in cessation of bleeding.

Frank hemorrhage or bleeding not controlled simply with local measures is a life-threatening event. Airway embarrassment through hematoma formation in soft tissues and malignant shock from extreme volume loss are sequelae of uncontrolled hemorrhage. Surgical intervention may be indicated to dissect, locate the vessel, and ligate it. Interventional radiography may also be performed to embolize the damaged vessel. Late complications of embolization are arterial venous shunts, aneurysm, and localized tissue ischemia, although these are less likely in the head and neck, given vascular redundancy.

If anatomic barriers such as bone cortices are violated, then the adjacent soft tissue is susceptible to injury. Rich *et al.*[30] grouped arterial injuries into five classifications: transection, laceration, contusion, spasm, and arteriovenous fistula. Of all reported arterial injuries, 85–90% were noted to be lacerations or transections.[30]

In the maxilla, the anterior portion typically has labial or buccal concavities superior to the alveolar crest. In the posterior maxilla the greater palatine artery, a descending branch of the external carotid artery emerges from the greater palatine canal at or near the junction of the maxilla and sphenoid bones. Anatomically, that corresponds to a point distal to the second molar near the junction of the alveolar process and the palatal vault. The artery may be at risk of violation when the anatomy is not respected.

Regarding the mandible, other than the inferior alveolar nerve, it is the contents of the floor of the mouth that are susceptible to injury. Anterior and posterior mandible may have concavities that are not palpable and can only be appreciated with imaging such as CT or CBCT. Contents of the floor of mouth that are at risk include the submandibular duct, ducts of the sublingual glands, and the lingual artery and its branches. The lingual artery arises from the external carotid artery at the level in the neck of the greater horn of the hyoid bone. It passes deep to the hyoglossus muscle and then into the floor of the mouth. The major branches are the hyoid artery and the sublingual artery, which are given off before the artery enters the confines of the tongue. It is the sublingual artery and its branches that are at risk from the surgical misadventure. The medial mandibular branch of the sublingual artery provides blood supply to the lingual aspect of the anterior mandible. It is found adjacent to the cortex and may also provide perforating arteries through the cortex. Those too are susceptible to damage.

One can imagine a twist drill or bone tap used to prepare the osteotomy venturing outside the bony confines and traumatizing the tissues immediately adjacent to the cortex. Use of preoperative imaging, such as those mentioned earlier, will reveal concavities and other anatomic variations. Use of a probe during site preparation may reduce this potentially catastrophic complication. Careful inspection of the osteotomy before stepping up to the next sized twist drill may reveal cortex compromise before greater damage occurs. A periodontal probe can investigate all aspects of the osteotomy and quickly discern cortex breach. Many implant companies also provide probes for sounding the bone.

Errant implant position

The surgeon may find, on radiographic examination or postoperative visit, that the implant is no longer in its original position. Several factors may contribute to this complication, the most obvious being lack of initial stability. The patient may also initiate movement of the implant with noncompliance. Forceful chewing, bruxism without using a guard, or intentional efforts to displace can all unseat the implant from its initial position. The sinus is the most common repository for the misplaced implant in the maxilla. In the mandible, the typically dense type I or II cortical bone usually resists undue forces. If the quantity of the cortical bone is reduced, the implant may be displaced inferiorly into the cancellous spaces. When faced with a displaced implant, the surgeon must determine the best approach for retrieval. Access for removal with a minimal disruption of anatomy is critical for overall success. Once the implant is retrieved, a critical assessment is needed to determine whether another implant can be placed, if grafting should be performed, or if implant treatment should be abandoned in favor of an alternate therapy (Figure 7.11).

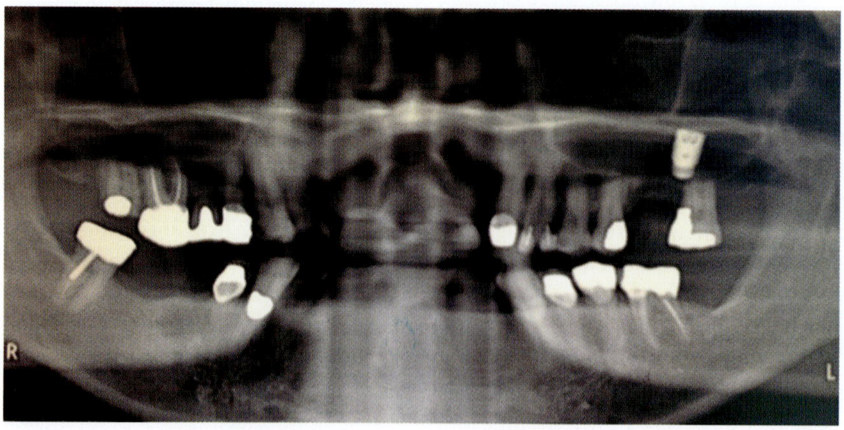

Figure 7.11 Implant displaced into the maxillary sinus.

Loss of integration/implant loosening

Primary, or initial, stability is paramount for implant success. Lack of initial stability virtually assures failure and the savvy surgeon will remove the implant and graft the area as a prelude to reimplantation. If there is enough bone present and adjacent structures are not at risk, a larger-diameter implant may be considered for immediate placement. Many factors and theories abound as causes for late loss of integration. Excess cement extruding into the peri-implant soft tissue provides chronic irritation and an ideal substrate for bacteria. Traumatic occlusion may also eventually overwhelm successful integration in the presence of inflammation. Occult infection, such as that remaining after endodontic therapy, has also been implicated. Periodontal health of adjacent teeth is another factor contributing to implant success. A comprehensive approach to the patient's dental health and needs is critical for an accurate prognosis. It is the practitioner with a nonholistic view of the patient needs who may be faced with unexpected complications.

Errors in positioning

Proper positioning of the implant in all three axes, buccal–lingual, mesiodistal, and apical–coronal, is essential for a good esthetic result. This is especially critical in the esthetic zone. The restoring dentist, in collaboration with a talented laboratory technician, may overcome some errors in implant placement, but not all. The head of the implant is ideally located 3 mm below the adjacent cementoenamel junction (CEJ), centered in the edentulous space mesiodistally, at least 2 mm palatal to the facial bone and emerging at or near the cingulum of the restoration (for screw-retained restorations). Tissue biotype, hard and soft tissue defects, and condition of adjacent teeth all impact the location of the implant as well as the long-term esthetic results. Thin biotype soft tissues are more likely to reveal errors in implant location than thick. A low smile line may mercifully hide what might be an otherwise poor esthetic result.[31]

Patient compliance

An open communication between patient and practitioner is a *sine qua non* for dependable compliance in the different stages of treatment. It appears that patients comply less with treatment directives when they feel that their clinician has not complied with acknowledgment of their needs. With that being said, it is quite difficult to appreciate and understand patients' priorities and unspoken agenda during the short initial interview and examination appointment. Patients will reveal what they want their audience to know or what they think their practitioner wants to know. Spoken priorities and unspoken priorities may be at odds with one another. Patients' stated desire to rid themselves of a troublesome tooth may in fact cover their high esthetic demands. Patients might also be looking for a scapegoat for their overarching psychosocial issues. Recapitulation and restating their comments and questions are but one method of active engagement and confirmation.

A comprehensive informed consent is always beneficial for offering the patient a customized cost, benefit, and risk analysis, as well as sorting out responsibility in the event of a complication. Careful screening by the treatment team may uncover trends, behavior patterns, or habits that can increase the likelihood of complications. Patients with occult habits, such as smoking, bruxism, and excessive alcohol consumption, may present as someone with no potential risk factors. A frank discussion with the patient prior to surgery will disclose risks associated with these habits.

Upon successful completion of the implant procedure and after patients are discharged, their activities, behavior, and habits largely control short- and long-term success. Patients' ability and willingness to comply with both preoperative and postoperative instructions are paramount to successful treatment. In a work-up for implant or preimplant surgery, there is invariably a deluge of information that may overwhelm the patient. That list of "dos and don'ts" may serve to confuse not inform them. Consistent instructions given over time in multiple formats (verbal, visual, print) may improve patient compliance.

Activities will likely need to be modified during the immediate postoperative period. Patients may minimize or trivialize the importance of activity restriction, not wanting to interfere with their daily routines. Work-related activity and exercise for health and fitness must be modified in the immediate recovery period as well. Patients who perform manual labor will need greater restrictions than those who have sedentary jobs.

Diet modification to encourage atraumatic mastication will reduce patient-generated loss of primary stability. Recommending a diet where everything ingested is "cut easily with a fork" or softer during the healing period can help avoid the "food-as-a-weapon" potential. Direct counseling, repeating the mantra of soft diet, providing written postoperative instructions, and close active follow-up/recall may prevent patients from straying to an inappropriate diet.

Careful but gentle hygiene is critical to suture and soft-tissue integrity. Avoiding the surgical site(s) with toothbrush, water pick, floss, and toothpicks is seemingly obvious but bears repeating to the patient. Rinsing with an antimicrobial solution is an atraumatic method of maintenance. It is extremely disappointing for the careful surgeon, who after a successful implant surgery, sees the patient for a postoperative visit only to discover early loss of sutures with soft-tissue flap dehiscence. Patients are typically uncomfortable and looking for a "reason why". Gentle, nonaccusatory questions regarding diet, hygiene habits, and activities will frequently uncover an event that coincides with the complication.

Conclusion

An educated and compliant patient with a tailored treatment plan and thoughtful execution of that plan will reduce the incidence of complications. When complications arise, as inevitably they will, timely and appropriate intervention is necessary to rectify the issue at hand. Postoperative follow-ups are an essential part of treatment. It is during those visits that complications will declare themselves, from patient reporting, direct observation, and/or imaging. Corrective action may run the gamut from watchful waiting, as in the presence of inflammation, to medical management, as in the presence of infection. Implant removal and site rehabilitation may be needed to arrest an ongoing complication. Whatever the complication, open and clear communication coupled with reassurance of the surgeon's willingness to "see this through" will help to assuage the patient's anxiety and fear regarding the unexpected occurrence. It cannot be overstated how clear, open, and empathetic communication is critical to the remedy and the patient's perception of success. The most talented surgeon will not be viewed as successful if he or she is unable or unwilling to engage the patient in an honest and informative dialogue.

References

1. Todescan S, Lavigne S, Kelekis-Cholakis A. Guidance for the maintenance care of dental implants: clinical review. *J Can Dent Assoc* 2012; **78**: c107.
2. Iqbal MK, Kim S. For teeth requiring endodontic treatment, what are the differences in outcomes of restored endodontically treated teeth compared to implant supported restorations? *Int J Oral Maxillofacial Implants* 2007; **22**(suppl): 96–116.
3. Seddon H. A classification of nerve injuries. *Br Med J* 1942; **2**(4260): 237–239.
4. Sunderland S. A classification of peripheral nerve injuries producing loss of function. *Brain* 1951; **74**(4): 491–516.
5. MacKinnon S, Dellon A. *Classification of Nerve Injuries as the Basis of Treatment*. New York: Theime Medical Publishers 1988; 35–63.
6. Bedrossian E. *Implant Treatment Planning for the Edentulous Patient*. St. Louis: Mosby Elsevier 2011; 69–79.
7. Misch C, Crawford E. Predictable mandibular nerve location – a clinical zone of safety. *Int J Oral Implantol* 1990; 7(1): 37–40.
8. Massey ND, Galil KA, Wilson TD. Determining position of the inferior alveolar nerve via anatomical dissection and micro-computed tomography in preparation for dental implants. *J Can Dent Assoc* 2013; **79**: d39.
9. Hagen QH. Pathophysiology of peripheral nerve injury during regional anesthesia. *Reg Anesth Pain Med* 2008; **33**(5): 435–441.
10. Hillerup S, Jensen RH, Ersboll BK. Trigeminal nerve injury associated with injection of local anesthetics. *J Am Dent Assoc* 2011; **142**(5): 531–539.
11. Renton T, Yilmaz Z. Managing iatrogenic trigeminal nerve injury: a case series and review of the literature. *Int J Oral Maxillofac Surg* 2012; **41**(5): 629–637.
12. Nerve Injuries. Trigeminal Foundation (Internet). Available from: http://trigeminalnerve.org.uk/professional-resources/manage-nerve-injuries/
13. Siemonow M, Estenmann-Klein M. *Plastic and Reconstructive Surgery*. London: Springer-Verlag 2010; 523–538.
14. *Mosby's Medical Dictionary*, 8th edn. Elsevier 2009.
15. Ariji Y, Kuroki T, Moriguchi S, *et al.* Age changes in the volume of the human maxillary sinus: a study using computed tomography. *Dentomaxillofac Radiol* 1994; **23**(3): 163–168.
16. Oh E, Kraut RA. Effect of sinus membrane perforation on dental implant integration: a retrospective study in 128 patients. *Implant Dent* 2011; **20**(1): 13–16.
17. Worthington P. Injury to the inferior alveolar nerve during implant placement: a formula for protection of the patient and clinician. *Int J Oral Maxillofac Implants* 2004; **19**(5): 731–734.
18. Danza M, Zollino I, Avantaggiato A, *et al.* Distance between implants has a potential impact of crestal bone resorption. *Saudi Dent J* 2011; **23**(3): 129–133.
19. Tarnow D, Cho S, Wallace S. The effect of inter-implant distance on the height of inter-implant bone. *J Periodontol* 2000; **71**(4): 546–549.
20. Porter J, Fraunhofer J. Success or failure of dental implants? A literature review with treatment considerations. Online, *General Dentistry*: Nov/Dec 2005.
21. Romanos G. Periosteal releasing incision for successful coverage of augmented sites. A technical note. *J Implantol* 2010; **36**(1): 25–30.
22. Merriam-Webster Online Dictionary (Internet); Springfield, Ma 2015. Bleeding, Hemorrhage. Available from: http://www.merriam-webster.com
23. Boyles S. Surgery patients unaware of herbal risk. WebMD Health News: April 16, 2009 Available from: http://webmd.com
24. On the Pulse News. Daily aspirin helpful to heart patients, not healthy individuals. (Internet) June 8, 2009. Available from: http://heartandstroke.com/site/apps/ninet/content2.aspx?c+ikIQLcMWJ+E&b=3485821&ct=7065257
25. Cutlip D. Antiplatelet therapy after coronary stenting 2015 (updated 2015 Jun 08). Available from: http://www.update.com
26. Visentin GP, Liu CY. Drug induced thrombocytopenia. *Hematol Oncol Clin North Am* 2007; **21**(4): 685–696.
27. Barwell J. Acquired platelet function disorder. 2012 Jul 16. Available from: http://www.healtline.com/health/acquired-platelet-function-defect
28. Review of hemostatic agents used in dentistry. Dentistry Today (Internet) 2005 March Available from: http://www.dentistry today. com/oral-medicine/oral surgery/1538-sp-1459248816
29. Collaplug (package insert). Plainsboro, NJ: Integra LifeSciences Corp 2001.
30. Farndale RW, Sixma JJ, Barnes MJ, *et al.* The role of collagen in thrombosis and hemostasis. *J Thromb Haemost* 2004; **2**(4): 561–573.
31. Al-Sabbagh M. Implants in the esthetic zone. *Dent Clin N Am* 2006; **50**(3): 391–407.

CHAPTER 8
Failure in Osseointegration

Kumar C. Shah[1], S. Andrew Chapokas[2], and Sreenivas Koka[3]
[1] University of California Los Angeles School of Dentistry, Los Angeles, California, USA
[2] San Diego, California, USA
[3] Loma Linda University School of Dentistry, Loma Linda, California, USA

Introduction

Successful osseointegration is the result of a state of "osseosufficiency", where the net contribution of the patient (host), the implant, and the clinician combine to promote and perpetuate osseointegration.[1] Following on, when an insufficient state results, the interface between host bone and an implant deteriorates and experiences "osseoseparation" (Table 8.1). In this chapter, we discuss the roles of patient, implant, and clinician as they relate to osseosufficiency, osseoseparation, and failure of osseointegration. In particular, we challenge the dogma that "implants fail" and ask all clinician scholars to ask themselves, "Do implants really fail?" in the way they are purported to behave. Or, in reality, are implants "retrieved", normally as a consequence of a combined set of events far more dependent upon the behavior of the patient and the clinician than of the implant? Perhaps our desire to find someone or something to blame when an implant is retrieved predisposes us to blame the one element that cannot answer back – the implant. In this chapter, we discuss in detail key attributes of patients, clinicians, and implants that are associated with failure in osseointegration.

Patient factors

In order for dental implants to remain "healthy" and in function, it is clear that direct bone apposition is required with minimally inflamed soft tissue surrounding the transmucosal interface. Although a certain amount of marginal bone loss may be tolerated, progression of bone loss may pose a serious threat to implant longevity. Criteria for implant success have been defined with a need for a reliable presence of bone around dental implants.[2] More recently, the previous nomenclature for peri-implant pathology has been challenged. Traditionally, inflammation with crestal bone loss around dental implants has been termed *peri-implantitis*. When gingival and/or mucosal inflammation exists, without bone loss, the term *peri-implant mucositis* is used. As the mechanisms for peri-implant pathology have been evolving, application of new terminology has been suggested.[1,3] Osseosufficiency best describes the process whereby osseointegration is maintained. When the soft tissue and bone–implant interfaces are compromised, osseoseparation has been used as a replacement of the term peri-implantitis.[4] Differentiation between primary and secondary peri-implantitis has been offered to clarify whether or not infection was considered as the primary cause for peri-implant bone loss or not, respectively.[3] Regardless of the terms used, new insight to peri-implant disease will be described that may entirely change the way that we understand the processes of developing, maintained, and lost osseointegration.

Several risk factors for peri-implantitis and marginal bone loss have been proposed, and the primary theories have been classically considered to be infection or overloading of dental implants. However, it is controversial as to which mechanisms best explain changes in the inflammatory status and marginal bone loss around dental implants. Until recently, biomaterials, surgical hardware, and any other foreign material have been understood as inert bodies that have no specific effect on the immune system and/or surrounding tissues. Now, there has been a paradigm shift in the approach to investigating the causes of peri-implantitis and associated peri-implant marginal bone loss. Osseointegration is better understood as a foreign body equilibrium reaction that requires a series of complex mechanisms in order to avoid host rejection that may manifest as peri-implant marginal bone loss and soft tissue inflammation (Figure 8.1). Therefore, the immune system dynamically determines the fate of any implant within living tissues.[5,6] In order to understand osseointegration, both the biomaterials and host immune characteristics need to be addressed.

Foreign body reactions are characterized by granulomatous inflammation, which is a distinctive pattern of chronic inflammation that occurs for a limited number of infectious and noninfectious conditions. When a certain offender is difficult or

Evidence-based Implant Treatment Planning and Clinical Protocols, First Edition. Edited by Steven J. Sadowsky.

Companion website: www.wiley.com/go/sadowsky/implant

Table 8.1 Osseoseparation staging system.

Stage 0 osseoseparation
Implant is asymptomatic and immobile
"Nuisance gingivitis" may or may not be present
Marginal bone loss is minimal
Eligible for prosthodontic abutment service with a predictable esthetic outcome
Stage I osseoseparation
Implant is asymptomatic and immobile
Gingivitis may or may not be present
Eligible for prosthodontic abutment service, although marginal bone loss and minimal accompanying implant material exposure may preclude a satisfactory esthetic outcome
Readily managed with routine debridement and oral hygiene protocols
Additional clinical intervention is not required because of noncompromising site location, e.g., favorable circumoral lip morphology. Alternatively, minor prosthetic design alterations may be indicated
Stage II osseoseparation
Implant is asymptomatic and immobile
Gingivitis is often present
Frequently precludes esthetically satisfactory prosthodontic outcome since the amount of marginal bone loss also exposes implant threads
Favorable oral hygiene considerations or a satisfactory esthetic outcome cannot be achieved without secondary changes in prosthesis design or attempting secondary plastic gingival surgical interventions
Stage III osseoseparation
Bone loss location may be variable and often substantial, although the implant(s) remain(s) asymptomatic and immobile
Gingivitis almost invariably present
Only eligible for prosthodontic abutment service if resultant esthetic and oral hygiene concerns can be rectified by additional interventions
Treatment outcome and prognostic considerations (both patient- and dentist-mediated ones) frequently demand change(s) in the original treatment plan, including removal of the implant(s) and surgical site development
Stage IV osseoseparation
Implant is usually symptomatic and slight mobility is almost invariably present
Bone loss may present as either inconsequential or substantially so
Gingivitis may or may not be present Biologic failure of the osseointegration process has occurred (early failure) or has developed gradually on an osseoinsufficiency/time-dependent basis (late failure)

impossible to eradicate, a granuloma will typically form in attempt to contain it. As in other types of chronic inflammation, tissue injury and attempted repair coexist over long or indefinite periods of time. Macrophages are the dominant cell type in chronic inflammation, and are differentiated from the mononuclear phagocyte system.[7] It is widely understood that macrophages play a key role this process and have been stratified into two different phenotypes. M1 macrophages are reactive, phagocytic, and proinflammatory, whereas M2 macrophages are more involved in the simultaneous repair phases that occur during chronic inflammation.[8]

Blood monocytes traffic into connective tissue or certain organs such as the liver (Kupffer cells) and central nervous system (microglia). Furthermore, bone-specific macrophages called osteomacs, have been identified on or near periosteal surfaces forming a canopy-like structure over mature osteoblasts. Although it is unclear whether osteomacs play a role in bone remodeling, newer emerging data suggest that osteomac populations play a role in bone homeostasis. Osteomac expression of cytokines, such as transforming growth factor (TGF)-beta and ephrin B2, provide coupling signals that have been previously implicated in osteoclastic regulation of bone formation.[9]

Granulomatous reactions are categorized based on *two* different types of pathogenic responses. *Foreign body granulomas* develop in response to inert foreign bodies. Histologically, macrophages aggregate, transform into epithelial-like cells, and may later fuse to become multinucleated giant cells (Langerhans or foreign body type with no known functional difference at this time). Typically, the foreign body will be in the center of the granuloma, does not incite any specific immune response, and is too large to allow phagocytosis by macrophages. At the periphery of the granuloma, there is a layer of mononuclear leukocytes, consisting of mostly lymphocytes and occasionally plasma cells. On the other hand, *immune granulomas* are caused by agents that can induce a cell-mediated immune response. A more complex series of immunogenic reactions takes place whereby macrophages ingest foreign protein antigen and present it to antigen-specific T lymphocytes. This process results in a series of cellular interactions through the production of several proinflammatory cytokines, such as interleukin (IL)-2 and interferon (IFN)-gamma that ultimately increase the transformation of macrophages to epithelioid cells and multinucleated giant cells. The most common example of an immune granuloma occurs in association with *Mycobacterium tuberculosis*.[7]

Until recently, dental implants have only been considered as inert biomaterials having no specific immunological effects. It now seems that the contrary is the case. Histologic evidence demonstrates the presence of multinucleated giant cells regularly found at the bone–titanium interface. Even though this alone can justify the concept of osseointegration

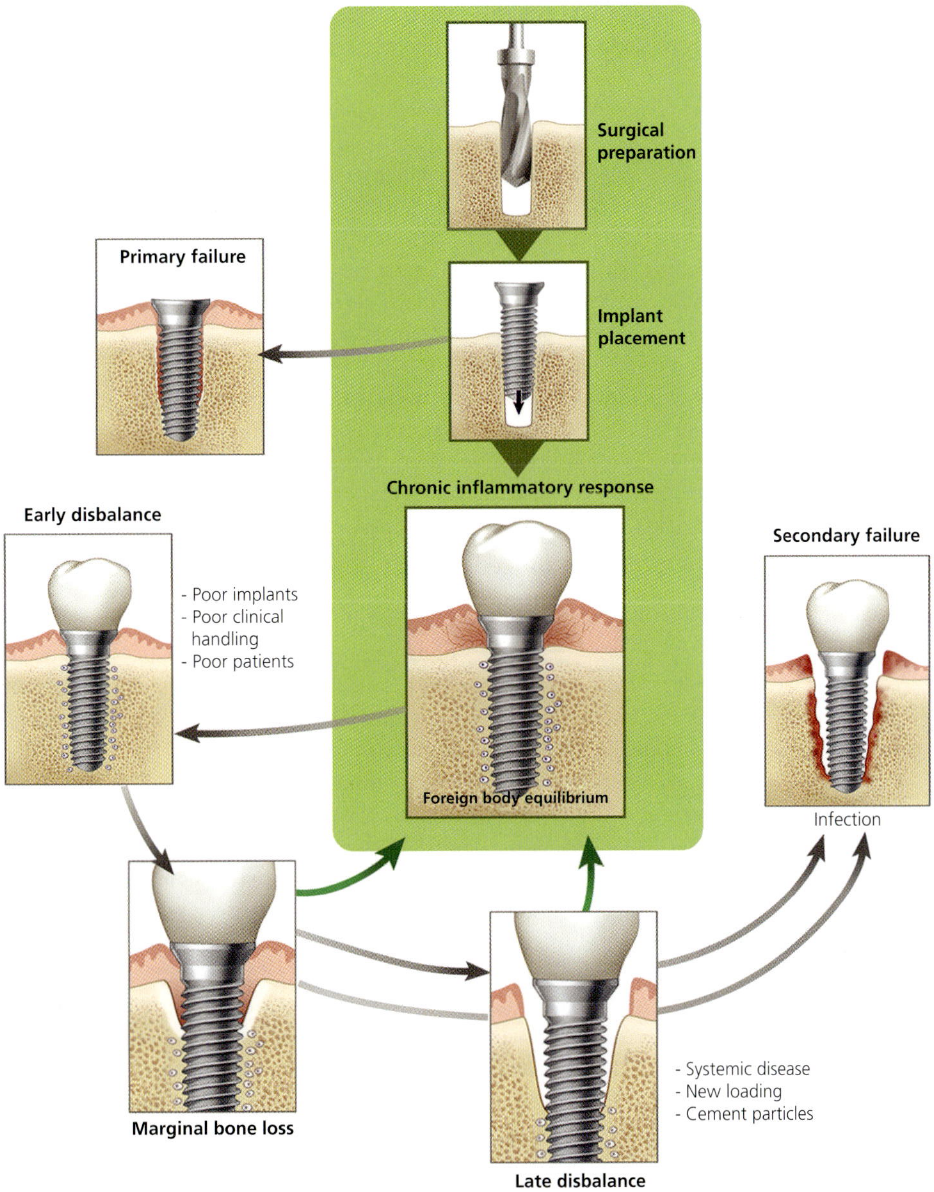

Figure 8.1 Foreign body equilibrium reaction. *Source:* © 2016, Chris Gralapp.

being a foreign body reaction, surface protein adsorption by titanium and other biomaterials has been demonstrated to have significant effects on the host response to further this concept. Certain proteins, such as fibrinogen, have been demonstrated to have hidden amino acid sequences that become exposed when adsorbed to a surface and/or denatured when compared to the soluble form.[10] When proteins are absorbed, they are unfolded and different antigenic sequences are exposed with the capability of inducing an entire host of molecular and cellular responses. The net result of these reactions can naturally have negative and/or positive effects.

Considering osseointegration as a dynamic series of complex host immune interactions, Albrektsson and colleagues[6] propose the following: 1) osseointegration is the result of a foreign body reaction that, with the right intensity in the inflammatory response, will balance itself out and allow for bone to grow on the implant surface; 2) similar to soft-tissue implants, which end up in poorly innervated and vascularized fibrous tissue, dental implants also become surrounded by condensed bone that is very poor in vascularization and innervation typical of a foreign body reaction that has reached equilibrium; and 3) this newly formed bone may be seen as a manner of shielding off the foreign entity from the tissues as a protective mechanism.[2]

Then, once an implant has "successfully" integrated, why does implant retrieval occur? What is the most plausible evidence? As mentioned previously, up until this time, infection and overloading have been the most accepted theories. However, there is no evidence of a primarily infection-driven reason for marginal bone loss around dental implants.[3] Some data exist to suggest that overloading of dental implants may result in marginal bone loss, but there is no evidence that suggests this is the sole factor when it is involved. There is most likely a disturbance in the foreign body equilibrium that changes the immunologic nature of the surrounding cells, resulting in marginal bone loss that is secondarily colonized by bacterial offenders.[5] This complex series of interactions can be initiated by a variety of biologic responses, including different dendritic cell phenotypes, autoimmune disorders, influence of medication, such as selective serotonin reuptake inhibitors (SSRIs), and even additional aseptic foreign body reactions to surrounding cement particles.[6,11–13] Further investigation and understanding of phenotypical variation in patients may provide better insight into the critical role of the immune system with regards to the fate of an implant in both the short and long term.

Implant factors

The dental literature exhaustively describes implant design variables that may influence osseointegration. Implant manufacturers have presented anecdotal clinical evidence suggesting clinical success with their implant systems. We will review some implant design variables and discuss how implant therapy is influenced by these variables.

Implant surface/coating

Since the introduction of the machined Branemark implant, multiple different roughened or micro-roughened implant surfaces have been introduced. For successful osseointegration, the biologic processes of blood clot formation, release of growth factors, and osteogenesis are paramount. A roughened surface improves the surface tension and wettability of the surface to plasma proteins. Consequently, platelets and growth factors from the fibrin clot attract migratory osteoprogenitor cells. Osteoprogenitor cells in the wound site initially deposit woven bone. Davies[14,15] described distance and contact osteogenesis, where, in distance osteogenesis, new bone is formed on the surface of old bone away from the implant surface, and contact osteogenesis is bone formation by those cells on the implant surface. When comparing distant and contact osteogenesis, implant surface characteristics preferentially influence contact osteogenesis.

Modification of machined titanium has been achieved via several mechanisms. Surfaces could be blasted with titanium grits, etched with acid, electrolytically modified, or be treated by any combination of these processes. Multiple studies have demonstrated that micro-roughened surfaces achieve superior osseointegration when measured using surrogates, such as torque removal force, bone appositional index, and gene expression, in addition to supporting evidence from clinical outcome studies. However, when roughened surfaces are exposed in the oral cavity, the propensity for increased plaque adherence could result in bone loss. This bone loss may be enhanced or expedited in certain categories of patients, especially smokers.

While there may be some microscopic differences in the bone–implant interface between various implant surfaces, there is still a lack of evidence to clearly demonstrate any superior implant surface. Many clinicians believe that using any one of a number of micro-roughened surface implants achieves initial clinical osseointegration. Following on, other factors assist in the maintenance of the osseosufficient state.

Implant dimensions

Implant length, diameter, and other design variables, like taper and thread pitch, are some of the factors that yield the biomechanical stability necessary for osseosufficiency. Nevertheless, early implant retrieval due to insufficient implant stability may occur.

Length

Short implants may integrate well when used in a delayed loading protocol approach. However, in cases of immediate load, short implants may not provide sufficient primary stability to prevent micromotion above 150 microns that could predispose to downward epithelial migration and fibrous encapsulation, leading ultimately to failure in osseointegration. While short machined implants have been demonstrated to have lower success rates, more recent systematic reviews have concluded that moderately roughened short implants (<10 mm) have similar peri-implant marginal bone loss as standard implants (10 mm or longer).[16] Splinting of short implants because of concerns regarding inordinate crown to implant ratios and ensuing marginal bone loss has not been shown to be essential when crown to implant ratios are up to 2.5:1.[17,18]

In immediate implant placement scenarios, longer implants are beneficial to engage the native bone beyond the apex in order to yield better initial stability.

Diameter

Implant diameter impacts short- and long-term implant success.[19] Previously, wider-diameter implants of 5 mm or 6 mm were used to achieve primary stability. When a regular-diameter implant is unstable, a wide implant can still engage the lateral bone in order to provide stability. However, in the presence of inadequate buccal plate dimensions, use of wide-diameter implants could lead to significant complications with some studies showing up to a 20% retrieval rate.[20,21] Nevertheless, when used in appropriate sites where there is bone available, naturally or after bone grating/augmentation, success rates of wide-diameter and regular-diameter implants are similar.[22–24]

Today, certain systems propose use of implants with an 8 or 9 mm diameter in fresh extraction sockets in the molar region and claim adequate primary stability in these sites.[25,26] However, long-term clinical data are lacking with these implants used for this clinical indication.

Implant design and thread patterns

Most of the implant systems available today are threaded and screw type. Pressed fit cylindrical implants are not popular any longer and will not be included in our discussion. The primary types of implant body type are parallel-sided and tapered implants. Parallel sides are generally regarded to be a little more forgiving in terms of osteotomy site preparation and the implant can generally be reversed out to place the platform at a more desired location apicocoronally. However, initial stability may not be sufficient for immediately loaded situations. In contrast, tapered implants may provide greater initial stability and may be suited better for placement in extraction sockets to engage the available bone.[27] Therefore, tapered implants are a common choice for immediate placement and/or immediate loading. Furthermore, some implants are designed to have a cutting and aggressive screw thread pattern in order to attain superior stability at the time of placement, and some implant systems have a micro-thread pattern on the coronal part of the implant.[28]

Implant platform

In recent years there has been major discussion regarding the implant and abutment platform. The "platform switch" concept was a serendipitous one. It is the situation where the restorative abutment platform is smaller than the implant platform. There are several different theories as to the reason for this benefit and clinical studies have demonstrated the benefit of the maintenance of the bone levels adjacent to the implant and in turn the corresponding peri-implant tissues. However, the relatively recent introduction of platform switching means that long-term studies are awaited.[29]

It has been proposed that the micro-gap may open and close microscopically during functional loading.[30] Whereas, a flat-top implant platform seems to be more susceptible to this opening and closing compared to a conical/tapered implant–abutment connection, flat-top designs may predispose to greater stress being applied to the abutment retaining screw with a resultant higher complications rate. Among other mechanical benefits of conical connections, like reduction of screw loosening and screw fracture, more load is transmitted directly to the implant and indirectly to the adjacent bone, although excess load could lead to implant fracture or bone loss if insufficient thought had been utilized during treatment planning. There appears to be better bone maintenance around implants with a conical type connection than flat-top implants.[31]

In summary, each manufacturer has responded to the marketplace demands by inordinate permutations of implant surface, design, and dimensions. This has challenged the clinician to not only select appropriate iterations for individual patient needs but has impacted the steepness of his/her learning curve. Here we have an unanticipated result from industry innovation.

Clinician factors

It is clear that the incidence of complications consequent to implant therapy is on the rise despite improving implant survival rates.[32] Of sufficient significance, numerous published papers and portions of scientific programs are devoted to the issue of "complications". Since complications can have far-reaching consequences, including restoration failure, implant retrieval, and loss of osseous or soft tissues yielding significant defects, the attention given to complications is understandable. However, in the context of the osseosufficiency model, most of the attention has focused on the dental implant, a little attention has been afforded the patient, and almost no attention has been placed on the clinician and consequent iatrogenic etiologies to implant retrieval. The surface presentation of implants to the host has certainly changed as machined surfaces have given way to treated surfaces to increase "roughness", and the microscopic presentation of a roughened implant is different to that of a polished implant. Nevertheless, despite a potpourri of connections and abutments and materials and digital technologies available, the dental implants of today are macroscopically the same as dental implants of 30 years ago – we are still using a metal screw-threaded implant with or without tapering walls. So if the implants are essentially similar and patients do not present with a different biological host response to that 30 years ago, why are implant complications so much more common? Could it be that the reason does not lie with the implant or with the patient, but with the clinician? Is the clinician engaged in providing implant therapy today different to the clinician engaged in providing implant therapy 30 years ago? In all likelihood, there are three clinician factors that impact the success of dental implant therapy: experience, knowledge, and competence. Patients of experienced, knowledgeable, and competent clinicians suffer few complications (Figure 8.2).

Experience/inexperience of clinician

Clinician experience level impacts clinical outcomes, and definitively so when interventional irreversible procedures are performed. Some call this scenario "the learning curve", a phenomenon first described by Herman Ebbinghaus, a psychologist. From other fields of study, the terms "experience curve", "improvement curve", and "progress curve" are used synonymously with learning curve.

The medical literature is replete with evidence indicating that many types of surgical intervention are sensitive to the learning

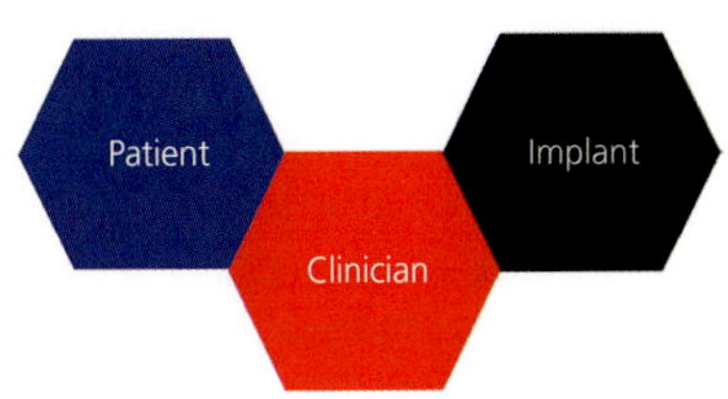

Figure 8.2 The osseosufficiency triad of clinician, patient, and implant.

curve concept. In some studies, clinical outcomes appear to be better, for example quicker healing time or lower complication rate and especially in more complex cases,[33–35] whereas in others the clinical outcomes are not better but the efficiency with which the procedure was completed on the day of surgery is improved, such as reduced operative time.[36,37] In some types of surgery, surgeon experience affects both clinical outcome and improves efficiency.[38,39] Improvements in clinical outcome enhance the quality of treatment and reduced operative time lowers the cost of treatment. Alone or in combination, the value of the care to the patient increases once a surgeon moves up the learning curve.

The dental literature does not offer many investigations of the effect of clinician experience, yet what is available parallels the findings observed in medicine, in that surgeon experience impacts clinical outcomes of dental implant therapy,[40–42] with better outcomes observed when more experienced clinicians are involved. *In vitro* investigation confirms that the experience level of the operator placing implants affects the accuracy of implant placement with significant differences observed between experienced and inexperienced operator groups, with regard to angular and horizontal error at the implant apex and the platform.[43] Nevertheless, the introduction of template-guided implant surgery appears to mitigate the effect of inexperience on the accuracy of implant placement since Scherer *et al.*[44] demonstrated that template-guided drilling yields significantly enhanced accuracy compared to freehand drilling, regardless of the clinical experience of the operator. However, the use of adjuncts to assist the surgeon does not exonerate the clinician from having the requisite skill, training, and awareness of how to handle complications that might occur.

In summary, experience of the surgeon placing implants influences the accuracy of implant placement and clinical outcomes. Moreover, the impact of restorative dentist or prosthodontist inexperience in treatment planning/provision and, consequently, on clinical outcomes remains poorly understood. However, the increase in the number of general dentists managing implant treatment modalities coupled with the marginalization of complete denture principles in the dental school curriculum has led to increasing iatrogenic problems when multiple dental landmarks are lost.

Competence/incompetence of clinician

Assessing the competence of a clinician in implant dentistry is, much like other elements of dentistry, challenging due to the lack of regulations. Although foundational procedures of dentistry are evaluated in state or regional board examinations and didactic and treatment planning knowledge evaluated in the National Dental Board examination process, there is no formal level of competence that must be attained before a dentist can place or restore dental implants. Indeed, the freedom to place and restore dental implants falls under the purview of a general dental license. Contributing to this scenario is the fact that implant dentistry is not a Commission on Dental Accreditation recognized dental specialty, so no guidelines mandating levels of exposure, familiarity, competence, and proficiency for each of the different aspects of implant dentistry are broadly accepted (http://www.ada.org/en/coda).

In the US, different dental specialties include dental implant placement and/or restoration. Prosthodontics, oral and maxillofacial surgery, periodontics, and endodotics all include language requiring some level of instruction in the educational standards for residency programs, with only the latter not demanding competence/proficiency in at least implant placement and/or implant restoration. Following on, to achieve board certification in these specialties requires demonstration of clinical skill through the presentation of patient treatment histories by examinees to the Board examiners of the respective specialties. There are currently no mandated competency or proficiency assessments for general dentists in the US.

Knowledge/ignorance of clinician

Many dental schools/colleges include implant dentistry in their curriculum to train general dentists. Therefore, a minimum level of knowledge is imparted to graduates. However, many practitioners placing and restoring implants began doing so after graduation from dental school. Training for these general dentists has come from voluntary attendance at educational programs that have widely differing degrees of scope in terms of curriculum content and clinical or *in vitro* exposure.

Dental specialty programs in prosthodontics, oral and maxillofacial surgery, periodontics, and endodontics all include education in implant dentistry. Since the specialties began teaching implant dentistry before general dentist students were taught implant dentistry, a larger percentage of the specialist population has received formal university- or hospital-based education in this field. For example, implant dentistry was widely taught in specialty programs in the US in the late 1980s. As a result, the dental specialist population is better-versed in implant dentistry than the general dentist population. Three professional organizations, the American Academy of Implant Dentistry, through its American Board of Oral Implantology/Implant Dentistry program, the International College of Oral Implantologists, through its Diplomate program, and the Academy of Osseointegration, through its Fellowship program, have sought to establish guidelines for a dentist to demonstrate fundamental knowledge of, or familiarity with, implant dentistry.

Although it must be recognized that there are general dentists who have committed to learning much about implant dentistry from reputable sources and who provide implant dentistry care of the highest quality, the median level of care by general dentists is likely lower than that provided by specialists. In this regard, implant dentistry is much like other dental fields where specialist care yields, on average, better outcomes than general dentist care. Orthodontic treatment outcomes[45] and endodontic treatment outcomes[46] appear to be different between general dentist and specialist groups, with specialist care yielding better outcomes. Recently published work also shows this pattern to be manifest in implant dentistry. Da Silva *et al.*[47] concluded that "implant survival and success rates in general dental practices may be lower than those reported in studies conducted in academic or specialty settings."

The concepts of osseosufficiency and osseoseparation lead us to propose a new way of thinking regarding success and failure of osseointegration. An example to support our contention comes from analyzing the "clustering" of implant retrievals. Historically, we have considered clustering to be a patient-based phenomenon, and it is likely true that there are patients who are not ideal biological candidates due to compromised osseous healing potential or other environmental factors.[48] However, there may also be a contributory role for the clinician – why do some clinicians experience a higher implant survival/success rates than others. Does the finding by Weyant *et al.*[49] that there is a 1.3 odds ratio of a second retrieval in a patient who has already experienced a first retrieval account for whether the surgeon was the same surgeon for all retrievals? Following on, if implants are retrieved at a higher rate when placed by some clinicians, this should be viewed as a form of clustering.

It is important to understand that most patients and most clinicians do well with most implants. Long-term success and survival data indicate that successful osseointegration is a routine outcome. Nevertheless, complications are presenting at a higher rate than previously seen. We propose, therefore, that the concept of osseosufficiency be applied in all treatment-planning discussions in order to determine whether the combined profile of patient–clinician–implant is one that predisposes to the desired success. The combination of certain patients being treated by certain clinicians who choose to use certain implants in a certain way may yield an undesirable outcome. As mentioned, the implant is the least influential and the clinician the most influential of the three factors.

Summary

Future investigation must start with seeking to understand the immunologic pathways that govern both maintenance and loss of dental implant osseointegration. This understanding will reveal clues that can enable more predictable patient-specific planning. Once the fundamentals of osseointegration are better understood after all these years of uncertainty, follow-up investigations may include a closer look at potential patient-related risk factors and complications associated with failed execution of proper surgical protocol/recommendations. Patient-related risk factors include evaluation of certain cytokines and systemic diseases that may predict expected changes in foreign body equilibrium reactions around dental implants. Additional efforts may be applied to evaluate current surgical guidelines, their consistency with the current scientific data, and how closely these instructions are followed by surgical operators.

Dental clinicians have long used the term "implant failure" to describe a situation where an implant is removed. In reality, in the vast majority of these unfortunate clinical outcomes, it is not the implant that fails. If anything, when considered alongside the patient and the clinician, the implant is the least variable and most predictable element of the three. It is a clever assignment of blame on the implant that our profession has undertaken. Other than those rare occasions when an implant fractures, an implant is better considered to be retrieved than to have failed. Patients and clinicians, alone or in combination, are far more likely the root cause of the variability that results in clinical treatment failure manifested by implant retrieval.

References

1. Koka S, Zarb GA. On osseointegration: the healing adaptation principle in the context of osseosufficiency, osseoseparation, and dental implant failure. *Int J Prosthodont* 2012: **25**(1): 48–52.
2. Albrektsson T, Zarb G, Worthington P, *et al.* The long-term efficacy of currently used dental implants: a review and proposed criteria for success. *Int J Oral Maxillofacr Implants* 1986; **1**(1): 11–25.
3. Qian J, Wennerberg A, Albrektsson T. Reasons for marginal bone loss around oral implants. *Clin Implant Dent Relat Res* 2012; **14**(6): 792–807.
4. Koka S. Osseoseparation and peri-implantitis: whates in a name? *Int J Prosthodont* 2015; **28**(1): 7.
5. Trindade R, Albrektsson T, Wennerberg A. Current concepts for the biological basis of dental implants: foreign body equilibrium and osseointegration dynamics. *Oral Maxillofac Surg Clin North Am* 2015; **27**(2): 175–183.
6. Albrektsson T, Dahlin C, Jemt T, *et al.* Is marginal bone loss around oral implants the result of a provoked foreign body reaction? *Clin Implant Dent Relat Res* 2014; **16**(2): 155–165.
7. Kumar V, Cotran RS, Robbins SL. *Pathologic Basis of Disease*, 8th edn. University of Chicago: Elsevier Health Sciences 2010.
8. Murray PJ, Wynn TA. Protective and pathogenic functions of macrophage subsets. *Nat Rev Immunol* 2011; **11**(11): 723–737.
9. Kular J, Tickner J, Chim SM, *et al.* An overview of the regulation of bone remodelling at the cellular level. *Clin Biochem* 2012; **45**(12): 863–873.
10. Tang L, Eaton JW. Fibrin(ogen) mediates acute inflammatory responses to biomaterials. *J Exp Med* 1993; **178**(6): 2147–2156.
11. Cutler CW, Jotwani R. Dendritic cells at the oral mucosal interface. *J Dent Res* 2006; **85**(8): 678–689.
12. Zaba LC, Fuentes-Duculan J, Eungdamrong NJ, *et al.* Identification of TNF-related apoptosis – inducing ligand and other molecules that distinguish inflammatory from resident dendritic cells in patients with psoriasis. *J Allergy Clin Immunol* 2010; **125**(6): 1261–1268.
13. Wu X, Al-Abedalla K, Rastikerdar E, *et al.* Selective serotonin reuptake inhibitors and the risk of osseointegrated implant failure: a cohort study. *J Dent Res* 2014; **93**(11): 1054–1061.
14. Davies JE. Understanding peri-implant endosseous healing. *J Dent Educ* **67**(8): 932–949.
15. Davies JE. Mechanisms of endosseous integration. *Int J Prosthodont* 1998; **11**(5): 391–401.

16. Monje A, Suarez F, Galindo-Moreno P, *et al.* A systematic review on marginal bone loss around short dental implants (<10 mm) for implant-supported fixed prostheses. *Clin Oral Implants Res* 2014; **25**(10): 1119–1124.
17. Malchiodi L, Cucchi A, Ghensi P, *et al.* Influence of crown–implant ratio on implant success rates and crestal bone levels: a 36-month follow-up prospective study. *Clin Oral implants Res* 2014; **25**(2): 240–251.
18. Blanes RJ. To what extent does the crown-implant ratio affect the survival and complications of implant-supported reconstructions? A systematic review. *Clin Oral Implants Reso* 2009; **20**.s4: 67–72.
19. Ortega-Oller I, Suárez F, Galindo-Moreno P, *et al.* The influence of implant diameter on its survival: a meta-analysis based on prospective clinical trials. *J Periodontol* 2014; **85**(4): 569–580.
20. Ivanoff C, Gröndahl K, Sennerby L, *et al.* Influence of variations in implant diameters: a 3- to 5-year retrospective clinical report. *Int J Oral Maxillofac Implants* 1999; **14**(2): 173–180.
21. Mordenfeld HM, Johansson A, Hedin M, *et al.* A retrospective clinical study of wide-diameter implants used in posterior edentulous areas. *Int J Oral Maxillofac Implants* 2004; **19**(3): 387–392.
22. Olate S, Lyrio MC, de Moraes M, *et al.* Influence of diameter and length of implant on early dental implant failure. *J Oral Maxillofac Surg* 2010; **68**(2): 414–419.
23. Krennmair G, Waldenberger O. Clinical analysis of wide-diameter frialit-2 implants. *Int J Oral Maxillofac Implants* 2004; **19**(5): 710–715.
24. Renouard F, Nisand D. Impact of implant length and diameter on survival rates. *Clin Oral Implants Res* 2006; **17**s2: 35–51.
25. Alsabeeha NH, DeSilva RK, Thomson WM, *et al.* Primary stability measurements of single implants in the middle of the edentulous mandible for overdentures. *Clin Implant Dent Rel Res* 2010; **21**(5): 563–566.
26. Vandeweghe S, Deferrerre R, Tschakaloff A, *et al.* Wide-body implant as an alternative for sinus lift or bone grafting. *Int J Oral Maxillofac Implants* 2011; **69**(6): e67–74.
27. Torroella-Saura G, Mareque-Bueno J, Cabratosa-Termes J, *et al.* Effect of implant design in immediate loading. A randomized, controlled, split-mouth, prospective clinical trial. *Clin Oral Implants Res* 2015; **26**(3): 240–244.
28. Ma P, Xiong W, Tan B, *et al.* Influence of thread pitch, helix angle, and compactness on micromotion of immediately loaded implants in three types of bone quality: a three-dimensional finite element analysis. *BioMed Res Int* 2014; 983103.
29. Herekar M, Sethi M, Mulani S, *et al.* Influence of platform switching on periimplant bone loss. *Implant Dentistry* 2014; **23**(4): 439–450.
30. Schwarz F, Hegewald A, Becker J. Impact of implant-abutment connection and positioning of the machined collar/microgap on crestal bone level changes: a systematic review. *Clin Oral Implants Res* 2013; **25**(4): 417–425.
31. Puchades-Roman L, Palmer RM, Palmer PJ, *et al.* A clinical, radiographic, and microbiologic comparison of Astra Tech and Brånemark single tooth implants. *Clin Implant Dent Rel Res* 2000; **2**(2): 78–84.
32. Pjetursson BE, Asgeirsson AG, Zwahlen M, *et al.* Improvements in implant dentistry over the past decade: comparison of survival and complication rates in older and newer publications. *Int J Oral Maxillofac Implants* 2014; **29**(Suppl): 308–324.
33. Kim CH, Kim HJ, Huh JW, *et al.* Learning curve of laparoscopic low anterior resection in terms of local recurrence. *J Surg Oncol* 2014; **110**(8): 989–996.
34. Schwaitzberg SD, Scott DJ, Jones DB, *et al.* Threefold increased bile duct injury rate is associated with less surgeon experience in an insurance claims database: more rigorous training in biliary surgery may be needed. *Surg Endosc* 2014; **28**(11): 3068–3073.
35. Shtein RM, Michelotti MM, Kaplan A, *et al.* Association of surgeon experience with outcomes of femtosecond LASIK. *Ophthalmic Surg Lasers Imaging* 2012; **43**(6): 489–494.
36. Anakwanze OA, Baldwin K, Milby AH, *et al.* Arthroscopic repair of large rotator cuff tears using the double-row technique: an analysis of surgeon experience on efficiency and outcomes. *J Shoulder Elbow Surg* 2013; **22**(1): 26–31.
37. Farach SM, Danielson PD, Chandler NM. Impact of experience on quality outcomes in single-incision laparoscopy for simple and complex appendicitis in children. *J Pediatr Surg* 2015; **50**(8): 1364–1367.
38. Spampinato MG, Arvanitakis M, Puleo F, *et al.* Assessing the learning curve for totally laparoscopic major-complex liver resections: a single hepatobiliary surgeon experience. *Surg Laparosc Endosc Percutan Tech* 2015; **25**(2): e45–50.
39. Cahill PJ, Pahys JM, Asghar J, *et al.* The effect of surgeon experience on the outcomes of surgery for adolescent idiopathic scoliosis. *J Bone Joint Surg* 2014; **96**(16): 1333–1339.
40. Preiskel HW, Tsolka P. Treatment outcomes in implant therapy: the influence of surgical and prosthodontic experience. *Int J Prosthodont* 1995; **8**(3): 273–279.
41. Lambert PM, Morris HF, Ochi S. Positive effect of surgical experience with implants on second-stage implant survival. *J Oral Maxillofac Surg* 1997; **55**(12 Suppl 5): 12–18.
42. Zoghbi SA, Alves de Lima LAP, Saraiva L, *et al.* Surgical experience influences 2-stage implant osseointegration. *J Oral Maxillofac Surg* 2011; **69**(11): 2771–2776.
43. Cushen SE, Turkyilmaz I. Impact of operator experience on the accuracy of implant placement with stereolithographic surgical templates: an in vitro study. *J Prosthet Dent* 2013; **109**(4): 248–254.
44. Scherer U, Stoetzer M, Ruecker M, *et al.* Template-guided vs. non-guided drilling in site preparation of dental implants. *Clin Oral Investig* 2015; **19**(6): 1339–1346.
45. Marques LS, Freitas Jr NDd, Pereira LJ, *et al.* Quality of orthodontic treatment performed by orthodontists and general dentists. *Angle Orthod* 2012; **82**(1): 102–106.
46. Alley BS, Kitchens GG, Alley LW, *et al.* A comparison of survival of teeth following endodontic treatment performed by general dentists or by specialists. *Oral Surg Oral Med Oral Pathol Oral Radiol Endod* 2004; **98**(1): 115–118.
47. Da Silva JD, Kazimiroff J, Papas A, *et al.* Outcomes of implants and restorations placed in general dental practices: a retrospective study by the Practitioners Engaged in Applied Research and Learning (PEARL) Network. *J Am Dent Assoc* 2014; **145**(7): 704–713.
48. Ekfeldt A, Christiansson U, Eriksson T, *et al.* A retrospective analysis of factors associated with multiple implant failures in maxillae. *Clin Oral Implants Res* 2001; **12**(5): 462–467.
49. Weyant RJ, Burt BA. An assessment of survival rates and within-patient clustering of failures for endosseous oral implants. *J Dent Res* 1993; **72**(1): 2–8.

CHAPTER 9

Implant Restoration of the Partially Edentulous Patient

Steven J. Sadowsky
University of the Pacific Arthur A. Dugoni School of Dentistry, San Francisco, California, USA

When the osseointegration concept was introduced to North America in 1982, it prompted a tectonic shift in how the completely edentulous patient could be restored to improve the quality of life of patients. No longer were compromised patients relegated to either highly invasive preprosthetic surgical procedures or tethered to a steady application of denture adhesive to function adequately. On the other hand, implant-supported restorations for the partially edentulous patient were slower to evolve and treatment designs were mired in broadly accepted tenets applicable to the natural tooth instead of an ankylosed root analog. Why else has there been such inertia to accept tilted implants, 2:1 crown-to-implant ratios, posterior cantilever fixed dental prostheses, short implants, nonsplinted posterior multiple units, and occlusal schemes that do not demand the absence of nonaxial contacts? Mark Twain said, "It's not what you don't know that gets you in trouble. It's what you know for sure that just ain't so." This chapter will address differential treatment planning decision-making criteria relevant to implant-borne prostheses for the partially edentulous patient.

An algorithm helpful to evaluate patient's candidacy and design preference in implant restorative treatment is a pyramid of diagnostic considerations (Figure 9.1). At the base of the pyramid is the best available evidence to establish prognosis. Chapter 1 offers the reader a map to navigate the literature in order to identify externally and internally valid studies. The second block is systemic factors. Chapter 2 delineates the absolute and relative contraindications to implant placement. The third block is local factors. These include four "F"s: field (spatial allowance), foundation (quantity/quality of bone, soft tissue biotype/morphology), facial esthetics (high/low lip line, lip support), and forces (parafunction, occlusal loading). The fourth block is patient-mediated factors. These also include 4 "F"s: financial considerations, forecast of treatment time, fixed splint vs. individual units, and fear of morbidity of treatment. Once the patient has been established as a candidate for dental implants, local and patient-mediated factors often dictate treatment decisions.

Local factors influencing implant therapy

The occlusocervical height of the residual alveolar ridge should be sufficient to accommodate a 7 mm long implant as documented in long-term studies, unless augmentation is planned.[1–3] In addition, the three-dimensional position of the implant has been shown to impact the bony and soft tissue contours which plays a prominent role in restorative success, especially in the esthetic zone.[4] There should be at least 2 mm of bone buccal to the implant on placement and approximately 1.5 mm proximal to the adjacent tooth, so a 4 mm diameter implant would require 7 mm interproximally (Figure 9.2).[4] The coronal–apical position of the implant should be approximately 2–3 mm apical to the mid-buccal cementoenamel junction of the adjacent teeth (Figure 9.3).[5] Crestal bone height discrepancies may be rectified before tooth extraction with orthodontic forced eruption. In the maxillary anterior sextant, a cement-retained crown may be designed because of the trajectory of bone and will require 1 mm of interarch space between the abutment and the antagonist tooth. On the other hand, if screw-retained crowns can be designed in this region, they will require at least 2 mm clearance between the implant platform and the opposing tooth in order to house the screw access in the cingulum area. This may be problematic in class II, division 2 jaw relations or patients with significant vertical overlap and minimal horizontal overlap (Figure 9.4a). When there is inadequate interarch space even for cement-retained implant prostheses, orthodontic intrusion is recommended (Figure 9.4b, c). In the posterior quadrants, a minimum of 5 mm of interocclusal space is required for screw-retained designs (Figure 9.5a, b) and 7 mm for cement-retained restorations (Figure 9.5c, d). With less than 5 mm of axial wall height

Evidence-based Implant Treatment Planning and Clinical Protocols, First Edition. Edited by Steven J. Sadowsky.

Companion website: www.wiley.com/go/sadowsky/implant

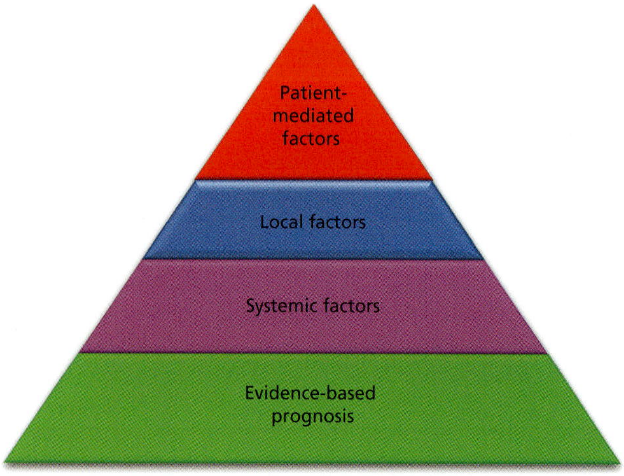

Figure 9.1 Pyramid of success when considering critical factors in diagnosis and treatment planning of implant prostheses.

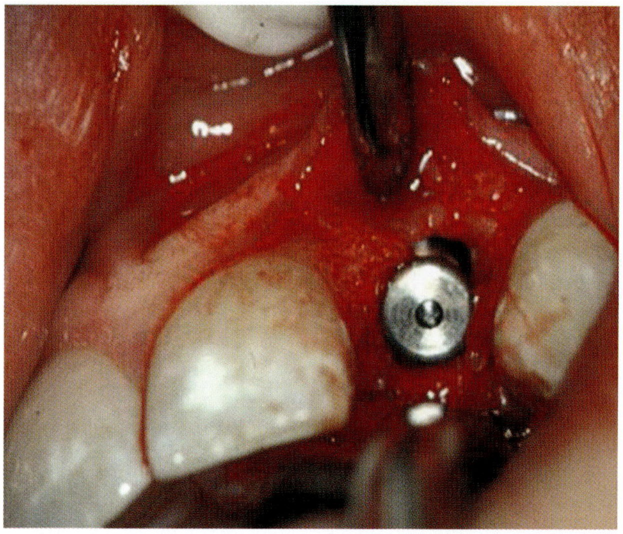

Figure 9.2 Placement of implant in horizontal plane with ≥2 mm bone facial to fixture. *Source:* Reproduced with permission from Charles Goodacre.

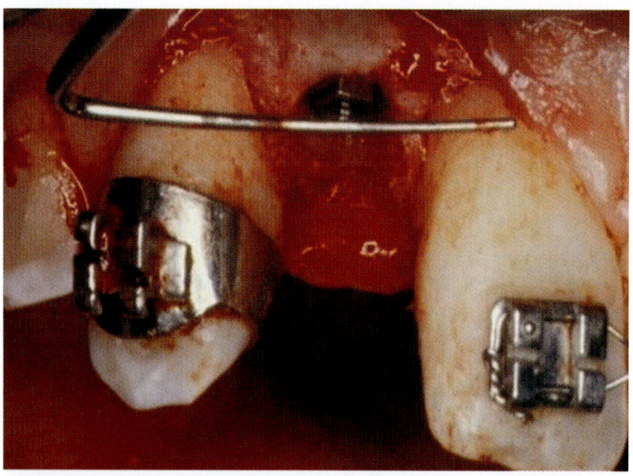

Figure 9.3 Placement of implant in frontal plane 2–3 mm apical to the adjacent teeth cementoenamel junction. *Source:* Reproduced with permission from Charles Goodacre.

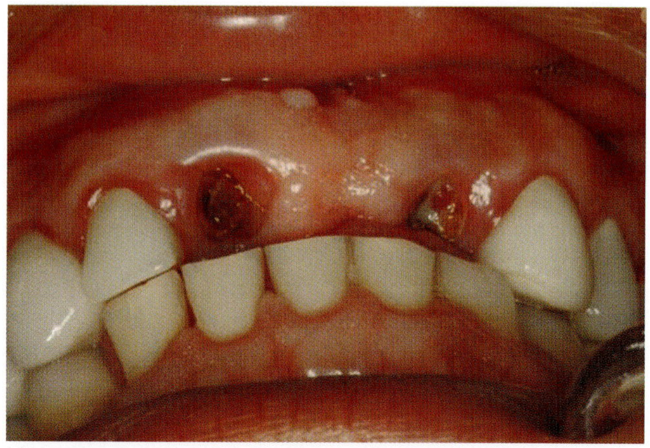

(a)

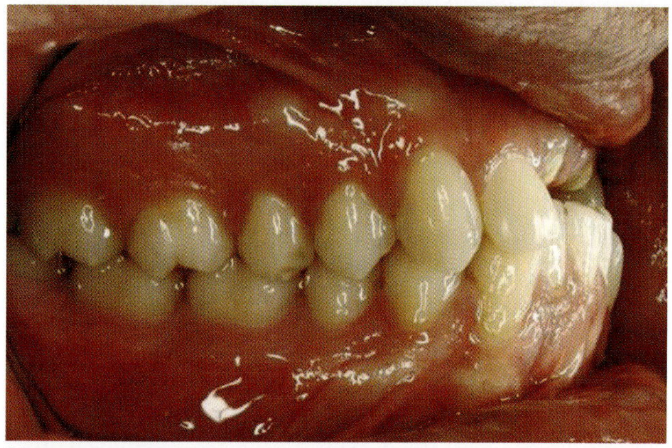

(b)

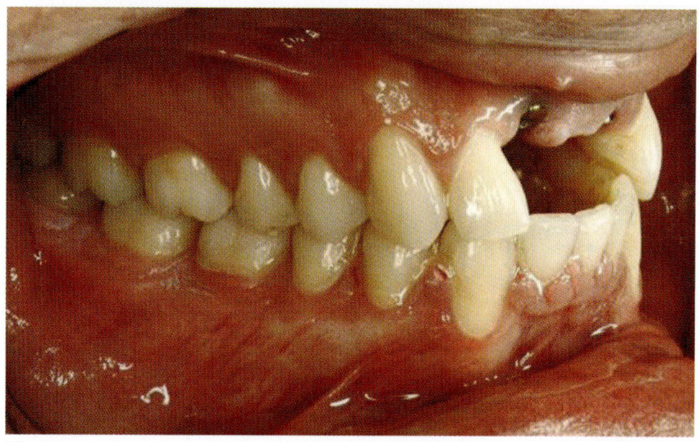

(c)

Figure 9.4 (a) Class II, division 2 jaw relation pre-empting replacement of decoronated roots with a screw-retained implant fixed dental prosthesis due to the lack of sufficient space for the screw-access housing. (b) Supraeruption of mandibular incisors encroaching on restorative space for implant prosthesis. (c) Orthodontic intrusion of mandibular incisors to accommodate maxillary anterior restorative requirements and harmonious crown morphologies.

for the abutment (Figure 9.5e), retention of the restoration is challenged. When any these aforementioned parameters cannot be achieved (Figure 9.6a), interceptive orthodontics (Figure 9.6b, c) has been instituted for space management and/or optimization of the occlusal plane in order to both retain and

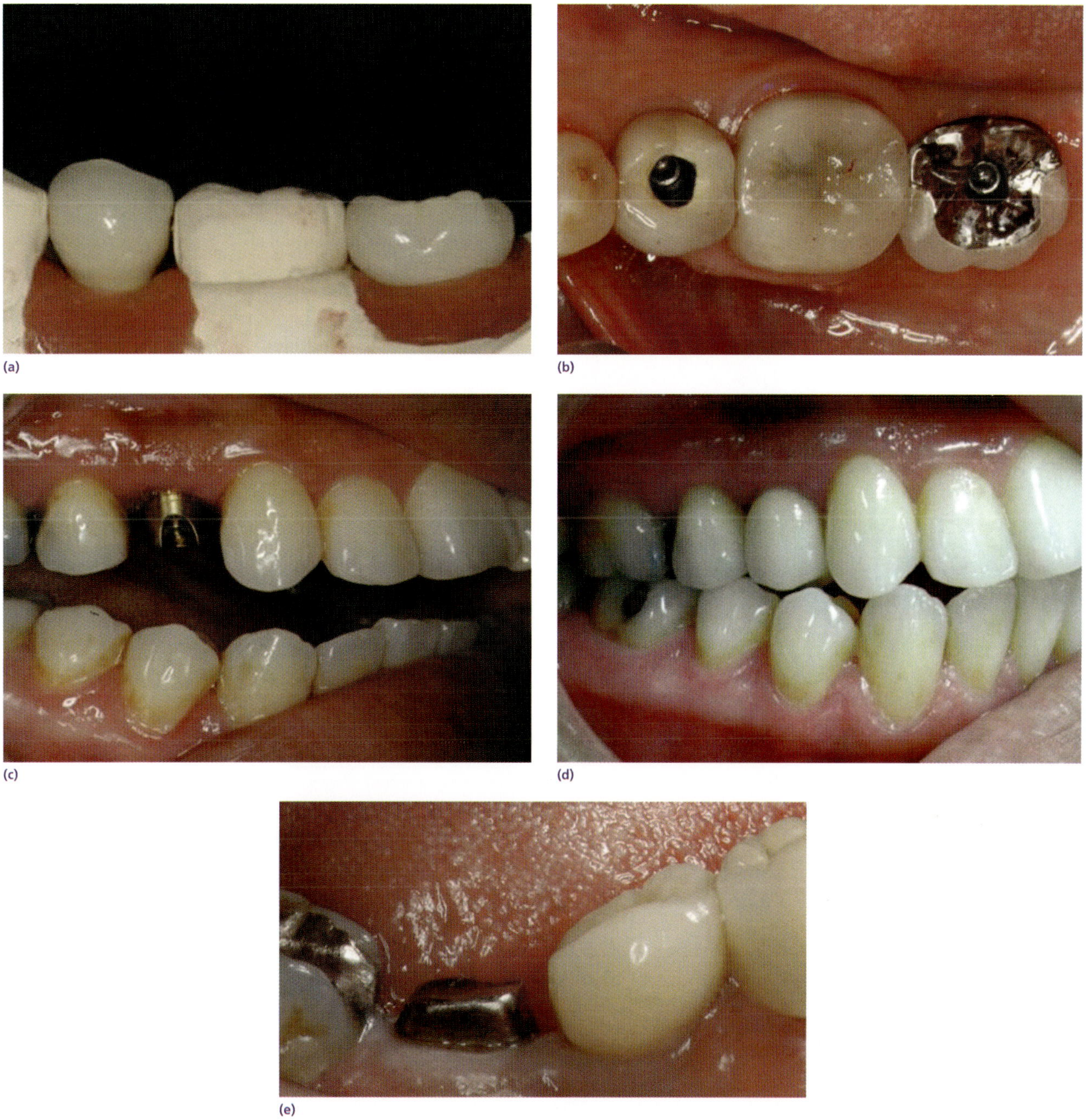

Figure 9.5 (a, b) Minimum of 5 mm interocclusal space is required for screw-retained restorations. (c) A minimum of 7 mm of interocclusal space is required for a cement-retained crown allowing at least 5 mm for abutment height. (d) Canine guidance or group function developed when restoring a posterior implant crown. (e) Implant not placed orthogonally with occlusal plane obviating the use of screw-retained design. However, restricted interarch space has compromised retention of a cement-retained prosthesis. Auxiliary retention using a lateral screw would be appropriate. *Source for* (a–d): Reproduced with permission from Carlos Eduardo Gonzales Espinoza.

maintain the restoration in harmony with excursions. Inadequate horizontal dimension of the bone has been addressed with guided bone regeneration, onlay/veneer grafting, ridge splitting, and ridge-preservation procedures.

Differences in gingival and osseous architecture have been documented widely and have been shown to exhibit a significant influence on restorative outcomes.[6,7] Thin gingival biotypes are highly sensitive to trauma and inflammation and have been reported to be associated with three times the marginal recession of thick biotypes after extraction (Figure 9.7).[8] The loss can be 1.5–2 mm over the first year, with the most loss occurring in the initial 3 months (Figure 9.8).[9] Ridge preservation should be considered for most thin biotypes.[10] On the other hand, if immediate placement of implants in thin biotypes is pursued,

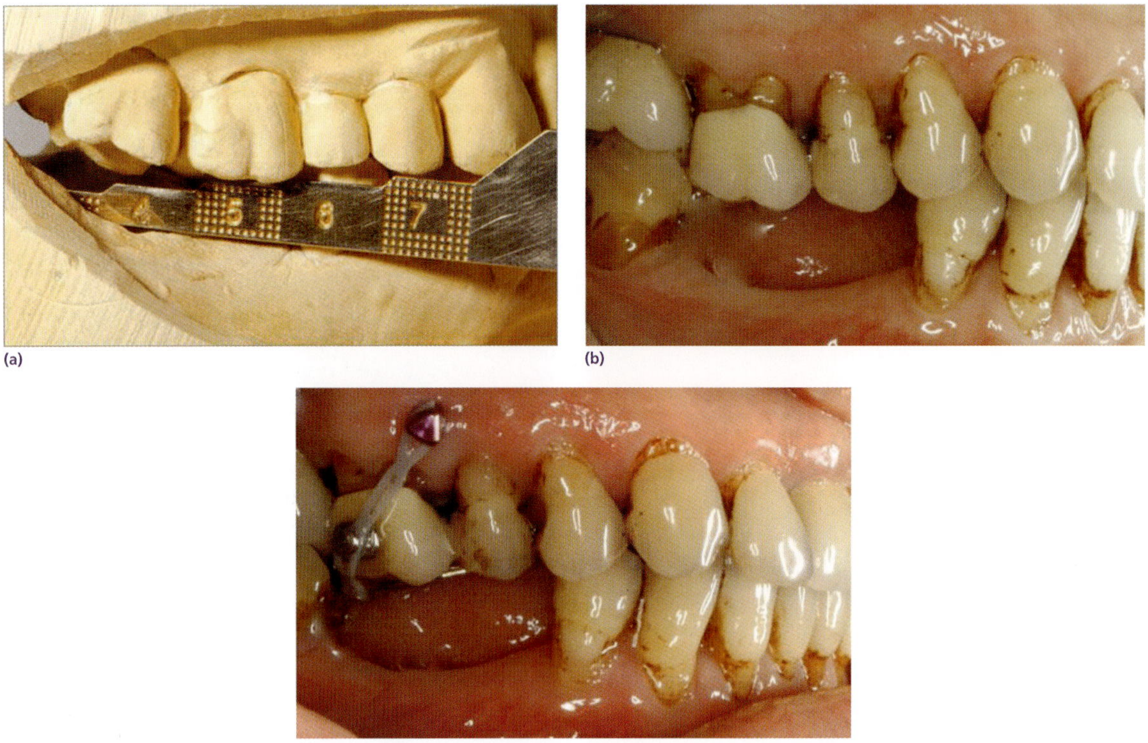

(a) (b) (c)

Figure 9.6 (a) Measurement of vertical space to assess interarch accommodation for screw- or cement-retained restorations. Despite the 5 mm allowance for a screw-retained restoration in this scenario, equilibration or restoration of antagonist teeth would be necessary to eliminate excursive interferences. (b) Supraeruption of maxillary second bicuspid and first molar influencing design of antagonist crown height and occlusal scheme in lateral excursions. (c) Use of buccal and palatal temporary anchorage devices (TADs) for intrusion with expected movement of 0.5–1 mm per month for adults.

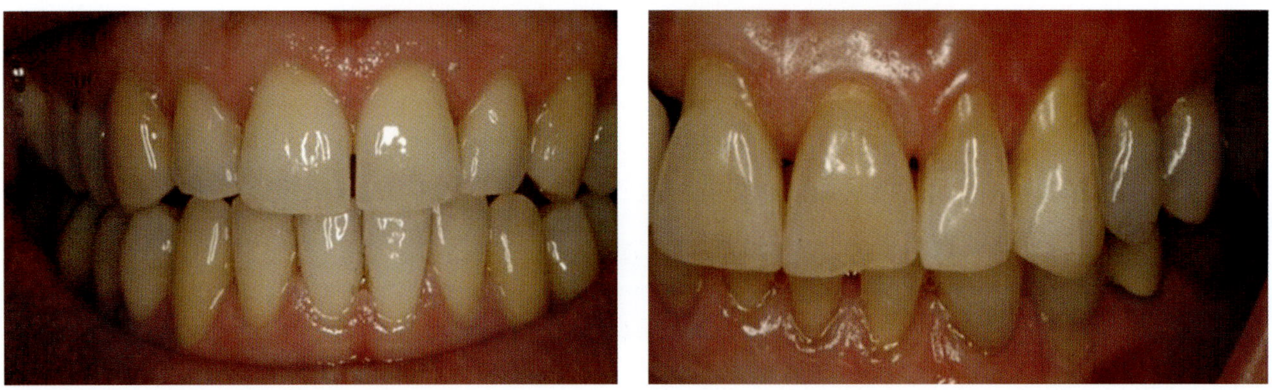

(a) (b)

Figure 9.7 (a) Thick gingival biotype, square tooth morphology, wide band of attached tissue, short papillae. (b) Thin gingival biotype, trigonal tooth morphology, narrow band of attached tissue, long papillae. *Source:* Reproduced with permission from Charles Goodacre.

there may be insufficient thickness in periodontal tissues to minimize alveolar resorption or lack of anchoring bone to ensure predictable stabilization.[10] The presence of a papilla between immediate single-tooth implants and adjacent teeth was significantly correlated with a thick flat biotype.[11,12] In fact, a 5-year prospective clinical study reported that the failure-free rate was 94% and 78% for maxillary central incisor metal–ceramic crowns with thick and thin biotype, respectively.[10] The main cause of failure was an esthetic problem.[13] In an effort to improve the esthetic outcome with thin gingival biotypes, subepithelial connective tissue grafting and specific implant and restorative planning have been recommended (Figure 9.9a–g). A change to a more palatal and apical implant placement with a straight-walled platform, 3–4 mm inter-implant space, use of concave abutment and crown profile, as well as platform switching may lead to greater success.[14,15] Two meta-analyses assessed the impact of platform switching on peri-implant bone changes, which revealed significantly less mean marginal bone loss (approximately 0.5 mm) at implants with a platform-switched compared to platform-matched implant–abutment configuration (Figure 9.10).[16,17] However, because of heterogeneity of the included studies, the results should be interpreted with caution.

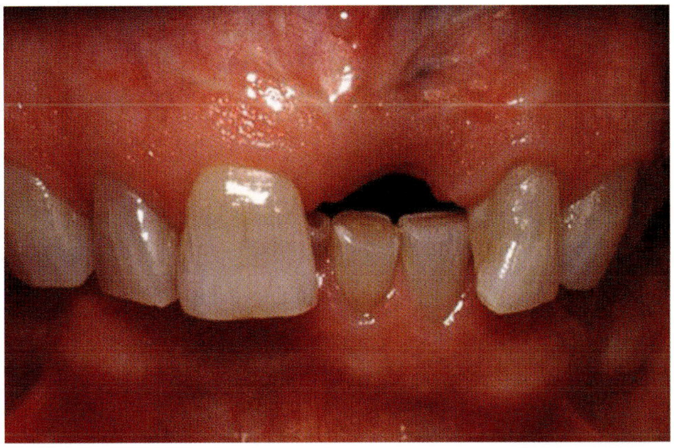

Figure 9.8 Extraction of central incisor on thin biotype without ridge-preservation procedure.

The presence of chronic periodontitis has been implicated in higher incidence of implant marginal bone loss and late failure, especially in cases of aggressive periodontitis without periodontal maintenance.[18,19] When patients with a history of periodontitis are well controlled, no link has been shown between their history and implant failure.[20] However, when a patient has had a previous implant failure, the risk of another failure increases by an odds ratio of 1.3.[21]

Finally, all adjunctive interceptive procedures involve additional risk factors that are patient, operator, and technique sensitive. A comprehensive treatment plan optimally weighs the risk, benefit, and cost of each treatment option.

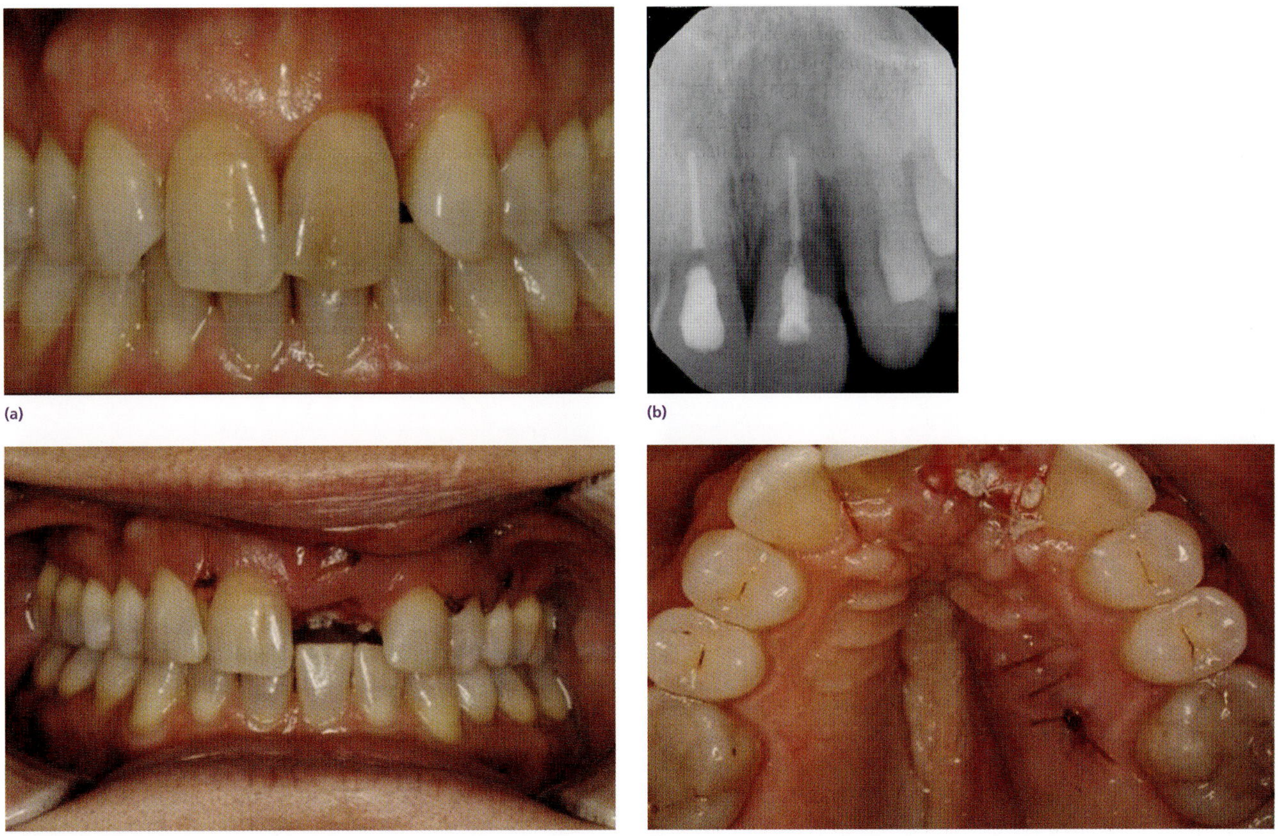

(a) (b) (c) (d)

Figure 9.9 (a) Maxillary left central incisor is unrestorable. (b) Periapical radiograph disclosing internal and external resorption. (c) Subepithelial connective tissue graft in conjunction with implant placement. (d) Palatal donor site for graft. (e) Resin-bonded bridge (facial view). (f) Resin-bonded bridge reinforced with orthodontic braided wire (palatal view). (g) Periapical radiograph of implant while integrating. (h) Patient with full smile with restoration in place.

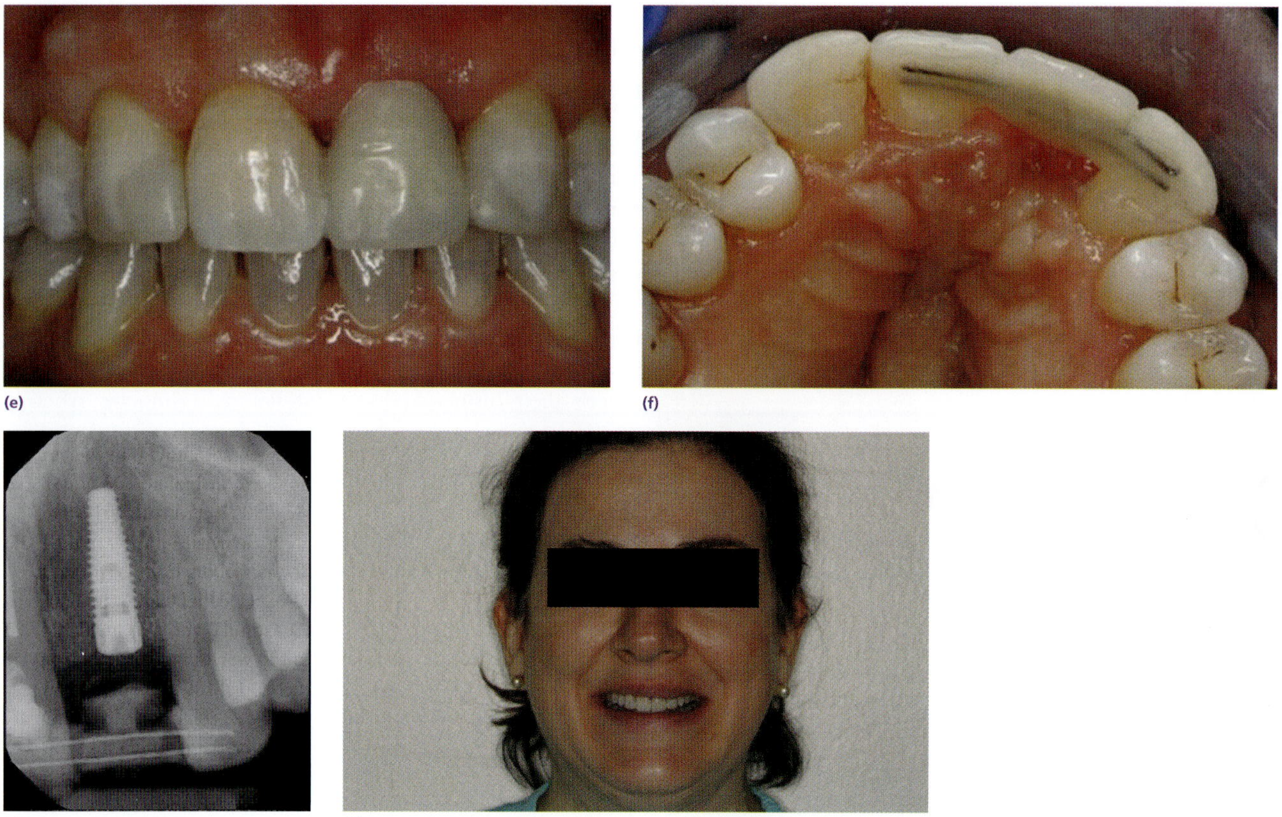

(e) (f) (g) (h)

Figure 9.9 (*Continued*)

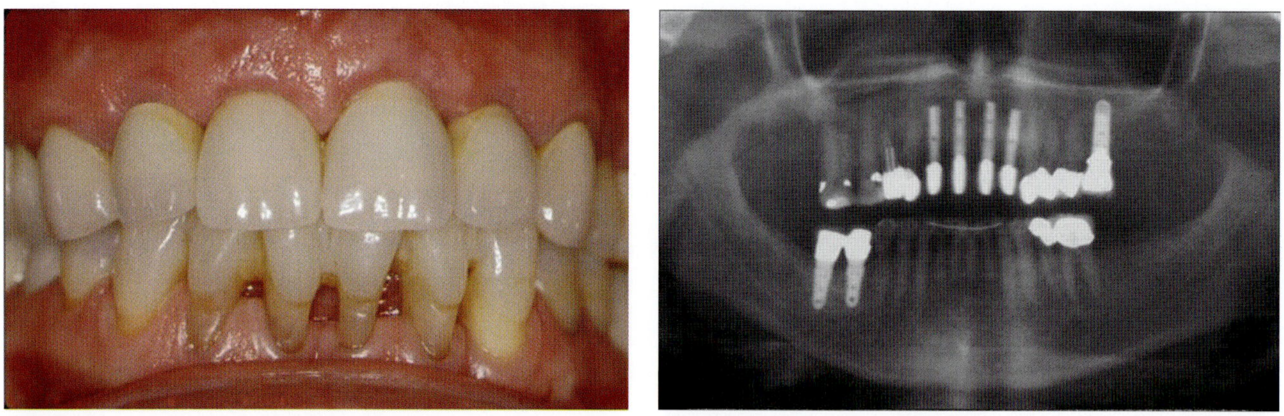

(a) (b)

Figure 9.10 **(a)** Individual porcelain fused to metal crowns on sites #7, 8, 9, 10 implants. **(b)** Platform-switched abutment design.

Indications for endodontic versus implant therapy

The decision to endodontically treat or retreat a tooth or extract and place an implant has been addressed in a number of systematic reviews.[22–24] Although similar high survival rates have been reported, the implant group has demonstrated almost fivefold higher incidence of postoperative complications.[25] However, the survival data vary with specific local factors which affect the prognosis of endodontic treatment. For example, Salehabi and Rotstein[26] assessed more than 1.4 million patients during an 8-year period and found, in the absence of apical periodontitis, the probability that initial endodontic treatment would keep the tooth disease-free was 92–98%, but the chance that a tooth with apical periodontitis would completely heal after initial treatment was 74–86% (Figure 9.11).

Odds of success of treatment were found to decrease by 14% for every 1 mm increase in the diameter of the preoperative lesion.[27] Tortuous root anatomy, and presence of calcifications or internal/external resorption also compromise prognosis, but with the aid of cone-beam computed tomography (CBCT), treatment results have improved (Figure 9.12).[28] Regarding orthograde retreatment, success was reduced if there was an alteration of the root canal morphology (47% as opposed to 86.8%, 2-year follow-up), presence of apical radiolucency, and adequate previous endodontic therapy (higher likelihood of extraradicular lesions, cystic lesions, and foreign body reactions).[29] For surgical retreatment, success reports vary widely (59–93%).[28,30,31] The following factors were identified as predictors of healing: absence of preoperative pain or signs, good density of the root canal filling, and a periapical lesion size of 5 mm or less. With regard to treatment-related factors, teeth treated with the use of an endoscope tended to have higher healed rates than teeth treated without the use of an endoscope.[32]

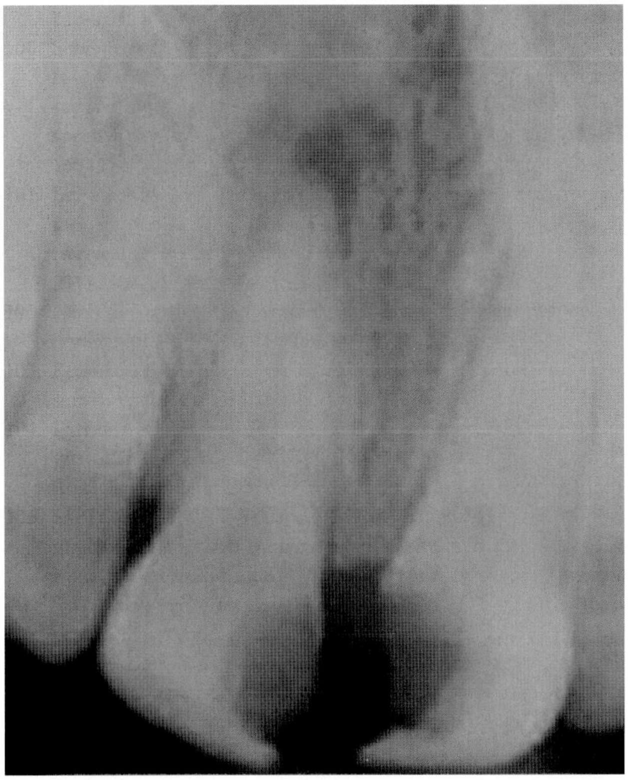

Figure 9.11 Approximately 10% reduced chance of complete healing after primary endodontic treatment for #8 compared to #9 because of apical radiolucency.

When deciding on endodontic treatment or replacement with an implant, the prosthetic restorability, periodontal support, caries index, strategic importance of the tooth, esthetic demands, cost/benefit/risk analysis, operator expertise, and patient preferences will weigh heavily. For example, the remaining coronal structure should allow for a 1.5–2 mm ferrule with at least 1 mm of dentinal thickness, otherwise forced eruption or crown lengthening (barring gingival scallop disharmony) is needed.[33]

An elongated epithelial attachment, which can be disclosed through sounding the midfacial bone, often does not create an esthetic blemish in the gingival contour. However, if the tooth is extracted without the preparation of orthodontic forced eruption, a soft/hard tissue dehiscence is likely. Therefore, this scenario would place a high premium on salvaging the natural tooth through endodontic (re)treatment.

The periodontal status of teeth considered for preservation has been stratified. Treatment of molars with class I furcation

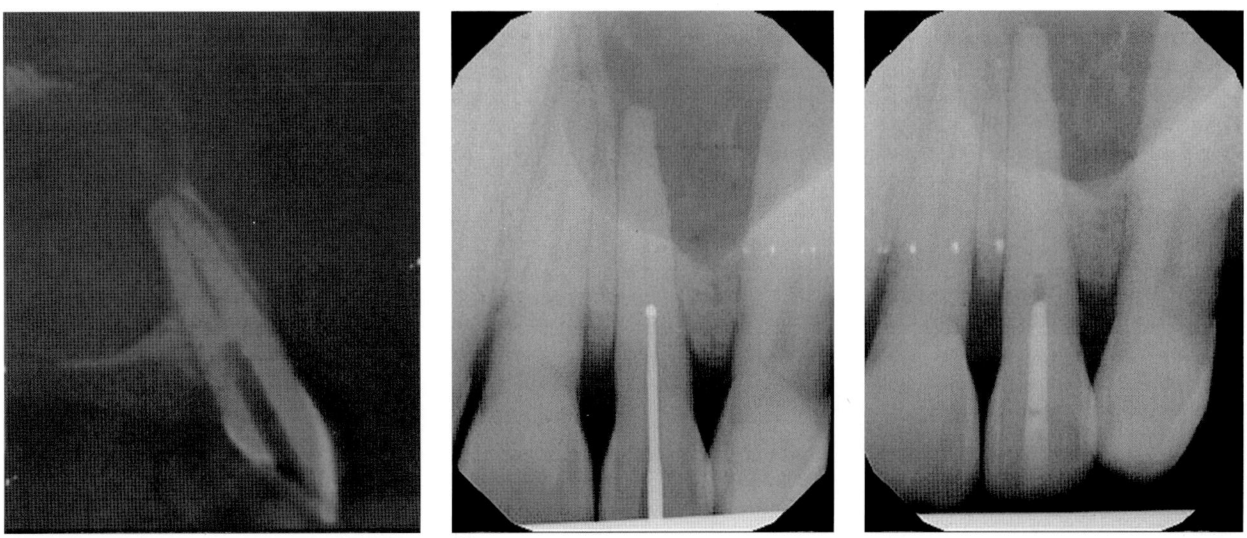

(a) (b) (c)

Figure 9.12 (a) Accuitomo scan of calcified canal of #10. (b) Gates-Glidden drill (Dentsply Tulsa Dental Specialties, Tulsa OK) accessing calcified blockage. (c) Completed obturation of #10. *Source:* Reproduced with permission from Ray Scott.

invasion with nonsurgical periodontal therapy was more cost effective than treatment with implant-supported crowns.[34] Samet *et al.*[35] have identified teeth with 6–8 mm pocket depth, 50% attachment loss, or class II furcation as questionable for retention. In a long-term study of up to 27 years with a mean of 11.5 years of follow-up, lack of compliance, smoking, and residual 6 mm post-periodontal treatment pocketing were risk factors for progression of tooth loss.[36] However, it is important to keep in mind when adequate periodontal treatment and maintenance are performed, a 10-year study tracking natural teeth with chronic or aggressive periodontitis (with an initial 50–70% attachment level) reported 88% survival of teeth.[37] As a consequence, the decision of tooth extraction, for periodontal reasons in favor of a dental implant, should be carefully considered in partially edentulous patients.

The use of adenosine triphosphate-driven bioluminescence has been demonstrated to be an effective innovative tool in enumerating the total bacteria count and oral *Streptococcus mutans*.[38] This enables the practitioner to assess a baseline reading and patient's commitment to oral hygiene to forecast long-term restorability of natural teeth. There may be a premium on endodontically (re)treating a tooth adjacent to an implant to preserve the interproximal bone (Figure 9.13), or an abutment which is part of a long-span fixed dental prosthesis. Additionally, esthetic demands may predicate salvaging a natural tooth. In these strategic scenarios, the patient should be apprised of the advantages of preservation and the importance of home-care maintenance for success.

When generalists perform endodontic therapy or implant surgery, there is a lower survival rate reported compared to specialists, with a greater discrepancy in implant outcomes.[39–41] Specifically, survival of implants placed by inexperienced clinicians was 73.0% as opposed to 95.5% by implant specialists.[42]

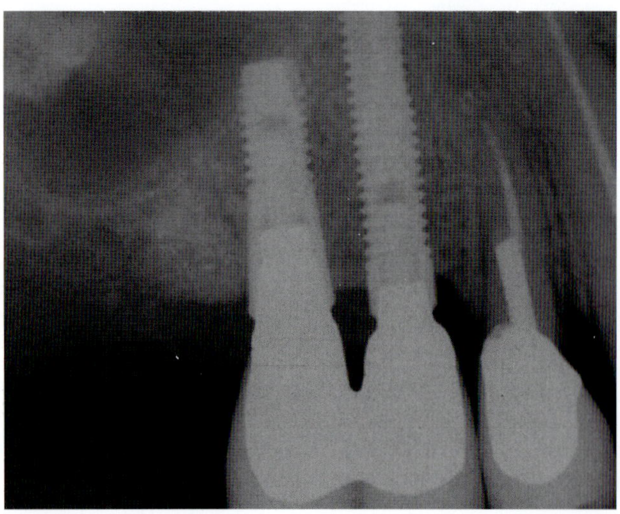

Figure 9.13 Interproximal bone preserved with natural tooth (#5) proximal to implant restoration, placing premium on retreatment of this tooth. *Source:* Reproduced with permission from Charles Goodacre.

A comparison of tooth survival rates after endodontic treatment by endodontic specialists vs. general practitioners, in a multicenter study consisting of 350 teeth that met the inclusion criteria, showed a difference of 98.1% vs. 89.7%.[43] Informed consents should include operator experience,[44] maintenance projections, esthetic and functional expectations, treatment cost/time comparisons, and impact of no treatment. An average treatment time estimate of an implant restoration on the maxillary arch is up to 250 days vs. 67 days for endodontic therapy.

In summary, when orthograde or surgical endodontic retreatment is indicated, the advent of dental operating microscopes, newer ultrasonic armamentaria, nickel–titanium rotary instrumentation, advanced electronic apex locators, thermoplastic gutta-percha delivery, mineral trioxide aggregate, and CBCT diagnostic tools have made this strategy the second line of defense before extraction and implant replacement.[45–48]

Indications for tooth-supported fixed dental prostheses versus single implant crowns

When comparing 10-year survival rates (approximately 89%) of tooth-supported fixed dental prostheses (FDPs) (Figure 9.14) and single implant crowns (SICs) (Figure 9.15), virtually no differences have been reported when metal–ceramic restorations were evaluated.[49] When the same investigators compared 5-year complication rates, conventional FDPs represented more biologic sequelae, such as loss of vitality, caries, and recurrent periodontitis, while SIC recorded more technical problems, such as loose abutment screws, veneer fracture, and loss of retention.

Despite high survival rates of metal–ceramic restorations, there has been a growing emphasis on evolving all-ceramic systems, driven by the debatable need for metal-free restorations. It is of note that 5-year follow-up studies have demonstrated lower survival rates of glass ceramic FDPs (e.g. lithium disilicate system), glass-infiltrated alumina FDPs (e.g. In-Ceram system), and densely sintered zirconia FDPs in comparison with metal–ceramic restorations.[50] The incidence of framework fractures was significantly higher for reinforced glass ceramic and infiltrated

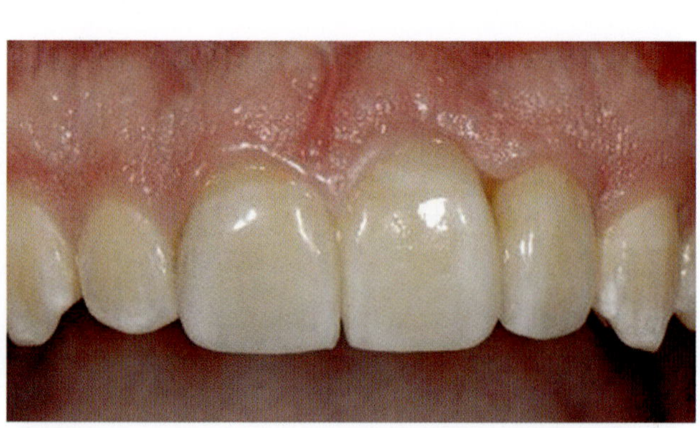

Figure 9.14 Three-unit fixed dental prosthesis replacing #8. *Source:* Reproduced with permission from Nicola Zitzmann, Basel, Switzerland.

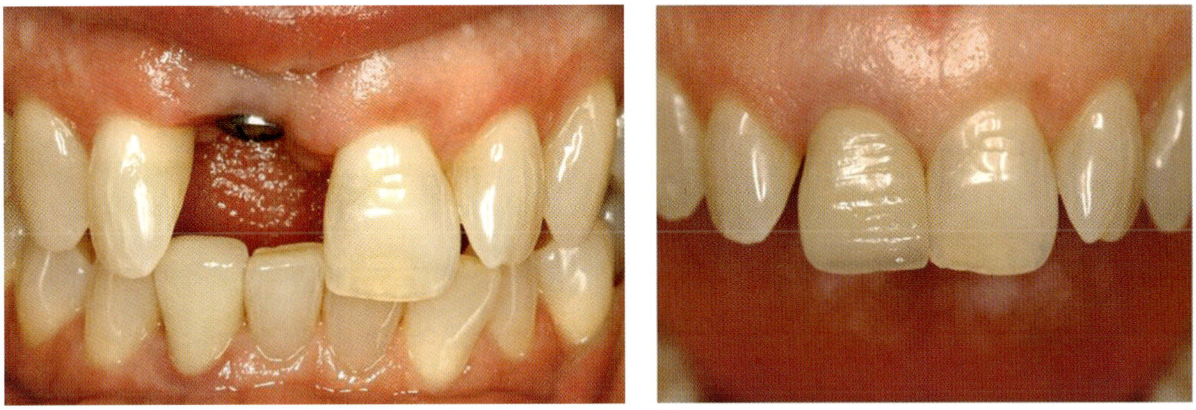

(a) (b)

Figure 9.15 (a) Healing abutment in #8 site. (b) Single implant crown replacing #8. *Source:* Reproduced with permission from Charles Goodacre.

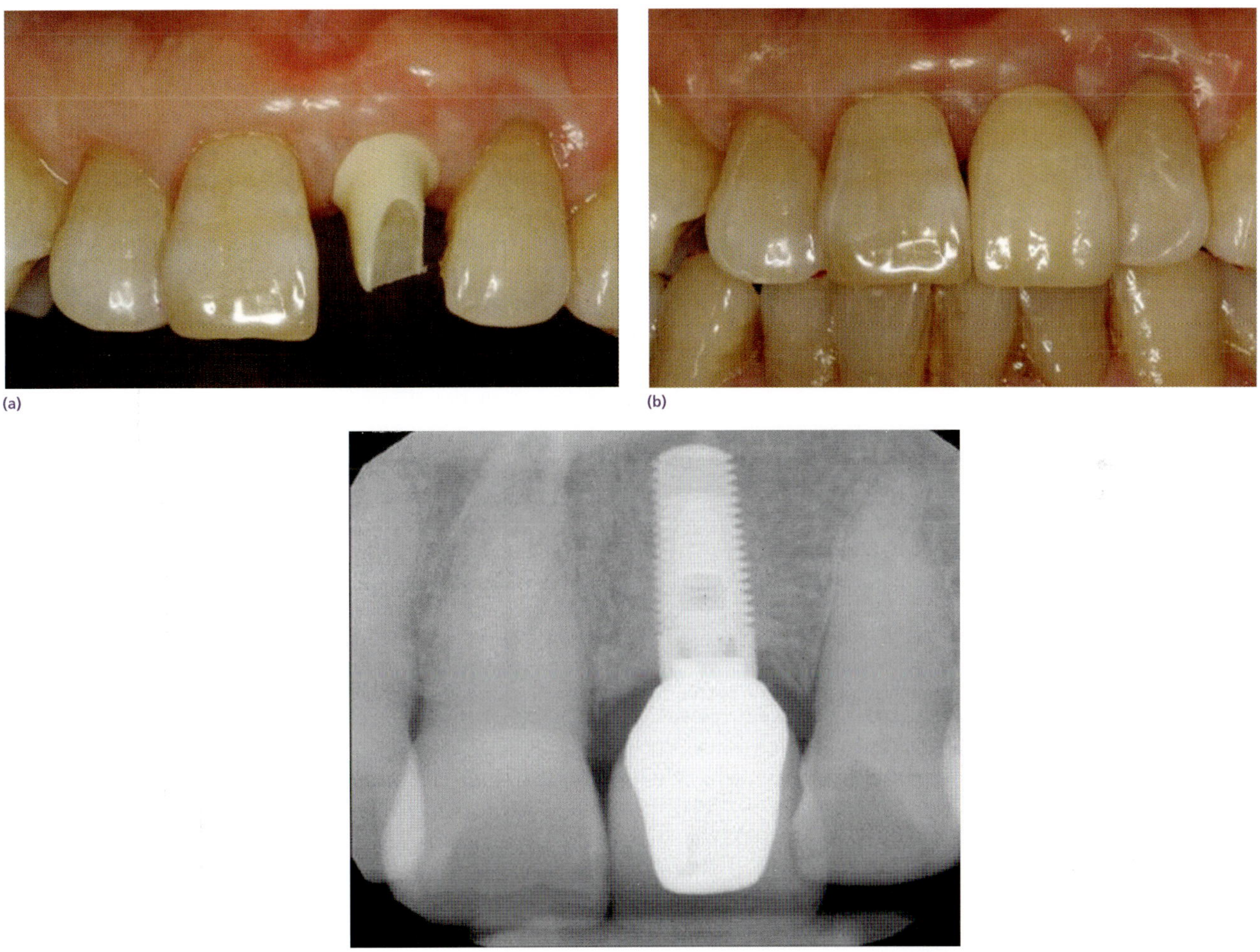

(a) (b) (c)

Figure 9.16 (a) Zirconia abutment affixed to implant in #8 site. (b) All-ceramic crown restoring #8. (c) Periapical radiograph. *Source:* Reproduced with permission from Carlos Eduardo Gonzales Espinoza.

glass ceramic FDPs, while the incidence for loss of retention and ceramic fractures was significantly higher for densely sintered zirconia FDPs compared to metal–ceramic FDPs. On the other hand, the performance of all-ceramic implant restorations supported by zirconium abutments versus metal–ceramic crowns on titanium abutments demonstrated no biologic or technical differences in complications with a 5-year follow-up (Figure 9.16).[51] One caveat in assessing the data on single implant crowns is that esthetic problems may be under-reported in as many as 60% of studies.[52,53] However, Zitzmann *et al.* focused in on the cost effectiveness of a three-unit tooth-borne FDP compared with a SIC in the anterior sextant. Their investigation revealed fewer complications and higher patient satisfaction for the implant restoration.[54] In addition, Walton,[55] in a 15-year study on over 300 patients, compared these two modalities and reported the estimated cumulative survival for SICs was significantly better than for three-unit FDPs when replacing anterior teeth. The complication rates of the FDPs and SICs were similar, but the economic burden for the FDPs was greater.

Given the aforementioned data, the optimal restorative design will be predicated on systemic,[56,57] local,[58] and patient-mediated factors.[59] Local factors to consider include caries index, periodontal condition of the teeth, the restorability or need for restoration of teeth bounding the edentulous span, the quality/quantity of bone of the prospective implant site, the indication for interdisciplinary care required to optimize the implant site, as well as the esthetic predictability of the conventional/implant regimens.[60,61] Patient-related factors include desire for either individual units or/and maintaining unrestored teeth, morbidity concerns especially with additional adjunctive care, and projected treatment time/cost differences. Single tooth implants have been projected to be financially commensurate with three-unit fixed dental prostheses, but 75–90% more costly than a similarly endodontically treated tooth, and require up to four times the number of days for treatment.[62]

Indications for implant-fixed dental prostheses and cantilevered fixed dental prostheses

When comparing studies before and after the year 2000, there has been a positive learning curve in the survival rate of not only single implant crowns but also multiple-unit implant-supported fixed dental prostheses (IFDPs).[63] The 5-year survival rate of IFDPs (Figure 9.17) has increased from 93.5% to 96.4%, but the incidence of complications is still high. For example, biologic problems, reported as peri-implant disease, soft tissue complications, marginal bone loss, fistula, or gingivitis, have slightly increased from 7.4% to 9.4% in newer studies.[63,64] These results may be in part due to better reporting. However, esthetic outcomes have improved in more recent investigations. The advent of wider application of zirconia-based ceramics and appreciation of biologic principles integral to a healthy and harmonious result appear to be responsible.[65–67] On the other hand, when assessing technical problems, IFDPs have about twice the incidence of veneer fracture (7.7%) than SICs in more recent studies. The risk of fracture of veneering material has been shown to increase with the size of the reconstruction, in addition to veneering ceramics for zirconia-based IFDP frameworks exhibiting higher chipping.[63] However, the use of slow cooling, more anatomically designed zirconia copings, sufficient thickness of veneer porcelain and minimum connector height of 3 mm may rectify this higher incidence of fracture. Occlusal guidelines have attempted to address the absence of proprioception recorded in implant- versus tooth-supported restorations by recommending light centric contacts and either the absence of or shared excursive contacts, although this is strictly empirical.[68] Abutment or screw loosening (4.0%) has been observed less in IFDPs than in SICs,[69] and has also shown a reduction of incidence in later investigations, perhaps due to the increasing use of internal connection implants[70] and the adoption of proper preload. It has been demonstrated *in vitro* that tightening the screw a second time within 10 seconds of initial recommended torque level has overcome 40% of the preload loss due to torsional relaxation of the screw shaft, embedment relaxation, and plastic deformation.[71,72]

Controversy has persisted regarding the decision to place one implant per crown instead of planning for an IFDP. Yi *et al.*[73] conducted a comparative retrospective study on three-unit IFDPs supported by two or three implants in posterior maxillary or mandibular partially edentulous patients (Figure 9.18). Results revealed 100% implant survival and no significant differences in complications with 63 patients observed with up to a 5-year follow-up. Salvi and Bragger[74] corroborated the absence of a link between complications and number of implants supporting the prosthesis. These clinical results address concerns of mechanical complications that have grown out of Rangert *et al.*'s work

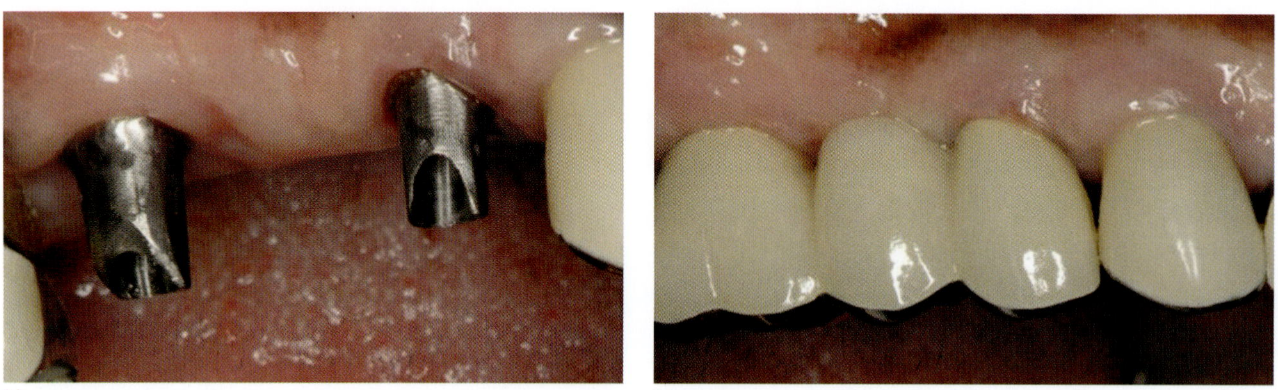

(a) (b)

Figure 9.17 (a) Titanium abutments to support a fixed dental prosthesis. (b) Porcelain-fused-to-metal implant fixed dental prosthesis.

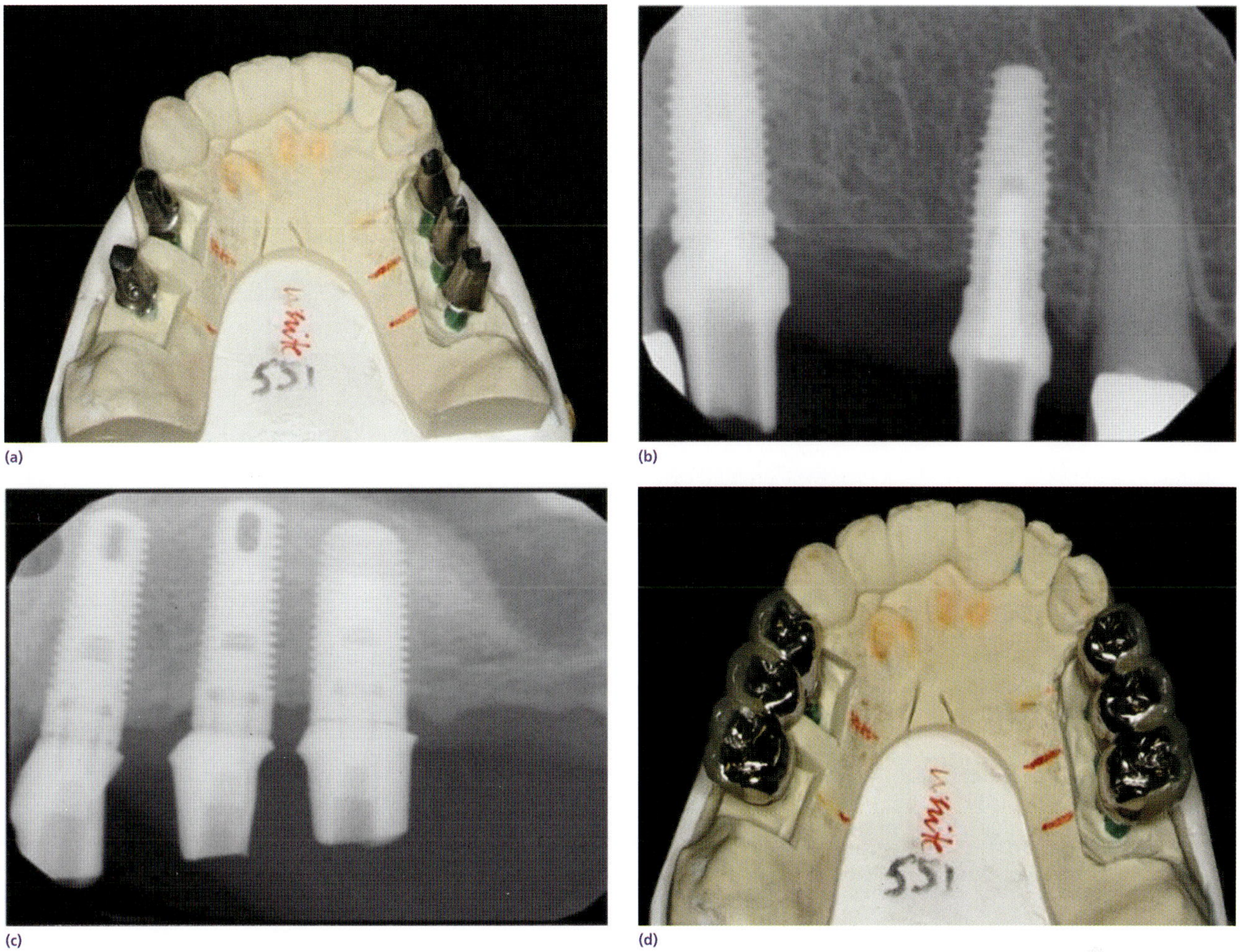

Figure 9.18 **(a)** Titanium abutments supporting posterior implant reconstruction. **(b)** Periapical radiograph of abutments affixed to implants which will support a fixed dental prosthesis. **(c)** Periapical radiograph of abutments affixed to implants which will support individual crowns. **(d)** Definitive restorations on master cast.

showing that a fixed prosthesis supported by three implants with an offset can reduce bending moments by 60%, compared to a linear array supported by two implants. However, a systematic review and a clinical study, with up to 18 years of follow-up, have borne out that *in vitro* analyses documenting significantly higher bending moment modeling do not necessarily lead to either bone loss or higher incidence of technical complications.[74,75] With regard to potential bone loss during function, if the microstrain units (<3000) remain within the adaptive window of the patient, nonaxial loading will not lead to microfracture.[76]

The decision to place two or three implants to support three crowns is best predicated on local factors. When anatomic limitations compromise the placement of three implants, while observing inter-implant (3 mm) and implant–tooth distances (1.5–2 mm), as well as acceptable-diameter implants (Figure 9.19a), two implants should be planned.[77,78] In addition, in order to manage papillae more predictably, a pontic versus a middle implant may provide an enhanced esthetic result. In most cases only an average 3.4 mm of papilla height can be expected to form over the inter-implant crest bone.[77,79] This is in contrast to more than 5 mm papilla height expected to form over the implant-pontic crest of bone. Finally, there is a cost saving to the patient by eliminating an implant placement. On the other hand, the three-implant design offers the facility of individual units when hygiene access is a priority for the patient, and a nonsplinted design is biomechanically sound. In addition, if there is a history of implant failure or there is questionable bony foundation, there may be a rationale for a three-implant splinted screw-retained prosthesis to allow for a ready-made prosthesis if an implant fails, either with a pontic in the central position or a cantilevered design (Figure 9.19b, c).

The use of tilted implants in the posterior quadrant to avoid either sinus augmentation (Figure 9.20) or the anatomic limitation presented by the inferior alveolar nerve has been documented in a number of studies.[80–82] Marginal bone level changes at axial- and nonaxial-positioned implants supporting FDPs, with over 5 years of observation, did not reach a statistical difference.[80] This was corroborated in another study with a range of angulation of the terminal implant between 20° and 50°.[82] Furthermore, a systematic review did not find higher incidence of mechanical complications with FDPs supported by both axial and tilted implants.[83]

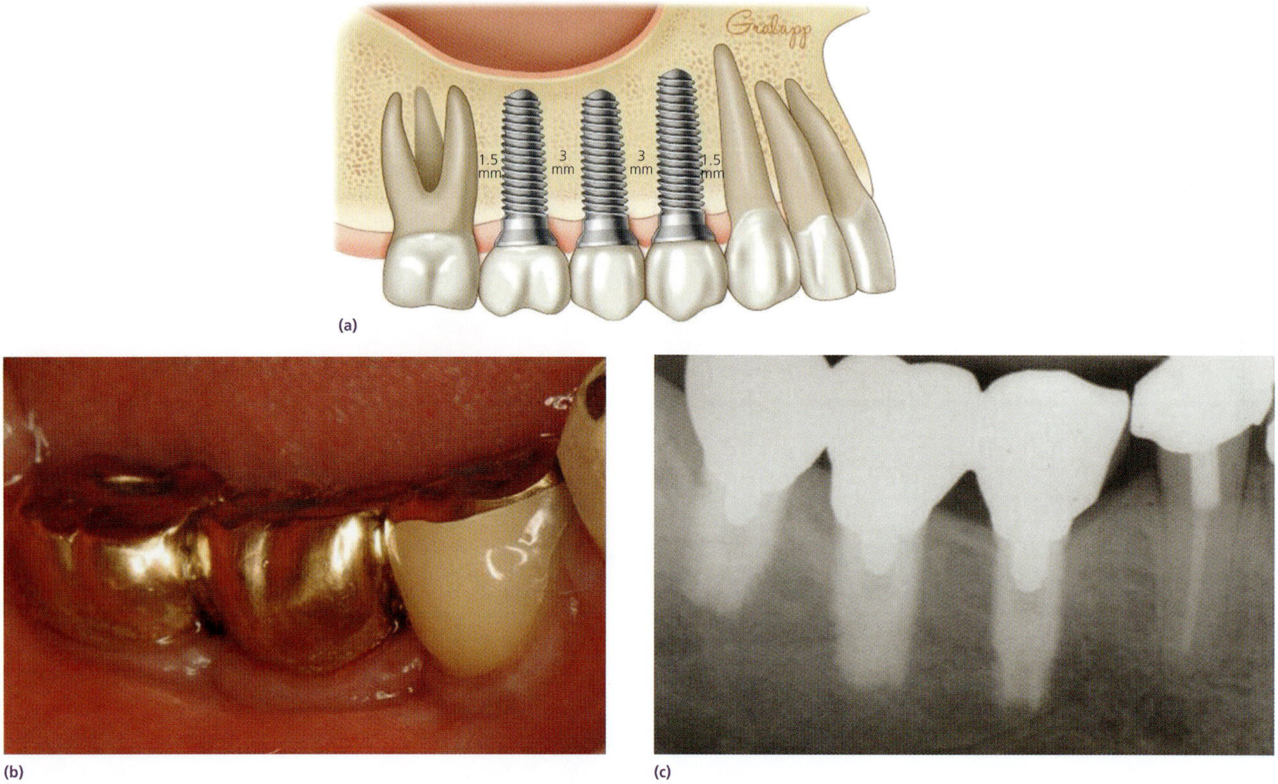

Figure 9.19 (a) Space analysis considering minimum mesiodistal requirements of inter-implant and implant–tooth distances for housing three implants. A three-unit fixed dental prosthesis supported by two implants is a viable alternative when space is at a premium. *Source:* © 2016, Chris Gralapp. (b) One implant per crown, screw-retained in a three-unit splint. (c) Periapical radiograph of three implants. If one fails, the prosthesis can be converted into a ready-made fixed dental prosthesis.

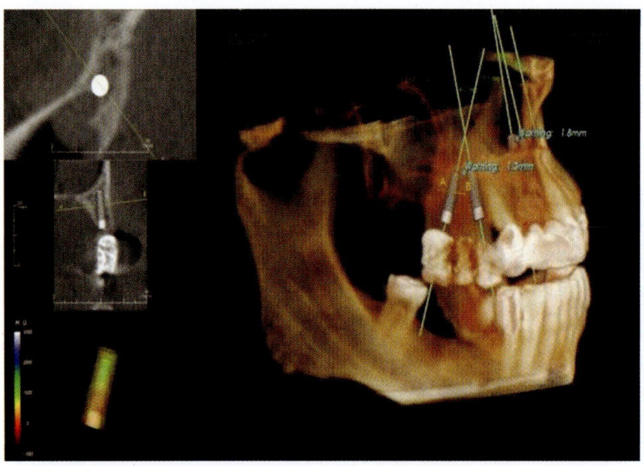

Figure 9.20 CBCT software planning for tilted implant fixed dental prosthesis design to avoid sinus grafting.

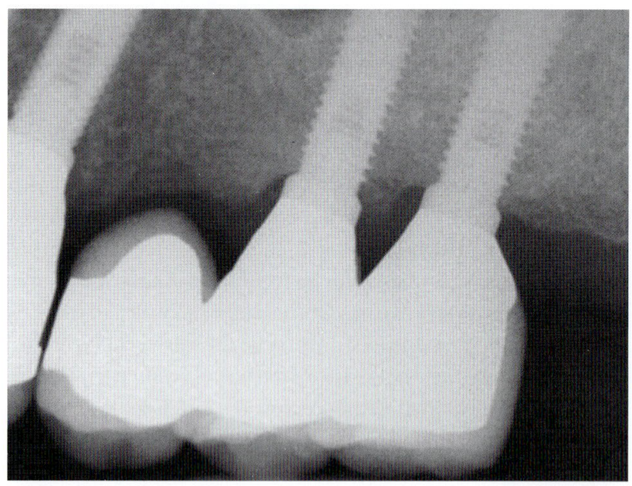

Figure 9.21 Implant cantilevered fixed dental prosthesis with marginal bone maintenance on implant proximal to cantilever. *Source:* Reproduced with permission from Charles Goodacre.

Long-term average survival of tooth-borne cantilever fixed dental prostheses has been reported to be 80.3% with a 10-year follow-up,[84–86] which may have influenced attitudes regarding implant cantilevered prostheses. While implant cantilevered prostheses have been documented with a 10-year survival of 88.9–100%,[49,87] clinicians have still been reluctant to plan treatment with this design. Despite high nonaxial loads on cantilevered implant-supported prostheses, marginal bone loss was unrelated to the length/location of cantilever and status of opposing dentition, unlike cantilever prostheses supported by the natural dentition (Figure 9.21).[88,89] Furthermore, both two- and three-unit posterior implant-supported cantilevered prostheses

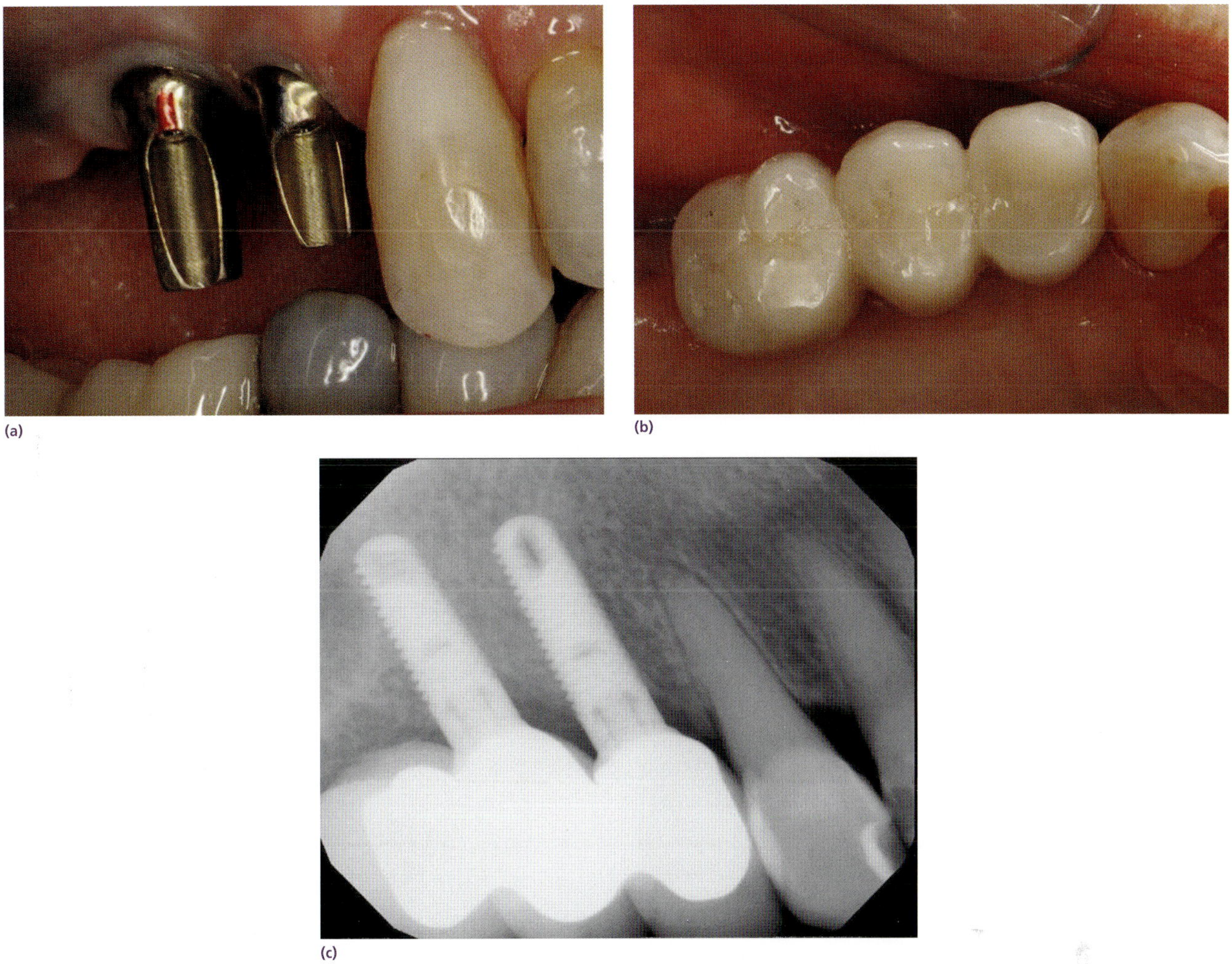

Figure 9.22 (a) Sufficient abutment length to retain a cantilever prosthesis. (b) Definitive three-unit porcelain-fused-to-metal cantilever prosthesis. (c) Periapical radiograph of cantilever prosthesis in (b).

have demonstrated high survival rates.[90,91] Anterior cantilevered implant prostheses may offer a solution to limitations of space, thin biotypes, or high smile lines. The most prevalent complications were technical problems, such as veneer fracture (10.3%), screw loosening (8.2%), and loss of retention (5.7%).[92] Therefore, patients with parafunction may be best treated with a metal occlusal design. When cement-retained cantilevered prostheses are selected, adequate crown-to-abutment ratio will safeguard against loss of retention (Figure 9.22).

Indications for splinting multiple implants

As in cantilevered implant prostheses, biases based on tooth-supported prostheses have influenced decision making regarding splinting multiple implant restorations, despite the absence of a periodontal ligament and the questionable need to improve the resistance to loading forces by altering the center of rotation of the splinted units.[93] A 10-year split-mouth design was conducted using posterior maxillary externally hexed implants with non-splinted units on the right side and splinted units on the left side.[94] Only 0.1 mm difference in marginal bone loss was found between the two groups. Norton[95] corroborated the maintenance of marginal bone levels with nonsplinted units on implants with internal connection in posterior jaws with up to a 7.5-year follow-up. The advantages of nonsplinted units are manifold (Figure 9.23). They allow for enhanced hygiene, easier passive fit reducing static forces,[96] eliminate the need for large quantities of ceramic and metal which may reduce the likelihood of framework/veneer fracture,[94] are easier to repair, and may be more esthetic in simulating natural teeth. With the aforementioned data in mind, the indications for splinting may include immediate function, high loading forces, compromised bony foundation, angled implants, and the use of short, narrow implants, and excessive effective crown lengths of at least 15 mm (Figure 9.24).[5,97] An additional consideration for splinting implants is the prospect of continual craniofacial growth into adulthood. Migration has been observed in partially edentulous patients with implant restorations after 20

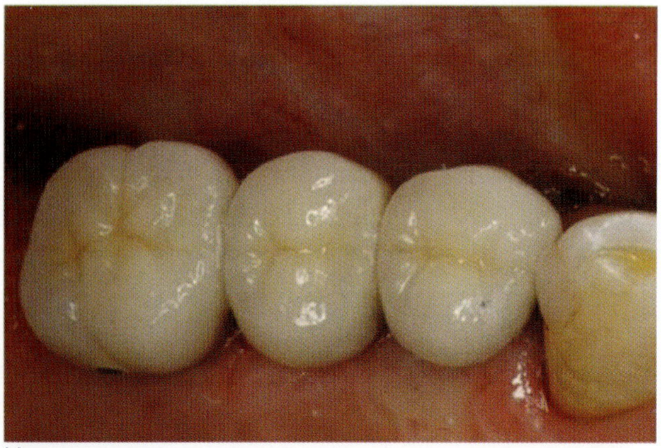

(a)

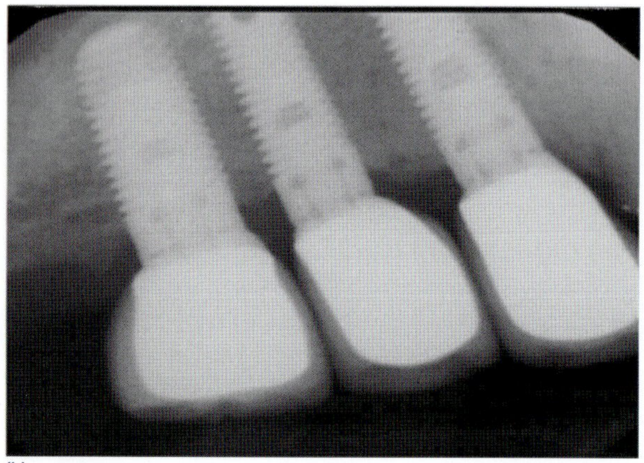

(b)

Figure 9.23 (a) Individual implant-supported crowns. (b) Periapical radiograph of unsplinted crowns.

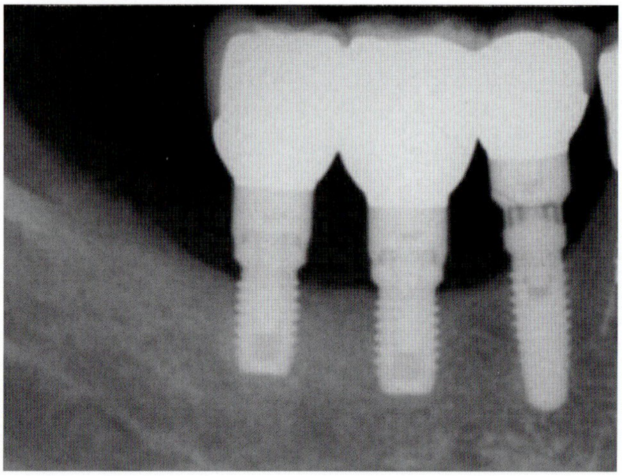

Figure 9.24 Splinted crowns with distal units approaching effective crown lengths of 15 mm. *Source:* Reproduced with permission from Charles Goodacre.

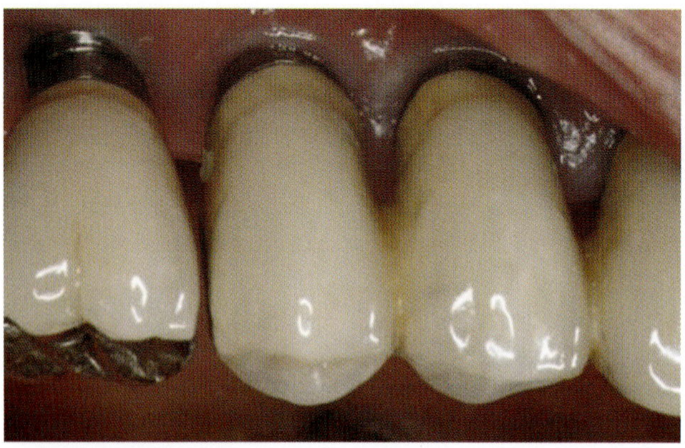

Figure 9.25 Opened interproximal contact between implant crowns due to continued craniofacial growth over 20 years of service.

years of follow-up.[98] This may include occlusal changes, opened contacts (Figure 9.25), and discrepancy of cervical gingival margin of implant restoration *vis à vis* the adjacent teeth. Surprisingly, reports of open contacts have ranged from 38–65% from 6 months to 12 years. This phenomenon was found in both screw- and cement-retained designs, more commonly on the mandible, and more frequently when the antagonist was a natural dentition rather than a removable prosthesis. Assessing the proximal walls of adjacent teeth to provide broad contact areas will not only limit food impaction in the gingival embrasure but also reduce the attrition where there is increased biting force. Night guards or retainers have also been recommended but the outcome has not been documented in the literature.

Indications for the selection of short implants

Teeth with greater than 1:1 crown-to-root ratios are considered compromised and that general assessment has influenced the caution that has accompanied short implants as an alternative to bone augmentation coupled with longer implants. However, multiple studies have clearly demonstrated no significant marginal bone loss with restorations when crown-to-implant (C:I) ratios were as high as 2.5:1.[91,99,100] Single crowns did not differ in implant-based success rates from splinted restorations.[99] Moreover, Lee *et al.* reported greater peri-implant bone loss in the maxilla when C:I was less than 1 compared to C:I greater than 1.[101] In addition, occlusal overload mimicked by supra-occlusal contacts in the absence of inflammation in animal studies has been shown to cause an anabolic effect on the bone.[102] Therefore, the main concern regarding short implants being subject to biomechanical loads above the physiological threshold of bone has not been borne out. While older studies reported a tendency of increased failure rate with short implants, these were with machined implants without a self-tapping surgical protocol and attention to bone quality.[103,104]

The impact of the data on short implants is the prospect of reducing the level of surgical invasiveness/morbidity, time, and cost investment for the patient seeking implants in atrophied native bone.[105] When comparing implants less than or equal to 8 mm in length with no grafting, to implants longer than 8 mm with sinus augmentation, there were three times the biological complications with the latter.[1,106] Furthermore, shorter than 8 mm medium-textured implants have demonstrated less bone loss after 5 years than longer implants in vertically augmented bone on the posterior mandible.[107] In summary, recent investigations, including randomized clinical trials with up to 5 years of observation, have reported implant success rates similar to those of long implants, offering patients conservative options in selected cases of native alveolar bone atrophy.[2,106,107]

Narrow-diameter implants

When horizontal crestal dimensions or spaces between adjacent teeth do not allow for a standard-diameter implant, narrow-diameter implants (NDIs) may preclude the need for augmentation or/and orthodontic intervention. This would be beneficial, especially for elderly patients, and patients with medical risks or/and financial limitations.[108,109] Implant survival rates (88.9–100%) of narrow-diameter implants (3.3–3.5 mm in load-bearing posterior regions, 3.0–3.25 mm in single tooth, low occlusal load-bearing areas) are well documented.[110] Unlike studies comparing short implants with standard implants in conjunction with augmentation, no similar methodology has been conducted for reduced-diameter implants. Clear analyses on associated risk factors with NDIs would be helpful to assess the influence of parafunction, bone quality, and prosthetic design (e.g. splinting vs. individual units).

Combined tooth- and implant-supported fixed dental prostheses

A prosthesis that is supported by an implant and a natural tooth may offer patients a conservative approach in scenarios where there are anatomic limitations to placing more than one implant, when one of two adjacent implants has failed, or a tooth adjacent to a two-tooth space requires coronal restoration. However, a systematic review tracking tooth- and implant-supported dental prostheses (TIFDP) over 10 years found a prosthetic survival rate of 77.8% (no significant differences in survival of tooth or implant abutments) as opposed to IFDPs with an 86.7% prosthetic survival rate.[49,111] Surprisingly, TIFDPs did not show a higher risk for biological or technical complications over 5 years when compared to either tooth- or implant-borne FDPs at 32%.[47,112,113] Even so, TIFDPs should be selected with specific local factors and design considerations in mind. Natural tooth abutments should be vital, periodontally sound, and have an orthogonal axis with the occlusal plane. A rigid connector should be designed, as intrusion has been shown to be mainly a factor (5.2%, 5-year incidence) with nonrigid connectors (Figure 9.26).[112,114,115] In summary, TIFDPs should be restricted to patients when anatomic or other patient-centered limitations would dictate a higher risk for an all-implant prosthetic design.

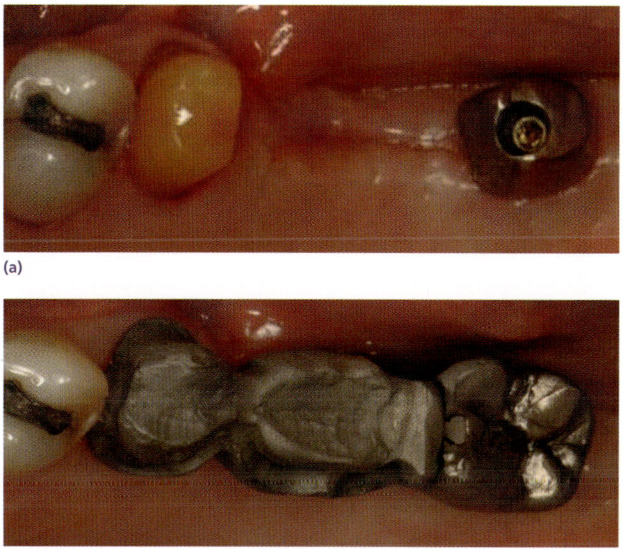

(a)

(b)

Figure 9.26 (a) Natural tooth and implant abutment supporting a mixed fixed dental prosthesis. (b) Framework design with nonrigid connector which has been linked to a 5-year, 5.2% incidence of intrusion of the natural tooth abutment.

Screw- versus cement-retained implant restorations

Originally when the UCLA abutment was introduced in the late 1980s, it afforded the practitioner the ability to mimic conventional tooth-borne restorations with a cement-retained prosthesis while offering more flexibility in the planning stage, and therefore this design was preferred by many clinicians. However, contrary to conventional wisdom, patients do not show preference for either a screw- or cement-retained prosthetic design.[116] Additionally, no significant differences have been reported for survival of either retention system with SICs or IFDPs as well as all-ceramic vs. all-metal abutments.[117] Although higher technical complications have historically been documented with screw retention, this is deceptive data.[118] When dissected out for all types of prosthetic reconstructions, veneer fracturing/chipping was statistically more prevalent for screw-retained designs, however the loss of retention and loosening of abutment were considerably more problematic for cement-retained designs, leading to overall higher technical maintenance.[119] In the same systematic review, biological complications were also significantly greater with cement-retained restorations. The presence of fistula/suppuration appears to be linked to cement extrusion which may lead to progressive bone loss.[120,121] Cement-retained prostheses also may be limited by the crown-to-abutment ratio and the increased taper of the abutment, due to excessive angle corrections. When only the minimum interocclusal space is available, cement debonding may be troublesome, especially in multiple-unit prostheses. It is paramount in this scenario to plan, in the presurgical phase, the positioning of the implant(s) consistent for screw retention. A hybrid design combining screw- and cement-retained abutments for a multiple-unit prosthesis offers improved retention as well as retrievability when one of the units can be screw-retained and the cemented unit is retained with temporary cement (Figure 9.27). When the anterior sextant teeth are missing

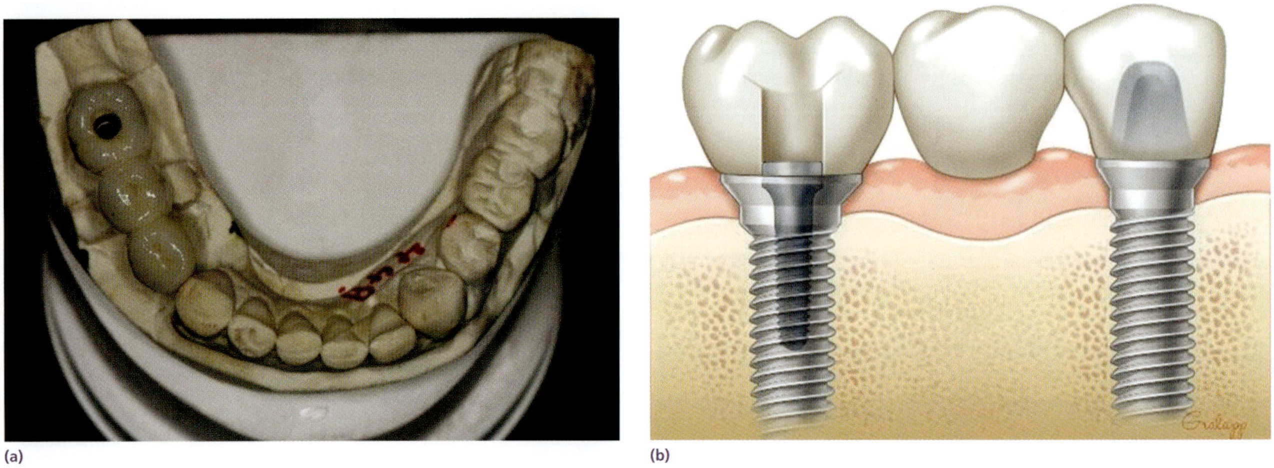

Figure 9.27 (a) Three-unit fixed dental prosthesis with screw-retained design on first molar and cement-retained design on first bicuspid. (b) Graphic depicting the "hybrid" design in Figure 9.26. *Source:* © 2016, Chris Gralapp.

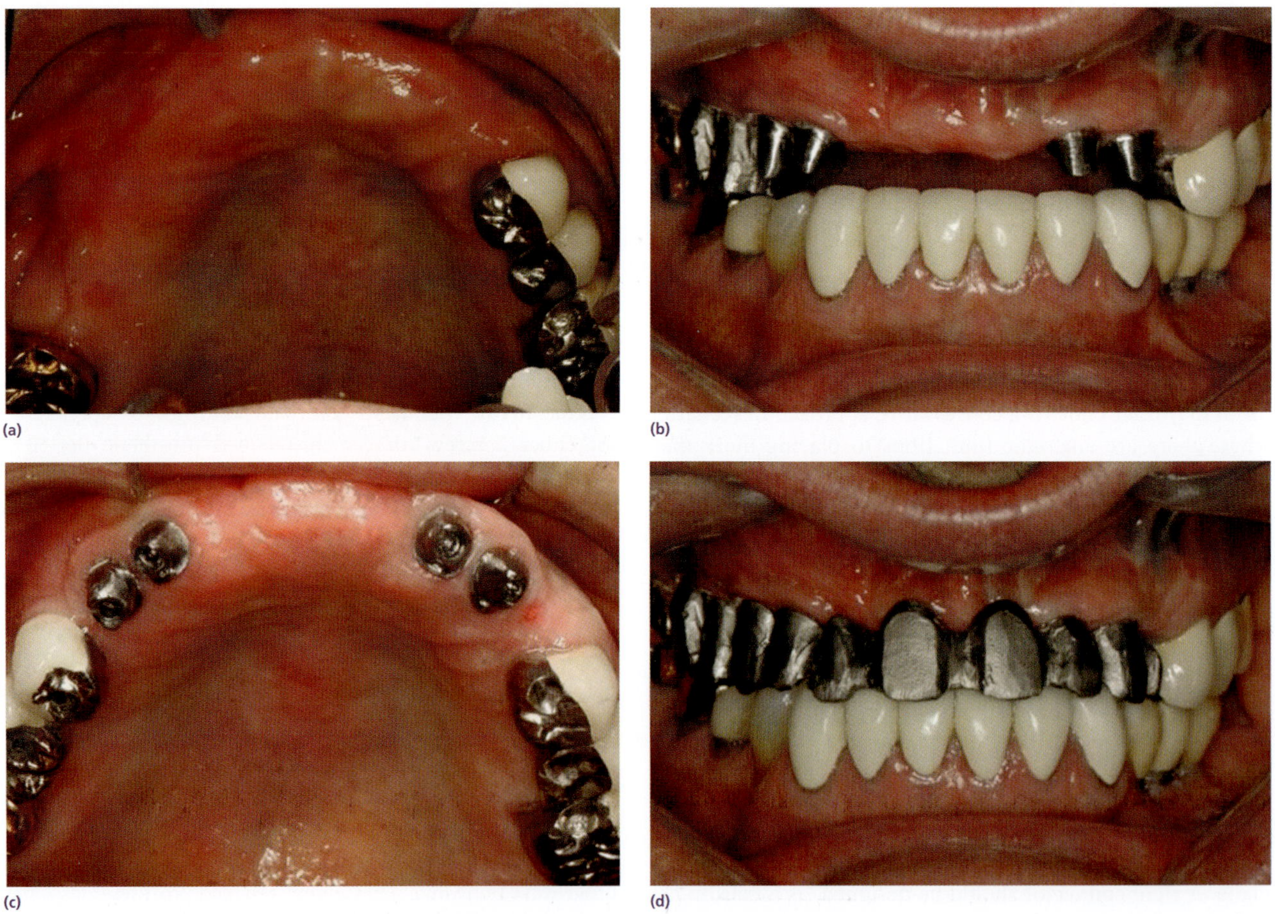

Figure 9.28 (a) Preoperative occlusal view of maxillary partially edentulous arch. (b) Frontal view of abutments for cement-retained cantilevered implant-fixed dental prosthesis design. (c) Occlusal view of abutments for cantilevered implant-fixed dental prosthesis with compromised retention due to both U-shaped arch and short abutments. (d) Frontal view of metal framework for cantilevered implant fixed dental prosthesis which demonstrated an anterior–posterior movement on try-in.

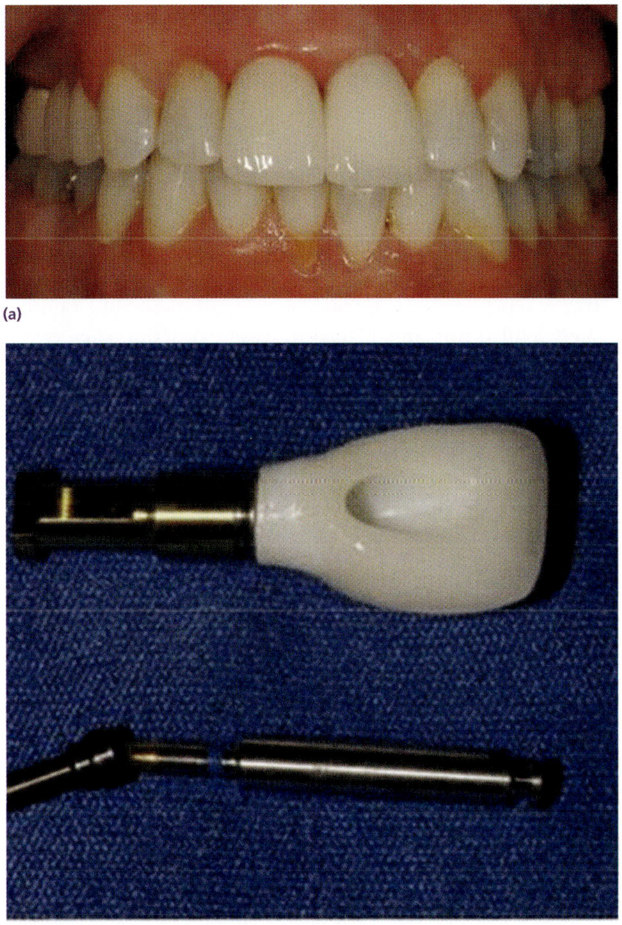

(a)

(b)

Figure 9.29 (a) Angulated Screw Channel design with Nobel Active implant system allowing offset of up to 25° implant axis to cingulum for a screw-retained zirconia crown. *Source:* Reproduced with permission from Brian Kucey. (b) Omnigrip screwdriver to torque screw at an oblique angle.

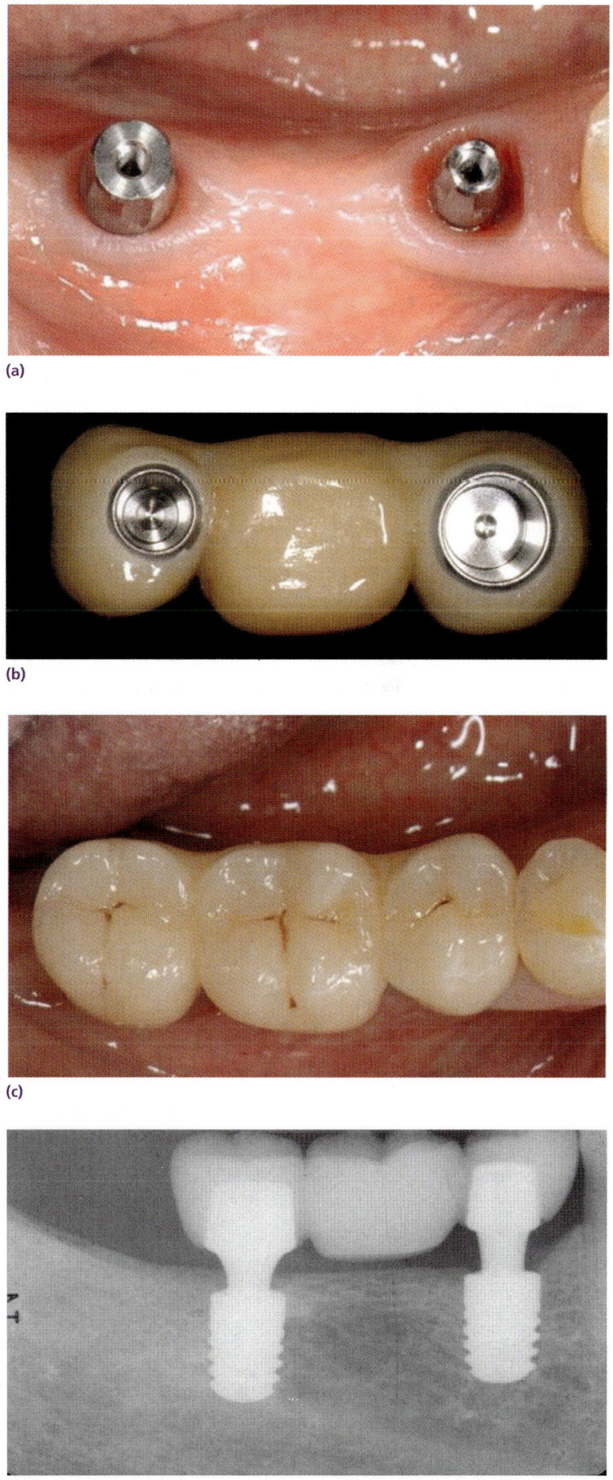

(a)

(b)

(c)

(d)

Figure 9.30 (a) Conometric design using frictional retention instead of cement for three-unit fixed dental prosthesis. (b) Intaglio of fixed dental prosthesis restoring (a). (c) Definitive three-unit fixed dental prosthesis. (d) Periapical radiograph of fixed dental prosthesis in c. *Source:* Reproduced with permission from Marco Degidi.

with a U-shaped arch, IFDPs may be best designed with three to four implants instead of two, when cement-retention is required, to prevent anterior–posterior flexing of the framework (Figure 9.28).

While the incidence of esthetic complications does not appear to be preferential to either retention design and has decreased in more recent studies, biologic and technical complications still loom high.[63] Despite the ease of fabrication, reduced cost, and familiarity with design, cement-retained restorations have higher complications and poor retrievability, making the screw-retained design a more advantageous alternative. However, when the bony trajectory is disparate from the long axis needed for a screw-retained restoration, an innovative design has been brought to market for a cement-free single implant crown (Figure 9.29). In addition, a conometric design has been developed to eliminate cement by using frictional resistance for retention (Figure 9.30).

Immediate loading and immediate implant placement protocols

The surface microtopography of dental implants has been found to be an important factor in the osteoblastic proliferation with titanium implants. Pathway analyses have demonstrated an upregulation of genes associated with signaling cascades relevant to bone healing, such as angiogenesis, osteoclastogenesis, and proteolysis, with moderately roughened implants.[122] This advent has influenced the clinical guidelines for the recommended time span between implant placement and delivery of the implant-supported restoration. Esposito *et al.*[123] have classified the loading protocols as follows:

- immediate loading: restoration connected to implant within 1 week post-placement;
- early loading: restoration connected to implant from 1 week to 2 months post-placement;
- conventional loading: restoration connected to implant after 2 months post-placement.

A number of outcomes has been analyzed in a meta-analysis on comparative loading protocols for SICs such as marginal bone loss, papilla level, midbuccal mucosal level, esthetic outcomes, and patient satisfaction, when implants are placed into a healed site.[124] Assuming careful clinical selection, operator expertise, and an initial insertion torque of >20 to 45 Ncm or an implant stability quotient (ISQ) of >60 to 65, without the need for adjunctive simultaneous augmentation, papilla height did not vary with immediate or conventional loading protocols. The other indices were inconclusive because of heterogeneity of studies or insufficient data. There remains controversy over the minimum insertion torque or ISQ needed to achieve osseointegration.[125,126] In posterior sites, multiple studies concluded implants placed in healed sites with either early or immediate loading did not show any differences in 5-year survival rates.[127] Van de Velde *et al.*,[128] in a split mouth RCT with an 18-month follow-up, compared early loading using conventional surgical protocol with immediate loading using a flapless, guided approach for implants placed in the posterior maxilla. Survival rates ranged between 97.2 and 100% for all implants. In addition, no statistical difference was found in the maxilla or mandible for immediate loading.[129] Further research is suggested for immediate loading protocols to be recommended as a standard procedure in partially edentulous patients with extended edentulous sites. Bone quality, primary insertion torque or ISQ values, the presence of smoking, parafunction, and compliance appear to be critical indices for decision making of immediate loading.[130]

High implant 5-year survival rates have been recorded when a nonfunctional (no centric/eccentric contacts) loaded immediate interim restoration is connected to an immediately placed implant in the esthetic zone (Figure 9.31).[131,132] A comparative retrospective study with a 6–7-year follow-up of immediately loaded implants placed in fresh extraction sites versus healed sites has revealed no statistical differences in success rates.[133] However, more granular patient-centered outcome measurements, such as pink and white esthetics are lacking.[134] A number of investigations have definite inclusion criteria dictating an immediate placement/loading protocol, such as thick tissue biotype and less than 4 mm of vertical loss of the buccal bone in relation to the palatal bone.[135,136]

Often when there is significant facial attachment loss, an immediate implant placement protocol has not been recommended (Figure 9.32b). However, a clinical alternative is to regenerate hard and soft tissues with orthodontic forced eruption or orthodontic forced extraction in preparation for immediate placement (Figure 9.32). The latter technique was evaluated on 32 hopeless teeth and was reported to demonstrate about 70% bone regeneration and 60% gingival regeneration, with an implant survival rate of 96%.[137] What was remarkable was the observation that the residual attachment level (type I–V) was not a limitation, only the interarch space (Figure 9.33). Light (15–50 g) continuous forces placing vertical steps on light wires producing 0.5–1 mm extrusion per month, with a month rest period between activations has been recommended. Orthodontic adjunctive care has been undertaken commonly to prepare implant sites for root proximity, occlusal revamping, mesiodistal spacing, and gingival scalloping of adjacent teeth. However, implant site development to change the crestal bone topography, although first reported over 20 years ago,[138] has recently gained "traction". Whenever additional interceptive care is considered, it must be comprehensively discussed in the informed consent. The importance of operator expertise and patient compliance in the

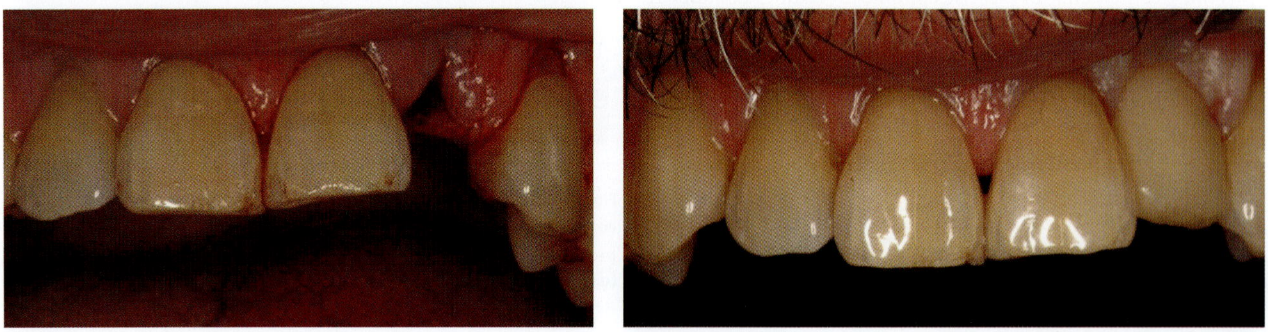

(a) (b)

Figure 9.31 (a) Extraction of root remnant #10 and immediate placement of implant. (b) Immediate provisional crown placement #10.

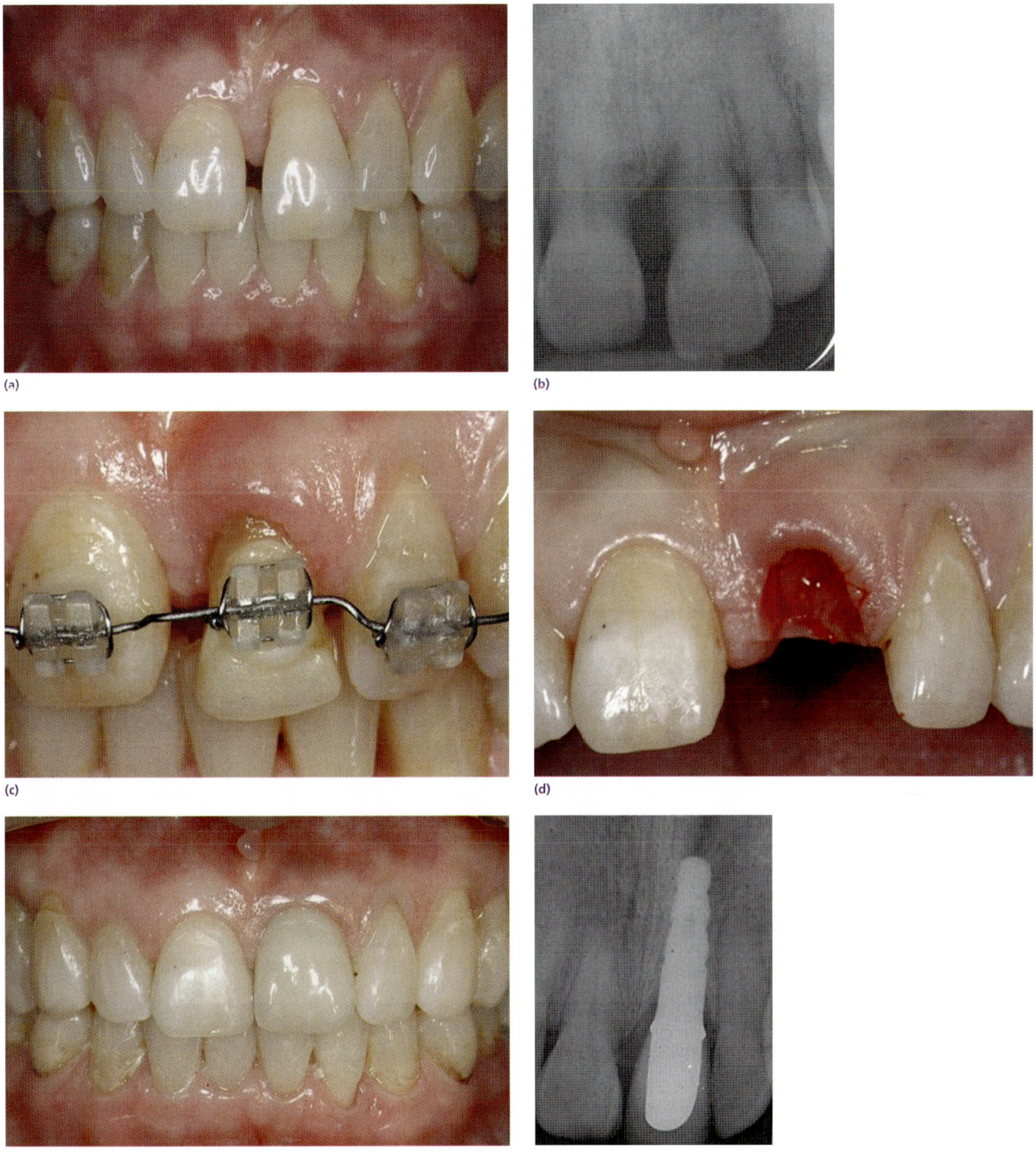

Figure 9.32 (a) Advanced periodontal attachment loss on #9. (b) Periapical radiograph. (c) Orthodontic forced extraction to level the crestal bone before implant placement. (d) Extraction of #9. (e) Definitive implant crown in place. (f) Periapical radiograph of (e).

entire scope of treatment involving immediate placement and provisional restoration cannot be overstated.

If the patient is not a candidate for orthodontic adjunctive care because of clinician-/patient-mediated concerns, should the extraction site be grafted in preparation for delayed implant placement? The sequela of tooth extraction is noted to be crestal bone loss, with width reduction in the coronal region of 2.7 mm as opposed to height reduction on the labial side of 1.9 mm.[139] When reviewing the literature on the effectiveness of alveolar ridge preservation following tooth extraction, in spite of considerable

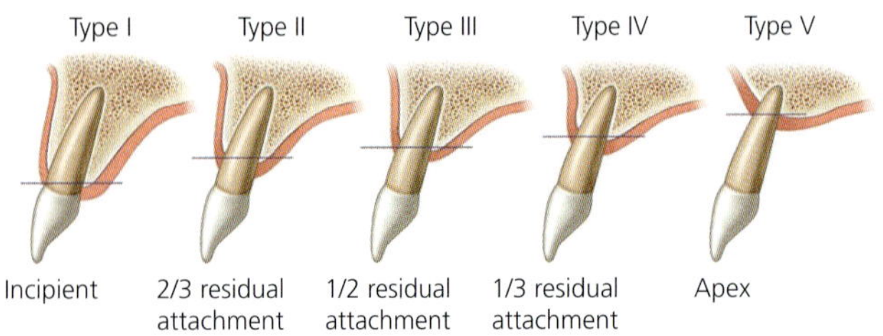

Figure 9.33 Spectrum of attachment loss (type I–V), all of which can capitalize on forced extraction to improve the bony housing for prospective implant placement as described in Amato *et al.* 2012.[137] *Source:* © 2016, Chris Gralapp.

heterogeneity, there appears to be consensus supporting ridge preservation.[140–142] These analyses did not show any clear benefit for one grafting material or the necessity of using a membrane. In addition, primary closure has not been shown to be essential.

Summary

It is the intent of the careful practitioner to restore the patient with the most conservative and enduring treatment. Counter-intuitive evidence in the field of implant rehabilitation for the partially edentulous patient has legitimized a number of prosthetic designs which may lower surgical risk, morbidity, cost, and, in some cases, treatment time. These newer approaches are changing both clinician- and patient-mediated factors.

References

1. Thoma DS, Zeltner M, Husler J, *et al.* EAO Supplement Working Group 4 - EAO CC 2015 Short implants versus sinus lifting with longer implants to restore the posterior maxilla: a systematic review. *Clin Oral Implants Res* 2015; **26**(Suppl 11): 154–169.
2. Nisand D, Picard N, Rocchietta I. Short implants compared to implants in vertically augmented bone: a systematic review. *Clin Oral Implants Res* 2015; **26**(Suppl 11): 170–179.
3. Esposito M, Pellegrino G, Pistilli R, *et al.* Rehabilitation of postrior atrophic edentulous jaws: prostheses supported by 5 mm short implants or by longer implants in augmented bone? One-year results from a pilot randomised clinical trial. *Eur J Oral Implantol* 2011; **4**(1): 21–30.
4. Bashutski JD, Wang HL. Common implant esthetic complications. *Implant Dent* 2007; **16**(4): 340–348.
5. Sadowsky SJ, Bedrossian E. Evidenced-based criteria for differential treatment planning of implant restorations for the partially edentulous patient. *J Prosthodont* 2013; **22**(4): 319–329.
6. Ochsenbein C, Ross S. A reevaluation of osseous surgery. *Dent Clin North Am* 1969; **13**(1): 87–102.
7. Kao RT, Pasquinelli K. Thick vs. thin gingival tissue: a key determinant in tissue response to disease and restorative treatment. *J Calif Dent Assoc* 2002; **30**(7): 521–526.
8. Evans CD, Chen ST. Esthetic outcomes of immediate implant placements. *Clin Oral Implants Res* 2008; **19**(1): 73–80.
9. Schropp L, Wenzel A, Kostopoulos L, *et al.* Bone healing and soft tissue contour changes following single-tooth extraction: a clinical and radiographic 12-month prospective study. *Int J Periodontics Restorative Dent* 2003; **23**(4): 313–323.
10. Kao RT, Fagan MC, Conte GJ. Thick vs. thin gingival biotypes: a key determinant in treatment planning for dental implants. *J Calif Dent Assoc* 2008; **36**(3): 193–198.
11. Lops D, Chiapasco M, Rossi A, *et al.* Incidence of inter-proximal papilla between a tooth and an adjacent immediate implant placed into a fresh extraction socket: 1-year prospective study. *Clin Oral Implants Res* 2008; **19**(11): 1135–1140.
12. Romeo E, Lops D, Rossi A, *et al.* Surgical and prosthetic management of interproximal region with single-implant restorations: 1-year prospective study. *J Periodontol* 2008; **79**(6): 1048–1055.
13. Tao J, Wu Y, Chen J, Su J. A follow-up study of up to 5 years of metal-ceramic crowns in maxillary central incisors for different gingival biotypes. *Int J Periodontics Restorative Dent* 2014; **34**(5): e85–92.
14. Fu JH, Lee A, Wang HL. Influence of tissue biotype on implant esthetics. *Int J Oral Maxillofac Implants* 2011; **26**(3): 499–508.
15. Rodriguez AM, Rosenstiel SF. Esthetic considerations related to bone and soft tissue maintenance and development around dental implants: report of the Committee on Research in Fixed Prosthodontics of the American Academy of Fixed Prosthodontics. *J Prosthet Dent* 2012; **108**(4): 259–267.
16. Strietzel FP, Neumann K, Hertel M. Impact of platform switching on marginal peri-implant bone-level changes. A systematic review and meta-analysis. *Clin Oral Implants Res* 2015; **26**(3): 342–358.
17. Atieh MA, Ibrahim HM, Atieh AH. Platform switching for marginal bone preservation around dental implants: a systematic review and meta-analysis. *J Periodontol* 2010; **81**(10): 1350–1366.
18. Safii SH, Palmer RM, Wilson RF. Risk of implant failure and marginal bone loss in subjects with a history of periodontitis: a systematic review and meta-analysis. *Clin Implant Dent Relat Res* 2010; **12**(3): 165–174.
19. Wen X, Liu R, Li G, *et al.* History of periodontitis as a risk factor for long-term survival of dental implants: a meta-analysis. *Int J Oral Maxillofac Implants* 2014; **29**(6): 1271–1280.
20. Garcia-Bellosta S, Bravo M, Subira C, *et al.* Retrospective study of the long-term survival of 980 implants placed in a periodontal practice. *Int J Oral Maxillofac Implants* 2010; **25**(3): 613–619.
21. Weyant RJ, Burt BA. An assessment of survival rates and within-patient clustering of failures for endosseous oral implants. *J Dent Res* 1993; **72**(1): 2–8.
22. Iqbal MK, Kim S. For teeth requiring endodontic treatment, what are the differences in outcomes of restored endodontically treated teeth compared to implant-supported restorations? *Int J Oral Maxillofac Implants* 2007; **22**(Suppl): 96–116.
23. Torabinejad M, Anderson P, Bader J, *et al.* Outcomes of root canal treatment and restoration, implant-supported single crowns, fixed partial dentures, and extraction without replacement: a systematic review. *J Prosthet Dent* 2007; **98**(4): 285–311.
24. Torabinejad M, Corr R, Handysides R, *et al.* Outcomes of nonsurgical retreatment and endodontic surgery: a systematic review. *J Endod* 2009; **35**(7): 930–937.
25. Doyle SL, Hodges JS, Pesun IJ, *et al.* Retrospective cross sectional comparison of initial nonsurgical endodontic treatment and single-tooth implants. *J Endod* 2006; **32**(9): 822–827.

26. Salehrabi R, Rotstein I. Endodontic treatment outcomes in a large patient population in the USA: an epidemiological study. *J Endod* 2004; **30**(12): 846–850.
27. Ng YL, Mann V, Gulabivala K. A prospective study of the factors affecting outcomes of nonsurgical root canal treatment: part 1: periapical health. *Int Endod J* 2011; **44**(7): 583–609.
28. Zitzmann NU, Krastl G, Hecker H, *et al.* Strategic considerations in treatment planning: deciding when to treat, extract, or replace a questionable tooth. *J Prosthet Dent* 2010; **104**(2): 80–91.
29. Gorni FG, Gagliani MM. The outcome of endodontic retreatment: a 2-yr follow-up. *J Endod* 2004; **30**(1): 1–4.
30. Naito T. Surgical or nonsurgical treatment for teeth with existing root filings? *Evid Based Dent* 2010; **11**(2): 54–55.
31. Song M, Shin SJ, Kim E. Outcomes of endodontic micro-resurgery: a prospective clinical study. *J Endod* 2011; **37**(3): 316–320.
32. Setzer FC, Shah SB, Kohli MR, *et al.* Outcome of endodontic surgery: a meta-analysis of the literature – Part 1: Comparison of traditional root-end surgery and endodontic microsurgery. *J Endod* 2010; **36**(11): 1757–1765.
33. Juloski J, Radovic I, Goracci C, *et al.* Ferrule effect: a literature review. *J Endod* 2012; **38**(1): 11–19.
34. Beikler T, Flemmig TF. EAO consensus conference: economic evaluation of implant-supported prostheses. *Clin Oral Implants Res* 2015; **26**(Suppl 11): 57–63.
35. Samet N, Jotkowitz A. Classification and prognosis evaluation of individual teeth – a comprehensive approach. *Quintessence Int* 2009; **40**(5): 377–387.
36. Salvi GE, Mischler DC, Schmidlin K, *et al.* Risk factors associated with the longevity of multi-rooted teeth. Long-term outcomes after active and supportive periodontal therapy. *J Clin Periodontol* 2014; **41**(7): 701–707.
37. Graetz C, Dorfer CE, Kahl M, *et al.* Retention of questionable and hopeless teeth in compliant patients treated for aggressive periodontitis. *J Clin Periodontol* 2011; **38**(8): 707–714.
38. Fazilat S, Sauerwein R, McLeod J, *et al.* Application of adenosine triphosphate-driven bioluminescence for quantification of plaque bacteria and assessment of oral hygiene in children. *Pediatr Dent* 2010; **32**(3): 195–204.
39. Spielman H, Schaffer SB, Cohen MG, *et al.* Restorative outcomes for endodontically treated teeth in the Practitioners Engaged in Applied Research and Learning network. *J Am Dent Assoc* 2012; **143**(7): 746–755.
40. Da Silva JD, Kazimiroff J, Papas A, *et al.* Outcomes of implants and restorations placed in general dental practices: a retrospective study by the Practitioners Engaged in Applied Research and Learning (PEARL) Network. *J Am Dent Assoc* 2014; **145**(7): 704–713.
41. Fonzar F, Fonzar A, Buttolo P, *et al.* The prognosis of root canal therapy: a 10-year retrospective cohort study on 411 patients with 1175 endodontically treated teeth. *Eur J Oral Implantol* 2009; **2**(3): 201–208.
42. Setzer FC, Kim S. Comparison of long-term survival of implants and endodontically treated teeth. *J Dent Res* 2014; **93**(1): 19–26.
43. Alley BS, Kitchens GG, Alley LW, *et al.* A comparison of survival of teeth following endodontic treatment performed by general dentists or by specialists. *Oral Surg Oral Med Oral Pathol Oral Radiol Endod* 2004; **98**(1): 115–118.
44. Lambert PM, Morris HF, Ochi S. Positive effect of surgical experience with implants on second-stage implant survival. *J Oral Maxillofac Surg* 1997; **55**(12 Suppl 5): 12–18.
45. Mortman RE. Technologic advances in endodontics. *Dent Clin North Am* 2011; **55**(3): 461–480, vii–viii.
46. Tsesis I, Rosen E, Schwartz-Arad D, *et al.* Retrospective evaluation of surgical endodontic treatment: traditional versus modern technique. *J Endod* 2006; **32**(5): 412–416.
47. Pennington MW, Vernazza CR, Shackley P, *et al.* Evaluation of the cost-effectiveness of root canal treatment using conventional approaches versus replacement with an implant. *Int Endod J* 2009; **42**(10): 874–883.
48. Derhalli M, Mounce RE. Clinical decision making regarding endodontics versus implants. *Compend Contin Educ Dent* 2011; **32**(4): 24–35; quiz 36.
49. Pjetursson BE, Bragger U, Lang NP, *et al.* Comparison of survival and complication rates of tooth-supported fixed dental prostheses (FDPs) and implant-supported FDPs and single crowns (SCs). *Clin Oral Implants Res* 2007; **18**(Suppl 3): 97–113.
50. Pjetursson BE, Sailer I, Makarov NA, *et al.* All-ceramic or metal-ceramic tooth-supported fixed dental prostheses (FDPs)? A systematic review of the survival and complication rates. Part II: Multiple-unit FDPs. *Dent Mater* 2015; **31**(6): 624–639.
51. Zembic A, Bosch A, Jung RE, *et al.* Five-year results of a randomized controlled clinical trial comparing zirconia and titanium abutments supporting single-implant crowns in canine and posterior regions. *Clin Oral Implants Res* 2013; **24**(4): 384–390.
52. Berglundh T, Persson L, Klinge B. A systematic review of the incidence of biological and technical complications in implant dentistry reported in prospective longitudinal studies of at least 5 years. *J Clin Periodontol* 2002; **29**(Suppl 3): 197–212; discussion 232–233.
53. Salinas T, Eckert S. Implant-supported single crowns predictably survive to five years with limited complications. *J Evid Based Dent Pract* 2010; **10**(1): 56–57.
54. Zitzmann NU, Krastl G, Weiger R, *et al.* Cost-effectiveness of anterior implants versus fixed dental prostheses. *J Dent Res* 2013; **92**(12 Suppl): 183S–188S.
55. Walton TR. An up-to-15-year comparison of the survival and complication burden of three-unit tooth-supported fixed dental prostheses and implant-supported single crowns. *Int J Oral Maxillofac Implants* 2015; **30**(4): 581–861.
56. Porter JA, von Fraunhofer JA. Success or failure of dental implants? A literature review with treatment considerations. *Gen Dent* 2005; **53**(6): 423–432.
57. Bornstein MM, Cionca N, Mombelli A. Systemic conditions and treatments as risks for implant therapy. *Int J Oral Maxillofac Implants* 2009; **24**(Suppl): 12–27.
58. Myshin HL, Wiens JP. Factors affecting soft tissue around dental implants: a review of the literature. *J Prosthet Dent* 2005; **94**(5): 440–444.
59. John V, Chen S, Parashos P. Implant or the natural tooth – a contemporary treatment planning dilemma? *Aust Dent J* 2007; **52**(1 Suppl): S138–150.
60. Belser UC, Schmid B, Higginbottom F, *et al.* Outcome analysis of implant restorations located in the anterior maxilla: a review of the recent literature. *Int J Oral Maxillofac Implants* 2004; **19**(Suppl): 30–42.
61. Buser D, Martin W, Belser UC. Optimizing esthetics for implant restorations in the anterior maxilla: anatomic and surgical considerations. *Int J Oral Maxillofac Implants* 2004; **19**(Suppl): 43–61.

62. Christensen GJ. Implant therapy versus endodontic therapy. *J Am Dent Assoc* 2006; **137**(10): 1440–1443.
63. Pjetursson BE, Asgeirsson AG, Zwahlen M, *et al.* Improvements in implant dentistry over the last decade: comparison of survival and complication rates in older and newer publications. *Int J Oral Maxillofac Implants* 2014; **29**(Suppl): 308–324.
64. Klinge B, Meyle J. Peri-implant tissue destruction. The Third EAO Consensus Conference 2012. *Clin Oral Implants Res* 2012; **23**(Suppl 6): 108–110.
65. Sailer I, Philipp A, Zembic A, *et al.* A systematic review of the performance of ceramic and metal implant abutments supporting fixed implant reconstructions. *Clin Oral Implants Res* 2009; **20**(Suppl 4): 4–31.
66. Chen ST, Buser D. Esthetic outcomes following immediate and early implant placement in the anterior maxilla – a systematic review. *Int J Oral Maxillofac Implants* 2014; **29**(Suppl): 186–215.
67. Yeung SC. Biological basis for soft tissue management in implant dentistry. *Aust Dent J* 2008; **53**(Suppl 1): S39–42.
68. Kim Y, Oh TJ, Misch CE, *et al.* Occlusal considerations in implant therapy: clinical guidelines with biomechanical rationale. *Clin Oral Implants Res* 2005; **16**(1): 26–35.
69. Krishnan V, Tony Thomas C, Sabu I. Management of abutment screw loosening: review of literature and report of a case. *J Indian Prosthodont Soc* 2014; **14**(3): 208–214.
70. Gracis S, Michalakis K, Vigolo P, *et al.* Internal vs. external connections for abutments/reconstructions: a systematic review. *Clin Oral Implants Res* 2012; **23**(Suppl 6): 202–216.
71. Byrne D, Jacobs S, O'Connell B, *et al.* Preloads generated with repeated tightening in three types of screws used in dental implant assemblies. *J Prosthodont* 2006; **15**(3): 164–171.
72. Cantwell A, Hobkirk JA. Preload loss in gold prosthesis-retaining screws as a function of time. *Int J Oral Maxillofac Implants* 2004; **19**(1): 124–132.
73. Yi YJ, Lee JY, Kim YK. Comparative clinical study of three-unit fixed partial prostheses supported by two or three implants. *Int J Oral Maxillofac Implants* 2013; **28**(4): 1110–1115.
74. Salvi GE, Bragger U. Mechanical and technical risks in implant therapy. *Int J Oral Maxillofac Implants* 2009; **24**(Suppl): 69–85.
75. Eliasson A, Eriksson T, Johansson A, *et al.* Fixed partial prostheses supported by 2 or 3 implants: a retrospective study up to 18 years. *Int J Oral Maxillofac Implants* 2006; **21**(4): 567–574.
76. Frost HM. Wolff's Law and bone's structural adaptations to mechanical usage: an overview for clinicians. *Angle Orthod* 1994; **64**(3): 175–188.
77. Tarnow D, Elian N, Fletcher P, *et al.* Vertical distance from the crest of bone to the height of the interproximal papilla between adjacent implants. *J Periodontol* 2003; **74**(12): 1785–1788.
78. Teughels W, Merheb J, Quirynen M. Critical horizontal dimensions of interproximal and buccal bone around implants for optimal aesthetic outcomes: a systematic review. *Clin Oral Implants Res* 2009; **20**(Suppl 4): 134–145.
79. Ishikawa T, Salama M, Funato A, *et al.* Three-dimensional bone and soft tissue requirements for optimizing esthetic results in compromised cases with multiple implants. *Int J Periodontics Restorative Dent* 2010; **30**(5): 503–511.
80. Koutouzis T, Wennstrom JL. Bone level changes at axial- and non-axial-positioned implants supporting fixed partial dentures. A 5-year retrospective longitudinal study. *Clin Oral Implants Res* 2007; **18**(5): 585–590.
81. Del Fabbro M, Ceresoli V. The fate of marginal bone around axial vs. tilted implants: a systematic review. *Eur J Oral Implantol* 2014; 7(Suppl 2): S171–189.
82. Barnea E, Tal H, Nissan J, *et al.* The use of tilted implant for posterior atrophic maxilla. *Clin Implant Dent Relat Res* 2015; doi: 10.1111/cid.12342. [Epub ahead of print]
83. Monje A, Chan HL, Suarez F, *et al.* Marginal bone loss around tilted implants in comparison to straight implants: a meta-analysis. *Int J Oral Maxillofac Implants* 2012; **27**(6): 1576–1583.
84. Hammerle CH, Ungerer MC, Fantoni PC, *et al.* Long-term analysis of biologic and technical aspects of fixed partial dentures with cantilevers. *Int J Prosthodont* 2000; **13**(5): 409–415.
85. Sundh B, Odman P. A study of fixed prosthodontics performed at a university clinic 18 years after insertion. *Int J Prosthodont* 1997; **10**(6): 513–519.
86. Karlsson S. Failures and length of service in fixed prosthodontics after long-term function. A longitudinal clinical study. *Swed Dent J* 1989; **13**(5): 185–192.
87. Becker CM. Cantilever fixed prostheses utilizing dental implants: a 10-year retrospective analysis. *Quintessence Int* 2004; **35**(6): 437–441.
88. Romeo E, Tomasi C, Finini I, *et al.* Implant-supported fixed cantilever prosthesis in partially edentulous jaws: a cohort prospective study. *Clin Oral Implants Res* 2009; **20**(11): 1278–1285.
89. Wennstrom J, Zurdo J, Karlsson S, *et al.* Bone level change at implant-supported fixed partial dentures with and without cantilever extension after 5 years in function. *J Clin Periodontol* 2004; **31**(12): 1077–1083.
90. Palmer RM, Howe LC, Palmer PJ, *et al.* A prospective clinical trial of single Astra Tech 4.0 or 5.0 diameter implants used to support two-unit cantilever bridges: results after 3 years. *Clin Oral Implants Res* 2012; **23**(1): 35–40.
91. Blanes RJ, Bernard JP, Blanes ZM, *et al.* A 10-year prospective study of ITI dental implants placed in the posterior region. II: Influence of the crown-to-implant ratio and different prosthetic treatment modalities on crestal bone loss. *Clin Oral Implants Res* 2007; **18**(6): 707–714.
92. Aglietta M, Siciliano VI, Zwahlen M, *et al.* A systematic review of the survival and complication rates of implant supported fixed dental prostheses with cantilever extensions after an observation period of at least 5 years. *Clin Oral Implants Res* 2009; **20**(5): 441–451.
93. Clelland NL, Seidt JD, Daroz LG, *et al.* Comparison of strains for splinted and nonsplinted implant prostheses using three-dimensional image correlation. *Int J Oral Maxillofac Implants* 2010; **25**(5): 953–959.
94. Vigolo P, Mutinelli S, Zaccaria M, *et al.* Clinical evaluation of marginal bone level change around multiple adjacent implants restored with splinted and nonsplinted restorations: a 10-year randomized controlled trial. *Int J Oral Maxillofac Implants* 2015; **30**(2): 411–418.
95. Norton MR. Multiple single-tooth implant restorations in the posterior jaws: maintenance of marginal bone levels with reference to the implant-abutment microgap. *Int J Oral Maxillofac Implants* 2006; **21**(5): 777–784.
96. Brunski JB. Biomechanical factors affecting the bone-dental implant interface. *Clin Mater* 1992; **10**(3): 153–201.
97. Anitua E, Pinas L, Begona L, *et al.* Long-term retrospective evaluation of short implants in the posterior areas: clinical results after 10-12 years. *J Clin Periodontol* 2014; **41**(4): 404–411.

98. Daftary F, Mahallati R, Bahat O, *et al.* Lifelong craniofacial growth and the implications for osseointegrated implants. *Int J Oral Maxillofac Implants* 2013; **28**(1): 163–169.
99. Malchiodi L, Cucchi A, Ghensi P, *et al.* Influence of crown-implant ratio on implant success rates and crestal bone levels: a 36-month follow-up prospective study. *Clin Oral Implants Res* 2014; **25**(2): 240–251.
100. Schneider D, Witt L, Hammerle CH. Influence of the crown-to-implant length ratio on the clinical performance of implants supporting single crown restorations: a cross-sectional retrospective 5-year investigation. *Clin Oral Implants Res* 2012; **23**(2): 169–174.
101. Lee KJ, Kim YG, Park JW, *et al.* Influence of crown-to-implant ratio on periimplant marginal bone loss in the posterior region: a five-year retrospective study. *J Periodontal Implant Sci* 2012; **42**(6): 231–236.
102. Naert I, Duyck J, Vandamme K. Occlusal overload and bone/implant loss. *Clin Oral Implants Res* 2012; **23**(Suppl 6): 95–107.
103. Renouard F, Nisand D. Impact of implant length and diameter on survival rates. *Clin Oral Implants Res* 2006; **17**(Suppl 2): 35–51.
104. Ekfeldt A, Christiansson U, Eriksson T, *et al.* A retrospective analysis of factors associated with multiple implant failures in maxillae. *Clin Oral Implants Res* 2001; **12**(5): 462–467.
105. Shi JY, Gu YX, Qiao SC, *et al.* Clinical evaluation of short 6-mm implants alone, short 8-mm implants combined with osteotome sinus floor elevation and standard 10-mm implants combined with osteotome sinus floor elevation in posterior maxillae: study protocol for a randomized controlled trial. *Trials* 2015; **16**: 324.
106. Lee SA, Lee CT, Fu MM, *et al.* Systematic review and meta-analysis of randomized controlled trials for the management of limited vertical height in the posterior region: short implants (5 to 8 mm) vs longer implants (>8 mm) in vertically augmented sites. *Int J Oral Maxillofac Implants* 2014; **29**(5): 1085–1097.
107. Felice P, Cannizzaro G, Barausse C, *et al.* Short implants versus longer implants in vertically augmented posterior mandibles: a randomised controlled trial with 5-year after loading follow-up. *Eur J Oral Implantol* 2014; **7**(4): 359–369.
108. Narby B, Kronstrom M, Soderfeldt B, *et al.* Changes in attitudes toward desire for implant treatment: a longitudinal study of a middle-aged and older Swedish population. *Int J Prosthodont* 2008; **21**(6): 481–485.
109. Carlsson GE, Omar R. The future of complete dentures in oral rehabilitation. A critical review. *J Oral Rehabil* 2010; **37**(2): 143–156.
110. Klein MO, Schiegnitz E, Al-Nawas B. Systematic review on success of narrow-diameter dental implants. *Int J Oral Maxillofac Implants* 2014; **29**(Suppl): 43–54.
111. Lang NP, Pjetursson BE, Tan K, *et al.* A systematic review of the survival and complication rates of fixed partial dentures (FPDs) after an observation period of at least 5 years. II. Combined tooth–implant-supported FPDs. *Clin Oral Implants Res* 2004; **15**(6): 643–653.
112. Pjetursson BE, Tan K, Lang NP, *et al.* A systematic review of the survival and complication rates of fixed partial dentures (FPDs) after an observation period of at least 5 years. *Clin Oral Implants Res* 2004; **15**(6): 625–942.
113. Bragger U, Aeschlimann S, Burgin W, *et al.* Biological and technical complications and failures with fixed partial dentures (FPD) on implants and teeth after four to five years of function. *Clin Oral Implants Res* 2001; **12**(1): 26–34.
114. Weber HP, Sukotjo C. Does the type of implant prosthesis affect outcomes in the partially edentulous patient? *Int J Oral Maxillofac Implants* 2007; **22**(Suppl): 140–172.
115. Block MS, Lirette D, Gardiner D, *et al.* Prospective evaluation of implants connected to teeth. *Int J Oral Maxillofac Implants* 2002; **17**(4): 473–487.
116. Sherif S, Susarla SM, Hwang JW, *et al.* Clinician- and patient-reported long-term evaluation of screw- and cement-retained implant restorations: a 5-year prospective study. *Clin Oral Investig* 2011; **15**(6): 993–999.
117. Sailer I, Muhlemann S, Zwahlen M, *et al.* Cemented and screw-retained implant reconstructions: a systematic review of the survival and complication rates. *Clin Oral Implants Res* 2012; **23**(Suppl 6): 163–201.
118. Nissan J, Narobai D, Gross O, *et al.* Long-term outcome of cemented versus screw-retained implant-supported partial restorations. *Int J Oral Maxillofac Implants* 2011; **26**(5): 1102–1107.
119. Wittneben JG, Millen C, Bragger U. Clinical performance of screw- versus cement-retained fixed implant-supported reconstructions – a systematic review. *Int J Oral Maxillofac Implants* 2014; **29**(Suppl): 84–98.
120. Wilson TG, Jr., Valderrama P, Burbano M, *et al.* Foreign bodies associated with peri-implantitis human biopsies. *J Periodontol* 2015; **86**(1): 9–15.
121. Wadhwani C, Rapoport D, La Rosa S, *et al.* Radiographic detection and characteristic patterns of residual excess cement associated with cement-retained implant restorations: a clinical report. *J Prosthet Dent* 2012; **107**(3): 151–157.
122. Vlacic-Zischke J, Hamlet SM, Friis T, *et al.* The influence of surface microroughness and hydrophilicity of titanium on the up-regulation of TGFbeta/BMP signalling in osteoblasts. *Biomaterials* 2011; **32**(3): 665–671.
123. Esposito M, Grusovin MG, Willings M, *et al.* Interventions for replacing missing teeth: different times for loading dental implants. *Cochrane Database Syst Rev* 2007(**2**):CD003878.
124. Benic GI, Mir-Mari J, Hammerle CH. Loading protocols for single-implant crowns: a systematic review and meta-analysis. *Int J Oral Maxillofac Implants* 2014; **29**(Suppl): 222–238.
125. Degidi M, Daprile G, Piattelli A. Primary stability determination by means of insertion torque and RFA in a sample of 4,135 implants. *Clin Implant Dent Relat Res* 2012; **14**(4): 501–507.
126. Park KJ, Kwon JY, Kim SK, *et al.* The relationship between implant stability quotient values and implant insertion variables: a clinical study. *J Oral Rehabil* 2012; **39**(2): 151–159.
127. Capelli M, Esposito M, Zuffetti F, *et al.* A 5-year report from a multicentre randomised clinical trial: immediate non-occlusal versus early loading of dental implants in partially edentulous patients. *Eur J Oral Implantol* 2010; **3**(3): 209–219.
128. Van de Velde T, Sennerby L, De Bruyn H. The clinical and radiographic outcome of implants placed in the posterior maxilla with a guided flapless approach and immediately restored with a provisional rehabilitation: a randomized clinical trial. *Clin Oral Implants Res* 2010; **21**(11): 1223–1233.
129. Schrott A, Riggi-Heiniger M, Maruo K, *et al.* Implant loading protocols for partially edentulous patients with extended edentulous sites--a systematic review and meta-analysis. *Int J Oral Maxillofac Implants* 2014; **29**(Suppl): 239–255.
130. Gapski R, Wang HL, Mascarenhas P, *et al.* Critical review of immediate implant loading. *Clin Oral Implants Res* 2003; **14**(5): 515–527.

131. Noelken R, Kunkel M, Jung BA, *et al.* Immediate nonfunctional loading of NobelPerfect implants in the anterior dental arch in private practice – 5-year data. *Clin Implant Dent Relat Res* 2014; **16**(1): 21–31.
132. Noelken R, Neffe BA, Kunkel M, *et al.* Maintenance of marginal bone support and soft tissue esthetics at immediately provisionalized OsseoSpeed implants placed into extraction sites: 2-year results. *Clin Oral Implants Res* 2014; **25**(2): 214–220.
133. Malchiodi L, Ghensi P, Cucchi A, *et al.* A comparative retrospective study of immediately loaded implants in postextraction sites versus healed sites: results after 6 to 7 years in the maxilla. *Int J Oral Maxillofac Implants* 2011; **26**(2): 373–384.
134. Grutter L, Belser UC. Implant loading protocols for the partially edentulous esthetic zone. *Int J Oral Maxillofac Implants* 2009; **24**(Suppl): 169–179.
135. Felice P, Pistilli R, Barausse C, *et al.* Immediate non-occlusal loading of immediate post-extractive versus delayed placement of single implants in preserved sockets of the anterior maxilla: 1-year post-loading outcome of a randomised controlled trial. *Eur J Oral Implantol* 2015; **8**(4): 361–372.
136. Esposito M, Barausse C, Pistilli R, *et al.* Immediate loading of post-extractive versus delayed placed single implants in the anterior maxilla: outcome of a pragmatic multicenter randomised controlled trial 1-year after loading. *Eur J Oral Implantol* 2015; **8**(4): 347–358.
137. Amato F, Mirabella AD, Macca U, *et al.* Implant site development by orthodontic forced extraction: a preliminary study. *Int J Oral Maxillofac Implants* 2012; **27**(2): 411–420.
138. Salama H, Salama M. The role of orthodontic extrusive remodeling in the enhancement of soft and hard tissue profiles prior to implant placement: a systematic approach to the management of extraction site defects. *Int J Periodontics Restorative Dent* 1993; **13**(4): 312–333.
139. Li B, Wang Y. Contour changes in human alveolar bone following tooth extraction of the maxillary central incisor. *J Zhejiang Univ Sci B* 2014; **15**(12): 1064–1071.
140. Horowitz R, Holtzclaw D, Rosen PS. A review on alveolar ridge preservation following tooth extraction. *J Evid Based Dent Pract* 2012; **12**(3 Suppl): 149–160.
141. Agarwal G, Thomas R, Mehta D. Postextraction maintenance of the alveolar ridge: rationale and review. *Compend Contin Educ Dent* 2012; **33**(5): 320–326.
142. Bartee BK. Extraction site reconstruction for alveolar ridge preservation. Part 1: rationale and materials selection. *J Oral Implantol* 2001; **27**(4): 187–193.

CHAPTER 10

Prosthodontic Considerations in the Implant Restoration of the Esthetic Zone

Ghadeer Thalji[1] and Sandra Al-Tarawneh[2]

[1] University of Illinois at Chicago College of Dentistry Chicago, Illinois, USA

[2] University of Jordan, Amman, Jordan

The esthetic zone can be defined as any dentoalveolar segment that is visible upon full smile from an objective standpoint. Subjectively, it has been defined as any dentoalveolar area of esthetic importance to the patient.[1] Unlike implant therapy in other segments of the oral cavity, implant treatment in the esthetic zone is one of the most intricate procedures in terms of creating harmonious gingival contours, and is often classified as advanced or complex according to the SAC classification.[2] Therefore, esthetic risk assessment analysis and determination of patients' expectations preoperatively are critical to successful implant therapy. Some of the challenging risk factors that make the case fall into the high-risk category for esthetic results include:[2–7]

- high lip line (high smile line, revealing the total cervicoincisal length of the maxillary anterior teeth and a contiguous band of gingiva);
- highly scalloped thin gingival biotype (more prone for recession compared to flat thick biotype);
- triangular shape of tooth crown;
- acute infection at implant site;
- bone level at adjacent teeth more than 6 mm to the contact point, which makes interdental papillary fill very difficult, if not impossible;
- restored adjacent teeth;
- an edentulous space of two or more teeth;
- soft tissue defect;
- vertical bone deficiency;
- adjacent implant restoration (inadequate inter-implant papilla);
- long junctional epithelium, low crest bony topography.

Esthetic risk factors should be recognized and explained to the patient before the initiation of implant therapy to avoid post-treatment disappointment that can occur from unmet high expectations; patient expectations are higher with implant restorations than with conventional prostheses.[8]

Achieving predictable long-term esthetics for an implant restoration requires a comprehensive multidisciplinary planning approach prior to surgical intervention and a restorative-driven approach. Patients' preoperative evaluation should include a comprehensive medical and dental history, diagnostic casts, photographs, site analysis, wax-up, and the necessary radiographs, which may include cone-beam computed tomography (CBCT) and virtual planning using suitable software. When a CBCT is selected, proper execution of the treatment plan is carried out through transfer of the virtual plan into real life through the surgical guide, and manipulation of the soft tissue architecture with the use of a properly designed interim restoration and, finally, the definitive restoration.

Adjunctive therapy, including orthodontics, additional restorative procedures, hard/soft tissue augmentation procedures, and/or periodontal therapy, should be considered and discussed with patients to optimize final treatment outcomes.

Examination and site analysis

A comprehensive evaluation of the site of interest is crucial and can provide a coherent guidance system for dental esthetics. A checklist for site analysis in the esthetic zone is included in Box 10.1.[1,9–14]

Diagnostic wax-up, radiographic guide fabrication, and three-dimensional imaging/virtual planning

Clinicians' objectives should be targeted to achieving predictable outcomes in the short and long term that respect the biological, functional, and esthetic requirements.[15] Ultimately, the desired tooth position must be the guide for final implant position. After performing a diagnostic wax-up that determines the position of the proposed gingival zenith (as it represents the most apical part of the clinical crown),[9,10] a radiographic guide can be

Evidence-based Implant Treatment Planning and Clinical Protocols, First Edition. Edited by Steven J. Sadowsky.

Companion website: www.wiley.com/go/sadowsky/implant

Box 10.1 Checklist for site analysis in the esthetic zone.

Gingival health
Width of facial keratinized mucosa
Arrangement, contour, and shade of adjacent teeth
Incisal edge configuration
Height of smile line
Lower lip line
Lip support
Smile symmetry
Midline and occlusal plane orientation
Balance of gingival levels
Gingival zenith position
Gingival morphotype (thin with highly scalloped gingiva, thick with shallow scalloped gingiva)
Interocclusal relationship (horizontal and vertical)
Dimension of the edentulous gap (mesiodistal gap dimension, single unit vs. multiple missing teeth)
Anatomy of the alveolar crest (horizontal bone deficiency, vertical bone deficiency)
Interdental contact location
Parameters affecting papillary tissue development (distance from proximal contact to interseptal bone, tooth to implant distance, inter-implant distance, platform switching)
Three-dimensional image analysis of CBCT obtained with a radiographic guide in place (adequate bone volume, anatomic structures, pathologies, axis of adjacent roots)

fabricated and a CBCT obtained with the radiographic guide in place, if a three-dimensional (3-D) scan is deemed necessary. This allows the proposed position of the definitive restoration to be related to the surrounding soft tissues and underlying bone. A decision can then be made whether the available bone foundation is sufficient or augmentation procedures will be needed (Figures 10.1 and 10.2). Ideally, a minimum of 2 mm of facial bone thickness is needed once the implant osteotomy has been prepared to minimize facial bone loss and consequent peri-implant soft tissue recession.[16] Grafting should be considered to obtain this amount of bone in cases where there was a deficiency upon site evaluation. Virtual planning may be followed by fabrication of CAD/CAM implant surgical guides which may enhance accuracy of implant placement (Figure 10.3). The use of surgical templates is of great importance for proper implant positioning.

Planning the implant position

Single-tooth implant restorations

Correct 3-D implant placement is critical for an esthetic treatment outcome. It is well known that biologic width around implants is slightly more than the average dentogingival complex dimension,[17–19] and the position of peri-implant mucosa attachment tends to be subcrestal compared to natural teeth where biologic width always forms supracrestally.[20] This makes maintaining or reforming the interdental papilla challenging and requires very careful planning for implant–tooth and inter-implant distance. Tarnow and colleagues[21] have shown that when the measurement from the interproximal coronal contact point to the crest of bone is 5 mm or less, the papilla is present almost 100% of the time. When the distance is 6 mm or greater, the papilla is present 50% of the time or less, and at 7 mm, the interdental space is completely filled about 25% of the time.[21] Hence, in the esthetic zone, the distance from alveolar crest to the adjacent tooth cementoenamel junction should be 3–5 mm to achieve the ideal implant location and appropriate space for the peri-implant sulcus to form.[20–23]

Control of the 3-D implant placement is a prerequisite for a pleasing mucosal margin level. This includes its position in the apicoronal, mesiodistal, and labiopalatal directions. This can be achieved by placing the implant abutment interface 3 mm apically from the gingival zenith and displacing it palatally by 2 mm.[9,10,24] Mesiodistally, it is recommended that a minimum distance of 1.5 mm be left between an implant and an adjacent tooth in order to maintain the bone and provide better esthetics.[25] However, recent studies have shown that, when using the platform-switching concept, it is possible to place the implant as close as 1 mm to the adjacent tooth without compromising crestal bone.[26–31]

Poor implant placement as a result of inadequate planning or poor execution of the plan can create significant esthetic complications. Placing the implant too deep or too facial might result in facial bone resorption and subsequent recession.[16] Placing the implant too shallow results in a visible metal margin, while placing the implant too palatal results in an improper emergence with a ridge. However, when planned according to the correct parameters, an esthetic result is more predictable (Figure 10.4).

Errors in the mesiodistal direction can substantially affect the generation of interproximal papillary support and bone crest resorption.[9,12] Additionally, special care should be placed on selection of proper implant size, based on site anatomy and the planned restoration.

Multiple missing teeth

Multiple missing teeth in the esthetic zone require a great deal of attention. Critical factors that must be considered include the number of implants used, inter-implant spacing, and angulation. Proper planning, with an ideal diagnostic wax-up and utilization of a surgical guide to avoid misplacement at embrasure sites, are a must. It is commonly observed that it is more difficult to create a papilla between two adjacent implants than it is to maintain or create a papilla between an implant and a natural tooth.[32] Tarnow and colleagues[21] reported a mean papillary height between two adjacent implants as 3.4 mm. Reduced inter-implant distance of less than 3 mm was shown to have a negative effect on the midproximal crestal bone levels. This is due to the extent of lateral bone loss. Maintaining a distance of more than 3 mm between two adjacent implants appears to preserve the interproximal bone peak and result in only 0.45 mm of resorption on average. In contrast, if the space between the

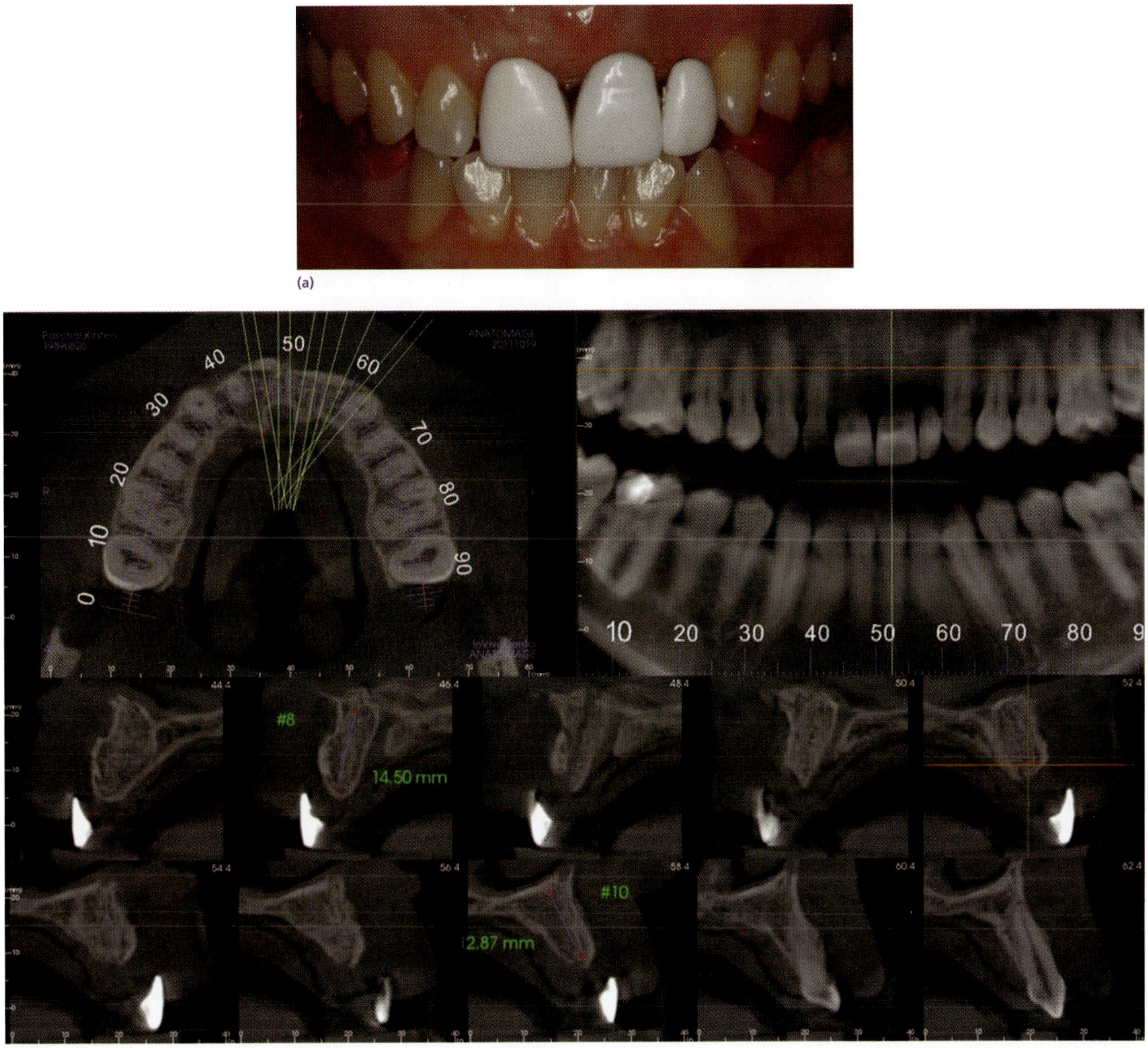

(a) (b)

Figure 10.1 (a) Radiographic guide fabricated using radiopaque teeth tried intraorally prior to obtaining CBCT. GC resin occlusal jig in place to allow separation of teeth and stabilize the patient during the process. (b) Sagittal section through site #9 shows the exact relation of the proposed final restoration position to the available bone bed demonstrating availability of bone for proper 3-D positioning of the fixture.

implants is 3 mm or less, average resorption of the interproximal bone peak increases to 1.04 mm, which compromises support for the inter-implant papilla.[31,32] Selective utilization of implants with a smaller diameter at the implant–abutment interface may be beneficial when multiple implants are to be placed in the esthetic zone, so that a minimum of 3 mm of bone can be retained between them.[32] In some cases involving multiple missing teeth, an implant-supported fixed dental prosthesis may be a more preferable choice through alternating implants and pontics in order to optimize soft tissue esthetics.[6] A greater projection of papilla may be seen around a pontic–pontic (6 mm) and implant–pontic (5.5 mm) than that between two implants (3.5 mm).[33]

Recent follow-up studies using new implant designs with internal conical connection and platform switching have shown that inter-implant bone levels can be maintained at similar levels when implants are placed at 2 mm or 3 mm inter-implant distances.[34–37] In cases where a significant amount of hard and soft tissue has been lost due to trauma or pathologies, it becomes imperative to plan for the use of pink ceramics or even the use of removable prostheses to compensate for the lost tissues.[38]

Anatomic factors

The presence of adequate bone and soft tissue volumes is crucial to achieving successful esthetic treatment outcome of dental implants in the anterior maxilla. Compromised esthetic outcomes,

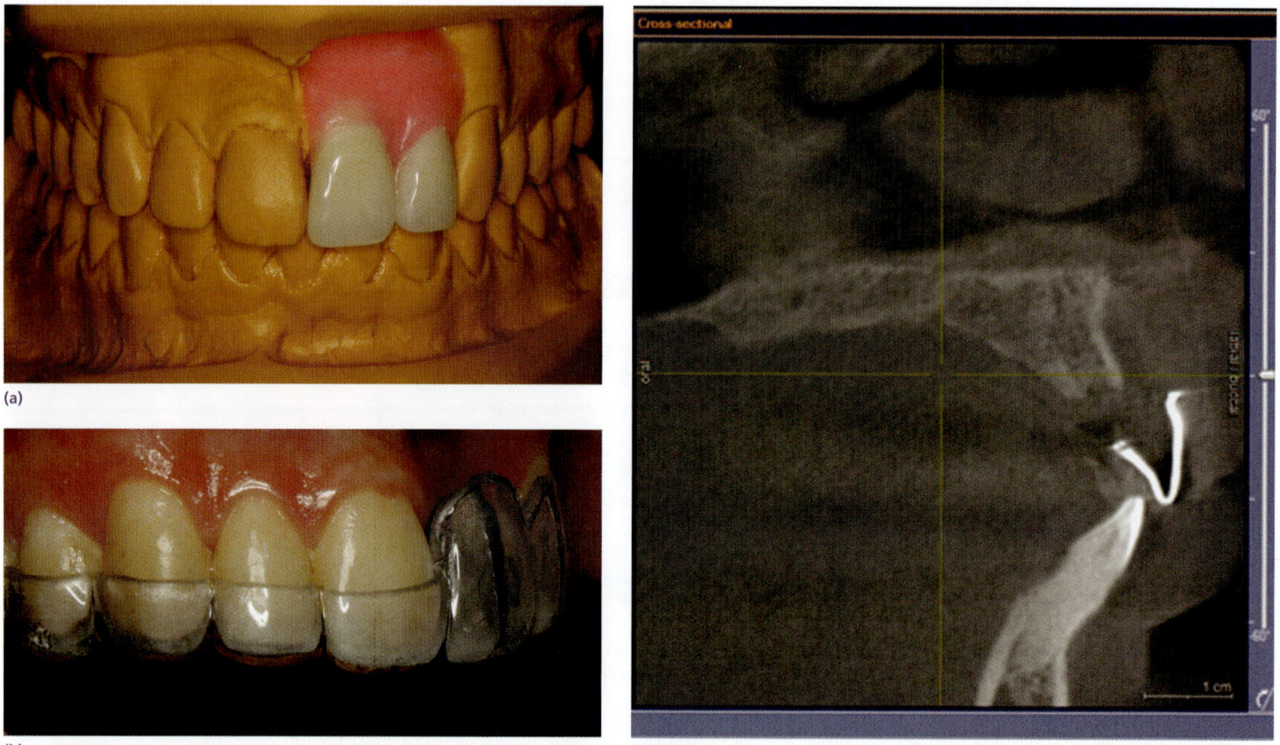

Figure 10.2 (a) Diagnostic wax-up for the proposed definitive restorations on maxillary left central and lateral incisors. (b) Radiographic guide fabricated using a vacuum template with lead foils centered on each tooth tried intraorally, demonstrating deficiency in facial bone in relation to the proposed definitive restoration position. (c) Sagittal section through the CBCT volume showing deficiency in facial bone that was noticed clinically in a quantifiable manner. In such a case, augmentation would be considered based on these findings.

due to the crest collapse that occurs following extraction, in particular during the first 3 months after the extraction,[34] is a major risk. A mean bone shrinkage of 3.79 mm horizontally and 1.24 mm vertically may occur following a tooth extraction in the maxilla.[35] Greater bone loss takes place at multiple adjacent extraction sites.[36] Ridge preservation can significantly limit the bone resorption process.[37,39] Jambhekar and colleagues[40] compared, in a systematic review, the clinical and histologic outcomes between various socket grafting procedures with the flapless extraction, after a minimum of 12 weeks of healing. The mean loss of buccolingual width at the ridge crest was lowest for xenografts (1.3 mm), followed by allografts (1.63 mm), alloplasts (2.13 mm), and sockets without any socket grafting (2.79 mm).[40] Despite the reduced bone loss with ridge preservation, bone remodeling still occurs, resulting in a buccal concavity, which may ultimately cause an esthetic discrepancy. The amount of dimensional changes occurring following tooth loss is influenced by local factors, including periodontal status, presence of dehiscence, and the type and fit of the interim prosthesis, as well as systemic factors, such as patient's general health and habits such as smoking. Preservation of the alveolar ridge dimension at both the hard and soft tissue level is critical to the functional and esthetic rehabilitation of missing teeth in the esthetic zone. Adequate soft tissue volumes may affect the soft tissue profile for the restorations. In addition, provision of proper hard tissue volume is necessary to allow placement of the dental implant as well as provide support of the soft tissues. There is a limit as to how much soft tissue can exist beyond the bone. The level of interdental papilla around single-tooth implants is mostly dependent on the marginal bone level at the adjacent teeth rather than the peri-implant marginal bone levels (Figure 10.5).[22,41,42]

More favorable soft tissue outcomes are seen at non-augmented sites than at augmented sites; this has been attributed to the scarring induced by additional surgical procedures rather than marginal bone levels, which are comparable at both sites.[43] Long-term studies have demonstrated that improvements in interdental papilla fill may occur over time following definitive prosthesis delivery.[44–46]

Patients with missing teeth may present with volumetric hard and soft tissue deficiencies in the vertical and buccolingual dimensions. Reconstruction of deficient tissues maybe ac-complished by surgical and/or prosthetic treatment approaches. Hard tissue reconstruction may be obtained using block bone graft, guided bone regeneration, and orthodontic tooth extrusion and distraction methods. Vertical bone augmentation is more challenging than horizontal augmentation.[47] Prosthetic methods include use of gingiva-colored prosthetic material and creation of a long proximal contact area (Figures 10.6 and 10.7).[48]

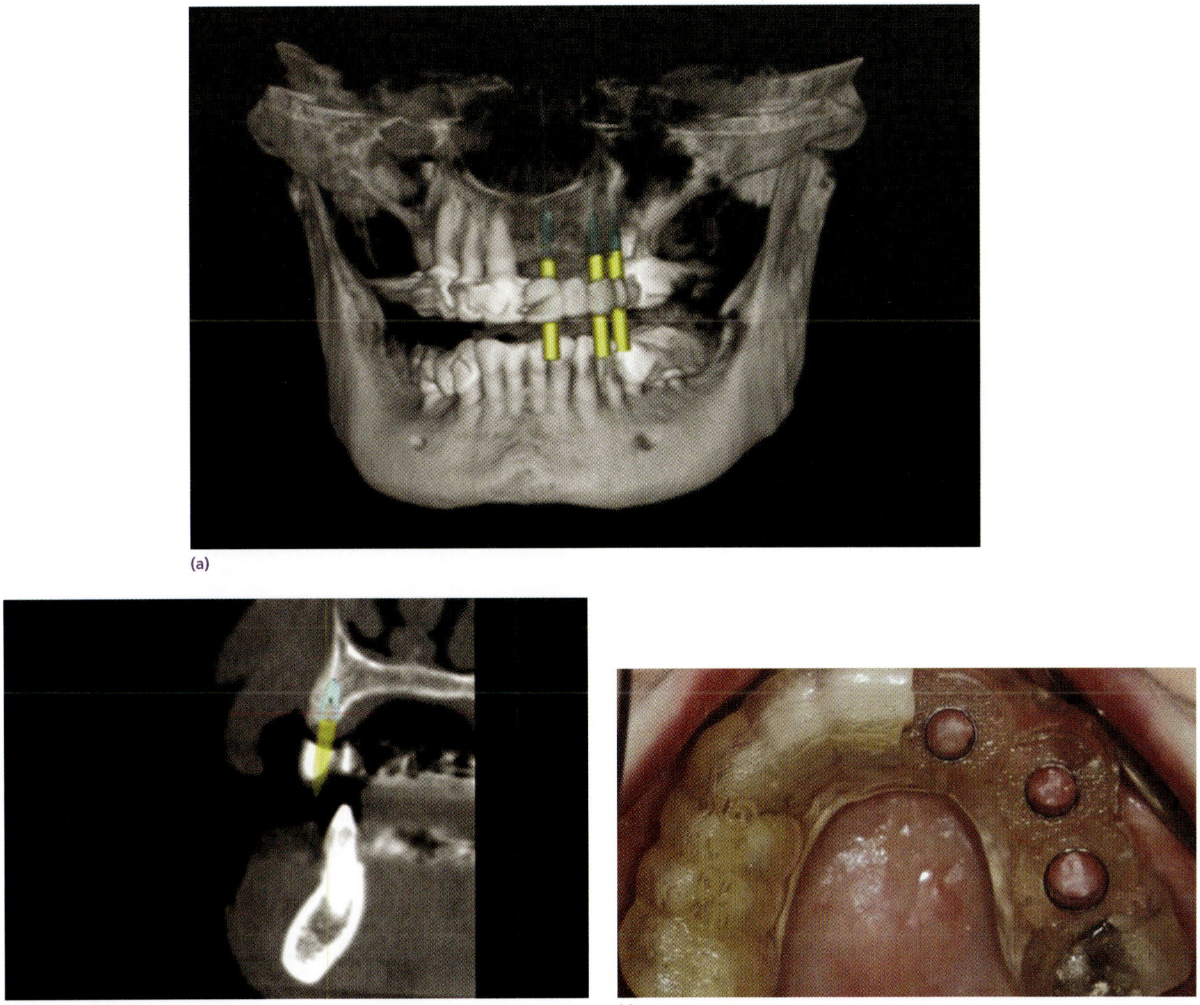

(a) (b) (c)

Figure 10.3 **(a)** Screen shot of the 3D view for virtual implant planning using Simplant Software. This is utilized to plan for implants at sites #9, 11, and 13. **(b)** Sagittal section that shows the long axis of implant planned at site #11. Planning was executed to allow for a screw-retained prosthesis. **(c)** Occlusal view of the teeth-supported CAD/CAM guide in place.

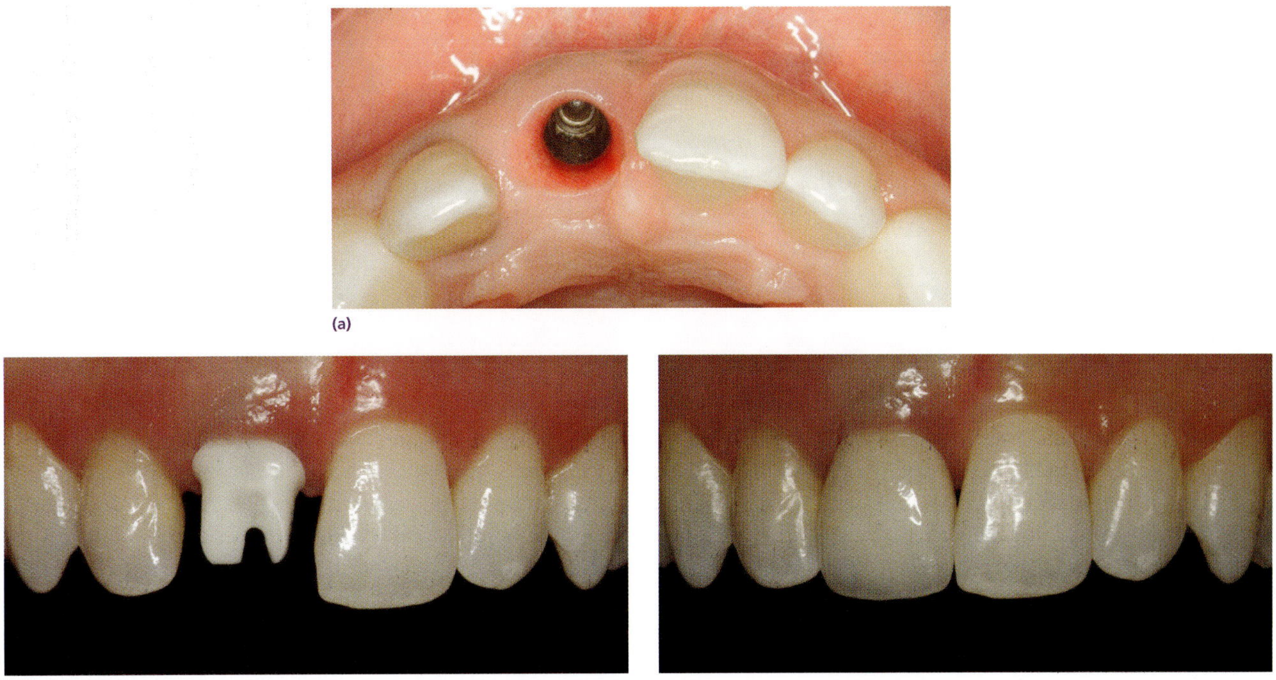

(a) (b) (c)

Figure 10.4 **(a)** Occlusal view of implant placed at site #8 demonstrating its facial and superficial misplacement. This creates a restorative challenge for providing a proper emergence profile and symmetrical midfacial gingival margin. **(b)** Facial view of zirconia abutment used to restore implant at site #8. Selection of zirconia was based on the patient's thin tissue biotype. **(c)** Facial view of definitive implant restoration. Asymmetrical gingival zenith has resulted from inadequate implant placement.

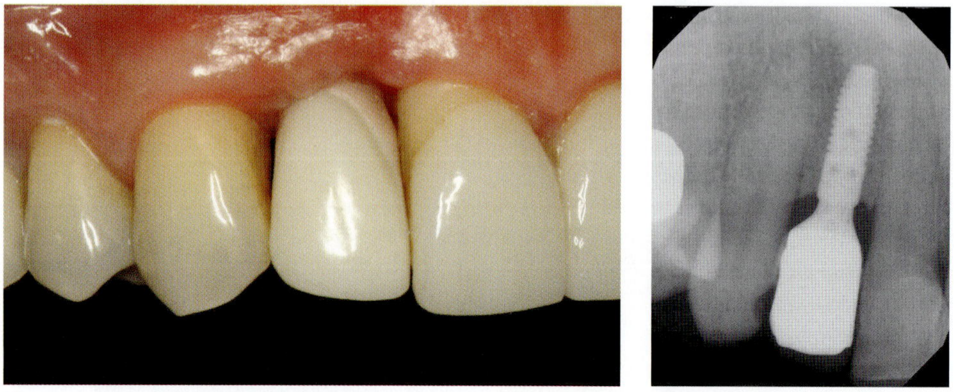

(a) (b)

Figure 10.5 (a) Facial view of implant crown at site #7 demonstrating deficient papillae on both the mesial and distal aspects. (b) Periapical radiograph at implant #7 demonstrating good marginal peri-implant bone levels but reduced levels on adjacent teeth. Soft tissue levels around single-tooth dental implants are affected by bone levels on adjacent teeth.

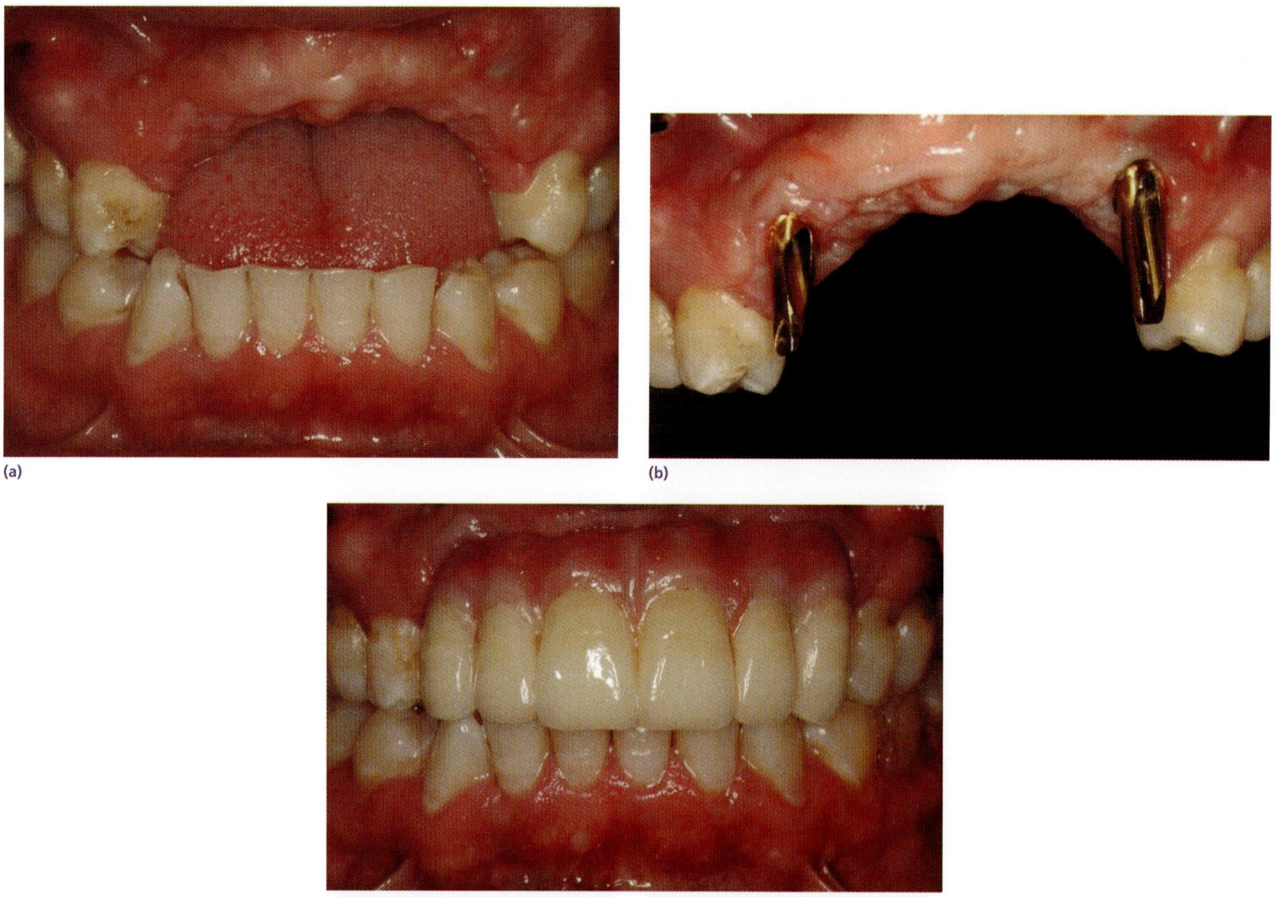

(a) (b) (c)

Figure 10.6 (a) Missing maxillary anterior teeth and deficient hard and soft tissues as a result of trauma; vertical augmentation would not be predictable. (b) The definitive abutments with gold hue in place. (c) The use of pink ceramics was a necessity to compensate for the lost tissues and provide an optimum esthetic result.

Advantages of prosthetic replacement of soft tissue include reduced morbidity associated with reconstructive surgeries, shortened treatment time, reduced treatment cost, and more predictable pink esthetics.[38] Currently available gingiva-colored prosthetic materials include acrylics, composite resins, or ceramics.[38,49,50] Use of gingiva-colored artificial materials, however, is technically demanding and requires skilled dental technicians. When this option is considered, bone reshaping to move the transition zone

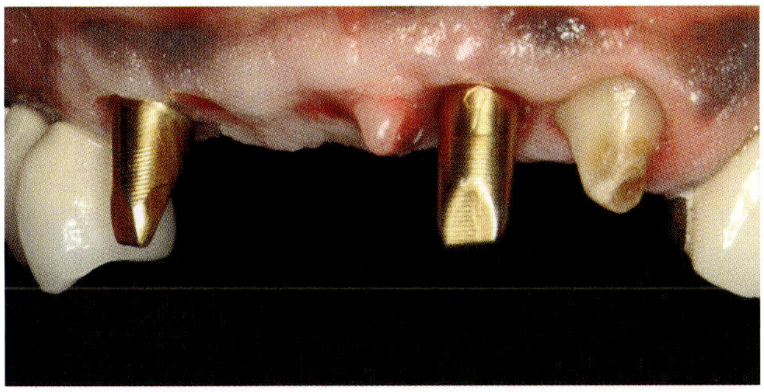

(a)

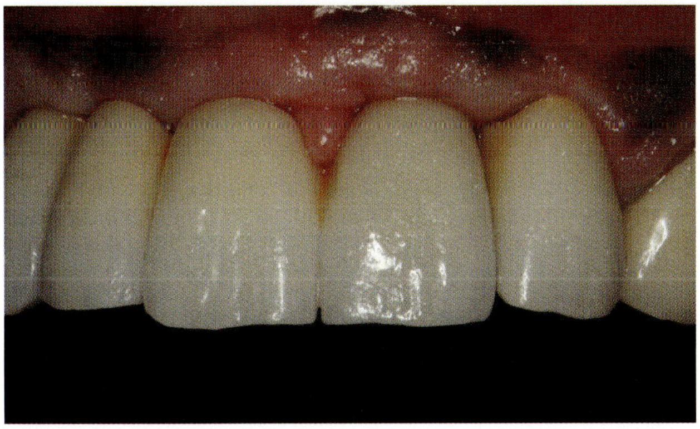

(b)

Figure 10.7 (a) A three-unit FDP adjacent to a natural tooth that needs a crown restoration. Custom abutments with gold hue are used to optimize esthetics. (b) Long proximal contacts were created to camouflage the short interdental papilla.

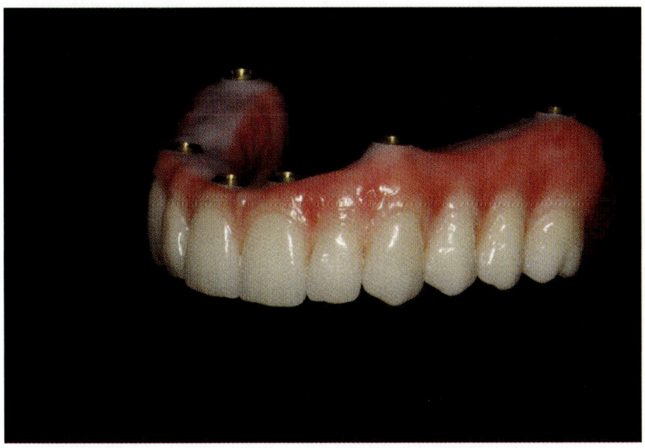

Figure 10.8 Lateral view of a full-arch monolithic zirconia prosthesis with artificial gingiva showing flat pontic design to facilitate hygiene.

(junction between the prosthesis and natural gingiva) beneath the lip perimeter and to create a flat ridge between the implants may be needed.[50] It is advised to use a flat pontic design as this allows for a smoother transition between the natural and prosthetic gingiva and permits better hygiene (Figure 10.8). Notable disadvantages include:

- high prosthetic maintenance, in particular when resins or acrylic materials are used – color instability and staining are inherent drawbacks of resin materials;
- more delicate oral hygiene is required;
- psychological factors related to negative patients' perception toward artificial gingiva.

Timing of implant placement

Timing of implant placement after tooth extraction can play an influential role in the esthetic zone. Post-extraction implant placement is referred to as type 1 (immediate implant placement), type 2 (early placement with soft tissue healing; 4–8 weeks), type 3 (early placement with partial bone healing; 12–16 weeks), and type 4 (late placement; more than 16 weeks).[51]

A major desirable advantage of immediate implant placement is shortening of the treatment course, which is preferable amongst patients. Other suggested potential biological benefits are enhanced esthetic outcomes, reduction of the patients' psychological trauma caused by loss of a front tooth, and preservation of the dimensions of the alveolar bone.[52] Clinical scientific documentation has shown, however, that this approach fails to completely prevent resorption of the alveolar ridge but may partially reduce its extent.[53,54] Bone dimensional alterations measured within the first year following immediate placement were reported as 1.07 mm of weighted mean buccal horizontal bone dimension reduction, 0.78 mm of buccal vertical bone dimension reduction, 0.62 mm of weighted mean palatal horizontal bone dimension reduction, and 0.50 mm of palatal vertical bone dimension reduction.[55] The initial thickness of the buccal alveolar plate is an important anatomic feature that can help predict the eventual outcome of implants placed immediately. Clinical data from CBCT studies suggest that the majority of patients have limited thickness of the buccal bone at the maxillary anterior region. Vera *et al.* reported a median buccal bone thickness of 1.03 mm at the midroot in the premolar area and 0.7 mm for the other anterior maxillary teeth.[56] Similarly, Wang *et al.*[57] demonstrated that 80% of anterior teeth and 40% of premolars exhibit a thin facial bone wall (<1 mm) and nearly 30% of sites had a bone wall thinner than 0.5 mm.

Nevertheless, the current available evidence demonstrates that esthetic outcomes may be achieved for single-tooth implants placed immediately. However, a greater variability in outcomes and a higher frequency of recession of more than 1 mm of the midfacial mucosa are seen compared to early implant placement (types 2 and 3).

A high level of technical competence and experience is needed in performing cases with immediate placement. Careful case selection is crucial to achieving successful esthetic outcome. Factors identified as influencing risk for recession include integrity of facial bone, tissue biotype, and facial implant malposition.[58] Use of CBCT can guide clinicians as to the best surgical approach (immediate or delayed approach) that should be undertaken.

The proceedings of the 5th International Team of Implantology Consensus Conference[59] recommended the following conditions should be satisfied for immediate implant placement:

- intact socket walls;
- facial bone wall at least 1 mm in thickness; a minimum distance of 2 mm between the implant platform and the inner surface of the facial socket wall should be present;
- thick soft tissue biotype;
- absence of acute infection;
- availability of bone apical and palatal to the socket to provide primary stability.

The surgical protocol followed in immediate implant placements should allow for atraumatic extraction procedures to preserve the facial bone plate. In addition, a flapless approach is recommended for immediate implants, primarily to reduce disruption of vascular supply to the periosteum. After the extraction, all granulation tissue must be removed and the implant placed with good primary stability to engage the palatal and apical aspects of the socket. Use of bone filler with a low substitution rate is recommended to compensate for the postextraction resorption at the facial gap.[60] In a retrospective cross-sectional cohort, Chu and coworkers[61] compared the changes in peri-implant soft tissue dimensions associated with immediate implant placement into anterior postextraction sockets for four treatment groups: no BGPR (no bone graft, no provisional restoration), PR (no bone graft, provisional restoration), BG (bone graft, no provisional restoration), and BGPR (bone graft, provisional restoration). The vertical distance of the peri-implant soft tissue was greater for grafted sites than for nongrafted ones (2.72 mm vs. 2.29 mm, $P < .06$). The facial soft tissue thickness at the gingival third also was greater for grafted than for nongrafted sites (2.90 mm vs. 2.28 mm, $P < .008$), and for sites with provisional restorations compared to sites without them (2.81 mm vs. 2.37 mm, $P < .06$), respectively.[61] Early implant placement (4–8 weeks) can provide an advantageous alternative to immediate implant placement, as it permits resolution of infection at the site and allows adequate soft tissue healing to take place.[62] However, longer healing periods should be considered, especially if initial implant stability is not foreseen.

Compared with conventional loading, immediate loading of single-implant crowns has been reported to be associated with a significantly higher risk of implant failure. Atieh *et al.*[63] reported a 5.07% increased risk based on a meta-analysis of five studies (95% confidence interval = 2.00–12.84%). Elevated risk for biological complications may arise due to local factors, such as bruxism, or systemic factors, such as general health, including those with wound-healing delays such as smoking, diabetes, and hyperparathyroidism.[64] Additional factors may include patient compliance and operator sensitivity.

Measures to evaluate esthetics around dental implants in the esthetic zone

Methods reported in the literature for assessment of esthetics around dental implants include both subjective and objective measures. Patient satisfaction depends on their perception and preference.

Objective measures of assessment of esthetics for dental implants include both the 1) implant-supported crown (shape and appearance – white esthetics) and 2) soft tissues surrounding the crown (pink esthetics). An esthetic implant restoration emulates the natural appearance of the missing teeth in form, size, texture, color, and translucency. Ninety percent of subjects display papillae in the anterior teeth and first premolars during enjoyment smiling regardless of gender.[65,66] Fill of interdental papilla, position of facial margin, and color and texture of the peri-implant mucosa all play a role in determining the esthetic outcome of dental implant restorations. Several indices are used in clinical studies to evaluate the esthetics of single-tooth implants (Table 10.1). The intra-observer reproducibility of pink esthetic score/white esthetic score (PES/WES) is relatively higher in comparison with the ICAI (Implant Crown Aesthetic Index).[71]

Table 10.1 Description of indices for assessment of single-tooth implant esthetics.

Papilla index; Jemt 1997[67]	Level of interproximal mucosa Most frequently used for esthetic evaluations	Mesial and distal papilla adjacent to the implant 0 = no papilla 1 = less than half of the papilla fills up the proximal space 2 = at least half of the papilla is present, but not all the way up to the contact point 3 = papilla fills up the entire proximal space 4 = papilla is hyperplastic
Implant Crown Esthetics Index (ICAI); Meijer *et al.* 2005[68]	Nine parameters: Dimension and form of the crown Labial peri-implant mucosa	Pink esthetics: labial margin, papillae, contour of the labial surface, color, and surface White esthetics: mesiodistal dimension, incisal edge position, labial convexity, color/translucency, and surface
PES – pink esthetics score; Furhauser *et al.* 2005[69] Modified PES; Belser *et al.* 2009[70]	Peri-implant mucosal features	Seven parameters; mesial and distal papilla, soft tissue level, contour, texture, alveolar process deficiency
White esthetics score; Belser *et al.* 2009[70]		Tooth form, outline/volume, color, surface texture, translucency, and characterization

Interim restorations

Different modalities of interim restorations have been described following teeth extractions, including removable partial dentures, vacuum-formed matrices with denture teeth, resin-bonded restorations with ovate pontics, screw-retained interim implant-supported restorations, and interim fixed dental prostheses when neighboring teeth need to be restored.[72] While removable partial dentures provide an easy, cost-efficient method, special care should be taken not to irritate and depress the underlying soft tissues, compromising the final esthetics outcome (Figure 10.9).

Use of interim implant-supported restorations in the esthetic zone with adequate emergence profiles is recommended to contour and shape the peri-implant soft tissues. Screw retention of the interim restorations is advisable as it eases modification of the soft tissue profiles if needed. Regardless, use of interim restorations remains strongly recommended as they permit assessment of esthetic parameters with the patient before the treatment is finalized. Duplication of the subgingival contours may be accomplished by retrofitting the interim to the master cast or with a custom impression coping (Figure 10.10).[73] The restorative dentist should pay special attention to providing optimal support for the soft issues to maintain the contour and shape of the mucosa. Excess pressure may lead to midfacial mucosal recession.[74]

Definitive restoration

Screw retention vs. cement retention

The choice for use of a screw-retained or a cement-retained restoration is dependent on the clinician's preference and the position of the implant. A critical aspect in the esthetic zone is controlling the emergence profile through proper design of the abutment and/or prosthesis.

If the screw access hole is located on the lingual aspect of the incisal edge, then a screw-retained restoration may be prescribed. New innovations with the Angulated Screw Channel (ASC) abutment and Omnigrip tooling allow a correction of an angle up to 25° off the axis of the implant, anywhere within a 360° range. In the anterior esthetic region this makes it possible to use screw-retained restorations where a buccal screw access point would previously have ruled them out. A major advantage for screw retention is retrievability and elimination of biological complications related to the presence of excess cement.

Abutments

The use of customized abutments rather than stock abutments in cemented restorations is preferred as they permit optimal support for the peri-implant tissues and positioning of the margins just below the gingival margin to allow access for cleaning excess cement. However, it is advisable that clinicians use minimal amounts of cement. Other techniques that have been prescribed to reduce excess cement include seating the restoration after placing the cement on the fitting surface on the abutment analog before cementing the restoration intraorally.[75] Abutments utilized in the esthetic zone include metal and zirconia. An often-reported problem of the use of titanium abutments has been the gray discoloration of the peri-implant mucosa in patients with a thin tissue biotype.[76]

Bressan and co-workers[77] demonstrated, using a spectrophotometric analysis of the color change of the peri-implant soft tissue with different materials, that while the color of the soft tissue around titanium implants differed significantly from the gingival color around natural teeth, no significant differences were present in the color performance of abutments made of gold and zirconium oxide. Ultimately, titanium abutments with nitride coatings that have a gold-shaded hue can be used as an alternative to ceramic abutments in cases with high esthetic demands (Figure 10.11).[78]

Alternatively, use of zirconia abutments must follow strict laboratory guidelines to avoid technical complications. Ceramic abutments should not be ground, abraded, or adjusted following sintering.[79] The zirconia abutments can be connected either internally to the implant as one piece by the abutment itself or via a secondary titanium metallic base. Preliminary *in vitro* data suggested that superior strength maybe achieved by means of internal connection via a secondary metallic component.[80] However, long-term *in vivo* data are still lacking.

Dental implants in the esthetic zone may be restored with either all-ceramic or metal–ceramic prostheses. Martin and coworkers[81] concluded in a recent systematic review based on available evidence that no significant difference can be established between both types of prostheses with regards to esthetic indices over short observation periods.

Maintenance and long-term complications

While implant treatment can provide a predictable and successful outcome in the short term, long-term clinical studies are scarce.[82] Complications presented with dental implants in the esthetic zone include technical, biological, and esthetic complications. Jung *et al.*[83] reported, in a recent systematic review, that the cumulative 5-year esthetic complication rate in single-tooth implants amounted to 7.1% (95% CI: 3.6–13.6%). Technical complications reached a cumulative incidence of 8.8% (95% CI: 5.1–15.0%) for screw loosening, 4.1% (95% CI: 2.2–7.5%) for loss of retention, and 3.5% (95% CI: 2.4–5.2%) for fracture of the veneering material after 5 years. A particularly troubling finding in long-term follow-up for implant restorations is their infraposition in relation to adjacent teeth. This presents with significant esthetic implications in the anterior zone (Figure 10.12).

Dierens *et al.*[84] demonstrated, in a retrospective study following implants in the esthetic zone, that the vast majority of cases (71%) were in infraposition after 16–22 years of function. This

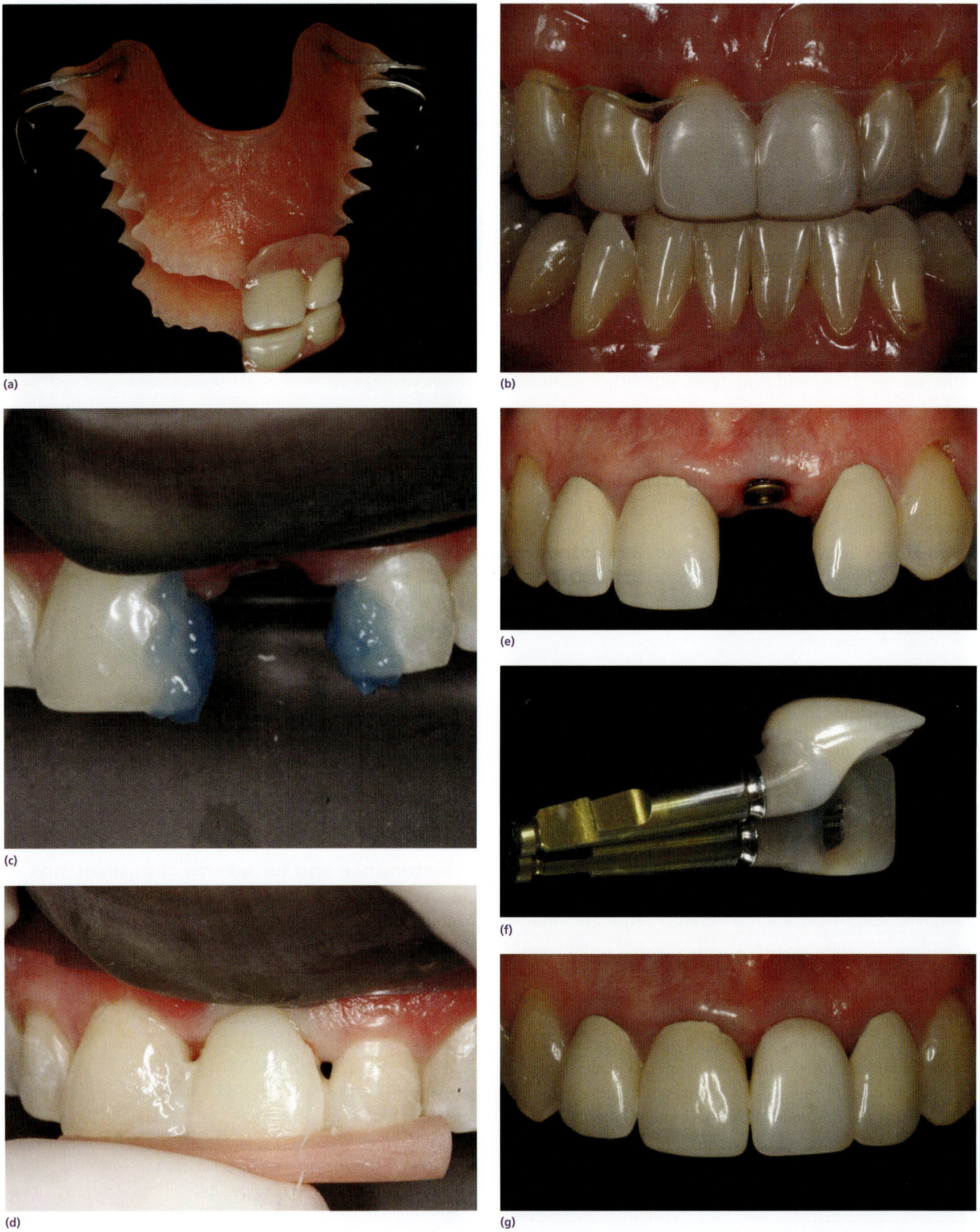

(a) (b) (c) (d) (e) (f) (g)

Figure 10.9 (**a**) The use of an acrylic partial denture as an interim prosthesis. (**b**) Essix retainer used an interim prosthesis by filling the area of missing teeth with Bis-Acryl material. (**c, d**) Bonding an interim restoration to adjacent teeth utilizing an index fabricated from the diagnostic wax-up. (**e–g**) The use of a screw-retained interim crown.

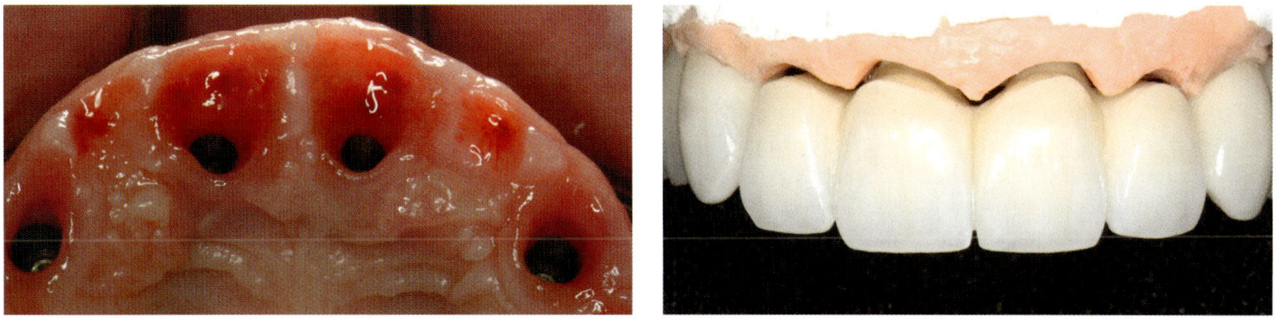

(a) (b)

Figure 10.10 (a) Occlusal view of the soft tissue contouring accomplished by use of a properly designed interim implant-supported prosthesis. (b) Duplication of soft tissue contours into the design of the definitive implant prosthesis.

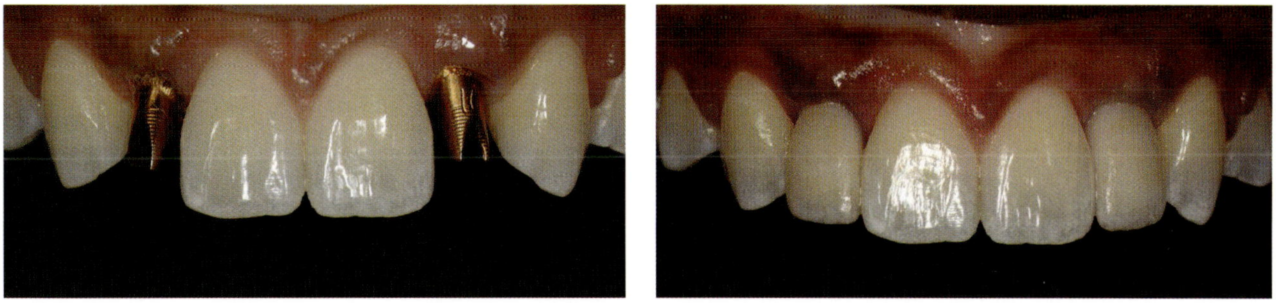

(a) (b)

Figure 10.11 (a) Facial view of gold-hue custom Atlantis abutments used to restore implants at sites #7 and 10. (b) Facial view of definitive implant crowns fabricated using lithium-disilicate (E-max press) at implants #7 and 10.

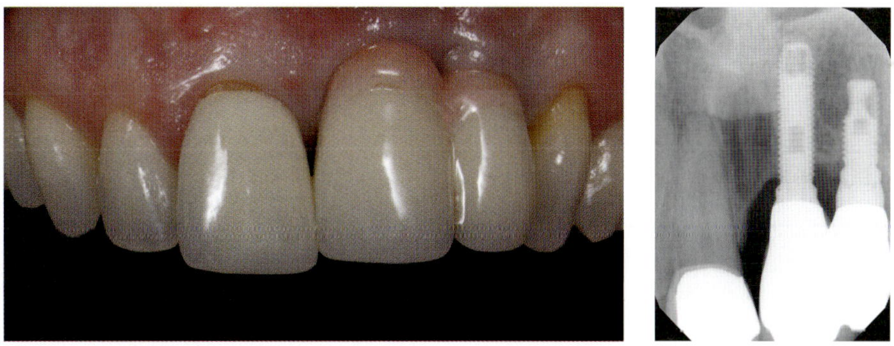

(a) (b)

Figure 10.12 (a) Facial view demonstrating discrepancy of the incisal edges of implant-supported prostheses at implants #9 and 10 with natural teeth (infra-occlusion). This creates a significant esthetic complication for patients in the anterior zone in the long-term. (b) Periapical radiograph for implants at sites #9 and 10 with splinted prostheses demonstrating some bone loss.

is in agreement with other studies by Bernard *et al.*[85] (100% of cases over an average 4.2 years of function), Chang and Wennstrom[86] (58% of cases after 8 years of function), and Jemt *et al.*[67] (60% of cases after a period of more than 15 years). In younger patients, alveolar bone growth cessation is important prior to anterior maxillary implant placement. This may be achieved by evaluation of sequential cephalometric radiographs over a 6–12-month time frame.[87] Nevertheless, the risk for implant infraposition is not limited to adolescents and young adults but may also occur in mature adults.[85,88,89]

Biological complications in dental implants in the esthetic zone may influence the esthetic outcome. These may include soft tissue recession, fistula, and mucosal inflammation (peri-implant mucositis and peri-implantitis). Facial soft tissue recession around single-tooth implants is an unfavorable esthetic complication that can occur. Patients with thin tissue biotype tend to be at higher risk. Prevention is considered the key approach, including adoption of techniques that preserve the soft and hard tissues, such as flapless surgery and papilla-preservation techniques.[90] The 3-D implant position has a predominant influence on the soft tissue responses. For example, facial deviations from the ideal implant position result in significantly worse implant esthetics.[91]

Resolution of this problem consists of a comprehensive evaluation of the etiology, that includes the 3-D implant position, restoration, and status of hard and soft tissue support, in addition to elimination of habits such as aggressive brushing and flossing for the area. Limited improvement with high variability in the outcome can be achieved using soft tissue augmentation procedures. It may be advantageous to perform restorative modifications of the abutment and crown contours in conjunction with the surgical approach. However, implant removal combined with hard and soft tissue augmentation should be considered as an option in certain cases.[59]

Summary

Esthetic rehabilitation of anterior implants is an intricate process. Comprehensive evaluation, site analysis, and careful planning are all essential elements for the success of this treatment modality. A restoratively driven protocol should be undertaken and treatment should be individually tailored to the patient based on present clinical findings and understanding of his/her expectations. Limitations and possible treatment complications must be discussed with patients at the initiation of the treatment to avoid misunderstandings and the need for revision/restitution at the end.

References

1. Belser U, Buser D, Higginbottom F. Consensus statements and recommended clinical procedures regarding esthetics in implant dentistry. *Int J Oral Maxillofac Implants* 2004; **19**(Suppl): 73–74.
2. Dawson A, Chen S, Buser D, *et al.* (eds). *The SAC Classification in Implant Dentistry*. Berlin: Quintessence 2009.
3. Kourkouta S. Implant therapy in the esthetic zone: Smile line assessment. *Int J Periodontics Restorative Dent* 2011; **31**(2): 195–201.
4. Al-Sabbagh M. Implants in the esthetic zone. *Dent Clin North Am* 2006; **50**(3): 391,407, vi.
5. Chang M, Wennstrom JL, Odman P, *et al.* Implant supported single-tooth replacements compared to contralateral natural teeth. crown and soft tissue dimensions. *Clin Oral Implants Res* 1999; **10**(3): 185–194.
6. Salama H, Salama MA, Garber D, *et al.* The interproximal height of bone: a guidepost to predictable aesthetic strategies and soft tissue contours in anterior tooth replacement. *Pract Periodontics Aesthet Dent* 1998; **10**(9): 1131–1141.
7. Kois JC. Predictable single-tooth peri-implant esthetics: five diagnostic keys. *Compend Contin Educ Dent* 2004; **25**(11): 895–900.
8. Allen PF, McMillan AS, Walshaw D. Patient expectations of oral implant-retained prostheses in a UK dental hospital. *Br Dent J* 1999; **186**(2): 80–84.
9. Cooper LF. Objective criteria: guiding and evaluating dental implant esthetics. *J Esthet Restor Dent* 2008; **20**(3): 195–205.
10. Cooper LF, Pin-Harry OC. "Rules of six" – diagnostic and therapeutic guidelines for single-tooth implant success. *Compend Contin Educ Dent* 2013; **34**(2): 94–101.
11. Belser UC, Buser D, Hess D, *et al.* Aesthetic implant restorations in partially edentulous patients – a critical appraisal. *Periodontol 2000* 1998; **17**: 132–150.
12. Buser D, Martin W, Belser UC. Optimizing esthetics for implant restorations in the anterior maxilla: anatomic and surgical considerations. *Int J Oral Maxillofac Implants* 2004; **19**(Suppl): 43–61.
13. Rodriguez AM, Rosenstiel SF. Esthetic considerations related to bone and soft tissue maintenance and development around dental implants: report of the committee on research in fixed prosthodontics of the american academy of fixed prosthodontics. *J Prosthet Dent* 2012; **108**(4): 259–267.
14. Spear FM, Kokich VG. A multidisciplinary approach to esthetic dentistry. *Dent Clin North Am* 2007; **51**(2): 487.
15. Hammerle CH, Cordaro L, van Assche N, *et al.* Digital technologies to support planning, treatment, and fabrication processes and outcome assessments in implant dentistry. summary and consensus statements. the 4th EAO consensus conference 2015. *Clin Oral Implants Res* 2015; **26**(Suppl 11): 97–101.
16. Levine RA, Huynh-Ba G, Cochran DL. Soft tissue augmentation procedures for mucogingival defects in esthetic sites. *Int J Oral Maxillofac Implants* 2014; **29**(Suppl):155–185.
17. Berglundh T, Lindhe J. Dimension of the periimplant mucosa. biological width revisited. *J Clin Periodontol* 1996; **23**(10): 971–973.
18. Cochran DL, Hermann JS, Schenk RK, *et al.* Biologic width around titanium implants. A histometric analysis of the implanto-gingival junction around unloaded and loaded nonsubmerged implants in the canine mandible. *J Periodontol* 1997; **68**(2): 186 -198.
19. Kan JY, Rungcharassaeng K, Umezu K, *et al.* Dimensions of peri-implant mucosa: an evaluation of maxillary anterior single implants in humans. *J Periodontol* 2003; **74**(4): 557–762.
20. Leblebicioglu B, Rawal S, Mariotti A. A review of the functional and esthetic requirements for dental implants. *J Am Dent Assoc* 2007; **138**(3): 321–329.
21. Tarnow DP, Magner AW, Fletcher P. The effect of the distance from the contact point to the crest of bone on the presence or absence of the interproximal dental papilla. *J Periodontol* 1992; **63**(12): 995–996.
22. Tarnow D, Elian N, Fletcher P, *et al.* Vertical distance from the crest of bone to the height of the interproximal papilla between adjacent implants. *J Periodontol* 2003; **74**(12): 1785–1788.
23. Garber DA, Salama MA, Salama H. Immediate total tooth replacement. *Compend Contin Educ Dent* 2001; **22**(3): 210–218.
24. Higginbottom F, Belser U, Jones JD, *et al.* Prosthetic management of implants in the esthetic zone. *Int J Oral Maxillofac Implants* 2004; **19**(Suppl): 62–72.
25. Vela X, Mendez V, Rodriguez X, *et al.* Crestal bone changes on platform-switched implants and adjacent teeth when the tooth-implant distance is less than 1.5 mm. *Int J Periodontics Restorative Dent* 2012; **32**(2): 149–155.
26. Stein AE, McGlmphy EA, Johnston WM, *et al.* Effects of implant design and surface roughness on crestal bone and soft tissue levels in the esthetic zone. *Int J Oral Maxillofac Implants* 2009; **24**(5): 910–919.
27. Urdaneta RA, Seemann R, Dragan IF, *et al.* A retrospective radiographic study on the effect of natural tooth-implant proximity and an introduction to the concept of a bone-loading platform switch. *Int J Oral Maxillofac Implants* 2014; **29**(6): 1412–1424.

28. Vela X, Mendez V, Rodriguez X, *et al.* Crestal bone changes on platform-switched implants and adjacent teeth when the tooth–implant distance is less than 1.5 mm. *Int J Periodontics Restorative Dent* 2012; **32**(2): 149–155.
29. Rodriguez AM, Rosenstiel SF. Esthetic considerations related to bone and soft tissue maintenance and development around dental implants: report of the committee on research in fixed prosthodontics of the american academy of fixed prosthodontics. *J Prosthet Dent* 2012; **108**(4): 259–267.
30. Vela-Nebot X, Rodriguez-Ciurana X, Rodado-Alonso C, *et al.* Benefits of an implant platform modification technique to reduce crestal bone resorption. *Implant Dent* 2006; **15**(3): 313–320.
31. Rodriguez-Ciurana X, Vela-Nebot X, Segala-Torres M, *et al.* The effect of interimplant distance on the height of the interimplant bone crest when using platform-switched implants. *Int J Periodontics Restorative Dent* 2009; **29**(2): 141–151.
32. Tarnow DP, Cho SC, Wallace SS. The effect of inter-implant distance on the height of inter-implant bone crest. *J Periodontol* 2000; **71**(4): 546–549.
33. Salama M, Ishikawa T, Salama H, *et al.* Advantages of the root submergence technique for pontic site development in esthetic implant therapy. *Int J Periodontics Restorative Dent* 2007; **27**(6): 521–527.
34. Schropp L, Wenzel A, Kostopoulos L, *et al.* Bone healing and soft tissue contour changes following single-tooth extraction: a clinical and radiographic 12-month prospective study. *Int J Periodontics Restorative Dent* 2003; **23**(4): 313–323.
35. Tan WL, Wong TL, Wong MC, *et al.* A systematic review of post-extractional alveolar hard and soft tissue dimensional changes in humans. *Clin Oral Implants Res* 2012; **23**(Suppl 5): 1–21.
36. Chen ST, Wilson TG Jr, Hammerle CH. Immediate or early placement of implants following tooth extraction: review of biologic basis, clinical procedures, and outcomes. *Int J Oral Maxillofac Implants* 2004; **19**(Suppl): 12–25.
37. Nevins M, Camelo M, De Paoli S, *et al.* A study of the fate of the buccal wall of extraction sockets of teeth with prominent roots. *Int J Periodontics Restorative Dent* 2006; **26**(1): 19–29.
38. Coachman C, Salama M, Garber D, *et al.* Prosthetic gingival reconstruction in a fixed partial restoration. part 1: introduction to artificial gingiva as an alternative therapy. *Int J Periodontics Restorative Dent* 2009; **29**(5): 471–477.
39. Barone A, Cornelini R, Ciaglia R, *et al.* Implant placement in fresh extraction sockets and simultaneous osteotome sinus floor elevation: a case series. *Int J Periodontics Restorative Dent* 2008; **28**(3): 283–289.
40. Jambhekar S, Kernen F, Bidra AS. Clinical and histologic outcomes of socket grafting after flapless tooth extraction: a systematic review of randomized controlled clinical trials. *J Prosthet Dent* 2015; **113**(5): 371–382.
41. Choquet V, Hermans M, Adriaenssens P, *et al.* Clinical and radiographic evaluation of the papilla level adjacent to single-tooth dental implants. A retrospective study in the maxillary anterior region. *J Periodontol* 2001; **72**(10): 1364–1371.
42. Nisapakultorn K, Suphanantachat S, Silkosessak O, *et al.* Factors affecting soft tissue level around anterior maxillary single-tooth implants. *Clin Oral Implants Res* 2010; **21**(6): 662–670.
43. Santing HJ, Raghoebar GM, Vissink A, *et al.* Performance of the straumann bone level implant system for anterior single-tooth replacements in augmented and nonaugmented sites: a prospective cohort study with 60 consecutive patients. *Clin Oral Implants Res* 2013; **24**(8): 941–948.
44. Schropp L, Isidor F. Papilla dimension and soft tissue level after early vs. delayed placement of single-tooth implants: 10-year results from a randomized controlled clinical trial. *Clin Oral Implants Res* 2015; **26**(3): 278–286.
45. Jemt T. Regeneration of gingival papillae after single-implant treatment. *Int J Periodontics Restorative Dent* 1997; **17**(4): 326–333.
46. den Hartog L, Meijer HJ, Stegenga B, *et al.* Single implants with different neck designs in the aesthetic zone: a randomized clinical trial. *Clin Oral Implants Res* 2011; **22**(11): 1289–1297.
47. Esposito M, Grusovin MG, Felice P, *et al.* Interventions for replacing missing teeth: horizontal and vertical bone augmentation techniques for dental implant treatment. *Cochrane Database Syst Rev* 2009;(**4**): CD003607.
48. Bidra AS, Chapokas AR. Treatment planning challenges in the maxillary anterior region consequent to severe loss of buccal bone. *J Esthet Restor Dent* 2011; **23**(6): 354–360.
49. Coachman C, Salama M, Garber D, *et al.* Prosthetic gingival reconstruction in fixed partial restorations. Part 3: laboratory procedures and maintenance. *Int J Periodontics Restorative Dent* 2010; **30**(1): 19–29.
50. Salama M, Coachman C, Garber D, *et al.* Prosthetic gingival reconstruction in the fixed partial restoration. Part 2: diagnosis and treatment planning. *Int J Periodontics Restorative Dent* 2009; **29**(6): 573–581.
51. Hammerle CH, Chen ST, Wilson TG, Jr. Consensus statements and recommended clinical procedures regarding the placement of implants in extraction sockets. *Int J Oral Maxillofac Implants* 2004; **19**(Suppl): 26–28.
52. Kan JY, Rungcharassaeng K, Lozada J. Immediate placement and provisionalization of maxillary anterior single implants: 1-year prospective study. *Int J Oral Maxillofac Implants* 2003; **18**(1): 31–39.
53. Araujo MG, Sukekava F, Wennstrom JL, *et al.* Tissue modeling following implant placement in fresh extraction sockets. *Clin Oral Implants Res* 2006; **17**(6): 615–624.
54. Araujo MG, Wennstrom JL, Lindhe J. Modeling of the buccal and lingual bone walls of fresh extraction sites following implant installation. *Clin Oral Implants Res* 2006; **17**(6): 606–614.
55. Lee CT, Chiu TS, Chuang SK, *et al.* Alterations of the bone dimension following immediate implant placement into extraction socket: systematic review and meta-analysis. *J Clin Periodontol* 2014; **41**(9): 914–926.
56. Vera C, De Kok IJ, Reinhold D, *et al.* Evaluation of buccal alveolar bone dimension of maxillary anterior and premolar teeth: A cone beam computed tomography investigation. *Int J Oral Maxillofac Implants* 2012; **27**(6): 1514–1519.
57. Wang HM, Shen JW, Yu MF, *et al.* Analysis of facial bone wall dimensions and sagittal root position in the maxillary esthetic zone: a retrospective study using cone beam computed tomography. *Int J Oral Maxillofac Implants* 2014; **29**(5): 1123–1129.
58. Chen ST, Buser D. Esthetic outcomes following immediate and early implant placement in the anterior maxilla – a systematic review. *Int J Oral Maxillofac Implants* 2014; **29**(Suppl): 186–215.
59. Morton D, Chen ST, Martin WC, *et al.* Consensus statements and recommended clinical procedures regarding optimizing esthetic outcomes in implant dentistry. *Int J Oral Maxillofac Implants* 2014; **29**(Suppl): 216–220.

60. Lau SL, Chow J, Li W, *et al.* Classification of maxillary central incisors – implications for immediate implant in the esthetic zone. *J Oral Maxillofac Surg* 2011; **69**(1): 142–153.
61. Chu SJ, Salama MA, Garber DA, *et al.* Flapless postextraction socket implant placement, part 2: The effects of bone grafting and provisional restoration on peri-implant soft tissue height and thickness – a retrospective study. *Int J Periodontics Restorative Dent* 2015; **35**(6): 803–809.
62. Chen ST, Wilson TG Jr, Hammerle CH. Immediate or early placement of implants following tooth extraction: review of biologic basis, clinical procedures, and outcomes. *Int J Oral Maxillofac Implants* 2004; **19**(Suppl): 12–25.
63. Atieh MA, Atieh AH, Payne AG, *et al.* Immediate loading with single implant crowns: a systematic review and meta-analysis. *Int J Prosthodont* 2009; **22**(4): 378–387.
64. Gapski R, Wang HL, Mascarenhas P, *et al.* Critical review of immediate implant loading. *Clin Oral Implants Res* 2003; **14**(5): 515–527.
65. Hu X, Nahles S, Nelson CA, *et al.* Analysis of soft tissue display during enjoyment smiling: Part 1 – caucasians. *Int J Periodontics Restorative Dent* 2013; **33**(1): e9–15.
66. Nelson K, Hu X, Nack C, *et al.* Analysis of soft tissue display during enjoyment smile. part II: elder caucasians. *Int J Periodontics Restorative Dent* 2014; **34**(4): 573–578.
67. Jemt T. Regeneration of gingival papillae after single-implant treatment. *Int J Periodontics Restorative Dent* 1997; **17**(4): 326–333.
68. Meijer HJ, Stellingsma K, Meijndert L, *et al.* A new index for rating aesthetics of implant-supported single crowns and adjacent soft tissues – the implant crown aesthetic index. *Clin Oral Implants Res* 2005; **16**(6): 645–649.
69. Furhauser R, Florescu D, Benesch T, *et al.* Evaluation of soft tissue around single-tooth implant crowns: the pink esthetic score. *Clin Oral Implants Res* 2005; **16**(6): 639–644.
70. Belser UC, Grutter L, Vailati F, *et al.* Outcome evaluation of early placed maxillary anterior single-tooth implants using objective esthetic criteria: a cross-sectional, retrospective study in 45 patients with a 2- to 4-year follow-up using pink and white esthetic scores. *J Periodontol* 2009; **80**(1): 140–151.
71. Tettamanti S, Millen C, Gavric J, *et al.* Esthetic evaluation of implant crowns and peri-implant soft tissue in the anterior maxilla: Comparison and reproducibility of three different indices. *Clin Implant Dent Relat Res* 2015. doi: 10.1111/cid.12306. [Epub ahead of print]
72. Holst S, Blatz MB, Hegenbarth E, *et al.* Prosthodontic considerations for predictable single-implant esthetics in the anterior maxilla. *J Oral Maxillofac Surg* 2005; **63**(9Suppl2): 89–96.
73. Higginbottom F, Belser U, Jones JD, *et al.* Prosthetic management of implants in the esthetic zone. *Int J Oral Maxillofac Implants* 2004; **19**(Suppl): 62–72.
74. Bishti S, Strub JR, Att W. Effect of the implant-abutment interface on peri-implant tissues: a systematic review. *Acta Odontol Scand* 2014; **72**(1): 13–5.
75. Dumbrigue HB, Abanomi AA, Cheng LL. Techniques to minimize excess luting agent in cement-retained implant restorations. *J Prosthet Dent* 2002; **87**(1): 112–114.
76. Jung RE, Sailer I, Hammerle CH, *et al.* In vitro color changes of soft tissues caused by restorative materials. *Int J Periodontics Restorative Dent* 2007; **27**(3): 251–257.
77. Bressan E, Paniz G, Lops D, *et al.* Influence of abutment material on the gingival color of implant-supported all-ceramic restorations: a prospective multicenter study. *Clin Oral Implants Res* 2011; **22**(6): 631–637.
78. Thalji G, Bryington M, De Kok IJ, *et al.* Prosthodontic management of implant therapy. *Dent Clin North Am* 2014; **58**(1): 207–225.
79. Wismeijer D, Bragger U, Evans C, *et al.* Consensus statements and recommended clinical procedures regarding restorative materials and techniques for implant dentistry. *Int J Oral Maxillofac Implants* 2014; **29**(Suppl): 137–140.
80. Sailer I, Sailer T, Stawarczyk B, *et al.* In vitro study of the influence of the type of connection on the fracture load of zirconia abutments with internal and external implant-abutment connections. *Int J Oral Maxillofac Implants* 2009; **24**(5): 850–858.
81. Martin WC, Pollini A, Morton D. The influence of restorative procedures on esthetic outcomes in implant dentistry: a systematic review. *Int J Oral Maxillofac Implants* 2014; **29**(Suppl): 142–154.
82. Dierens M, de Bruecker E, Vandeweghe S, *et al.* Alterations in soft tissue levels and aesthetics over a 16-22 year period following single implant treatment in periodontally-healthy patients: a retrospective case series. *J Clin Periodontol* 2013; **40**(3): 311–318.
83. Jung RE, Zembic A, Pjetursson BE, *et al.* Systematic review of the survival rate and the incidence of biological, technical, and aesthetic complications of single crowns on implants reported in longitudinal studies with a mean follow-up of 5 years. *Clin Oral Implants Res* 2012; **23**(Suppl 6): 2–21.
84. Dierens M, de Bruecker E, Vandeweghe S, *et al.* Alterations in soft tissue levels and aesthetics over a – 22 year period following single implant treatment in periodontally-healthy patients: a retrospective case series. *J Clin Periodontol* 2013; **40**(3): 311–318.
85. Bernard JP, Schatz JP, Christou P, *et al.* Long-term vertical changes of the anterior maxillary teeth adjacent to single implants in young and mature adults. A retrospective study. *J Clin Periodontol* 2004; **31**(11): 1024–1028.
86. Chang M, Wennstrom JL. Longitudinal changes in tooth/single-implant relationship and bone topography: an 8-year retrospective analysis. *Clin Implant Dent Relat Res* 2012; **14**(3): 388–394.
87. Levine RA, Huynh-Ba G, Cochran DL. Soft tissue augmentation procedures for mucogingival defects in esthetic sites. *Int J Oral Maxillofac Implants* 2014; **29**(Suppl): 155–185.
88. Thilander B, Odman J, Jemt T. Single implants in the upper incisor region and their relationship to the adjacent teeth. An 8-year follow-up study. *Clin Oral Implants Res* 1999; **10**(5): 346–355.
89. Misje K, Bjornland T, Saxegaard E, *et al.* Treatment outcome of dental implants in the esthetic zone: a 12- to 15-year retrospective study. *Int J Prosthodont* 2013; **26**(4): 365–369.
90. Oh TJ, Shotwell J, Billy E, *et al.* Flapless implant surgery in the esthetic region: advantages and precautions. *Int J Periodontics Restorative Dent* 2007; **27**(1): 27–33.
91. Furhauser R, Mailath-Pokorny G, Haas R, *et al.* Esthetics of flapless single-tooth implants in the anterior maxilla using guided surgery: Association of three-dimensional accuracy and pink esthetic score. *Clin Implant Dent Relat Res* 2015; **17**(Suppl 2): e427–433.

CHAPTER 11

Ceramic Materials in Implant Dentistry

Parag R. Kachalia
University of the Pacific Arthur A. Dugoni School of Dentistry, San Francisco, California, USA

Introduction

Over the last century, monumental improvements have occurred in dentistry and patients today have the ability to maintain their teeth for a lifetime, if they are healthy individuals and they are diligent with their overall oral health. In the event a single tooth or multiple teeth are lost, implant therapy can be utilized to restore the missing dentition. The challenge, however, is to fabricate an invisible replacement that will last for decades, given the growing esthetic demand and extended life expectancy. Since the introduction of endosseous implants, evidence-based documentation has reported high implant survival rates, but more recently there has been an emphasis on biological, technical, and esthetic success outcomes measurements. Unfortunately, esthetic success with metal-based restorations has not always been predictable. On the other hand, continual developments with all-ceramic materials have led to restorative alternatives that can satisfy specific hue, saturation, and light refraction/reflection needs while providing durability. However, the selection and management of these materials may be less forgiving than metal-based ceramics. This chapter will address the protocols for utilization of all-ceramic implant restorations. In addition, new materials utilizing the properties of resin and ceramics will also be discussed as they may show some promise in providing a dampening behavior and ease of reparability.

Materials

Dental ceramics have continued to improve over the last quarter century and ceramics are no longer restricted to only being used in the anterior sextant of the mouth. Over this period of time new developments have focused on creating ceramics that are biocompatible, durable, and esthetic. Ceramics have always had a high esthetic potential and well-trained ceramists have been able to create beautiful anterior restorations that blend seamlessly with the natural dentition. Unfortunately, in historical terms this beauty was not paired with strength. Dental ceramics have generally had low fracture toughness and traditional ceramics, such as feldspathic porcelain, were highly dependent on being fused to metal substructures in order to have intraoral success in the posterior aspect of the dentition.[1] Leucite- and alumina-based materials, such as IPS Empress (Amherst, NY) and Procera Alumina (Zurich, Switzerland) respectively, had come to market to combat some of the issues evident with feldspathic porcelain; however, advancements in leucite-based materials and alumina-based material have stagnated and the use of these materials in dentistry is clearly fading away.

Two key areas of evolution in ceramic dentistry have occurred, one is in the lithium disilicate arena and the other is in the zirconia arena. The primary reason for migration towards these materials is the fact that both materials can be utilized as either core materials or as monolithic materials that can be used in full contour. The ability to use these materials monolithically may help combat a significant portion of the chipping and fracture issues traditionally evident when ceramics are used as a veneering material.[2]

Lithium disilicate

The crystalline phase that forms in the manufacturing of this ceramic is lithium disilicate ($Li_2Si_2O_5$) and it accounts for approximately 70% of the total volume of glass.[3] The interlocked microstructure of lithium disilicate happens to occur in a random pattern and this is thought to give the material its ability to deflect cracks and minimize propagation. In fact, lithium disilicate exhibits a flexural strength of 350–400 Mpa, compared to the 160 MPa flexural strength of leucite glass. It also exhibits fracture toughness of approximately three times that of leucite glass. These properties allow this material to be used as a core that can be layered with veneering ceramic or as a material that can be used monolithically. The monolithic utilization of lithium disilicate appears to be most promising and, since

Evidence-based Implant Treatment Planning and Clinical Protocols, First Edition. Edited by Steven J. Sadowsky.

Companion website: www.wiley.com/go/sadowsky/implant

Ivoclar Vivadent's (Amherst, NY) introduction of IPS e.max in 2009, practitioners around the world have adopted this material and have had very good success in using the material for anterior and posterior full-coverage single-unit restorations, veneers, inlays, onlays, and selective three-unit fixed partial dentures, replacing a single anterior tooth or a first bicuspid.

The material is available as IPS e.max Press or IPS e.max CAD (Figure 11.1). IPS e.max Press utilizes a traditional lost wax technique and exhibits a flexural strength of 400 MPa. IPS e.max CAD is manufactured and sold in a partially crystalized state with a purple to bluish hue and has an initial flexural strength of 160 MPa. This partially crystallized state is used to allow for efficient milling and simple chairside adjustment during intraoral fitting. Once the restoration is placed into a porcelain firing oven with the proper cycles, a final crystallization occurs and the material achieves its final esthetic appeal as well as its greater flexural strength of 360 MPa. The crystals of both the IPS e.max Press and IPS e.max CAD are the same in composition; however, the length and size of these crystals are different, leading to a difference in fracture strength and fracture toughness. The fracture strength of IPS e.max Press is approximately 10% greater than its counterpart and its fracture toughness is approximately 20% greater than that of IPS e.max CAD.

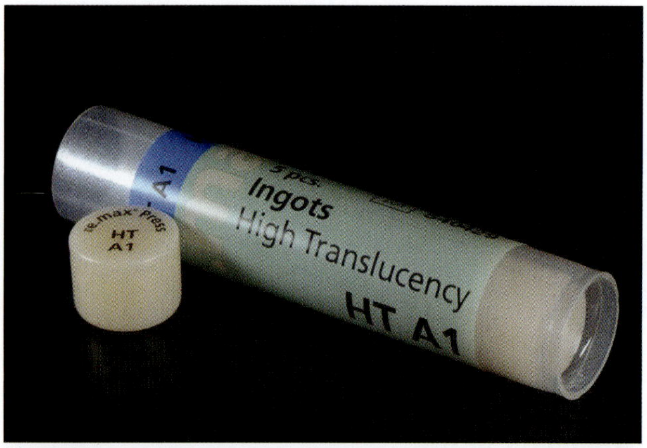

(a)

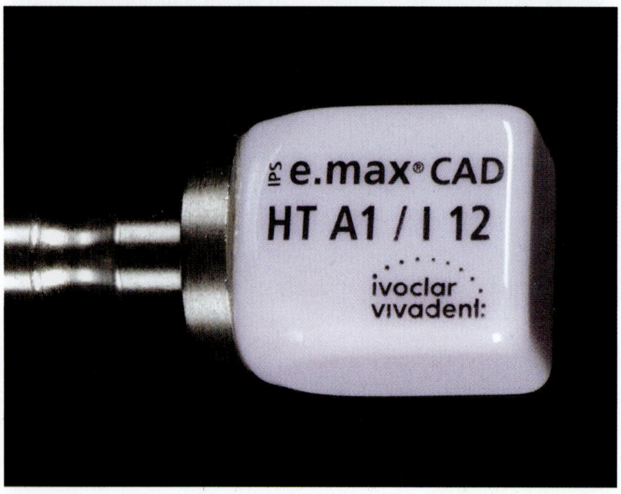

(b)

Figure 11.1 (a) IPS e.max pressable ingot. (b) IPS e.max CAD block.

Zirconia

In the general marketplace many types of zirconia are present; however, in dentistry 3% yttria-stabilized zirconia oxide is what is typically used in dental prostheses. Zirconia is used in dentistry because of its biocompatibility, favorable physical properties, and its appearance. The strength and esthetic benefits of zirconia allow it to be utilized as a replacement for traditional dental alloys. Over the last decade zirconia has been used quite extensively for single-unit, full-coverage extracoronal restorations as well as for fixed dental prostheses in the posterior dentition. Historically these areas were restored utilizing metal-based restorations; however, the strength of zirconia allows it to act as a viable tooth-colored alternative compared to traditional metal-based restorations. On the periodic table, zirconia is classified as a metal; however, in dentistry it is commonly classified as a ceramic due to its tooth-colored appearance. In order to maintain alignment with common perception and limit confusion zirconia will be discussed as though it is a ceramic. Zirconia's strength properties are considerably greater than those of feldspathic or glass ceramics. It can exhibit flexural strength properties up to 1200 MPa and fracture toughness K_{IC} values of 3.2 $MPam^{(1/2)}$.[4,5] This material is the most durable of all dental ceramics and its structural value derives from a phenomenon termed "transformation toughening". Transformation toughening occurs in zirconia due to the transformation of meta-stable tetragonal grains to stable monoclinic grains around the crack tip. This process is thought to limit crack progression in the material. These favorable physical properties paired with its relative tooth color have expanded zirconia's use in dentistry.

Zirconia first came to the dental market in the late 1990s and, for the first decade, it was only used as a dentin-colored core material to support veneering ceramic (Figure 11.2). In the early days of veneered zirconia restorations, numerous incidences of chipping and delamination of the veneering ceramic were being reported. These unusual occurrences were thought to be due to traditional feldspathic porcelain being used as a veneering ceramic and it having a different coefficient of thermal expansion than that of the zirconia core, but it was later demonstrated that residual stresses were introduced by fast cooling of the restorations upon removal from a porcelain furnace.[6,7] The clear benefit of placing a veneering ceramic onto a zirconia coping is that an esthetic restoration can be achieved while having similar properties and indications to a traditional metal–ceramic restoration. Veneering ceramic chipping or delaminating from a zirconia core is less prevalent today then in years past. There is emerging science to understand the etiology of these fractures using fractology, which has disclosed that failures originate below the occlusal surface because of hoop stresses and do not involve the interface.[8,9] This phenomenon underscores the importance of minimizing stresses

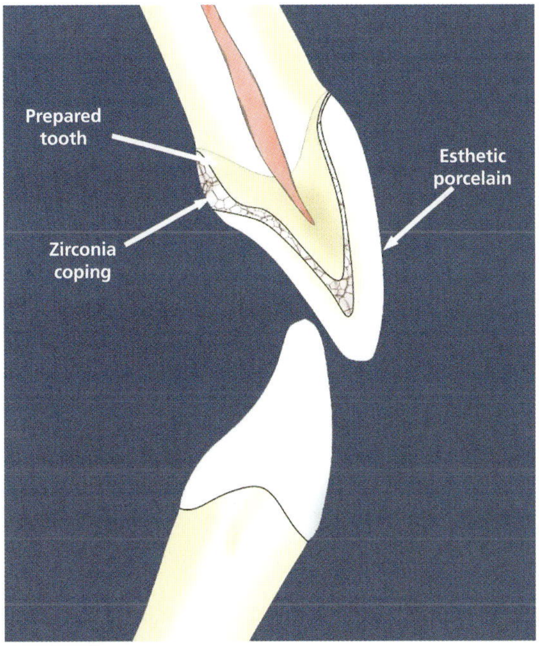

Figure 11.2 Cross-section of layered zirconia crown depicting zirconia and veneering porcelain. *Source:* Courtesy of Jeff Miles.

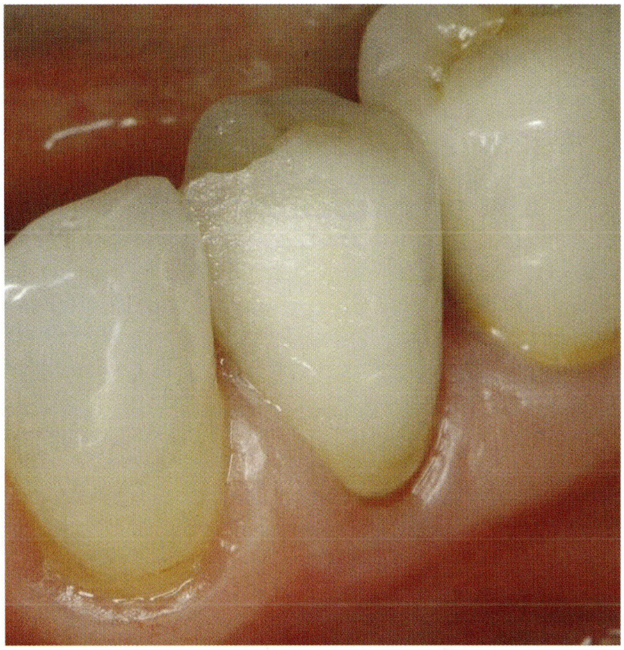

(a)

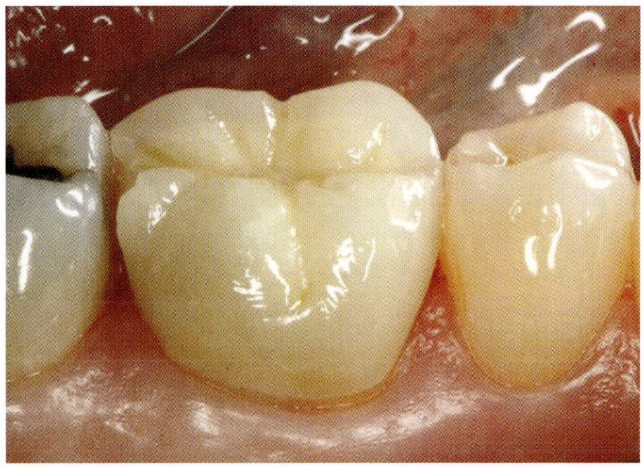

(b)

Figure 11.3 (**a**) Layered zirconia restoration with veneering ceramic fractured. *Source:* Reproduced with permission from Charles Goodacre. (**b**) Layered zirconia restoration with marginal ridge veneering ceramic fractured.

by eliminating axial wall binding and achieving sufficient occlusal thickness of the restoration.

The fabrication process has also undergone scrutiny. The improved performance of veneered zirconia restorations is due not only to the slow cooling process but also the use of anatomic copings,[10] as well as utilizing veneering ceramics that have been specifically developed to be applied directly to zirconia substructures. In fact, a study, which followed over 1000 of each zirconia-based and porcelain-fused crowns for more than 7 years, found that survival probabilities did not differ between the two and were independent of the molar or bicuspid site.[11] The improvements in veneered zirconia restorations have run parallel with the developments of utilizing zirconia as a monolithic material for both single-unit restorations as well as fixed dental prostheses.

The original concerns surrounding chipping of veneering ceramic (Figure 11.3) led researchers and material scientists down a path to see if zirconia could be utilized monolithically. The clear benefit of zirconia is that it offers a high flexural strength (800–1000 N), and a restoration made solely of this material may be able to hold up to the maximum occlusal forces.[12] The initial caveats of utilizing zirconia as a monolithic material were that the material may cause significant amounts of wear on the opposing dentition and the material would be too opaque to be considered an esthetic alternative to monolithic metal restorations. To address the concern of wear on the opposing dentition, numerous researchers have studied the impact monolithic zirconia may have on enamel, and it has been shown that, when monolithic zirconia is hand polished to a high luster, it has a similar wear rate on enamel as enamel has against itself.[13] In regard to the esthetic potential of monolithic zirconia restorations, new monolithic zirconia materials are coming to market that offer higher translucency levels that allow these types of restorations to be utilized on anterior teeth.[14] These more translucent materials are being achieved by altering the grain size of yttria-stabilized zirconia as well as the introduction of various trivalent oxides to the manufacturing process.[15,16]

The advances in glass-based ceramics as well as polycrystalline ceramics are allowing these materials to be used predictably on natural teeth and they should be considered as reasonable alternatives to traditional metal-based ceramics for implant restorations.

Abutments

If one is to restore an implant utilizing an abutment-based approach, this abutment will have an esthetic as well as a physical property impact on the complete implant restorative complex, if an all-ceramic restoration is to be prescribed. The trend over the last decade has been a move away from stock abutments towards customized CAD/CAM abutments. This change allows for an abutment that has optimal margin design, while allowing for appropriate retention and resistance form for each patient. The digital dental workflow, utilizing scanning and milling technologies, has allowed the cost of custom abutments to decrease substantially, making them more accessible for the average dental practice. CAD/CAM abutments are primarily produced utilizing titanium or yttria-stablized zirconia. Zirconia abutments have generally been considered in the esthetic zone because of their coloration; however, titanium abutments that have been gold anodized may also be considered in moderate esthetic areas, as they may offer some physical property advantages while providing reasonable esthetics (Figure 11.4).

Zirconia abutments

Zirconia abutments have been utilized in the anterior region as well as the premolar region with high survival rates and the annual failure rate appears to be similar to that of metal abutments.[17] Yttria-stablilized zirconia abutments have the clear advantage over titanium abutment in terms of esthetics. The ability to colorize zirconia abutments into various shades allows for better color of the periodontium as well as the coronal restoration (Figure 11.5). The typical gray appearance of the tissue overlying titanium abutments in patients with thin biotype can be mitigated with the use of zirconia abutments (Figure 11.6). In addition, zirconia abutments appear to have a benefit of less bacterial adhesion compared to titanium abutments, assuming a similar microgap.[18,19]

Zirconia abutments are available in either a pre-manufactured or stock form or in a patient-specific form. CAD/CAM zirconia abutments today are available in two variations. In the

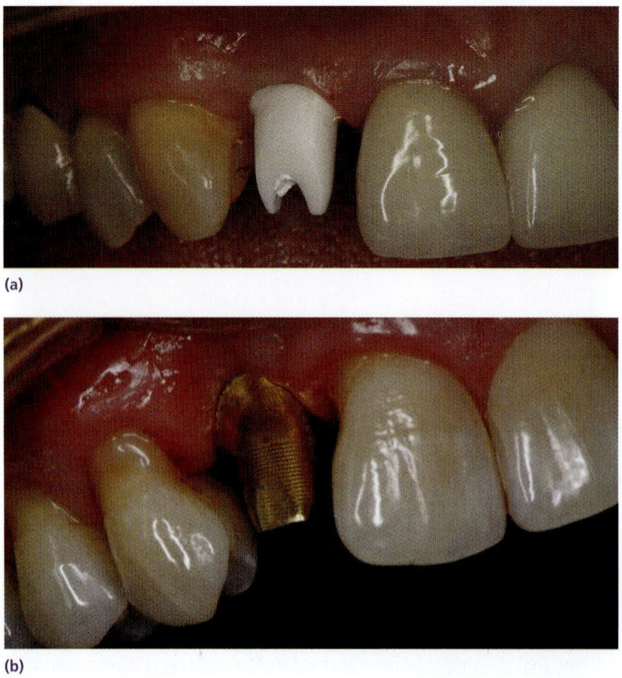

(a) (b)

Figure 11.4 (a) Zirconia CAD/CAM abutment in place. (b) Gold hue abutment in place.

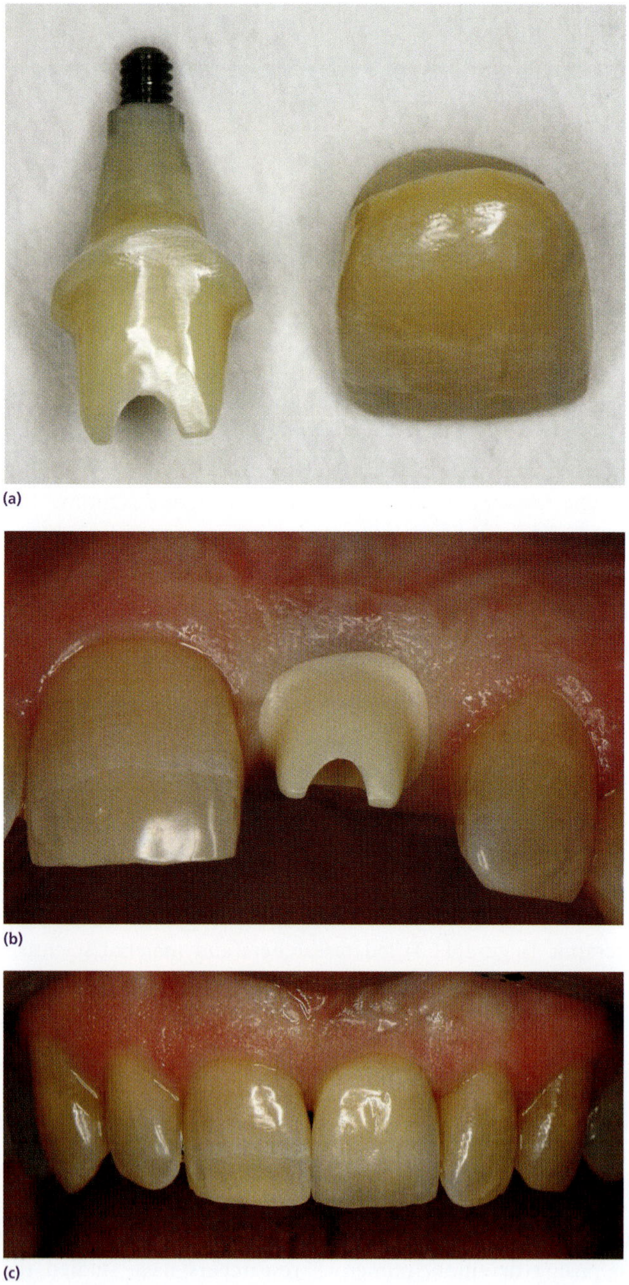

(a) (b) (c)

Figure 11.5 (a) Colorized zirconia abutment. (b) Zirconia abutment in place. (c) Definitive lithium disilicate crown in place. *Source:* Reproduced with permission from Charles Goodacre.

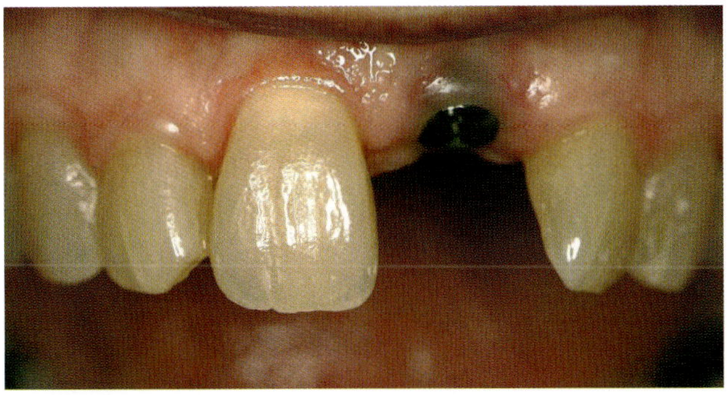

Figure 11.6 Grayish coloration in the gingiva from a titanium healing abutment. *Source:* Reproduced with permission from Charles Goodacre.

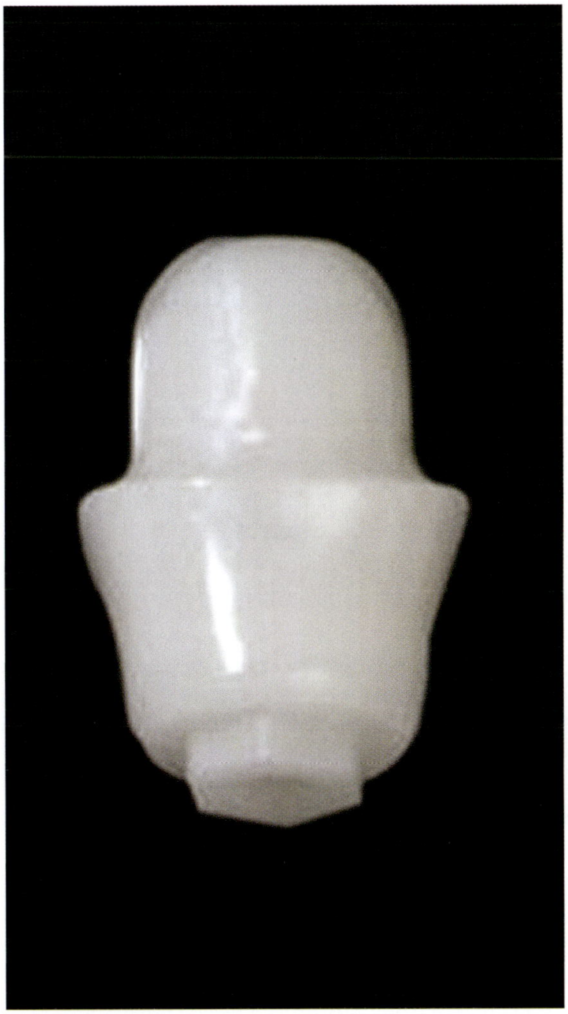

Figure 11.7 One-piece zirconia abutment.

first variant, a monolithic zirconia abutment is manufactured (Figure 11.7), and this abutment is directly seated to the implant fixture and retained with a titanium screw. These types of abutments are commonly referred to as one-piece abutments. In the second variant, a hybrid manufacturing process is accomplished. In this variant a zirconia abutment is manufactured and

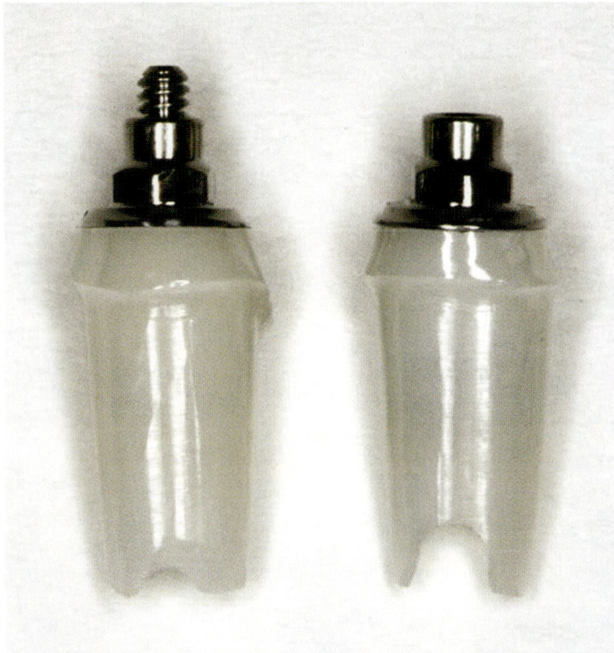

Figure 11.8 Two-piece zirconia abutment with titanium base. *Source:* Reproduced with permission from Charles Goodacre.

then adhered to a titanium base (Figure 11.8). This titanium base houses the channel for the screw and it is this titanium base that is in contact with the platform of the implant fixture. The benefit of the monolithic zirconia abutment is that it utilizes a relatively straightforward manufacturing process; however, there are some concerns appearing in the literature with respect to the connection point with the implant fixture.

The advantage of metal is that it can be highly machined to intricate shapes without sacrificing a substantial amount of strength, as opposed to zirconia.[20] As zirconia thins out, it becomes weak and has a tendency to fracture (Figure 11.9). This is further complicated as one-piece zirconia abutments are in direct contact with the implant fixture and the female connection point of the implant must properly match the male insert of the zirconia abutment. The less accurate fit of these abutments allows for a greater degree of micromotion to occur, and there is some concern that titanium implants can experience wear caused by the zirconia abutment.[21] This wear can lead to titanium debris contamination of the soft tissue. Additionally, fractures of this type of abutment have a tendency to be catastrophic.[22] If too high a force is applied to the zirconia–implant connection point, the abutment will not be salvageable.

Two-piece zirconia abutments have been developed to have the esthetic benefit of one-piece systems yet address the problematic aspects of titanium wear, micromotion, and catastrophic fractures. Two-piece abutments allow for a titanium-to-titanium connection to occur and for the connecting screw to be housed within a titanium channel. As an axial force is applied to these abutments, the force is concentrated at the level of the abutment

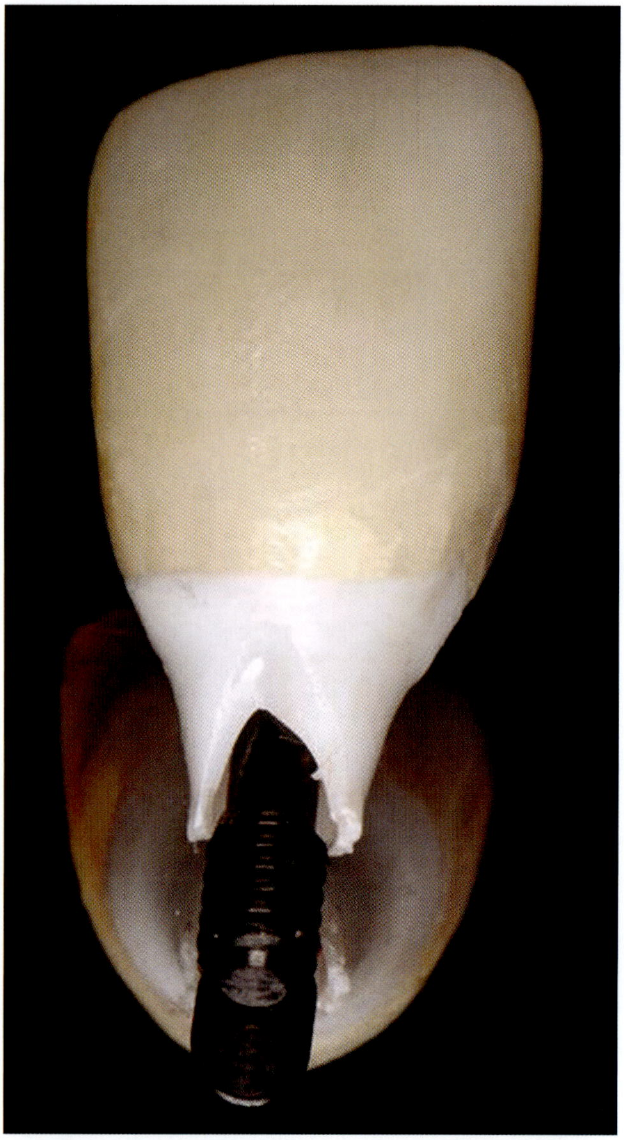

Figure 11.9 Fractured one-piece zirconia abutment. *Source:* Reproduced with permission from Charles Goodacre.

screw, as it is the weakest point.[20] This concentration of force allows a significantly higher fracture resistance compared to one-piece systems. As this screw is encased in a titanium sleeve, the connection point generally does not fracture, rather the retaining screw bends within the titanium sleeve. Chewing forces in an axial direction generally do not exceed 220 N[12] and studies show that two-piece zirconia abutments demonstrate fracture loads of approximately 290 N, while one-piece abutments demonstrate an ability to withstand fracture loads in the range of 230–250 N.[20] The fracture load of one-piece abutments is relatively close to the axial forces that occur in normal mastication, so this type of abutment should be used cautiously. In patients that exhibit high levels of bite force, maximum anterior forces can reach 400 N and posterior forces can reach 1000 N.[12] In these patients, a titanium abutment would be advantageous. This has given traction to development of an esthetic derivative.

Gold hue abutments

One clear advantage of titanium abutments is that they offer very high load-to-fracture rates, thus allowing them to be used anywhere in the mouth. In cases that have greater than 2 mm of tissue thickness, color and light reflection of soft tissue is not appreciably different between zirconia and titanium abutments.[23] The downside, however, is that the tissue can appear gray if the patient has a thin biotype. Another potential downside of titanium abutments is that they can cause a grayish appearance to the final restoration if a ceramic restoration is to be used on top of the titanium abutment. One consideration in moderate esthetic demand areas is to use a titanium abutment that has been opaqued with porcelain (Figure 11.10) or coated with titanium nitride. In the latter instance, the coating effect gives the titanium abutment a gold hue, allowing it to blend more naturally under the soft tissue, and it provides a warmer stump shade for all-ceramic restorations compared to traditional gray titanium abutments. The combination of gold hue abutments and ceramic restorations can be especially useful in the canine to bicuspid area. The dentition in this area tends to undergo a greater amount of occlusal force and these teeth also tend to be more opaque then incisors; therefore, high translucency in these areas is generally not mandatory in order to achieve esthetic harmony. When considering the influence of zirconia or gold-hue titanium abutments on peri-implant soft tissue, after 2 years of service, the abutment type was not critical.[24]

Lithium disilicate abutments

Companies are experimenting with lithium disilicate implant abutments, but neither clinical studies nor *in vitro* fatigue data are available to date.

Single-unit crowns and fixed dental prostheses

Anterior restorations

The most critical area of one's smile is the maxillary anterior zone and in this region the optical properties of the overlying ceramics should be combined with proper abutment selection in order to achieve a harmonious result. Generally speaking, zirconia abutments provide the proper optical foundation upon which ceramic restorations can be placed. One key benefit of zirconia is that the abutment can be colorized to mimic traditional dentin shading. Assuming that a zirconia restoration has been selected, the overlying ceramic restoration can be a glass-based ceramic or a polycrystalline ceramic. New materials are coming to the market that may add future options; however, at this time, materials in these two categories allow technicians to deliver proper esthetics and reasonable physical properties to withstand average occlusal forces.

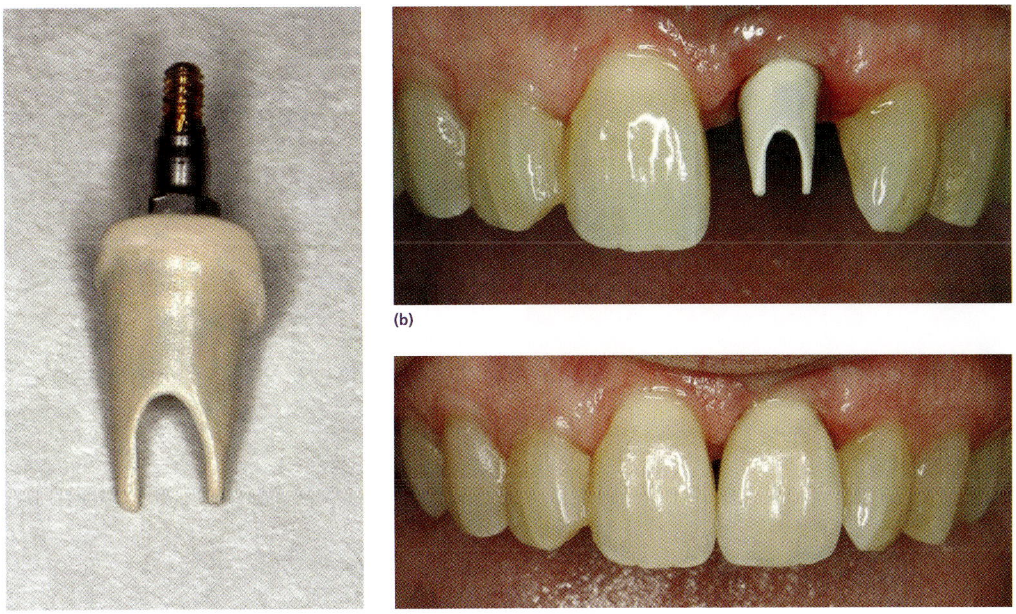

(a) (b) (c)

Figure 11.10 (a) Opaqued titanium abutment. (b) Opaqued titanium abutment in place. (c) Lithium disilicate crown in place. *Source:* Reproduced with permission from Charles Goodacre.

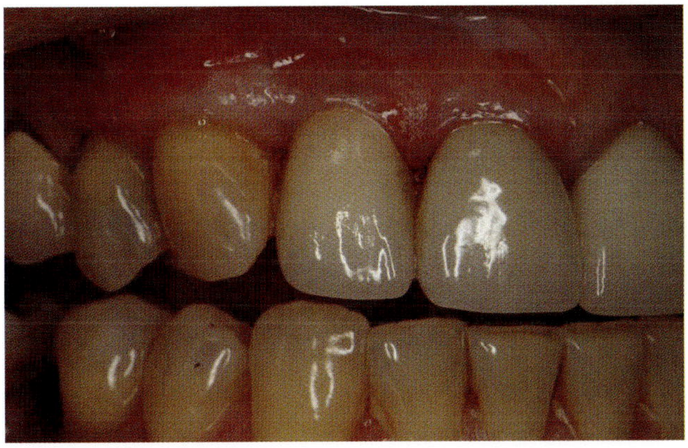

Figure 11.11 Lithium disilicate crown #7 on zirconia abutment.

Glass-based ceramics

In the glass-based ceramic category the market has shifted away from ceramic restorations classified as feldspathic and leucite-reinforced ceramics to those ceramics that are categorized as lithium disilicate-based ceramics. In the esthetic zone, lithium disilicate can be utilized in a true monolithic manner (Figures 11.4a and 11.11) to provide optimal strength, or it can be cut back and stacked for improved color characterization and translucency. The area in which the restoration is cut back and stacked with veneering porcelain tends to be weaker than the underlying lithium disilicate, and these areas are more susceptible to fractures. Both monolithic and layered lithium disilicate restorations have very good survival rates; however, it should be noted that in a study that evaluated over 15 000 single-unit full-coverage restorations over a 4-year span on natural teeth, layered restorations had a failure rate of 1.83% and monolithic restorations had a failure rate of 0.91%.[25] In the referenced study, failure included any fracture of the restorative material that required a remake of the restoration. These survival rates demonstrate that, while the risk of failure is low for both types of restoration, layered restorations should be reserved for cases that require enhanced esthetics. In terms of implant dentistry, survival is dependent on both the overlying ceramic and the abutment. When lithium disilicate is used in conjunction with two-piece zirconia abutments, the axial preparation depth utilized on these abutments impacts the total load to failure. The properties of zirconia are maximized when it is used in larger dimension; therefore, care must be taken to create overlying restorations with proper esthetic and functional properties without negatively impacting the underlying abutment. Fracture loads of anterior lithium disilicate restorations bonded to zirconia abutments have been shown to be 20–25% greater for 0.5 mm axial preparations than for 0.9 mm axial preparations.[26]

Polycrystalline ceramics

Another restorative material that can be considered in the anterior zone is a veneered zirconia restoration. The only concern with this type of restoration is that chipping of the veneering ceramic is still a possibility. One key benefit of veneered zirconia restorations in implant dentistry is that these restorations tend to be more opaque and this higher opacity may be a benefit. The higher opacity of zirconia restorations affords the ability to utilize these crowns in conjunction with traditional titanium abutments or gold anodized abutments (Figures 11.4b and 11.12). These restorations may not be the most esthetic; however, they may be very acceptable for many patients. Veneered zirconia

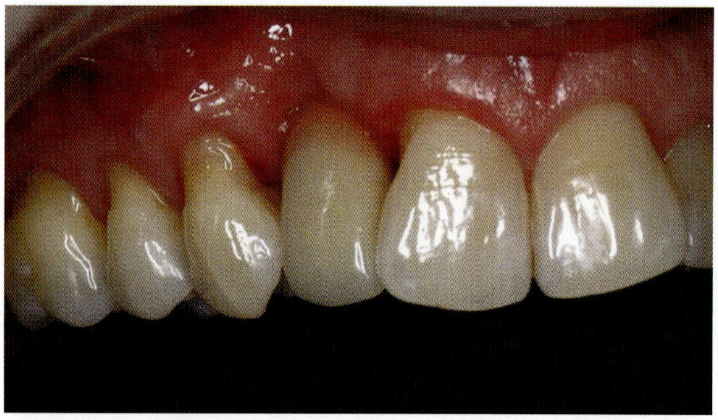

Figure 11.12 Zirconia crown on gold hue abutment in #7 position.

restorations on titanium abutments are able to withstand high loads without experiencing fractures of the crown, given these are not aftermarket components.[27] Unfortunately, this ability to withstand heavy occlusal load may come at a cost. When heavy loads are placed onto these restorations the neck of the implant can actually undergo distortion.[28] This distortion theoretically could lead to a catastrophic failure requiring replacement of the implant. However, the forces that are reached in laboratory testing rarely happen clinically in the anterior portion of the dentition. There is an important distinction in significance at the bench and in the clinic.

Posterior single-unit restorations

In the posterior aspect of the dentition occlusal loads tend to be greater; therefore, esthetics must also be blended with optimal physical properties. In the bicuspid region, treatment options tend to mimic those that were discussed for anterior therapy; however, in the molar region alternative ceramic and abutment combinations can be considered. Generally speaking, titanium abutments should be selected in the molar region, as high occlusal loads tend to put zirconia abutments at risk and esthetic needs tend not to be as high.[12] The blend of proper physical properties and reasonable esthetics can be achieved with monolithic zirconia restorations mixed with titanium abutments.

Glass ceramics

In the glass ceramic category, lithium disilicate restorations can be prescribed as monolithic restorations. As discussed earlier, these restorations provide high esthetic value and, in the posterior aspect of the dentition, reasonable esthetics can be achieved without having to cut back restorations and adding a layering ceramic. In the bicuspid regions of patients that have higher esthetic needs, monolithic lithium disilicate can be paired with two-piece zirconia abutments (Figure 11.13). In the molar region of patients with moderate to low occlusal loads this material can be paired with gold hue titanium abutments. If an opaque ingot of lithium disilicate is selected, it can also be paired with traditionally colored titanium abutments.

Polycrystalline ceramics

In the molar region, monolithic zirconia restorations can be considered for their high strength and relative esthetic value. In the early days of monolithic zirconia restorations, the restorations tended to be very opaque and offered very low esthetic value; however, these restorations were considered reasonable alternatives to traditional metal restorations. Monolithic zirconia restorations have become very popular, as practitioners have searched for a material that is considered strong yet has a more economical cost structure when compared to metallic restorations. Gold has been appreciated as a biocompatible and durable material with wear rates similar to those of enamel for many years; however, as gold prices quadrupled between 2005 and 2011, practitioners began to search for alternatives. In addition, many patients demand natural-looking restorations and the acceptance of metallic restorations has decreased over the years.

Since their initial introduction into the marketplace, monolithic zirconia restorations have performed very well both on the natural teeth and as implant restorations and, during this time, the restorations have also become more esthetically pleasing (Figure 11.14). Unlike layered restorations, no veneering ceramic is placed on these restorations; therefore, chipping tends not to be a concern when these restorations are placed in occlusal function. In fact, the load that can be placed in a laboratory setting on monolithic zirconia restorations before they fail greatly exceeds the masticatory force of healthy young adults.[12] The disadvantage of this material continues to be the inability to adjust and repair with ease. This has led to innovative work in the realm of nano-filled composite resins.

Hybrid ceramics/nano-ceramics: a future direction?

As chairside milling has increased in popularity, many manufacturers have developed materials that can be efficiently milled yet maintain reasonable strength, gloss, and esthetics, as well as facile adjustability and repairability. The goal of these materials is to combine the properties of ceramics and resins, and they therefore have been termed hybrid ceramics or nano-ceramics. Presently they can be classified as an improved particle-filled resin composite. Products in this category include Lava Ultimate by 3M (St. Paul, MN), Cerasmart by GC (Alsip, IL) (Figure 11.15), and Vita Enamic by Vita (Yorba Linda, CA). To date there is limited *in vivo* research available with regard to success of these materials in clinical practice. An *in vitro* study evaluated the mechanical properties of polymer-based CAD/CAM milling blocks. The results were encouraging as they exhibited high flexural strength and smoother margins than the ceramic counterparts. One concern with traditional resin-based materials is that they tend to have low wear resistance and these materials also have lower flexural strength. The new hybrid ceramics and nano-ceramics are claimed to have better wear resistance then traditional resin-based material. In a recent *in vitro* study resin "nano-ceramic"

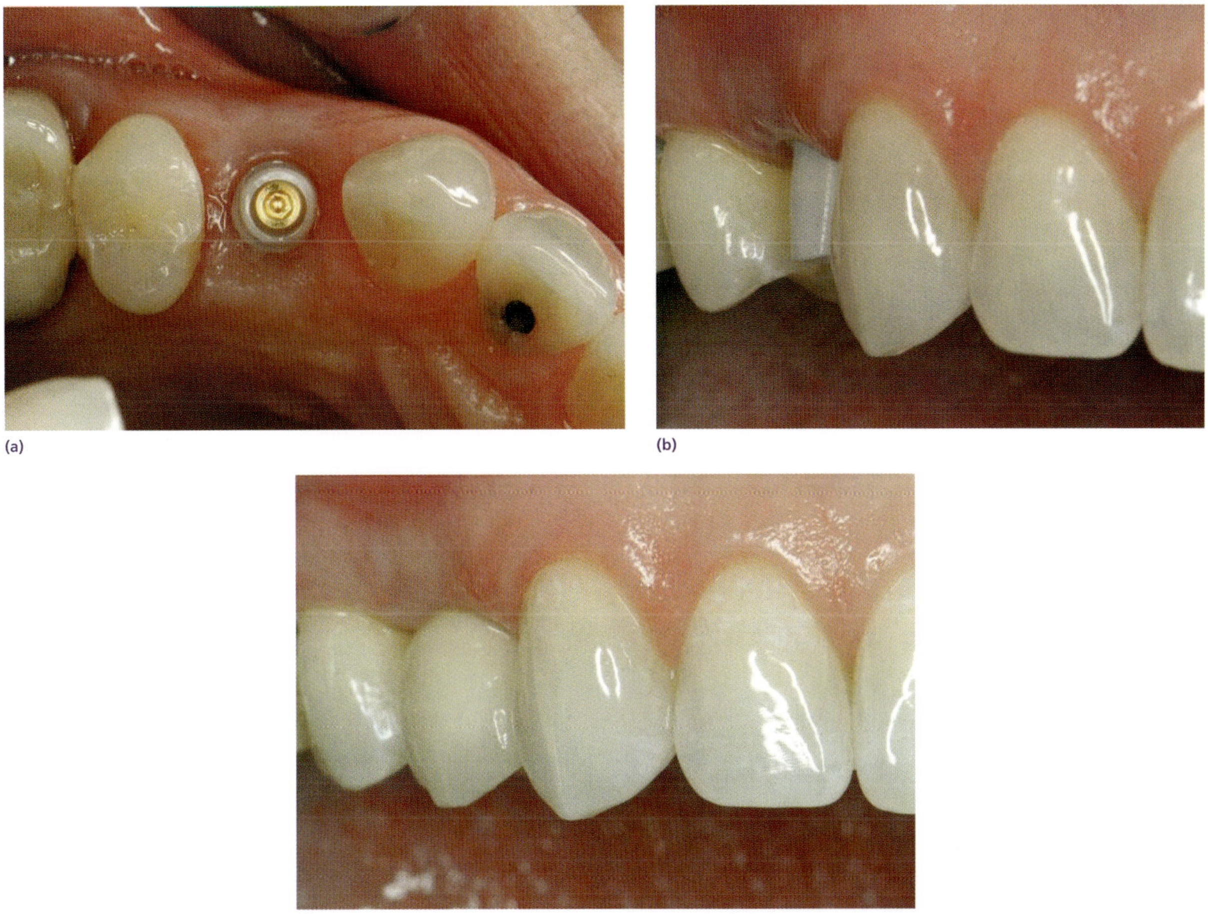

Figure 11.13 (a) Zirconia two-piece abutment #5 (occlusal view). (b) Zirconia abutment #5 (facial view). (c) Monolithic lithium disilicate crown in place (#5).

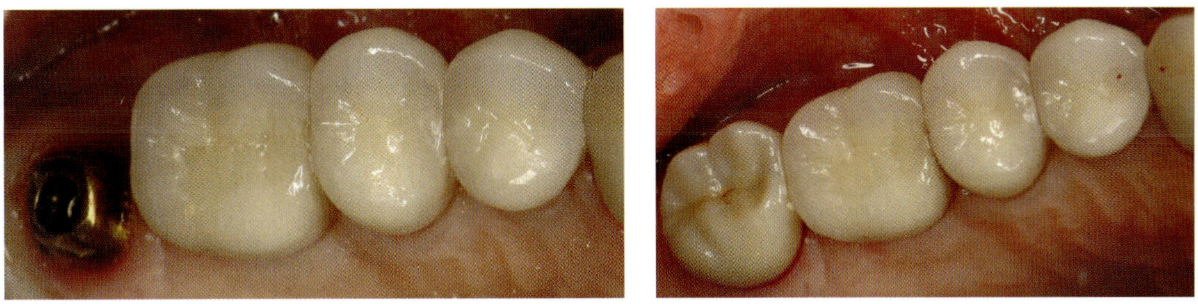

Figure 11.14 (a) Gold hue abutment #2. (b) Monolithic zirconia crown #2 in place.

crowns (3M's Lava Ultimate) cemented to titanium abutments with self-adhesive cement survived the normal range of masticatory forces over 5 years of simulated chewing.[29] However, 3M ESPE has taken this material off the market for complete coverage crowns. A greater level of research is needed to develop these new-age materials to achieve the physical and esthetic goals of an ideal restoration as well as the impact on time of repairs.

Fixed dental prostheses

If a clinician chooses to utilize an all-ceramic restoration for an implant-borne fixed dental prosthesis, essentially three options exist today. These options are lithium disilicate, monolithic zirconia, and veneered zirconia. The decision to utilize a given material should be dependent upon the span of the prosthesis, esthetic needs, and estimated occlusal load. As discussed earlier, the most esthetic result can generally be obtained by combining

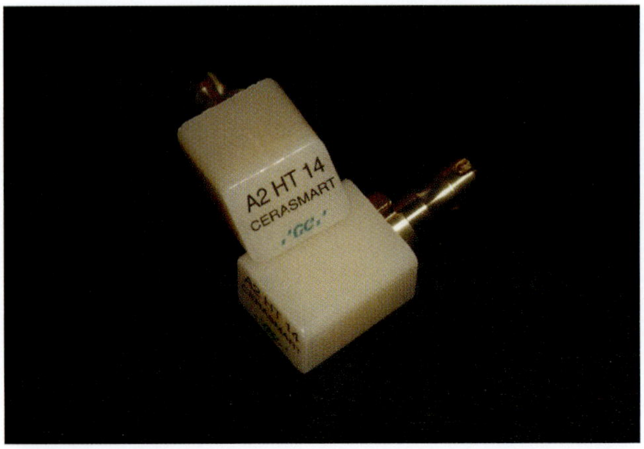

Figure 11.15 Cerasmart milling block.

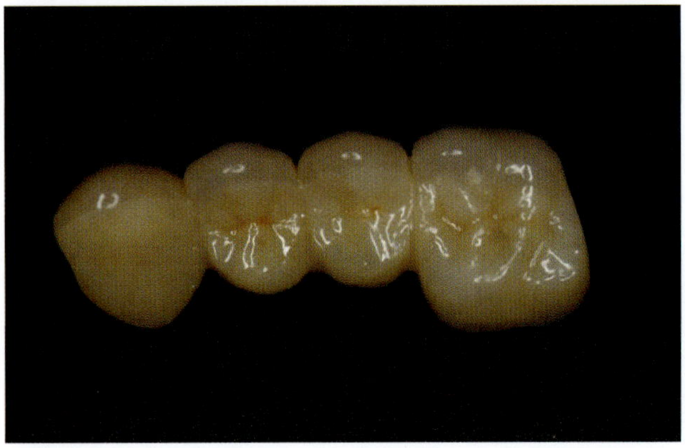

Figure 11.16 Partially veneered zirconia fixed dental prosthesis.

lithium disilicate restorations with zirconia abutments; however, lithium disilicate restorations should be used cautiously as the material of choice for a fixed dental prosthesis. Lithium disilicate restorations can be utilized in a three-unit span to replace a single anterior tooth or a first bicuspid and should not be used in larger spans or to replace a molar. The manufacturer also states that cantilever restorations are contraindicated. In addition, the manufacturer recommends that the pontic should be less than 11 mm in width in the anterior region and less than 9 mm in width in the canine and bicuspid regions. Furthermore, it is recommended that the connector dimension should also be a minimum of 16 mm^2 and the vertical aspect of this measurement is most critical.[30]

If a larger span or posterior fixed dental prosthesis is to be placed, zirconia should be considered. Monolithic zirconia is well suited for limited posterior spans as well as for full-arch rehabilitation. In posterior spans, reasonable esthetics can be achieved to closely match any adjacent natural dentition, and in full-arch cases the restoration can be properly stained and colorized to achieve esthetic harmony. Partially veneered zirconia restorations may offer an alternative option to three-unit lithium disilicate anterior restorations or metal–ceramic cantilever restorations, as well as providing a more esthetic alternative to monolithic zirconia restorations in the posterior segment. Practitioners can choose to use a hybrid approach in these cases, so that full-contour zirconia is used in all areas that are in function as well as all nonesthetic areas, and veneering ceramic is placed on top of the zirconia core in more esthetic areas (Figure 11.16).

Summary

Ceramic materials have evolved exponentially over the last 20 years and these materials can be used predictably in all aspects of the mouth. Practitioners must understand that all full-ceramic restorations are not created equal and that these restorations must be properly paired with the appropriate abutment to achieve long-term success.

References

1. Sailer I, Makarov NA, Thoma DS, *et al.* All-ceramic or metal ceramic tooth-supported fixed dental prostheses (FDPs)? A systematic review of the complication and survival rates. Part 1: single crowns (SCs). *Dent Mater* 2015; **31**(6): 603–623.
2. Lameira DP, Silva WA, Silva FA, *et al.* Fracture strength of aged monolithic and bilayered zirconia-based crowns. *Biomed Res Int* 2015; 418641. doi: 10.1155/2015/418641.epub 2015 Oct 21.
3. Kang SH, Chang J, Son HH. Flexural strength and microstructure of two lithium disilicate glass ceramics for CAD/CAM restorations in the dental clinic. *Restor Dent Endod* 2013; **38**(3): 134–140.
4. Tong H, Tanaka CB, Kaizer MR, *et al.* Characterization of three commercial Y-TZP ceramics produced for their high-translucency, high-strength and high-surface area. *Ceram Int* 2016: **42**(1 Pt B): 1077–1085.
5. Harada K, Shinya A, Yokoyama D, *et al.* Effect of loading conditions on the fracture toughness of zirconia. *J Prosthodont Res* 2013; **57**(2): 82–87.
6. Benetti P, Kelly JR, Sanchez M, *et al.* Influence of thermal gradients on stress state of veneered restorations. *Dent Mater* 2014; **30**(5): 54–63.
7. Choi JE, Waddell JN, Swain MV. Pressed ceramics onto zirconia. Part 2: indentation fracture and influence of cooling rate on residual stress. *Dent Mater* 2011; **27**(11): 1111–1118.
8. Scherrer SS, Quinn GD, Quinn JB. Fractographic failure analysis of a Procera AllCeram crown using stereo and scanning electron microscopy. *Dent Mater* 2008; **24**(8): 1107–1113.
9. Scherrer SS, Quinn JB, Quinn GD, *et al.* Failure analysis of ceramic clinical cases using qualitative fractology. *Int J Prosthodont* 2006; **19**(2): 185–192.
10. Larsson C. Zirconium dioxide based dental restorations. Studies on clinical performance and fracture behavior. *Swed Dent J Suppl* 2011; **213**: 9–84.
11. Ozer F, Mante FK, Chiche G, *et al.* A retrospective survey on long-term survival of posterior zirconia and porcelain-fused-to-metal crowns in private practice. *Quintessence Int* 2014; **45**(1): 31–38.
12. Okiyama S, Ikebe K, Nokubi T. Association between masticatory performance and maximal occlusal force in young men. *J Oral Rehab* 2003; **30**(3): 278–282.
13. Janyavula S, Lawson N, Cakir D, *et al.* The wear of polished and glazed zirconia against enamel. *J Prosthet Dent* 2013; **109**(1): 22–29.

14. Sulaiman TA, Abdulmajeed AA, Donovan TE, *et al.* Optical properties and light irradiance of monolithic zirconia at variable thicknesses. *Dent Mater* 2015; **31**(10): 1180–1187.
15. Zhang F, Vanmeensel K, Batuk M, *et al.* Highly-translucent, strong and aging-resistant 3Y-TZP ceramics for dental restoration by grain boundary segregation. *Acta Biomater* 2015; **16**: 215–222.
16. Zhang Y. Making yttria-stabilized tetragonal zirconia translucent. *Dent Mater* 2014; **30**(10): 1195–1203.
17. Sailer I, Philipp A, Zembic A, *et al.* A systematic review of the performance of ceramic and metal implant abutments supporting fixed implant reconstructions. *Clin Oral Implants Res* 2009; **20**(Suppl 4): 4–31.
18. Nakamura K, Kanno T, Milleding P, *et al.* Zirconia as a dental material: a systematic review. *Int J Prosthodont* 2010; **23**(4): 299–309.
19. Nasciemento CD, Pita MS, Fernandes FH, *et al.* Bacterial adhesion on the titanium and zirconium abutment surfaces. *Clin Oral Implants Res* 2014; **25**(3): 337–343.
20. Gehrke P, Johannson D, Fischer C, *et al.* In vitro fatigue and fracture resistance of one- and two-piece CAD/CAM zirconia implant abutments. *Int J Oral Maxillofac Implants* 2015; **30**(3): 546–554.
21. Klotz MW, Taylor TD, Goldberg AJ. Wear at the titanium–zirconia implant abutment interface: a pilot study. *Int J Oral Maxillofac Implants* 2011; **26**(5): 970–975.
22. Guazzato M, Albakry M, Ringer SP, *et al.* Strength, fracture toughness and microstructure of a selection of all ceramic materials. Part II Zirconia-based dental ceramics. *Dent Mater* 2004; **20**(5): 449–454.
23. Van Brakel R, Noordmans HJ, Frenken J, *et al.* The effect of zirconia and titanium implant abutments on light reflection of the supporting soft tissues. *Clin Oral Implants Res* 2011; **22**(10): 1172–1178.
24. Ferrari M, Cagidiaco MC, Garcia-Godoy F, *et al.* Effect of different prosthetic abutments on peri-implant soft tissue. A randomized controlled clinical trial. *Am J Dent* 2015; **28**(2): 85–89.
25. Sulaiman TA, Delgado AJ, Donovan TE. Survival rate of lithium disiclate restorations at 4 years: a retrospective study. *J Prosthet Dent* 2015; **114**(3): 364–366.
26. Joo HS, Yang HS, Park SW, *et al.* Influence of preparation depths on the fracture load of customized zirconia abutments with titanium insert. *J Adv Prosthodont* 2015; **7**(3): 183–190.
27. Yilmaz B, Salaita LG, Seidt JD, *et al.* Load to failure of different titanium abutments for an internal hexagon implant. *J Prosthet Dent* 2015; **114**(4): 513–516.
28. Bijjargi S, Chowdhary R. Stress dissipation in the bone through various crown materials of dental implant a 2-D finite element analysis. *J Investigat Clin Dent* 2013; **4**(3): 172–177.
29. Awada A, Nathanson D. Mechanical properties of resin-ceramic CAD/CAM restorative materials. *J Prosthet Dent* 2015; **114**(4): 587–593.
30. Raigrodski AJ. Contemporary materials and technologies for all-ceramic fixed partial dentures: a review of the literature. *J Prosthet Dent* 2004; **92**(6): 557–562.

CHAPTER 12

Cement-Retained Implant Restorations: Problems and Solutions

Chandur P.K. Wadhwani
Loma Linda University School of Dentistry, Loma Linda, California, USA

Dental practitioners have a preference for the cement-retained implant-supported restoration,[1–3] essentially because it is more like the traditional tooth-borne crown and bridge restorations with which they are familiar. Developed primarily to overcome issues with esthetics and occlusion, it also has benefits related to cost, potential for a better passive fit when dealing with a multiple-unit prosthesis,[4] and reduced chair time. Although dentists reported a preference for using cemented implant restorations, patients when surveyed did not appear to have any definite preference.[5]

Along with the reported benefits of using cemented implant restorations, a number of concerns emerged, for example there has been no technique for predictable removal and salvage of the restoration to access the abutment screw.[6,7] Then, as implant therapy grew and popularity of cemented prostheses increased, implant site health issues started to emerge. For example, the influence on the type of implant restoration used and the general health of the surrounding soft tissues has been studied. Weber *et al.*[5] conducted a prospective multicenter study on 152 implants placed in the maxillary anterior region. They concluded the peri-implant soft tissues responded more favorably to screw-retained crowns than to cement-retained crowns. A recent systematic review also concluded that cement-retained reconstructions exhibited more technical and biological complications compared with screw-retained reconstructions.[8] Pauletto *et al.*[9] reported on complications associated with excess cement around crowns on osseointegrated implants in 1999, a series of four case studies. Tomson *et al.*[10] and others[11–16] followed suit with more case reports on issues relating to excess cement and peri-implant disease.

Wilson[17] evaluated 42 implants in 39 patients that showed signs of inflammation (peri-implant mucositis or peri-implantitis) and reported a positive link between excess cement and peri-implant disease. This endoscopic study found excess residual cement associated with 81% of diseased sites. While the removal of the cement resulted in healing in most instances, further intervention was required in almost 25% of the cases. Most alarmingly, the time for the disease to be discovered varied from 4 months to almost 9.5 years after the crown was cemented. In January 2013 the American Academy of Periodontics, under the direction of the task force on peri-implantitis, developed a position paper elucidating risk factors. Residual excess cement was highlighted as an etiological factor.[18]

Cemented restorations and issues related specifically to dental implants

The dental community has been using cemented restorations on natural teeth for well over 100 years[19] with minor issues, provided the pulp and periodontal status are healthy. It is often questioned "why should it be when we use the same cement materials, with the same type of crown, place it with the same techniques for the implant restoration, adverse effects are reported which could potentially lead to the implant being lost?"

Tooth versus implants: biology

Implants have a very different mechanism of attachment to both the bone and the surrounding soft tissues compared with the natural tooth.[20] A tooth crevice has keratinized epithelium at the base of the gingival sulcus, whereas an implant does not. The junctional epithelium is adherent and less permeable and has a high capability to regenerate around a tooth. Apical to the junctional epithelium lies the soft connective tissue attachment. The periodontium of a healthy tooth has a major advantage over the peri-implant tissues in that the supracrestal collagen fiber bundles exist. Some of these insert directly into living cementum on the root surface of the tooth (Figure 12.1). This robust tooth–tissue interface has evolved over millions of years and serves as a seal to protect this area; it is highly protective against the ingress of bacteria and insult from trauma. Also, the arrangement of the periodontal fiber

Evidence-based Implant Treatment Planning and Clinical Protocols, First Edition. Edited by Steven J. Sadowsky.

Companion website: www.wiley.com/go/sadowsky/implant

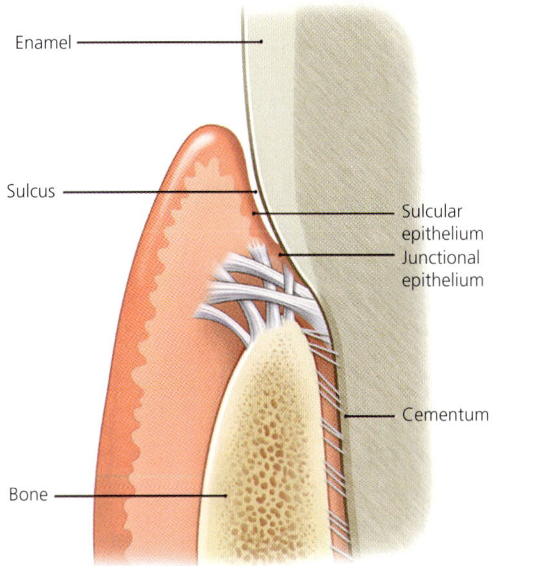

Figure 12.1 Biological attachment of a natural tooth. Connective tissue fibers insert into the root apical to the junctional epithelium. *Source:* © 2016, Chris Gralapp

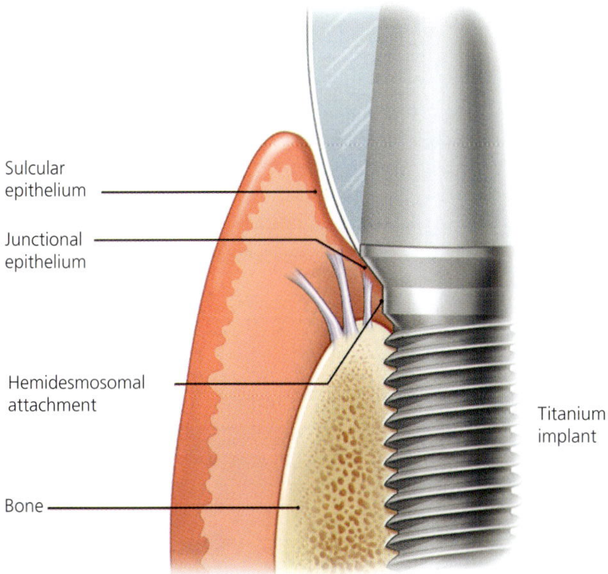

Figure 12.2 Biological attachment to a dental implant. There is no insertion of connective tissue fibers into the implant surface. *Source:* © 2016, Chris Gralapp

bundles results in a compartment-like structure around the tooth which limits the spread of periodontal disease. By comparison, there is no cementum associated with the dental implant, so no direct collagen fiber insertion exists. Circumferential fibers that encircle the dental implant are present, behaving somewhat as a scar "cuff" that maintains the tissues in close apposition to the implant (Figure 12.2). This arrangement provides only one compartment that exists 360° around the implant. The single compartment around an implant explains why the associated

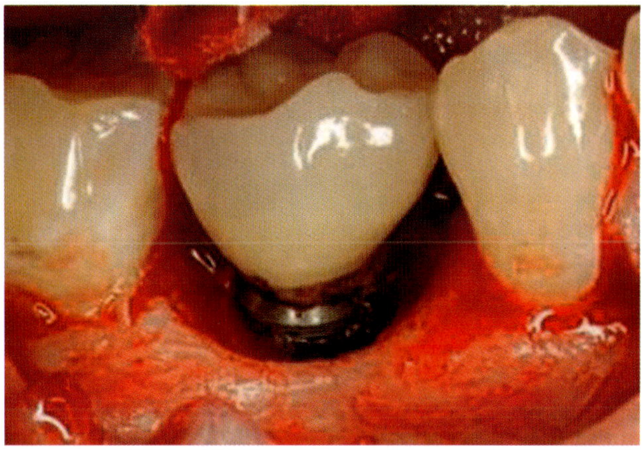

Figure 12.3 Example of Implant site with residual excess cement and associated peri-implantitis. Note the generalized "crater" pattern of bone loss relates to the character of the biological attachment. *Source:* Reproduced with permission from Ken Akimoto, periodontist.

inflammatory responses are generalized (Figure 12.3) rather than localized, as in the case of a tooth. The implant site that develops through healing within a few days is far more fragile, because the implant to soft tissue attachment mechanism is more of a cellular adhesion, being hemidesmosomal in nature.

As a consequence, the connective tissue adhesion at implants is considered as having a poor mechanical resistance,[21] with some authors considering that the mucosa at implants can hardly be qualified as "attached".[22]

Implant depth and cement margin depth

In health, the implant–soft tissue attachment tends to occur at deeper levels when compared with the soft tissue attachment in the natural dentition. The platform of an implant, which is commonly flat topped, is frequently related to the facial crest of the soft tissues and is intentionally placed 3 mm deep to facilitate an emergence profile for the abutment and restoration. Where papillae exist, the flat top of the implant may now be located 5–7 mm deep to the crest of soft tissues.[23] Maintaining and cleaning deeper than 4 mm is impossible with routine scaling instruments,[24] and the microbiota at deeper sites tends to favor Gram-negative bacteria, the type that are known to cause peri-implant diseases.[25,26] The depth of the implant site and associated bacterial challenge might contribute to a predisposition for a disease process, especially with residual excess cement.

When preparing the natural tooth for a cement-retained restoration the cement finish line is rarely placed deeper than 0.5 mm into a healthy gingival sulcus, which is still considered a compromise.[27,28] The prepared margins follow the outline of the gingival crest, moving more coronally to follow the outline of the papillae and remaining supragingival tissue wherever possible.[29,30]

Cement extrusion from the margin site during seating an implant crown can present problems with the ability to detect and remove this foreign material. Although anecdotal recommendations of 1–3 mm[31,32] have been made regarding the

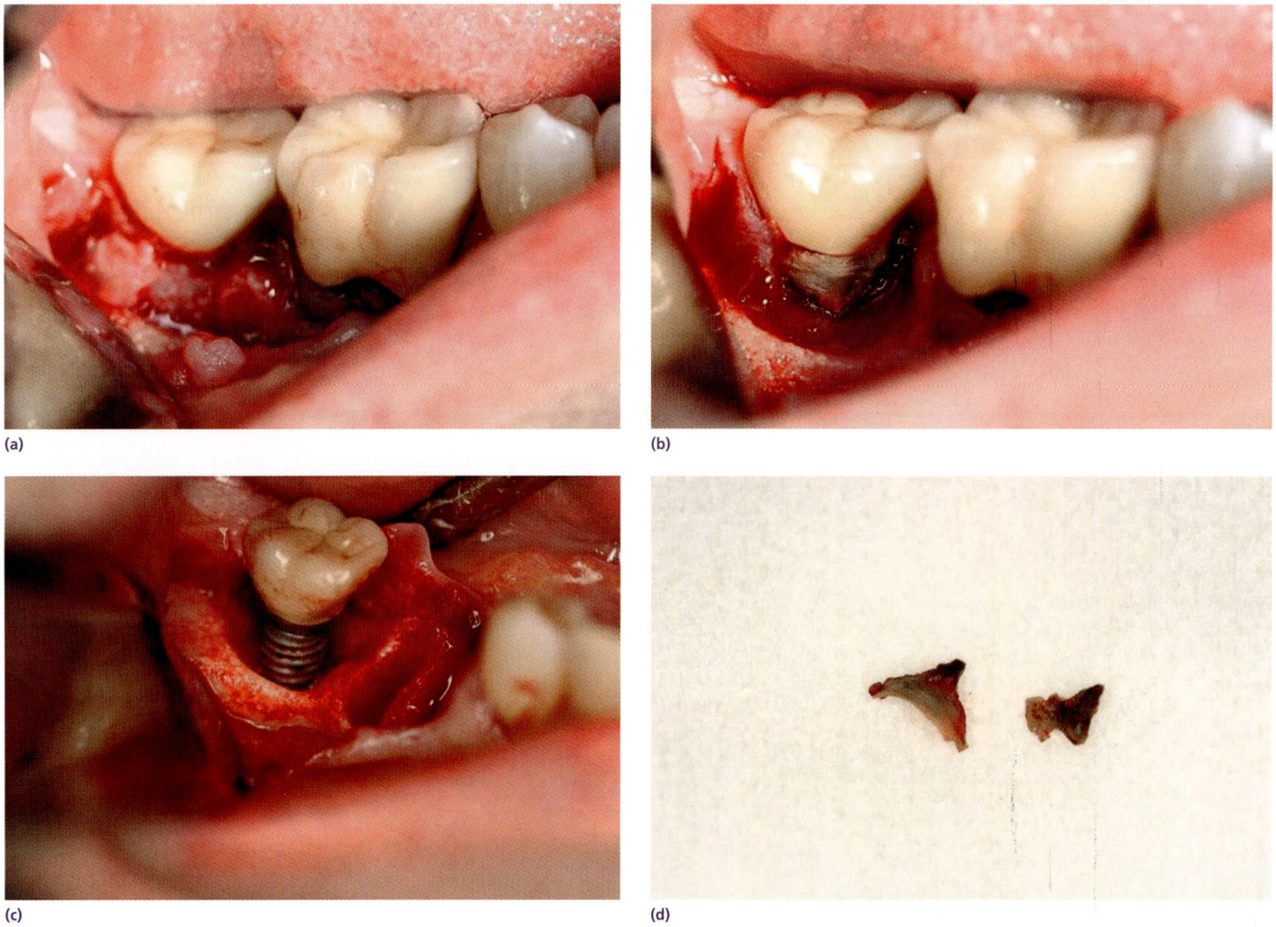

Figure 12.4 Series of photographs indicating the bone loss associated with an implant and residual excess cement and deep soft tissue cement margin. **(a)** Presenting with inflammation of the soft tissues. **(b)** Full-thickness flap elevation – granulation tissue and cement evident. **(c)** Cement removed from implant and tissues. **(d)** Cement remnants. *Source:* Reproduced with permission from Franc Audia, OMS.

acceptable depth a cemented margin may be placed relative to the tissue level, this has only recently been evaluated. The influence of the cementation margin position with respect to the amount of undetected cement was reported by Linkevicius *et al.*[33] In a prospective clinical study they compared cement margin sites that were: equal with tissue level, 1 mm subgingival, 2 mm subgingival, and 3 mm subgingival. Although remnants were found at all depths, the cement average on the implant abutment and crown was ten times more when comparing equigingival to 1 mm subgingival. Statistically significant differences existed among the four groups: with the deeper the position of the margin, the greater the amount of undetected cement was discovered. The conclusions of the study indicated that, ideally, cement margins on implant abutments should always be visible for intraoral cementation.

The disease processes associated with residual excess cement are not understood. For example, it has not been determined if a threshold volume of cement extrusion is required, the location the cement reaches, or if the flow characteristics of the cement are individual or combined factors. The cement itself may also play an etiological role with microbial interactions, foreign body reactions, corrosion, and allergy (Figures 12.4 and 12.5).

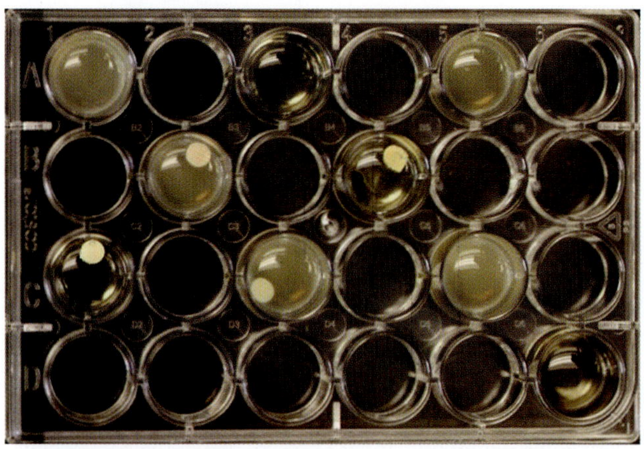

Figure 12.5 Example of test wells following 2 days of anaerobic incubation. *F. nucleatum* with four test cements, positive and negative controls are included in test. Note control wells – they contain no cement. The clear wells are the negative control (sterile). *Source:* Ravel *et al.*, 2015.[40] Reproduced with permission of John Wiley & Sons.

Cement interactions: specific issues with implants

Microbial growth

The cementation of dental restorations is considered by many to be a simple unskilled task requiring little if any thought; in fact, the process is often delegated. Dental cements have been exclusively developed for teeth and as such have attributes such as antimicrobial agents, fluoride release, and adhesion properties all aimed at the natural tooth structures, where caries and bonding to dentin are demanding issues.[34] Implants do not suffer from the effects of caries, nor do they have a structure based in dentin or enamel, so many of the properties desirable for the natural tooth are superfluous when considering dental implant restorations; in fact many of the properties optimized for a cement used for a natural tooth can be detrimental to an implant.[35,36]

Many studies have been undertaken to evaluate the antimicrobial effects of cements, however, they have been directed exclusively at how the materials behave in the presence of *Streptococcus mutans* and *Lactobacillus acidophilius*, which are the cariogenic microbes.[34,37–39] There is little, if any, relevance for the implant restoration, where the effects of microbes that may result in peri-implant disease are completely different and these should be the prime focus.

Raval and Wadhwani *et al.*[40] designed a study with the periodontal department of the University of Washington to determine the interaction of implant luting cements and oral bacteria linked to peri-implant disease. Specific luting cements were exposed to peri-implant disease-producing microbes. The five luting cements that were tested were as follows:

- zinc oxide–eugenol (TempBond Original, TB; Kerr, Orange, CA, USA);
- eugenol-free zinc oxide (TempBond Non- Eugenol, TBNE; Kerr);
- zinc orthophosphate (Fleck's, FL; Keystone Industries, Cherry Hill, NJ, USA);
- methacrylate-based resin (Premier Implant Cement [PIC; Premier, Plymouth Meeting, PA, USA] and Multilink Implant [ML; Ivoclar Vivadent Inc., Amherst, NY]).

Disks 5 mm in diameter were made from each cement, under carefully controlled conditions to prevent contamination. The disks were made with similar surface configurations to be macroscopically smooth. A planktonic growth evaluation used bacterial species of *Aggregatibacter actinomycetemcomitans*, *Fusobacterium nucleatum*, and *Porphyromonas gingivalis*, grown individually in modified TYK broth (trypticase soy broth, yeast extract, vitamin K) in test wells. The concentration of bacteria was standardized for each test with measurements made using an optical spectrometer, which related the opacity of the broth, such that the greater the broth opacity the greater the microbial content. Statistically significant differences were found among the cement groups, with TempBond Original consistently providing results no different to the media alone at the $P < .05$ significance level. The results for *A. actinomycetemcomitans* (Aa), *F. nucleatum* (Fn), and *P. gingivalis* (Pg) are consistent in this respect (Figure 12.6).

A second part of this study involved how these anaerobic Gram-negative microbes grew as a biofilm on the test cement disks. Here the cement disks were removed from the TYK and bacterial solutions, washed with a sterile solution of TYK, and also agitated to remove the more adhered bacteria. The resulting solution was used to coat agar plates then incubated for 4 days anaerobically. Colony-forming units (CFUs) were recorded for each bacterium–cement combination. This experiment was repeated three times. The biofilm test was used to compare the cement that inhibited the planktonic growth the most (TB) to the one that inhibited the least (ML). Again contrasting results were obtained, with TempBond Original consistently giving no CFU counts, and Multi-Link implant cement giving CFUs too numerous to count (these were greater than 5000 in many instances) (Figure 12.7).

This simple but enlightening study indicated that cement selection should be considered with respect to how it may impact the environment in which it is being placed. This is particularly relevant for a patient who is periodontally susceptible, as these patients present a greater risk of peri-implant disease.[18] Consistent with this is the observation that in most peri-implantitis cases, the composition of the flora is similar to that of the subgingival flora of chronic periodontitis.[25,26]

It has also been demonstrated that the bacteria in cases of partially edentulous implants may be more pathogenic (especially Gram-negative rods and spirochetes) than in the fully edentulous case, indicating a possible seeding mechanism from tooth pocket to implant crevice.[28] The cements that performed the best overall within this study had the common element of zinc. Zinc is known to be highly effective as an antimicrobial and eugenol is also well known for its anti-inflammatory, anti-oxidative, and antimicrobial pharmaceutical properties; the combination of these two components is likely the reason for the effectiveness of TempBond Original.

Host response: foreign body reaction

Histopathological evaluation of the soft tissues associated with failed implants has found cement particles within the soft tissue specimens.[41,42] Residual cement may act as a nidus for both acute and chronic inflammatory cells, which in turn may elicit a cascading autoimmune destructive process. Further studies have identified the types of cement that have been found within the tissues using scanning electron microscopy coupled to energy dispersive X-ray spectral analyzers, capable of determining the composition of the foreign material encountered.[43]Using commercially available cements as a standard, the particles in each biopsy specimen could be associated with one of the commercial cements with a level of probability ranging between 0.79–1. Table 12.1 shows the results of 19 soft tissue biopsy specimens related to implant failure where

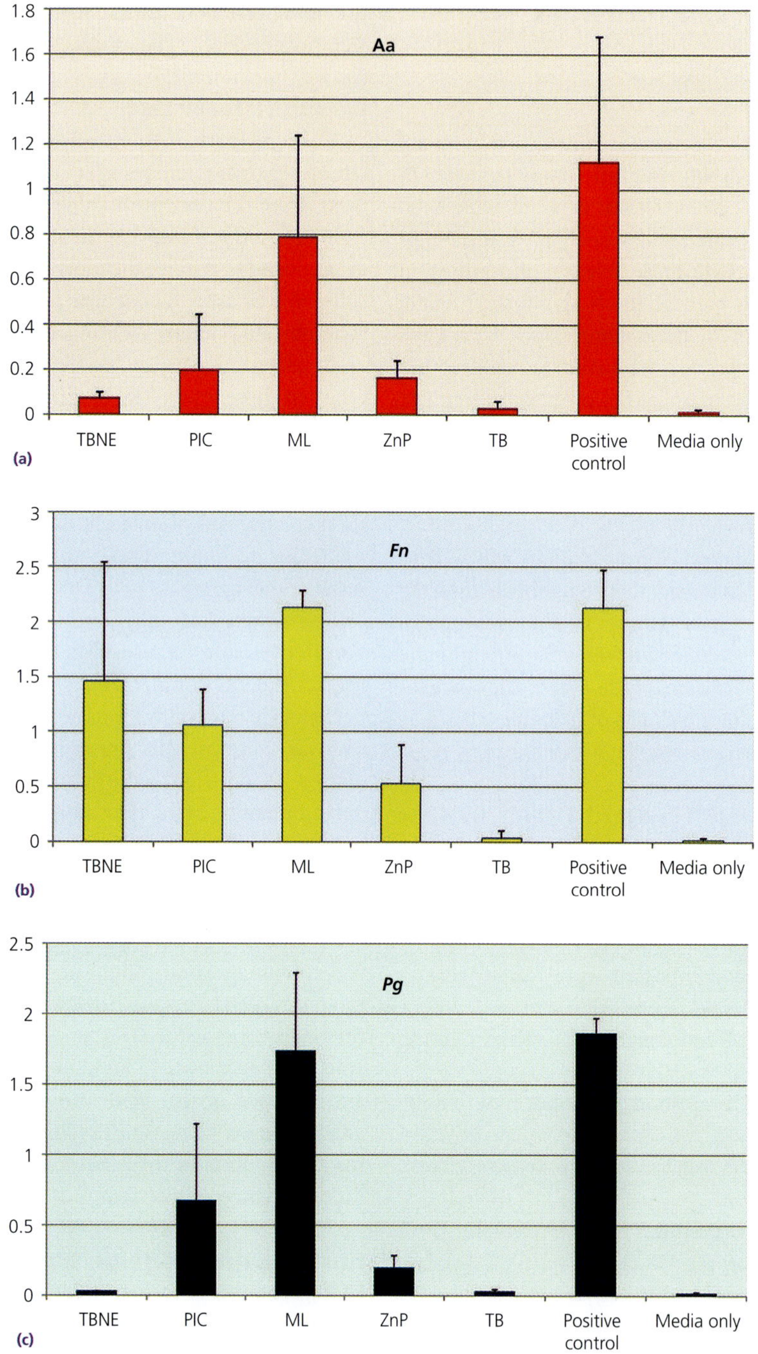

Figure 12.6 Planktonic growth measurement on different cements by opacity test (OD 600) values. **(a)** *Aggregatibacter actinomycetemcomitans – Aa.* **(b)** *Fusobacterium nucleatum – Fn.* **(c)** *Porphyromonas gingivalis – Pg.* FL, Fleck's Cement; ML, Multilink Implant; PIC, Premier Implant Cement; TBNE, Temp-Bond Non-eugenol; TBO, TempBond Original. Positive control (media with bacteria, no cement) and negative control (sterile media) also shown.

residual excess cement particles were detected; the cements were identified and quantified.

The study concluded that the particles found in human soft tissue biopsy specimens around implants affected by peri-implant disease occurred with a variety of cements. No data quantified the individual amounts of cement found within the tissues, which could be a confounding factor.

The question how the cement particles became embedded within the tissues is speculative. It may have resulted from the time the crown was initially seated: with sufficient force the mass of liquid cement could have disrupted the fragile hemidesmosomal attachment of the epithelium to the implant. It may have resulted during clean up, with the dislodgement of the set particles being forced into the tissues.

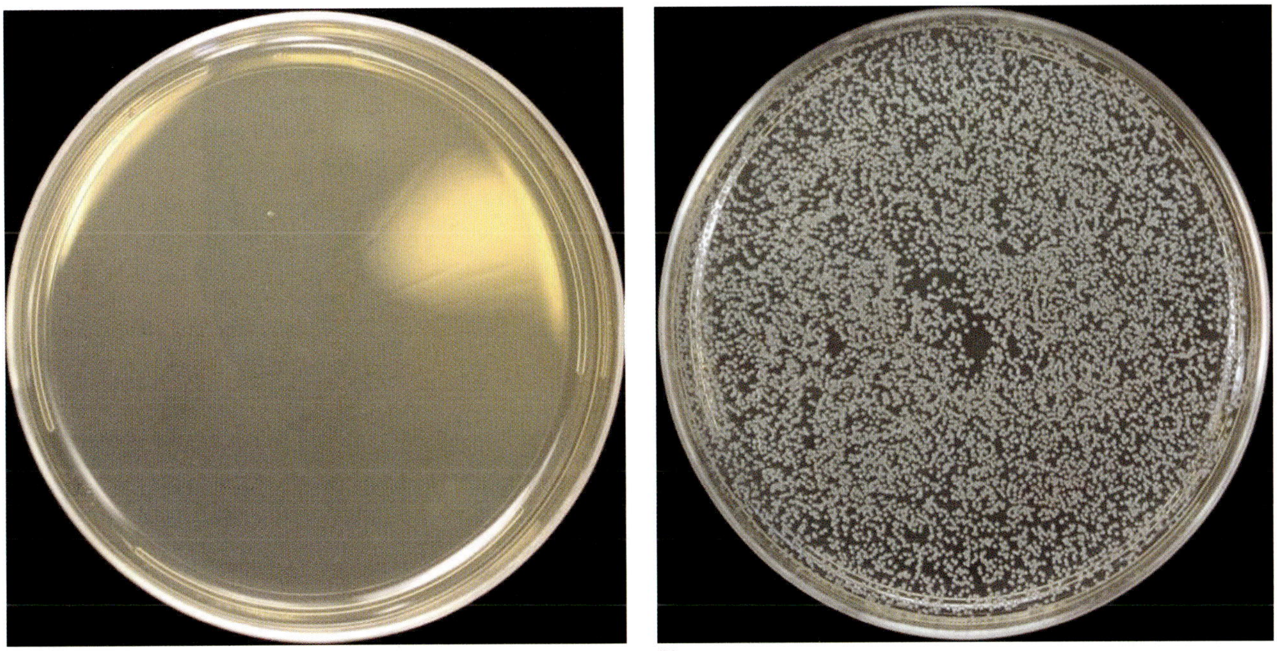

Figure 12.7 Examples of agar plates with colony-forming units (CFUs) obtained from cement disks sampled for *Aggregatibacter actinomycetemcomitans* biofilm growth. (a) No CFUs (TempBond Original). (b) CFUs >5000 and too numerous to count (Multilink). *Source:* Raval *et al.*, 2015.[40] Reproduced with permission from John Wiley & Sons.

Table 12.1 Cement types identified in 19 soft tissue biopsy samples of failed, removed implants.

Cement brand and nomenclature	Manufacturer	Number of cases (19 biopsy specimens)
Telio CS Cem Implant (Telio)	Ivoclar Vivadent (Amherst, NY)	**7**
TempBond clear with triclosan (TB)	Kerr Sybron Dental Specialties (Orange, CA)	1
Premier® Implant Cement (PIC)	Premier (Plymouth Meeting, PA)	4
RelyX™ Unicem 2 Self-Adhesive Resin Cement (Relyx1)	3M ESPE (St. Paul, MN)	4
Intermediate Restorative Material (IRM)	Dentsply (Waltham, MA)	3

Host response: allergic response

Dental cement manufacturers continue to develop cements based to a large degree on their retentive capabilities. As noted previously, cements have evolved from use with natural teeth, where the primary elements involved are dentin and enamel. Resin-modified glass ionomers (RGMI) have become popular due to their ability to adhere chemically to dentin and the potential for fluoride release. In 2010 an estimated 73% of dental schools also used this material as the definitive medium for cementing restorations to implants,[44] which interestingly followed a similar pattern for cement selection for teeth (Figure 12.8). One of the constituents of the RMGIs is hydroxyethyl methacrylate (HEMA).[45] This material is extremely irritating to the tissues to the extent that the material safety data sheet (MSDS) advises that gloves and other mucosal tissue, such as eyes, be barrier protected when it is used. With the natural tooth, where preparation finish lines are supragingival and isolation with rubber dam is feasible, this presents no real issue. However, with implants, barrier protection is more difficult to achieve, the epithelial attachment adheres poorly, is more permeable, and may be more susceptible to the effects of chemicals leaching out from materials.

Corrosion

Much of the success of dental implants relates to the relatively low corrosive susceptibility of the materials involved. Titanium appears well suited to the oral environment under most conditions.

However, recent reports have found a reactive issue with some materials commonly found in dental cements.[35,46,47] Fluoride, the ubiquitous anti-caries agent, is known, in some forms, to corrode titanium.[48] One study found that several cements containing the fluoride ion, under acidic conditions, caused pitting corrosion when in contact with titanium (Figure 12.9).[49] Corrosive elements are generally undesirable as the surface alterations produce an increased adhesion to peri-implant disease-producing

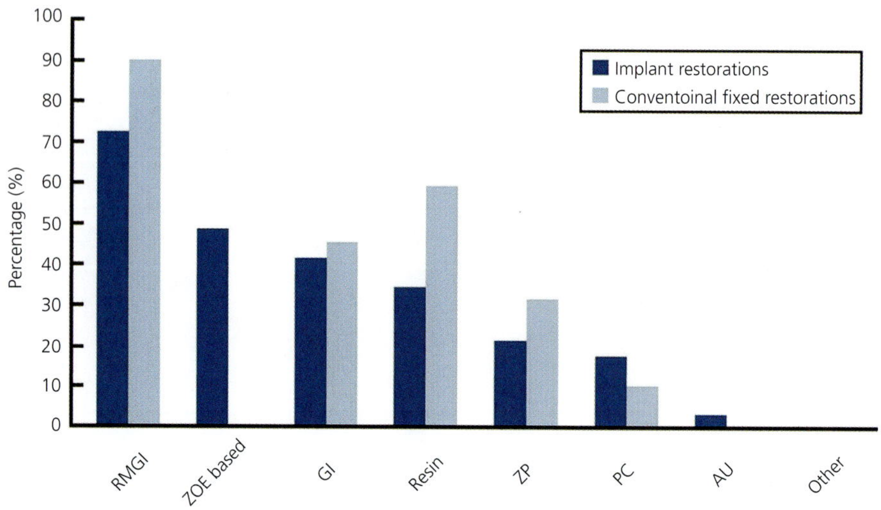

Figure 12.8 Data graph on definitive cements used for implant and tooth restorations by USA dental schools. (RMGI, resin modified glass ionomer; ZOE, zinc oxide eugenol; GI, glass ionomer; ZP, zinc phosphate; PC, polycarboxylate; AU, acrylic urethane). *Source:* Tarica *et al.*, 2010.[44] Reproduced with permission from Elsevier.

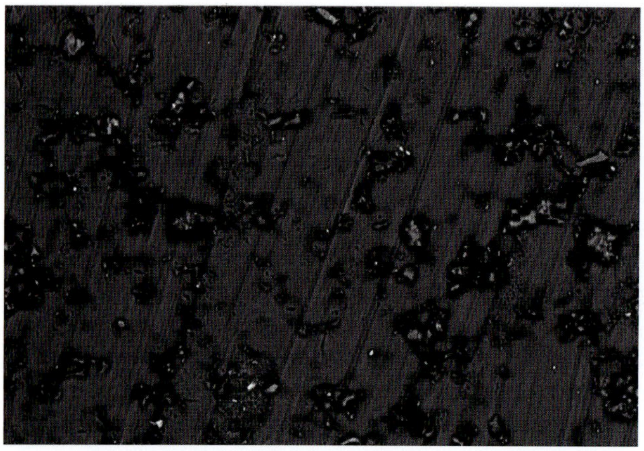

Figure 12.9 Scanning electron microscope image of the surface of a turned titanium alloy disk – the machined marks are visible as concentric lines. The surface shows pitting corrosion after the application of Durelon cement. This surface pitting perpetuates the corrosion over the electrochemically active heterogeneous surface.

anaerobic bacteria,[50] and also result in reactive oxidative species being produced by the host.[51] The inflammatory response produced may be one mechanism that results in peri-implant disease. The cements identified as producing the conditions for corrosion include some polycarboxylates and some glass ionomer cements.[49,52] Durelon (3M-ESPE) alludes to this problem in the Instructions For Use (IFU),[49] which is of interest as 17% of US dental schools[44] admit to using it on implant restorations. This indicates the IFU are not being followed or may not even be read.

To date, no ideal implant luting cement exists, all have the potential to cause issues. However, the prudent clinician will evaluate carefully the material used, will elevate the cement margin to be readily accessible to cleaning, and have a good biological understanding of the limitations of the dental implant.

Luting material selection

Desirable properties for implant cements include ease of clean up and removal of excess cement; studies have indicated this to be especially challenging with resin cements.[53] The greater the retentive properties a cement has for titanium the more difficult it will be to remove. Also, the greater the mechanical retention of a given cement to the implant materials used, the more difficult it will be to clean excess cement from them. Table 12.2 outlines some of the more appropriate properties required of implant cements and compares these to cement properties more ideal for natural teeth. Desirable properties such as the noncorrosive nature and antimicrobial properties have been discussed. Excellent radiographic density is also a valuable asset for an implant cement (Figure 12.10).[13,54]

Many cements used for implant restoration are poorly radiopaque, which compounds the issue of detection. It is imperative that the restorative dentist select a cement that is highly radiopaque to allow for detection in cases where extrusion of cement is suspected (Figure 12.11). Currently no minimum standard exists for cements. As a general recommendation the cement should have at least a 300% radiopacity compared to a standard aluminum guide. The importance of early detection and removal of this foreign material early enough cannot be over emphasized, as this may prevent the disease process from becoming established and allow for full resolution of the site to occur.[17,55] Post-cementation radiographs should be standard protocol, and practitioners need the ability to recognize the radiographic characteristic effects of implant cement extrusion.

Having a good rationale for implant luting material selection is part of the issue. The clinician must also understand how the cement flows, based upon parameters such as cement loading site, amounts required, and implant abutment design.

Table 12.2 Some considerations for material selection specific to teeth and implants for cemented restorations.[36]

	Implant restoration	Natural tooth
Substructure	Metal, ceramic, acrylic	Dentin, enamel
Biologic tissue association	Peri-implant tissues	Periodontal tissues, pulp
Primary disease issue	Peri-implant disease	Caries, pulpal, periodontal
Restoration finish line	1–2 mm below the gingival crest – often deeper	1 mm below in anterior esthetic sites, often above free gingival margin elsewhere
Cement margin	May or may not follow scallop of gingival tissues	Preparation follows gingival tissue
Need for cement seal	Questionable	Desired (prevent caries)
Anticaries agent	May be detrimental	Desirable
Corrosion	Possible corrosion of titanium	Not applicable
Radiopacity	Should be highly radiopaque	Similar to dentin
Microbial challenge	Bacteria found in peri-implant sites	*Streptococcus mutans*, *Lactobacillus* (caries producers)

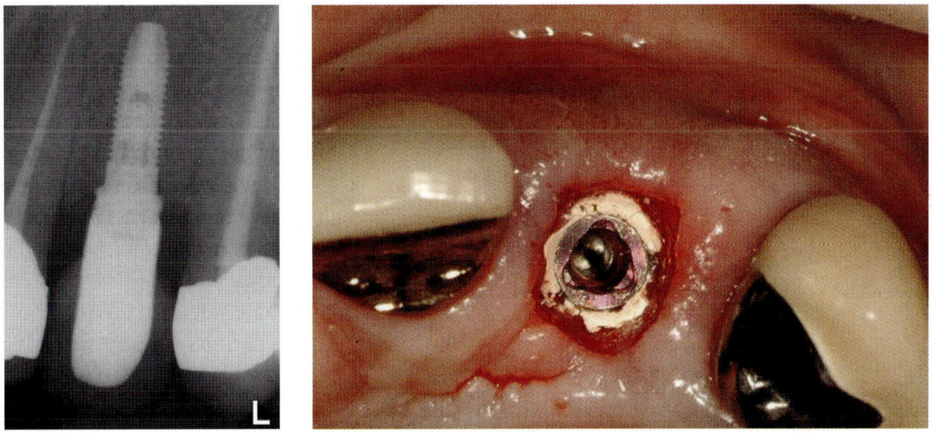

(a) (b)

Figure 12.10 (**a**) Radiograph made after crown cementation indicates residual excess cement. (**b**) The crown has been removed along with the abutment, residual excess cement is obvious.

One common procedure in restorative dentistry is the use of luting cements, which for many dentists occurs on a daily basis. As ubiquitous as cementing a crown is, it appears that most dentists have little if any idea where to place the cement and how much is required. The impact of this lack of understanding compromises cement removal and may cause pathologic sequelae (Figure 12.12). A survey of over 400 dentists exemplifies this problem. Wadhwani *et al.*[56] found little consistency in the site application of cement when intended for an implant crown as well as how much cement is placed within the crown compared to an ideal amount required.

The participants were shown a Power Point presentation with an image of a crown and an abutment. A polycarbonate crown, sachet of cement, and mixing and application instruments, including a brush, flat plastic, and a probe type, were provided. The subjects were instructed to consider the crown was the definitive restoration and asked to mix the cement and load the crown as they would in a real clinical situation. No further instructions were provided. The cement within the crowns was allowed to set with the crowns held in a clamp and collected (Figure 12.13).

Evaluating the application techniques, three basic types were recognized: gross, where the cement was simply loaded within the intaglio of the crown; brush application, where the brush strokes were identifiable; and a selective site application at the margin of the crown (Figure 12.14). An "ideal" amount of cement was calculated, assuming the abutment:crown relief space was 40 μm. This equated to 3% of the total crown volume. By comparing the weight of the crowns loaded with cement with the weight of the crowns prior to cement application, the amount of cement used was recorded and charted (Figure 12.15). The survey demonstrated that, in the majority of cases, an amount of cement far in excess of that required was being placed within the crown. The conclusion from the study was that, for a common technique, vast differences existed, with no real protocols.

Implant restorative cementation: developing clinical protocols

The problems associated with cement selection and use have been discussed, indicating the differences between the restoration of the natural dentition and the implant restoration.

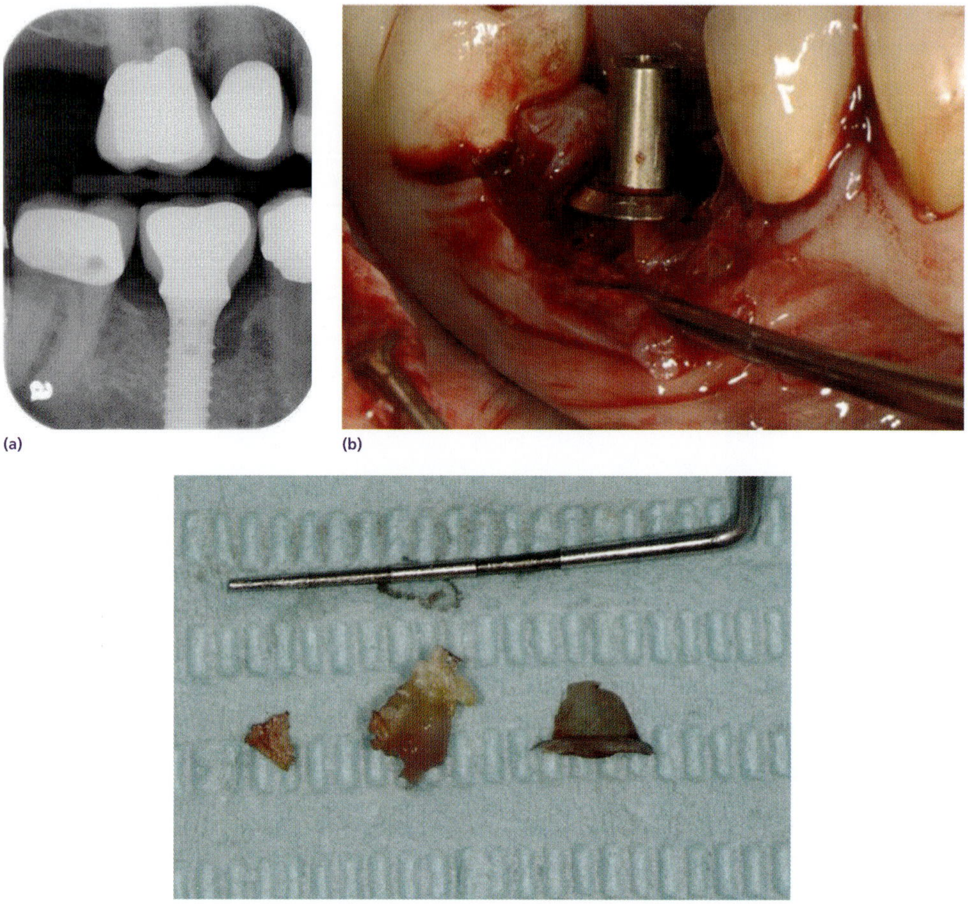

(a) (b) (c)

Figure 12.11 (a) Radiograph indicating crater-effect bone loss. No indication of cement. (b) Surgical flap exposes residual excess cement. This poorly radiopaque cement has similar radiopacity to air. (c) Cement remnants against periodontal probe indicating size of material removed.

Controlling the flow of the cement during the process of seating the restoration is yet another key element in prevention of residual excess cement extrusion.

Cement flow can be readily demonstrated with models.[57] One facsimile designed by the author is to use clear plastic drinking beakers that have a similar "flat top" cone shape and angle of convergence (Figure 12.16) as a standard implant abutment, with a material to mimic cement, such as shaving foam. This provides an easy learning tool in evaluating cement flow direction as it relates to position the cement is placed.

A demonstration of how cement flow is affected by the site the cement is applied shows that if the cement is placed around the margin of the crown, the cement flows upward initially, toward the occlusal surface, then it flows toward the margins of the crown (Figure 12.17). This is very different from the phenomenon of when the cement is placed in the occlusal aspect of the crown, where the cement becomes compressed and resists seating (Figure 12.18).

While the beakers provide a nice visual effect they cannot be well controlled for experimental purposes, for which the author elicited the help of industrial engineers (CD-adapco, Bellevue, WA) that use state-of-the-art computational fluid dynamics software (Star-CCM^{+}).[58,59] The project is currently underway with initial results having been reported and compared to real-life models for validation. Scanned abutment digital images of abutments and crowns (Figure 12.19) are converted to superimposing three-dimensional virtual engineering models (Figure 12.20). These models comprise essentially of a piston (abutment) seated within a chamber (crown) with a fluid dispersion (cement) being evaluated as a complete system and using highly sophisticated computer programs, run on powerful "supercomputers". The cement material properties are mathematically calculated to represent the non-Newtonian flow character. Non-Newtonian behaviour includes shear thining under pressure, which is subject to variables such as speed of seating the crown, the form of the abutment/crown, relief space, and volumes used.

It is the hope that by understanding how the cement actually works in this system, which can be considered to mimic a piston being driven into a chamber with fluid, the system can be reverse-engineered to make it more efficient and reduce the likelihood of inducing cement extrusion. Using these simulations, cement

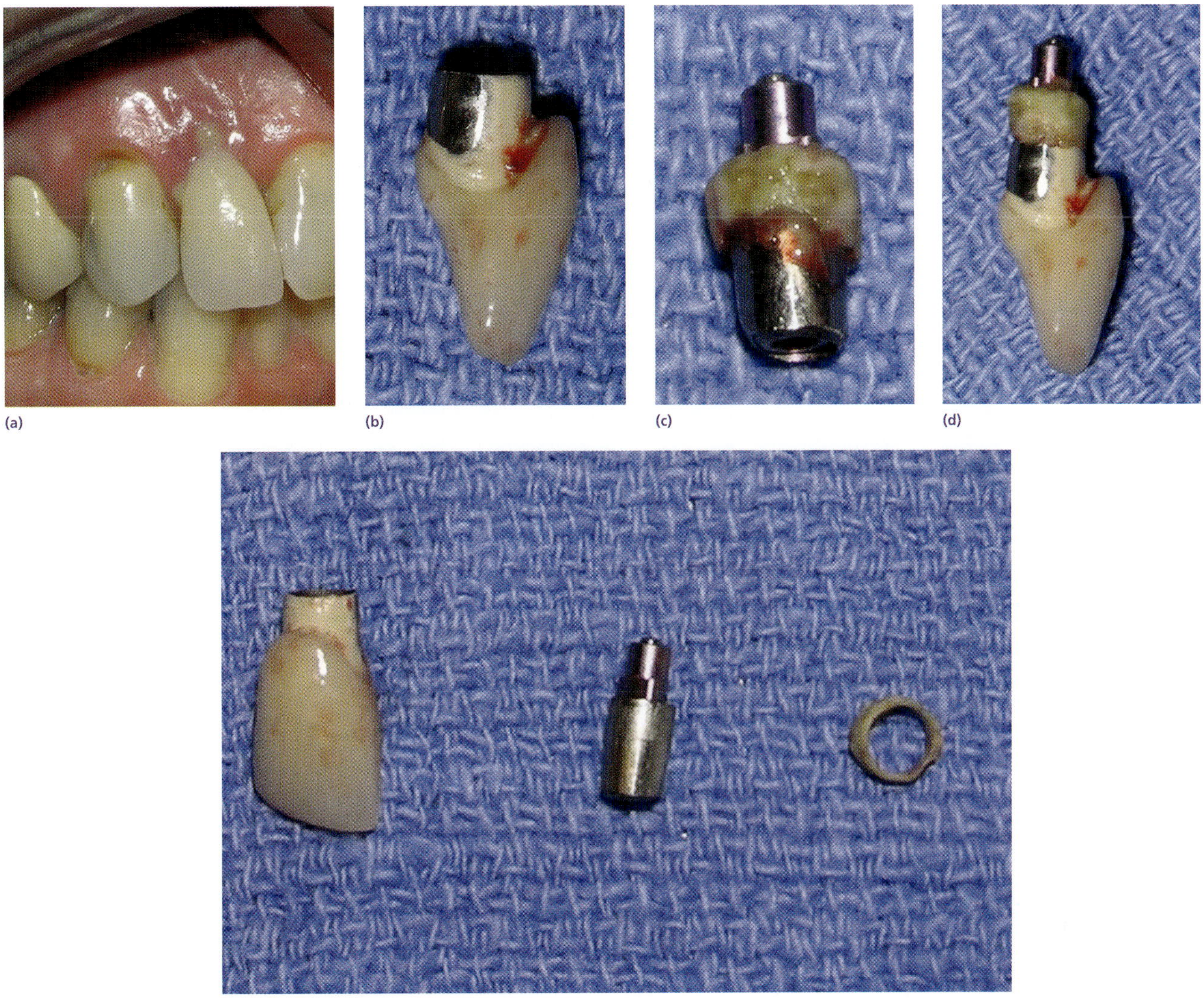

(a) (b) (c) (d) (e)

Figure 12.12 (a) Implant crown with peri-implantitis, suppuration is seen. (b) Crown removed, poorly contoured. (c) Abutment removed with cement residue present. (d) Crown reseated on abutment showing deep margins and lack of control of cement. (e) Crown, abutment, and residual cement. *Source:* Reproduced with permission from Jaden Erwin, periodontist.

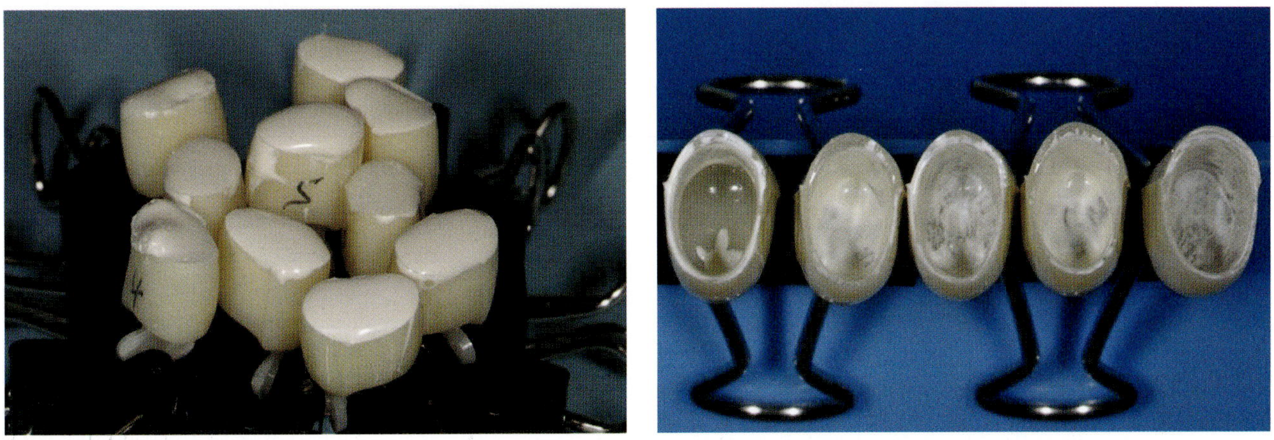

(a) (b)

Figure 12.13 Actual examples of cement application techniques and amounts. (a) Overfilled beyond the margins of the crown. (b) Underfilled with insufficient amount of cement.

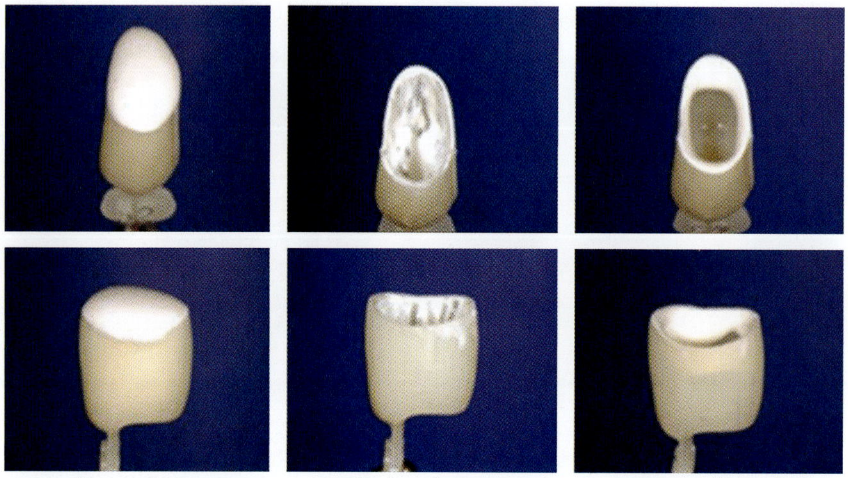

Figure 12.14 Examples of the application techniques: gross application, brush application, margin application.

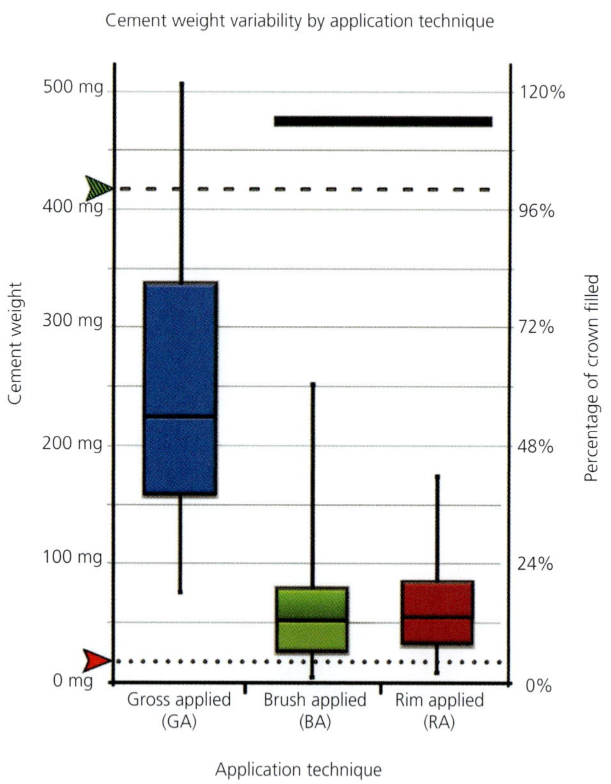

Figure 12.15 Box plots of the application techniques and the quantity of cement loaded. The median, 25th and 75th percentile, as well as highest and lowest value range are shown. The horizontal line above the box plots indicates no significant differences (P>.05). The lower arrowhead and dotted line indicates "ideal" cement lute quantity given a 40 μm relief space. The upper arrow and dashed line indicate maximum intaglio cement fill (used as the control).

flow can be imaged using two-dimesional frames that allow the flow to be evalauted, with air and cement being exchanged. It becomes apparent that protocols can be developed on where to place the cement (Figure 12.21), how much to use, how rapidly the crown is seated, and optimizing the abutment design (Figure 12.22). The system even allows the evaluation of the cement extrusion velocity, which can be used to determine if the thrust of cement could disrupt the hemidesmosomal soft tissue attachment (Figure 12.23).

With further investigation into the design and character of cementation, it is likely that protocols will be readily available in the near future. It is also envisaged that implant companies will start to use these techniques in their design of abutments and crowns, rather than relying on the shape of tooth preparations that were developed 50 years or more ago.

Other clinical solutions to the cement extrusion issue include maintaining a supragingival margin on the abutment, allowing cement extrusion to be carefully controlled. Linkevicius *et al.*[33] have shown that the safest site for a cemented implant abutment margin is supragingival. One method of producing an esthetic margin is to press a ceramic supragingival margin directly to the abutment (Figure 12.24a, b).[59] This type of abutment modification has an added advantage that hydrofluoric acid etching, silane application, and resin bonding protocols will bond the crown ceramic margin to the abutment margin (Figure 12.24c).[60] The result is a highly esthetic restoration where the margin can be hidden or made to appear as a cervical restoration (Figure 12.25). The supragingival margin also allows for the use of a barrier of Teflon (PTFE) tape to protect the soft tissues coming into contact with cement and other chemicals).[61,62]

A piece of sterilized PTFE tape approximately 2 cm in length is used, with a small rubber dam hole punched into the center. This is slipped onto the abutment, taking extreme care not to encroach onto the implant connection site, or crown margin site of the abutment (Figure 12.26a). The abutment is placed onto the implant and the screw torqued as recommended by the manufacturer. The barrier "bib" can be seen to protect the soft peri-implant tissues, yet not overlap the abutment/crown margin (Figure 12.26c). During the cementation

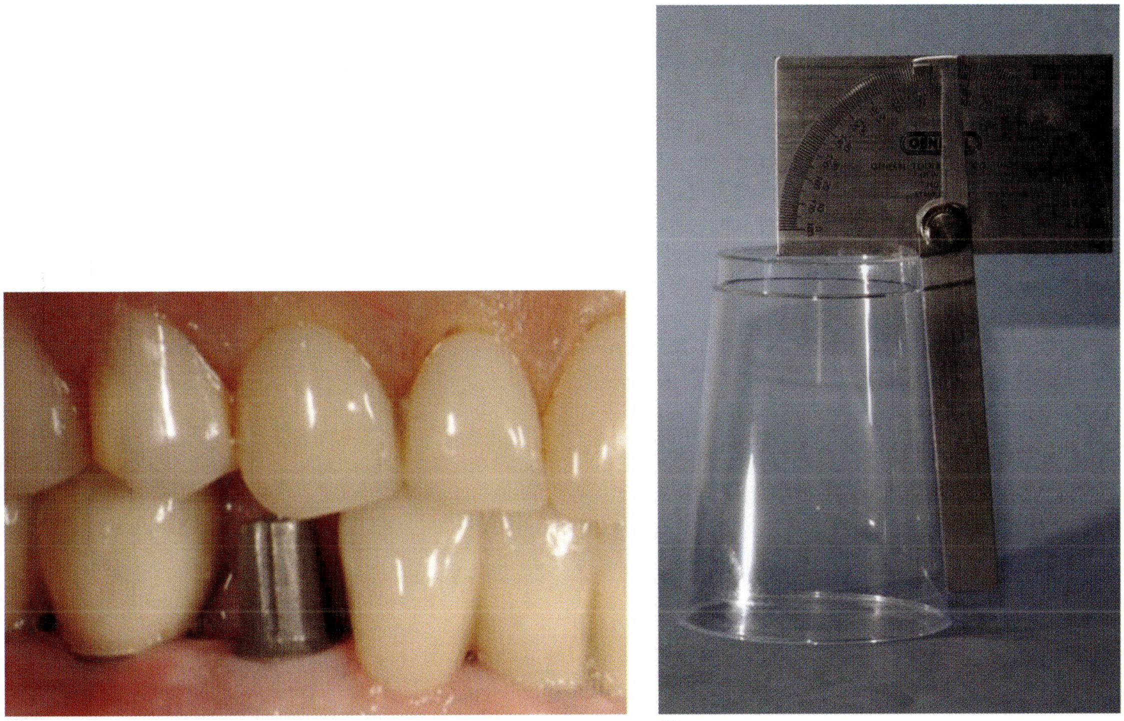

(a) (b)

Figure 12.16 An implant abutment **(a)** has a similar occlusal taper to this clear plastic drinking beaker **(b)**. The beakers are designed to seat one on top of another mimicking a crown seated onto an implant abutment.

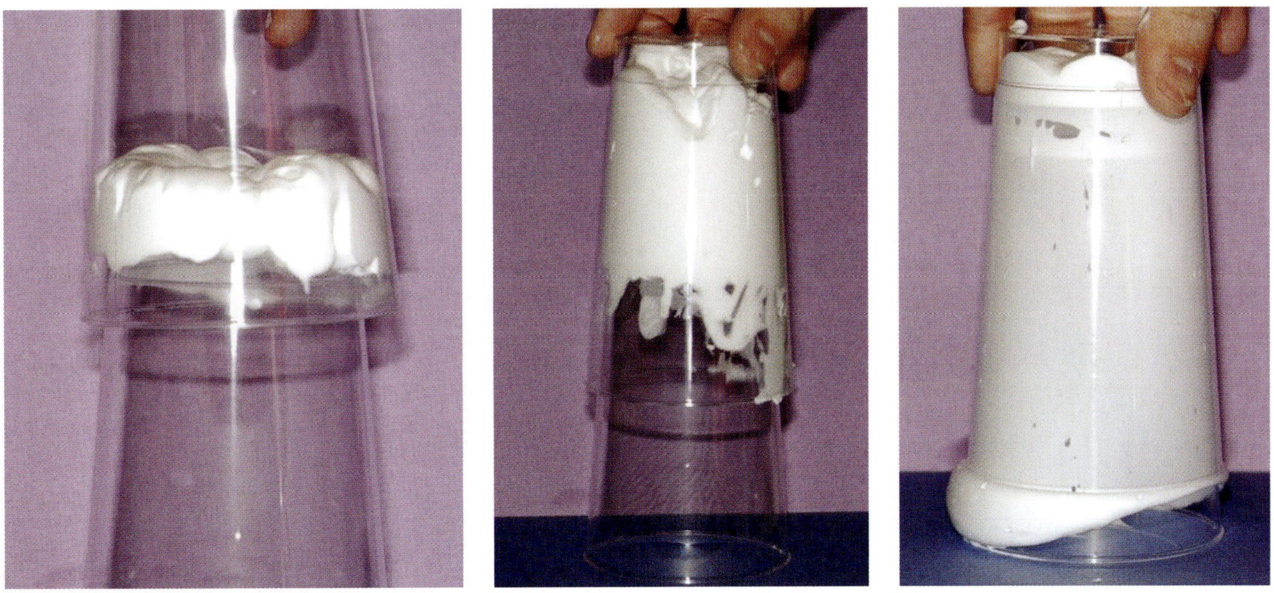

(a) (b) (c)

Figure 12.17 **(a)** Cement (shaving foam) placed at the crown margin. **(b)** The crown seats easily with little resistance and the cement flow is toward the occlusal. **(c)** At fully seating a minimal amount of cement extrusion is noted and the lute space fill is complete.

process the soft tissues are protected, and the site remains uncontaminated by peri-implant crevicular fluid that affects setting of cements (Figure 12.26d). Once the cement has set, the PTFE is simply removed along with any excess material (Figure 12.26e).

Other techniques available with the use of cement are cement pre-extrusion devices, such as the copy abutment technique.[63] Here a copy of the intaglio of the crown or cemented prosthesis is made, first by placing a layer of PFTE against the inside (intaglio) of the crown (Figure 12.27a). This has two important functions.

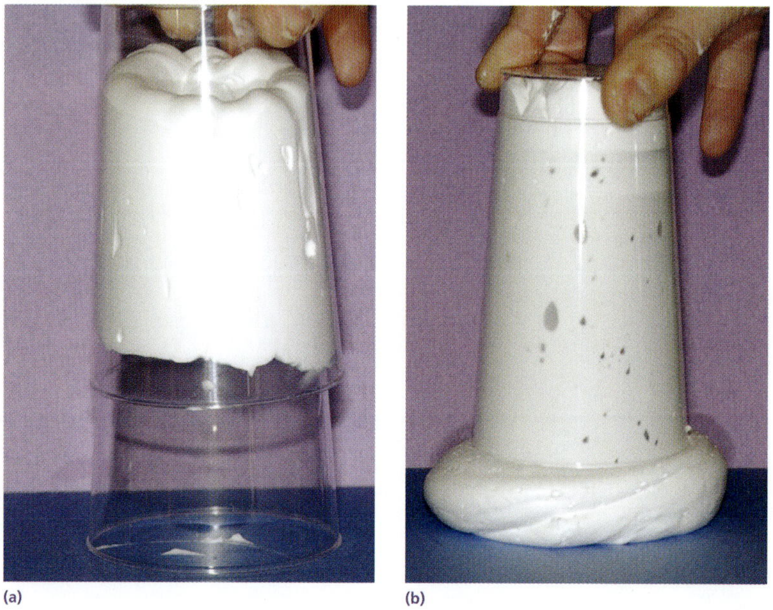

Figure 12.18 (a) The cement is gross applied. (b) A large excess is extruded through the margin.

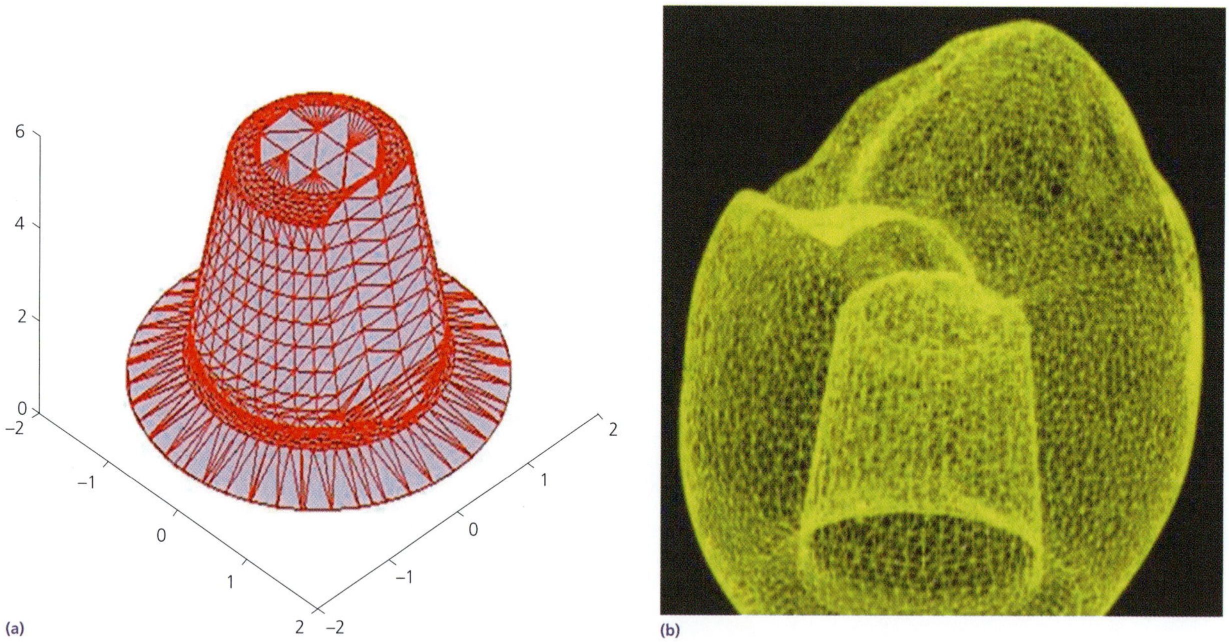

Figure 12.19 Copy scanned and digitized abutment (a) and crown (b) virtual models for the computational fluid dynamics study.

First, it produces a 50 μm spacer that will give close to the required volume of cement. It should be remembered that most implant restorations are fabricated with a 40–50 μm luting space. Second, it prevents the intaglio of the crown getting contaminated with the polyvinyl siloxane (PVS) material.

To aid the placement of the PTFE, first coat the intaglio of the crown with pure petroleum jelly, then using a brush carefully adapt the PTFE so it adheres to the internal surface (Figure 12.27b, c). Using a fast-setting polyvinyl siloxane (PVS) material (e.g. Blu-Mousse, Parkell) with a fine tip extruder, completely fill the internal aspect of the lined crown (Figure 12.27d) with the aim to capture the crown margins as much as possible. Continue expressing the PVS until a handle is formed (Figure 12.27e). Allow to set, then remove the copy die, remove and discard the PTFE layer (Figure 12.27f), and thoroughly clean out the intaglio of the crown, ensuring all the petroleum jelly is removed. Inspect the copy die, it should resemble the inside of the crown, yet be smaller in dimension (Figure 12.27g).

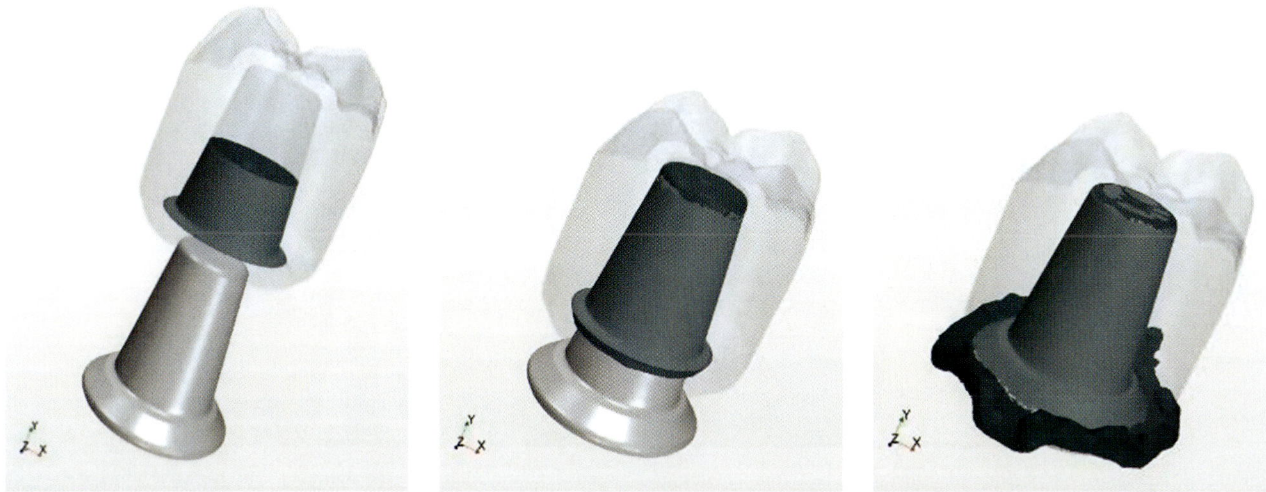

(a) (b) (c)

Figure 12.20 Series of stills taken from real-time simulations. **(a)** Crown with cement loaded at the crown margin start of process. **(b)** Crown being seated with cement flow. **(c)** Complete seating indicating flow and excess cement extrusion. *Source:* Reproduced with permission from CD-adapco.

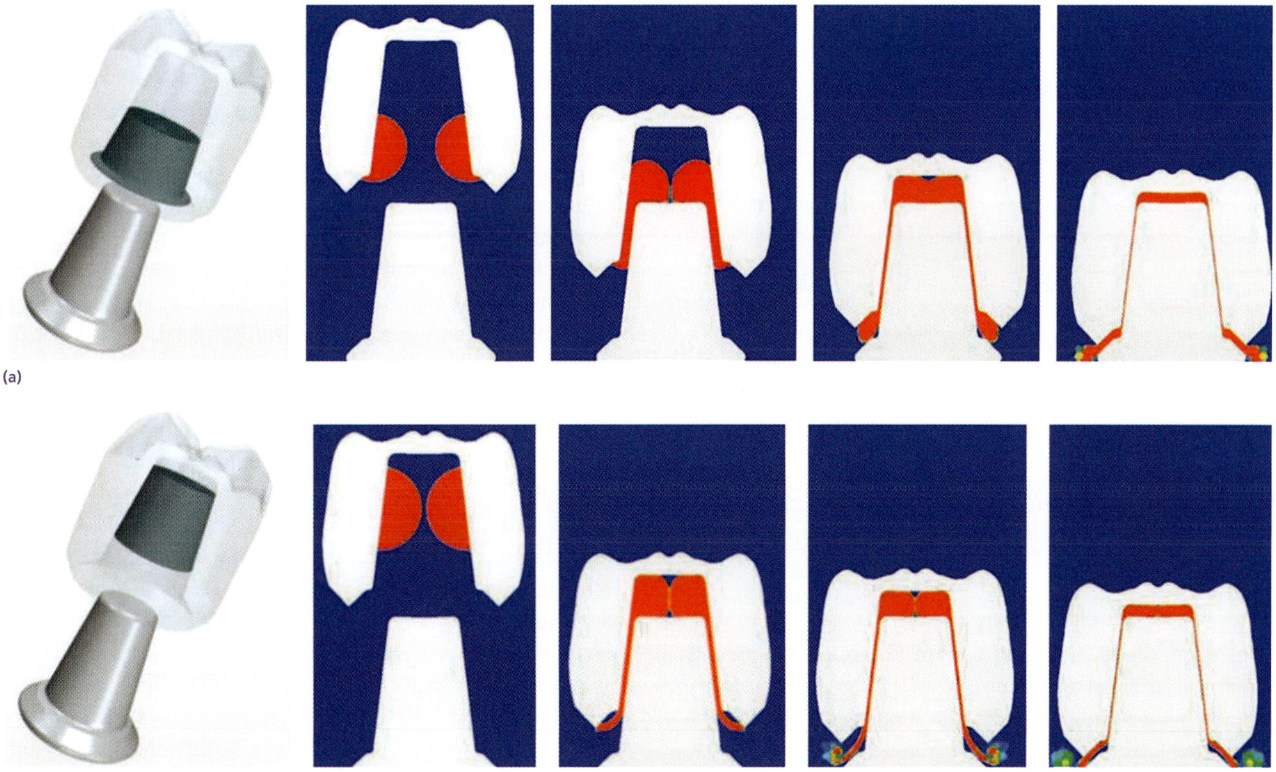

(a)

(b)

Figure 12.21 Computer simulation relating to cement application site. Cement (red) exchanged for air (blue). Both simulations have the same parameters except site of application. **(a)** Cement placed at the margin crown site. **(b)** Cement placed more occlussaly. Note how the margin fill differs and how the cement extrudes from the crown **(b)** before it fully seats. *Source:* Reproduced with permission from CD-adapco.

When the restoration is ready to be cemented, attach the original abutment to the implant in the usual manner and with the appropriate torque. The crown can be gross filled with cement, the PVS copy abutment is seated firmly into the crown, resulting in the extrusion of excess material (Figure 12.27h). The clean up extraorally is followed by inspection of the internal surface, where a uniform layer of cement, 50 μm thick, should exist. The crown is then cemented as usual, with minimal clean up, and provided all other parameters, such as cement margin height, control of seating forces, and speed of seating, are

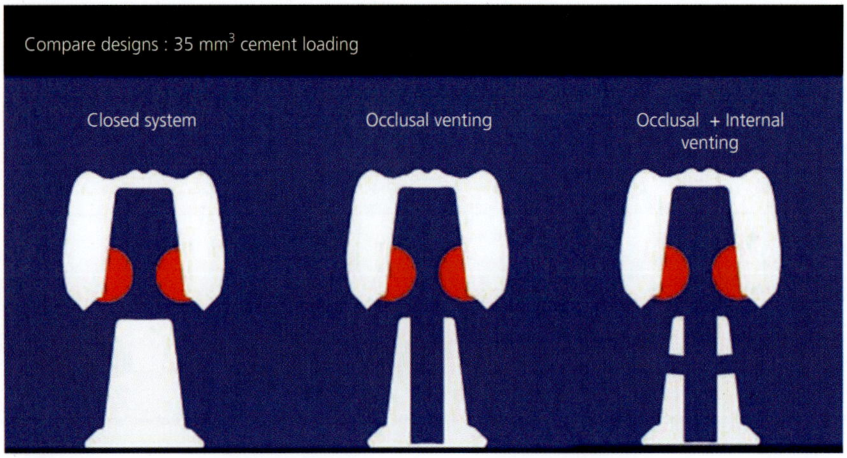

Figure 12.22 Computer simulation with different implant abutment designs – closed off abutment, leaving the abutment screw-access channel open, internal venting. *Source:* Reproduced with permission from CD-adapco.

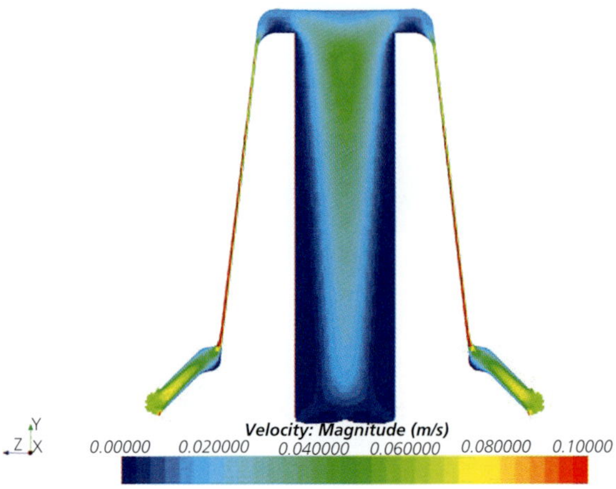

Figure 12.23 The velocity of cement extrusion can also be determined. This relates to the extrusion forces induced at the margin. Such information can determine if the hemidesmosomal attachment will be disrupted as the cement is forced out of the system. The different colors relate to velocity. *Source:* Reproduced with permission from CD-adapco.

controlled, the likelihood of cement extrusion into the tissues should be minimized (Figure 12.27i). The technique is also suitable for multiple joined restorations such as an implant-supported fixed dental prosthesis (Figure 12.28).

Other ways to control cement flow involve abutment modifications. The concept here is to alter the shape of the abutment so that an increase in cement held within the system results in a reciprocating reduction of cement extrusion. It was apparent that the US dental schools[44] and implant component manufacturers directed clinicians to completely occlude the screw-access channel of the abutment. This site, if left partially unfilled (the screw head protected with a spacer), could act as a receptacle for cement during seating of the restoration.

The first publication on this concept of abutment internal cement retention involved a subtractive method suitable for metal abutments, the internal vented abutment (IVA) modification.[64] Two holes, 180° apart, are placed within the walls of the abutment. The screw head is covered and protected with a small pellet of PTFE, and cement is forced into the screw-access channel. Whenever the screw channel is not sealed, there is the potential to allow cement to fill this space. Simply leaving the screw-access channel open as an "open abutment" (OA) or leaving open and adding internal vent holes within the abutment walls (IVA) (Figure 12.29) provided a significant reduction in cement extrusion out through the margin site, compared to the closure of the abutment (CA) (Figure 12.30). Although this was somewhat anticipated, what was not, were the differences seen when comparing the OA with the IVA extrusion amounts. When the OA was compared to the IVA, a difference in flow was observed (Figure 12.31). The OA was never completely filled, compared to the IVA where cement was directed to completely occlude the space available. This accounted not only for the reduction of cement extrusion, but also provided a significant increase in force required to dislodge the crown. Hence, manipulation of flow had a gross effect on crown retention (Figure 12.32).[65]

The IVA had proven to change cement flow by subtractive methods suitable with metal; however, a large number of restorations use zirconia-based materials. Placing vent holes within such structures would weaken them, so a different form of modification was devised.

The effect of modifying the screw-access channels of zirconia implant abutments on the cement flow pattern and retention of zirconia restorations was investigated by using an abutment insert (Figure 12.33).[66] In this experiment, the tip of a syringe was placed into the screw head of the abutment screw but did not project out of the screw channel. When an insert was placed within the abutment (IA) it altered the performance of the cement, increasing the force required to dislodge the restoration compared to closing off the abutment (CA) and leaving it open (OA) (Figure 12.34).

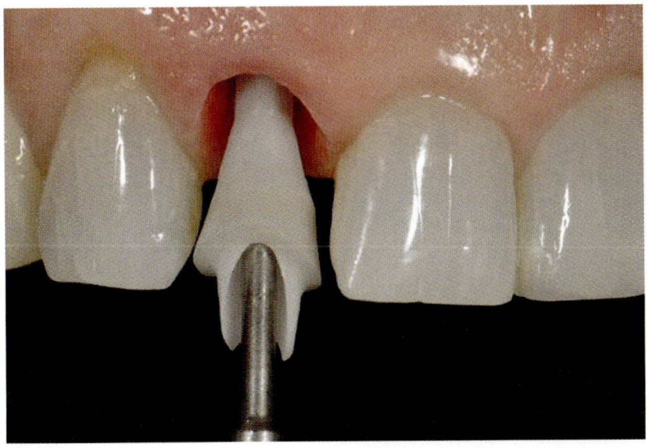

(a)

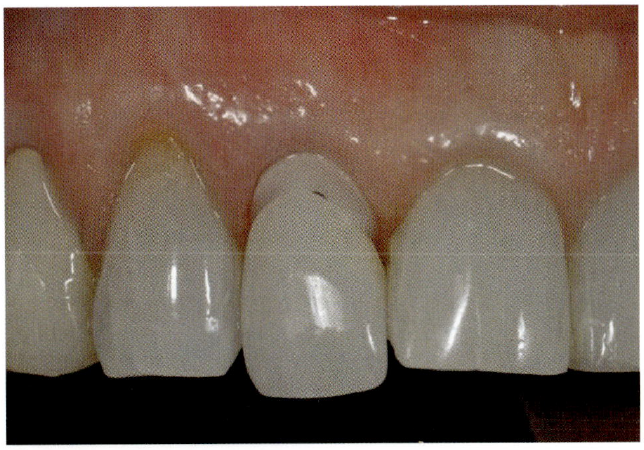

(b)

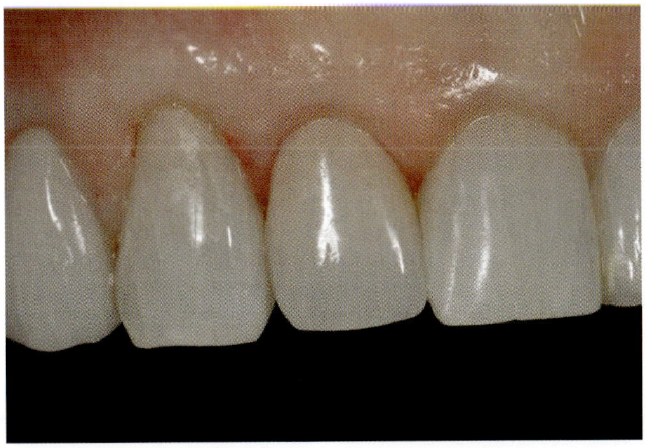

(c)

Figure 12.24 (**a**) CAD/CAM zirconia abutment with a porcelain margin added. (**b**) Supragingival margin design, with the ability to be directly bonded to the reciprocating margin of the crown. (**c**) Bonded margin-to-margin crown and abutment.

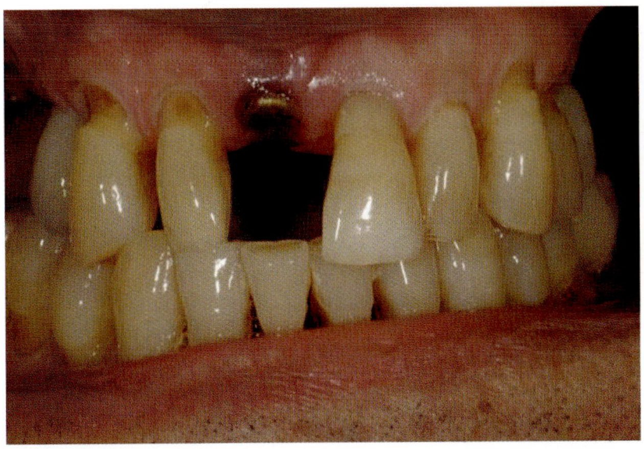

(a)

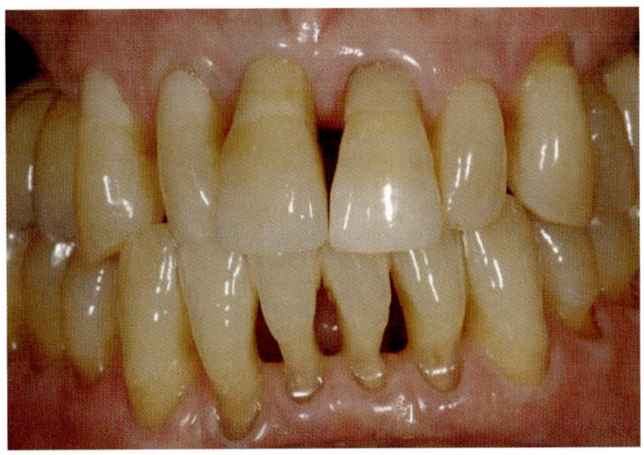

(b)

Figure 12.25 Implant site. (**a**) Porcelain abutment margins may be added to mimic a restoration. (**b**) This margin is several millimeters from the gingiva, and is highly esthetic.

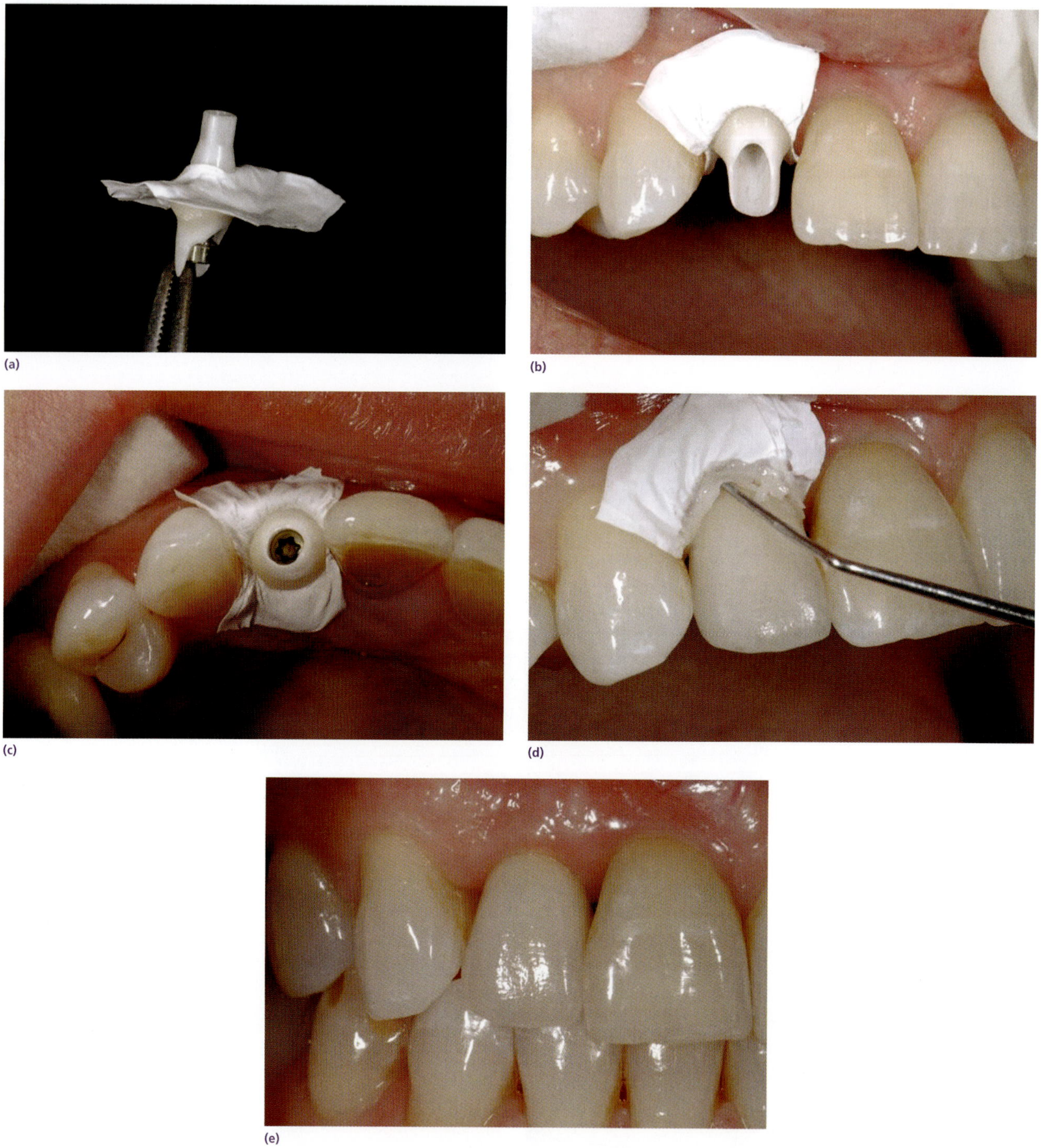

(a) (b) (c) (d) (e)

Figure 12.26 (a) Supragingival margins allow barrier protectors (PTFE bib) to be used. It must be away from the implant screw and cement margin site so as not to be trapped. (b, c) Bib protects the soft tissues and helps maintain a dry field for bonding. (d) Excess cement and bib easily removed. (e) Final restoration.

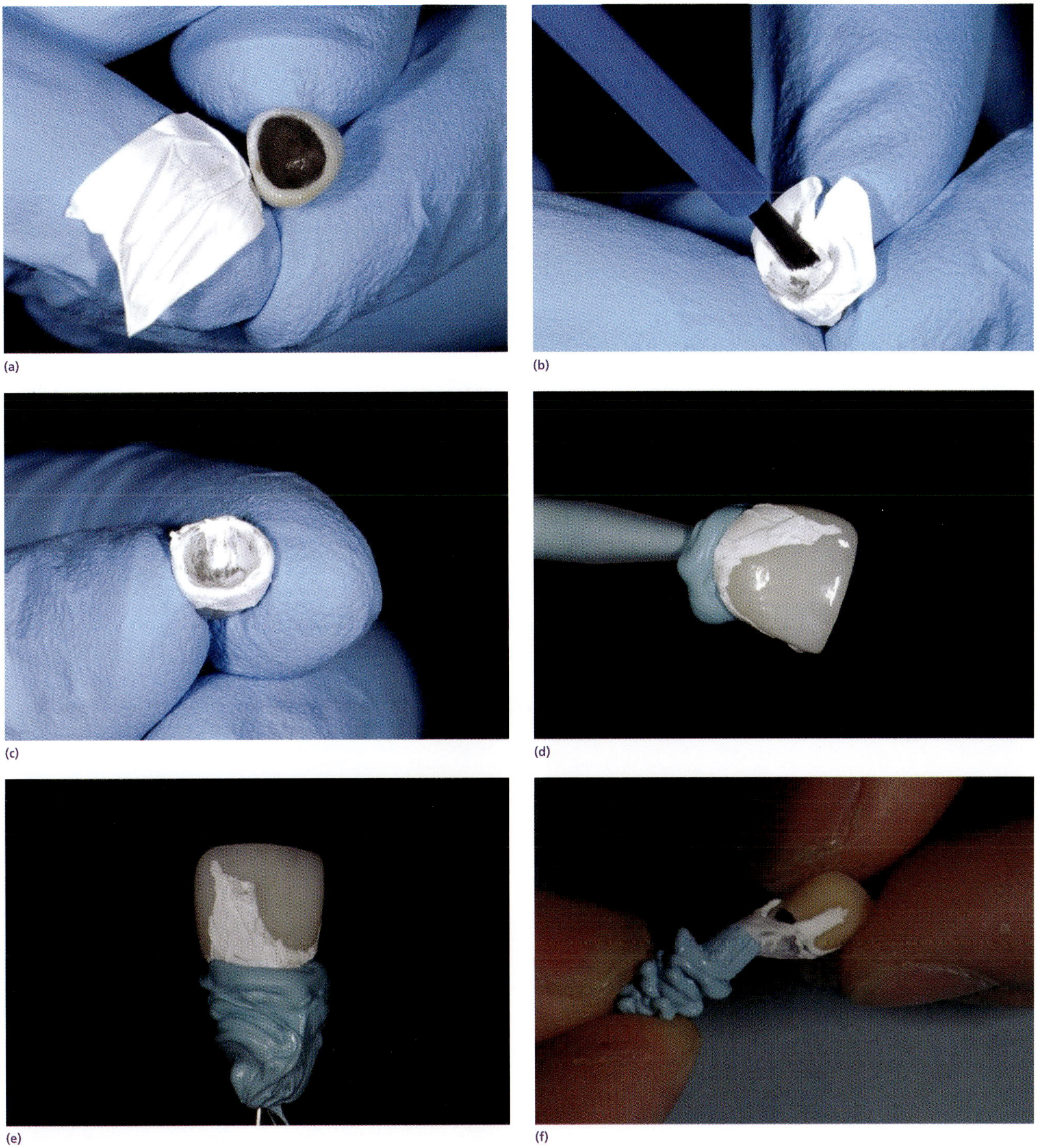

Figure 12.27 Copy abutment technique. (**a**) Crown intaglio coated with petroleum jelly and PTFE tape. (**b**) Brush used to assist adaptation of the PTFE lining. (**c**) The PTFE well adapted to the inside of the crown. (**d**) The crown with PTFE spacer being filled with PVS material. (**e**) Base extended after abutment replica formed. (**f**) PVS abutment and base removed from crown. (**g**) Once removed the copy abutment (smaller by 50 μm in all dimensions than the intaglio of the crown) is seen next to the original abutment. (**h**) The copy PVS abutment pushed into the crown with cement being extruded extraorally. (**i**) the crown is seated with minimal clean up (note tissue blanching is from abutment).

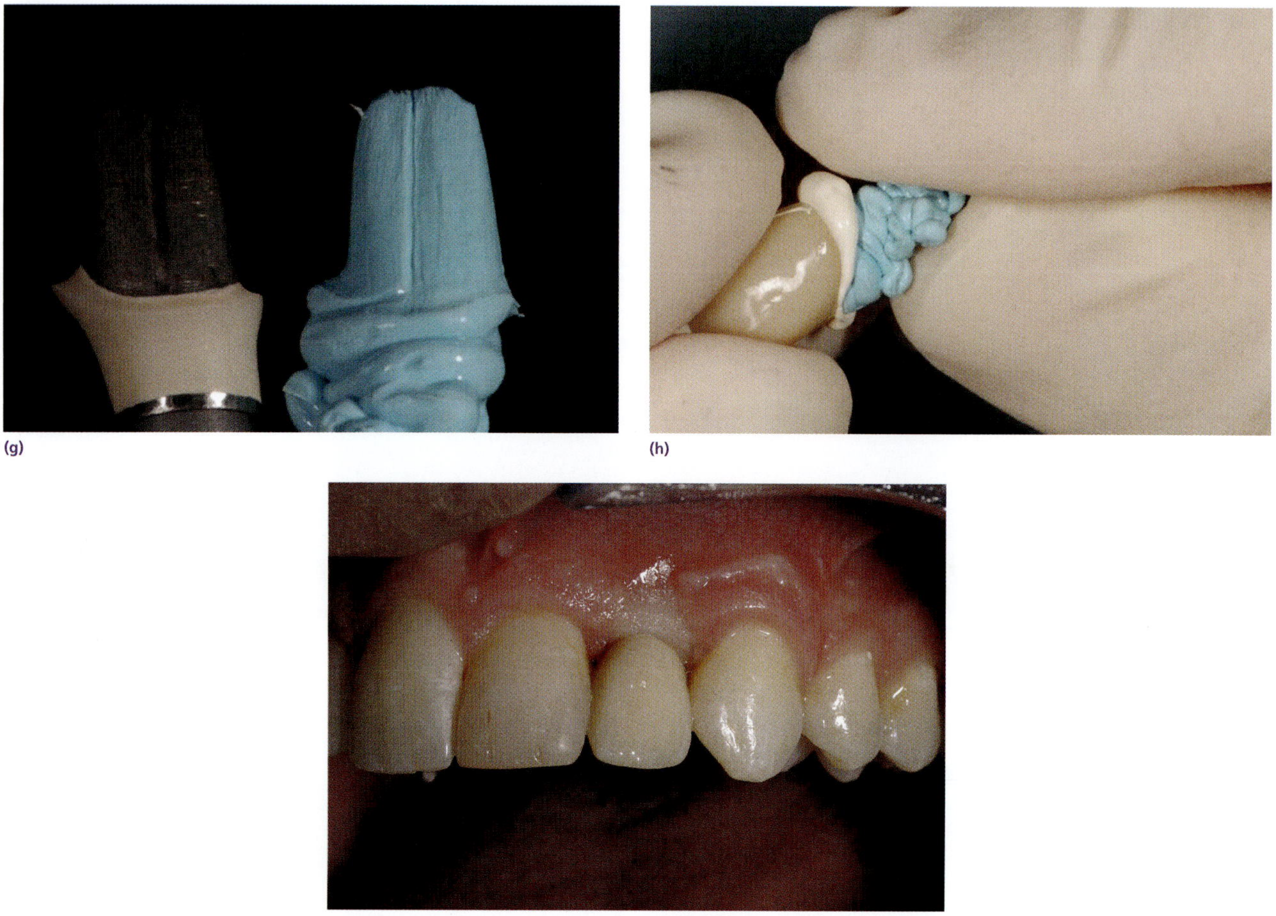

(g) (h) (i)

Figure 12.27 (*Continued*)

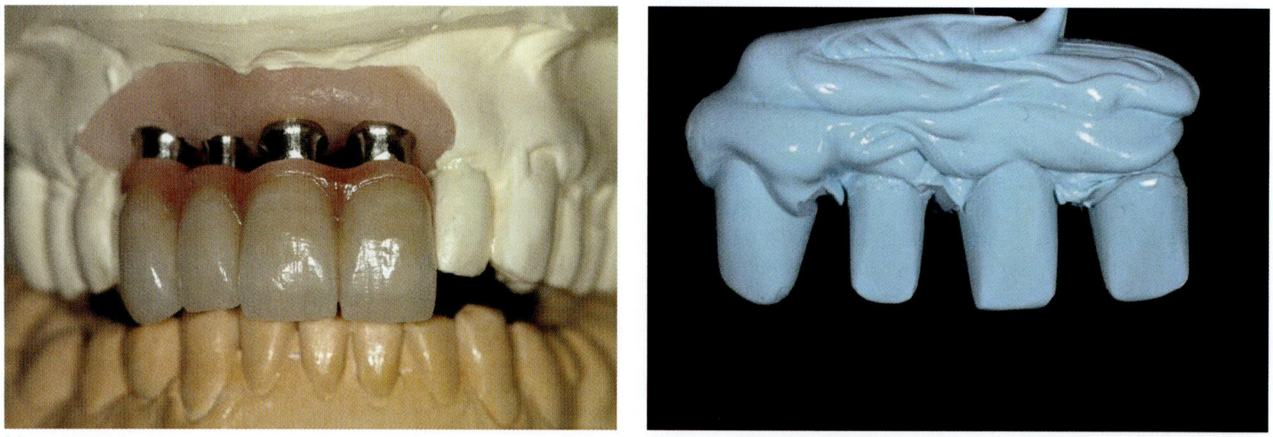

(a) (b)

Figure 12.28 (a) Multi-unit cemented prosthesis on cast. (b) PVS copy abutment for use prior to cementation.

On removal of the zirconia crowns, the cement flow patterns were evaluated, with the site of cement fracture suggesting that where the cement flowed during seating (how far within the abutment screw channel) had an effect on margin extrusion and resulted in modifications with the restoration retention (Figures 12.35, 12.36 and 12.37). Understanding this helps the clinician control both these variables.

The above studies indicate the ability to alter cement flow by abutment modifications that are beneficial with respect to cement-extrusion and crown-retention effects. Although

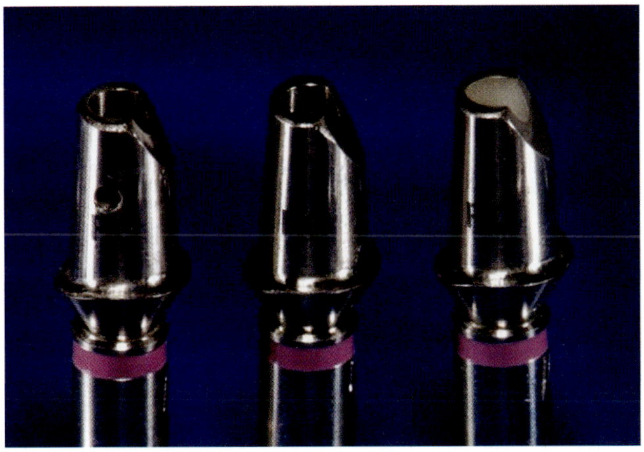

Figure 12.29 Left to right. Internal vented abutment (IVA), open abutment (OA), closed abutment (CA).

further scientific investigation is required, these seemingly easy steps can help the clinician.

Many other techniques exist that can potentially reduce cement extrusion and the clinician can decide which is the most appropriate. Alternatively, screw-retained restorations may be chosen, especially if the surgical planning and placement has provided the ideal implant location. Although clinicians claim that esthetics and occlusal management are problematic, the skilled laboratory technician can readily overcome these issues, especially with the materials available today.[67] One technique is to use a hybrid cemented–screw-retained crown. This provides a relatively inexpensive solution by combining a cemented crown with a stock abutment (Figure 12.38a). The crown is cemented onto the abutment extraorally and cleaned of excess cement (Figure 12.38b). A screw-access hole is produced

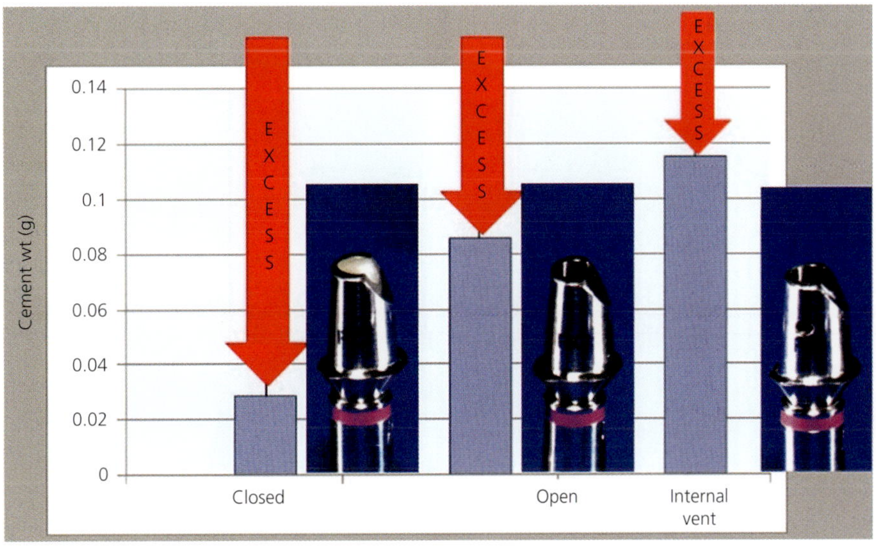

Figure 12.30 Comparison of cement amount extruded/retained internally to abutment when similar amounts are used. Red arrow indicates amount of excess cement extruded out, blue column amount retained within the crown/abutment system. More excess is seen when there is no internal venting.

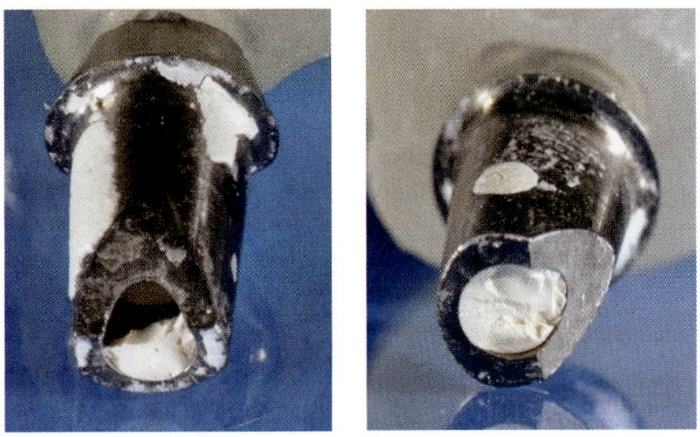

(a) (b)

Figure 12.31 Cement flow pattern in abutments. (a) OA air entrapment. (b) IVA with complete fill.

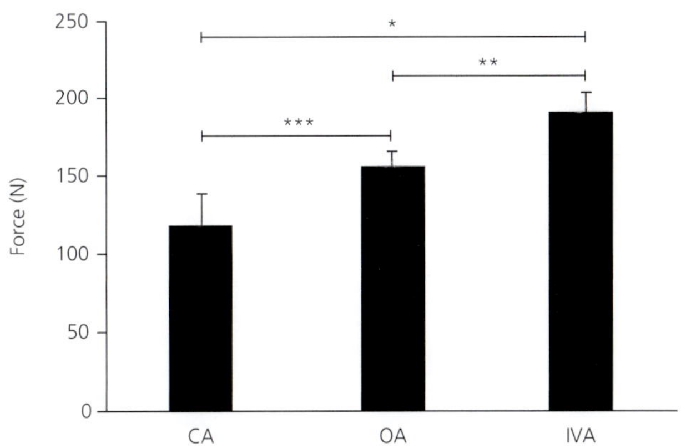

Figure 12.32 Graph indicating retentive force of cemented crown according to abutment design (CA, closed abutment; OA, open abutment; IVA, internal vented abutment). Statistical analysis, *P<.001, **P<.01, ***P<.05.

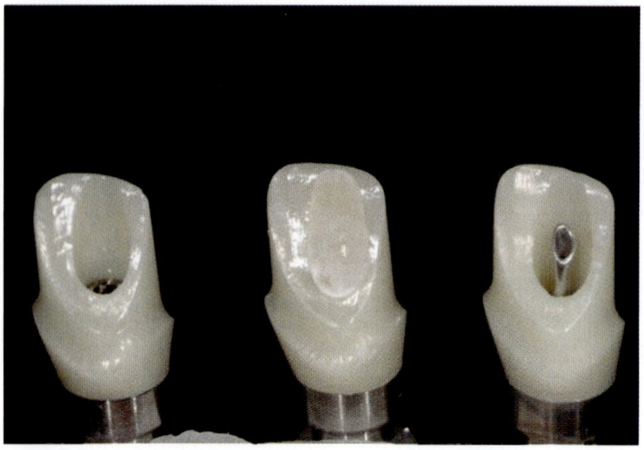

Figure 12.33 Esthetic zirconia abutments with modifications from study. Left to right: open abutment (OA), closed abutment (CA), insert abutment (IA).

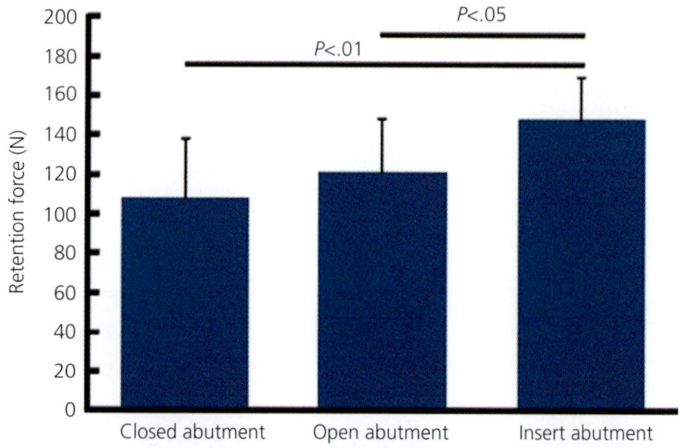

Figure 12.34 Graph showing effect on retention of the zirconia crown according to modification seen in Figure 12.33.

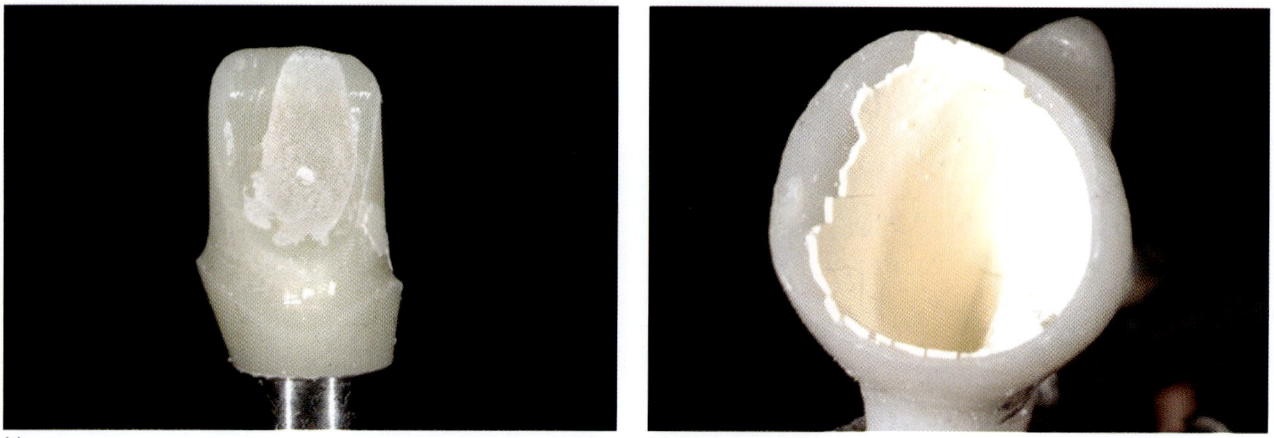

(a) (b)

Figure 12.35 Cement fracture pattern after removal of the crown. (a) CA – very little cement remained. (b) Cement remains within the crown.

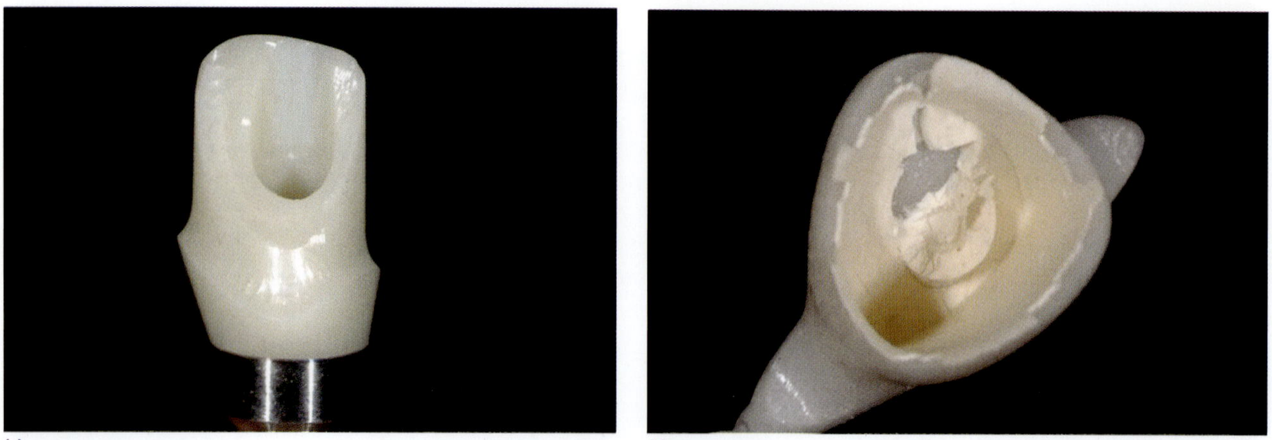

(a) (b)

Figure 12.36 Cement fracture pattern with the zirconia OA group. (a) Minor amount of cement seen on abutment. (b) The cement failed to fill the screw-access hole completely, an air void is noted inside the crown.

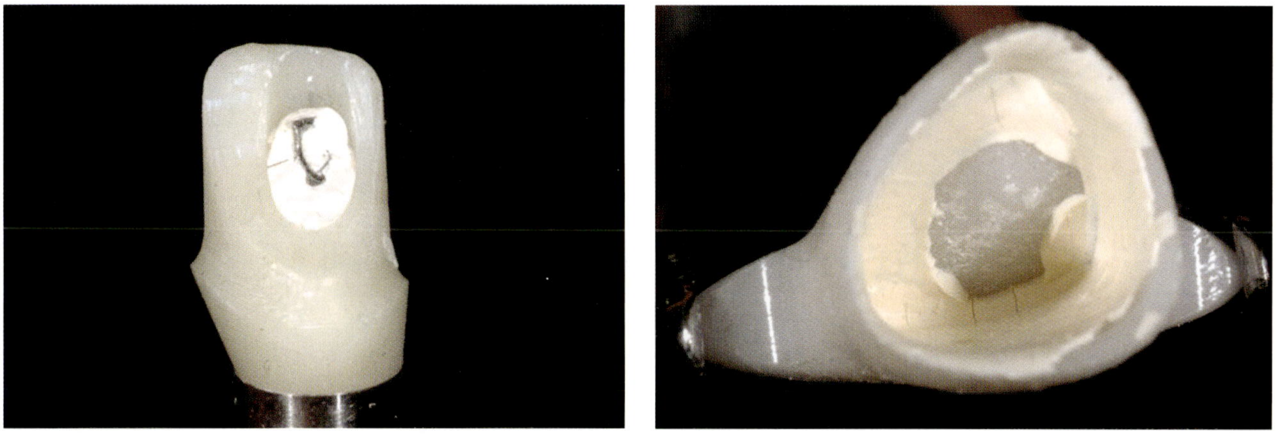

(a) (b)

Figure 12.37 Cement fracture in IA group. **(a)** Cement internalized and filling the screw locking into the insert. **(b)** The cement fracture is very different to other groups (OA, CA).

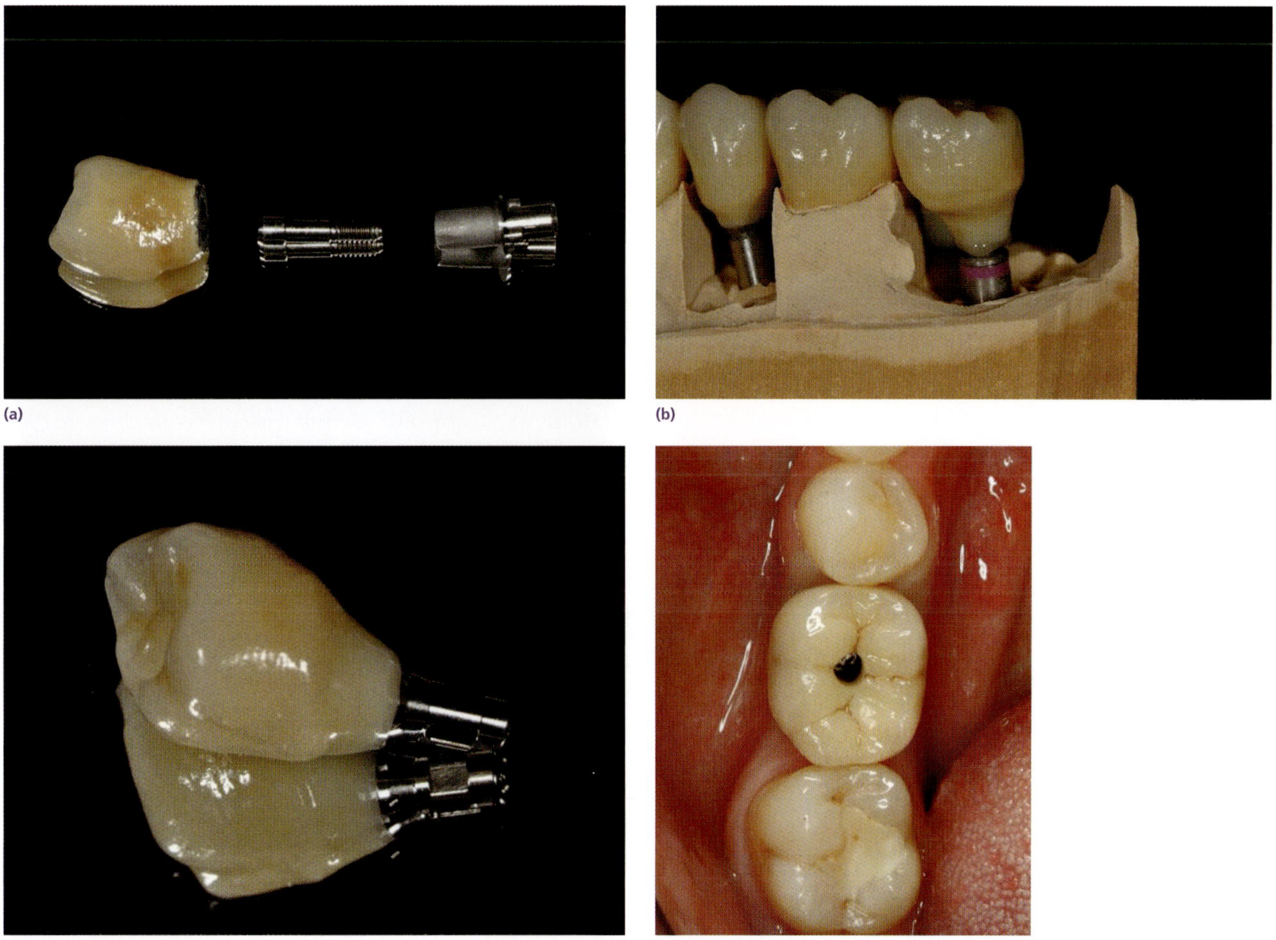

(a) (b) (c) (d)

Figure 12.38 **(a)** Components of cement–screw-retained restoration – crown with occlusal hole, abutment screw, titanium base. **(b)** Titanium base attached to implant analog on the cast. **(c)** Controlled cementation of crown to titanium base. **(d)** Cement–screw-retained restoration delivered to implant. *Source:* Courtesy of Dr Tomas Linkevičius.

either by drilling into the crown or having a pre-prepared screw-access hole in the crown, which allows this hybrid restoration to be attached to the implant with a screw (Figure 12.38c, d).[68] One concern using stock abutments is that the hybrid design requires consideration when fabricating the crown. Careful consideration to porcelain support is required, also being a two-piece (crown and abutment cementation) introduces potential failure within the cement layer unless the

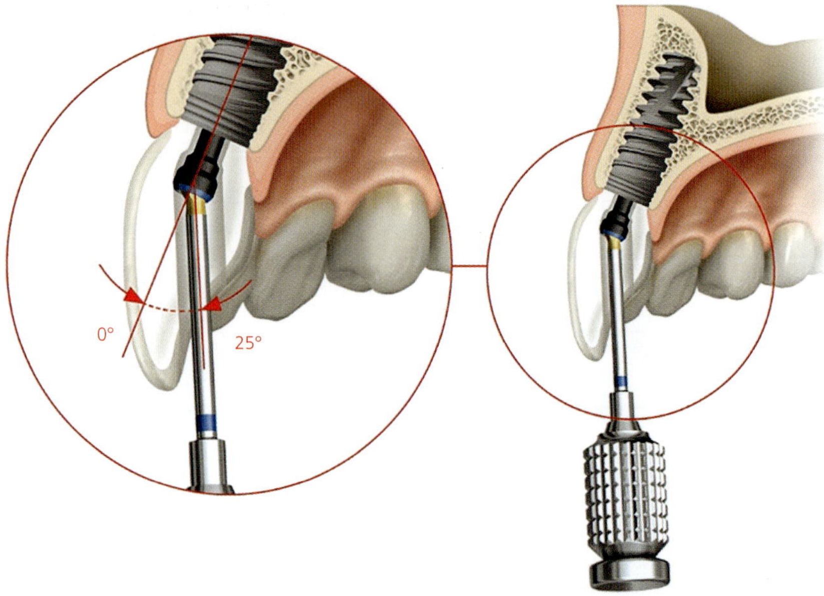

Figure 12.39 Angulated Screw Channel abutment (NobelBiocare, Switzerland) is a zirconia CAD/CAM abutment: it allows angle deviations up to 25°.

abutment height, surface area, and other resistance and retention features are considered.

Some manufacturers are aware of the issues with residual excess cement and its effect on implant health. They have developed abutments that allow angle changes that can be used when straight-line screw access would compromise the restorative outcome (Figure 12.39).[69]

Conclusion

The exact mechanisms that result from residual excess cement leading to peri-implant disease have not been fully elucidated. The need to understand biological interactions between cements and peri-implant microbes, potential for foreign body reactions, corrosion effects, and allergic responses to materials is more important now than previously thought. Unlike natural teeth, where little regard is given to cement selection or techniques involved, implants require a greater understanding of the biological and physical determinants that affect them. Protocols need to be established that include careful monitoring of the implant site, as the disease linked to cement extrusion may take years and up to a decade before any signs or symptoms develop. It should also be clear that when residual excess cement is found related to the implant site, it must be considered undesirable and the restorative dentist take responsibility. Alternatives exist that require no cement, these should be considered at the planning and surgical stages with a team approach – the surgeon, restorative dentist, and dental laboratory technician all working together to provide the best treatment possible for their patient.

References

1. Da Silva JD, Kazimiroff J, Papas A, *et al.* Practitioners Engaged in Applied Research and Learning (PEARL) Network Group. Outcomes of implants and restorations placed in general dental practices: a retrospective study by the Practitioners Engaged in Applied Research and Learning (PEARL) Network. *J Am Dent Assoc* 2014; **145**(7): 704–713.
2. Hebel KS, Gajjar RC. Cement-retained versus screw-retained implant restorations: achieving optimal occlusion and esthetics in implant dentistry. *J Prosthet Dent* 1997; **77**(1): 28–35.
3. Taylor TD, Agar JR. Twenty years of progress in implant prosthodontics. *J Prosthet Dent* 2002; **88**(1): 89–95.
4. Guichet DL, Caputo AA, Choi H, *et al.* Passivity of fit and marginal opening in screw- or cement-retained implant fixed partial denture designs. *Int J Oral Maxillofac Implants* 2000; **15**: 239–246.
5. Weber HP, Kim DM, Ng MW, *et al.* Peri-implant soft-tissue health surrounding cement- and screw-retained implant restorations: a multi-center, 3-year prospective study. *Clin Oral Implants Res* 2006; **17**(4): 375–379.
6. Alfaro MA, Papazoglou E, McGlumphy EA, *et al.* Short-term retention properties of cements for retrievable implant-supported prostheses. *Eur J Prosthodont Restor Dent* 2004; **12**(1): 33–37.
7. Chaar MS, Att W, Strub JR. Prosthetic outcome of cement-retained implant-supported fixed dental restorations: a systematic review. *J Oral Rehabil* 2011; **38**(9): 697–711.
8. Wittneben JG, Millen C, Brägger U. Clinical performance of screw- versus cement-retained fixed implant-supported reconstructions – a systematic review. *Int J Oral Maxillofac Implants* 2014; **29**(Suppl): 84–98.
9. Pauletto N, Lahiffe BJ, Walton JN. Complications associated with excess cement around crowns on osseointegrated implants: a clinical report. *Int J Oral Maxillofac Implants* 1999; **14**(6): 865–868.

10. Tomson PL, Butterworth CJ, Walmsley AD. Management of peri-implant bone loss using guided bone regeneration: a clinical report. *J Prosthet Dent* 2004; **92**(1): 12–16.
11. Gapski R, Neugeboren N, Pomeranz AZ, *et al.* Endosseous implant failure influenced by crown cementation: a clinical case report. *Int J Oral Maxillofac Implants* 2008; **23**(5): 943–946.
12. Korsch M, Obst U, Walther W. Cement-associated peri-implantitis: a retrospective clinical observational study of fixed implant-supported restorations using a methacrylate cement. *Clin Oral Implants Res* 2014; **25**(7): 797–802.
13. Wadhwani C, Rapoport D, La Rosa S, *et al.* Radiographic detection and characteristic patterns of residual excess cement associated with cement-retained implant restorations: a clinical report. *J Prosthet Dent* 2012; **107**(3): 151–157.
14. Shapoff CA, Lahey BJ. Crestal bone loss and the consequences of retained excess cement around dental implants. *Compend Contin Educ Dent* 2012; **33**(2): 94–101.
15. Linkevicius T, Puisys A, Vindasiute E, *et al.* Does residual cement around implant-supported restorations cause peri-implant disease? A retrospective case analysis. *Clin Oral Implants Res* 2013; **24**(11): 1179–1184.
16. Callan DP, Cobb CM. Excess cement and peri-implant disease. *J Implant Adv Clin Dent* 2009; **1**: 61–68.
17. Wilson TG Jr. The positive relationship between excess cement and peri-implant disease: a prospective clinical endoscopic study. *J Periodontol* 2009; **80**(9): 1388–1392.
18. Peri-implant mucositis and peri-implantitis: a current understanding of their diagnoses and clinical implications. *J Periodontol* 2013; **84**(4): 436–443.
19. Christensen GJ. Clinical and research advancements in cast-gold restorations. *J Prosthet Dent* 1971; **25**(1): 62–68.
20. Hermann JS, Buser D, Schenk RK, *et al.* Biological width around titanium implants. A physiologically formed and stable dimension over time. *Clin Oral Implant Res* 2000; **11**(1): 1–11.
21. Ikeda H, Yamaza T, Yoshinari M, *et al.* Ultrastructural and immunoelectron microscopic studies of the peri-implant epithelium-implant (Ti-6Al-4V) interface of rat maxilla. *J Periodontol* 2000; **71**(6): 961–973.
22. Rompen E. The impact of the type and configuration of abutments and their (repeated) removal on the attachment level and marginal bone. *Eur J Oral Implantol* 2012; **5**(Suppl): S83–90.
23. Sadan A, Blatz MB, Bellerino M, *et al.* Prosthetic design considerations for anterior single-implant restorations. *J Esthet Restor Dent* 2004; **16**(3): 165–175.
24. Stambaugh RV, Dragoo M, Smith DM, *et al.* The limits of sub-gingival scaling. *Int J Periodontics Restorative Dent* 1981; **1**(5): 30–41.
25. Mombelli A, Décaillet F. The characteristics of biofilms in peri-implant disease. *J Clin Periodontol* 2011; **38**(Suppl 11): 203–213.
26. Bumgardner JD, Adatrow P, Haggard WO, *et al.* Emerging antibacterial biomaterial strategies for the prevention of peri-implant inflammatory diseases. *Int J Oral Maxillofac Implants* 2011; **26**(3): 553–560.
27. Lang NP, Berglundh T; Working Group 4 of Seventh European Workshop on Periodontology. Periimplant diseases: where are we now? Consensus of the Seventh European Workshop on Periodontology. *J Clin Periodontol* 2011; **38**(Suppl 11): 178–181.
28. Goldberg PV, Higginbottom FL, Wilson TG. Periodontal considerations in restorative and implant therapy. *Periodontol 2000* 2001; **25**: 100–109.
29. Silness J. Periodontal conditions in patients treated with dental bridges 3. The relationship between the location of the crown margin and the periodontal condition. *J Periodontal Res* 1970; **5**(3): 225–229.
30. Valderhaug j, Birkeland JM. Periodontal conditions in patients 5 years following insertion of fixed prostheses. Pocket depth and loss of attachment. *J Oral Rehabil* 1976; **3**(3): 237–243.
31. Andersson B, Odman P, Lindvall AM, *et al.* Cemented single crowns on osseointegrated implants after 5 years: results from a prospective study on CeraOne. *Int J Prosthodont* 1998; **11**(3): 212–218.
32. Belser UC, Buser D, Hess D, *et al.* Aesthetic implant restorations in partially edentulous patients – a critical appraisal. *Periodontol 2000* 1998; **17**: 132–150.
33. Linkevicius T, Vindasiute E, Puisys A, *et al.* The influence of the cementation margin position on the amount of undetected cement. A prospective clinical study. *Clin Oral Implants Res* 2013; **24**(1): 71–76.
34. Hill EE, Lott J. A clinically focused discussion of luting materials. *Aust Dent J* 2011; **56**(Suppl 1): 67–76.
35. Wadhwani CP. Peri-implant disease and cemented implant restorations: a multifactorial etiology. *Compend Contin Educ Dent* 2013; **34**(7): 32–37.
36. Wadhwani CP, Schwedhelm ER. The role of cements in dental implant success, Part I. *Dent Today* 2013; **32**(4): 74–78.
37. Hicks J, Garcia-Godoy F, Donly K, *et al.* Fluoride-releasing restorative materials and secondary caries. *Dent Clin North Am* 2002; **46**(2): 247–276.
38. Klai S, Altenburger M, Spitzmüller B, *et al.* Antimicrobial effects of dental luting glass ionomer cements on *Streptococcus mutans. ScientificWorldJournal* 2014; **23**: 807086.
39. Rohilla M, Pandit IK, Srivastava N. Why the carioprotective potential of luting cements crucial? *J Indian Soc Pedod Prev Dent* 2009; **27**(4): 219–223.
40. Raval NC, Wadhwani CP, Jain S, *et al.* The interaction of implant luting cements and oral bacteria linked to peri-implant disease: an in vitro analysis of planktonic and biofilm growth – a preliminary study. *Clin Implant Dent Relat Res* 2015; **17**(6): 1029–1035.
41. Ramer N, Wadhwani C, Kim A, *et al.* Histologic findings within peri-implant soft tissue in failed implants secondary to excess cement: report of two cases and review of literature. *N Y State Dent J* 2014; **80**(2): 43–46.
42. Wilson TG Jr, Valderrama P, Burbano M, *et al.* Foreign bodies associated with peri-implantitis human biopsies. *J Periodontol* 2015; **86**(1): 9–15.
43. Burbano M, Wilson TG, Valderrama P, et al. Characterization of cement particles found in peri-implantitis human biopsies. *Int J Oral Maxillofac Implants* 2015; **30**(5): 1168–1173.
44. Tarica D, Alvarado VM, Truong ST. Survey of United States dental schools on cementation protocols for implant crown restorations. *J Prosthet Dent* 2010; **103**(2): 68–79.
45. Nicholson JW, Czarnecka B. The biocompatibility of resin-modified glass-ionomer cements for dentistry. *Dent Mater* 2008; **24**(12): 1702–1708.
46. Wadhwani CP, Piñeyro AF. Implant cementation: clinical problems and solutions. *Dent Today* 2012; **31**(1): 56–62.
47. Rodrigues DC, Valderrama P, Wilson TG, *et al.* Titanium corrosion mechanisms in the oral environment: a retrieval study. *Materials* 2013; **6**(11): 5258–5274.

48. Noguti J, de Oliveira F, Peres RC, *et al.* The role of fluoride on the process of titanium corrosion in oral cavity. *Biometals* 2012; **25**(5): 859–862.
49. Wadhwani C, Chung KH. Bond strength and interactions of machined titanium-based alloy with dental cements. *J Prosthet Dent* 2015; **114**(5): 660–665.
50. Barão VA, Yoon CJ, Mathew MT, *et al.* Attachment of *Porphyromonas gingivalis* to corroded commercially pure titanium and titanium-aluminum-vanadium alloy. *J Periodontol* 2014; **85**(9): 1275–1282.
51. Tsaryk R, Kalbacova M, Hempel U, *et al.* Response of human endothelial cells to oxidative stress on Ti6Al4V alloy. *Biomaterials* 2007; **28**(5): 806–813.
52. Horasawa N, Marek M. Effect of fluoride from glass ionomer on discoloration and corrosion of titanium. *Acta Biomater* 2010; **6**(2): 662–666.
53. Agar JR, Cameron SM, Hughbanks JC, *et al.* Cement removal from restorations luted to titanium abutments with simulated subgingival margins. *J Prosthet Dent* 1997; **78**(1): 43–47.
54. Wadhwani C, Hess T, Faber T, *et al.* A descriptive study of the radiographic density of implant restorative cements. *J Prosthet Dent* 2010; **103**(5): 295–302.
55. Akimoto K, Schuler RF. Treatment options related to cement contamination and repair of lesions. In: Wadhwani C (ed). *Cementation in Dental Implantology: An Evidence-Based Guide.* Heidelberg: Springer Science 2015; 177–197.
56. Wadhwani C, Hess T, Piñeyro A, *et al.* Cement application techniques in luting implant-supported crowns: a quantitative and qualitative survey. *Int J Oral Maxillofac Implants* 2012; **27**(4): 859–864.
57. Wadhwani CP, Chung KH. The role of cements in dental implant success, Part 2. *Dent Today* 2013; **32**(6): 46–51.
58. Wadhwani C, Goodwin S, Chung KH. Cementing an implant crown: a novel measurement system using computational fluid dynamics approach. *Clin Implant Dent Relat Res* 2016; **18**(1): 97–106.
59. Goodwin S, Chung KH, Wadhwani C. Something to smile about: using simulation to improve dental implants. *Dynamics Design Exploration* 2014; **37**: 9–12.
60. Wadhwani CP, Piñeyro A, Akimoto K. An introduction to the implant crown with an esthetic adhesive margin (ICEAM). *J Esthet Restor Dent* 2012; **24**(4): 246–254.
61. Hess TA. A technique to eliminate subgingival cement adhesion to implant abutments by using polytetrafluoroethylene tape. *J Prosthet Dent* 2014; **112**(2): 365–368.
62. Wadhwani CP. Clinical solutions: PTFE. In: Wadhwani C (ed). *Cementation in Dental Implantology: An Evidence-Based Guide.* Heidelberg: Springer Science 2015; 147–150.
63. Wadhwani C, Piñeyro A. Technique for controlling the cement for an implant crown. *J Prosthet Dent* 2009; **102**(1): 57–58.
64. Wadhwani C, Piñeyro A, Hess T, *et al.* Effect of implant abutment modification on the extrusion of excess cement at the crown-abutment margin for cement-retained implant restorations. *Int J Oral Maxillofac Implants* 2011; **26**(6): 1241–1246.
65. Wadhwani C, Hess T, Pineyro A, *et al.* Effects of abutment and screw access channel modification on dislodgement of cement-retained implant-supported restorations. *Int J Prosthodont* 2013; **26**(1): 54–56.
66. Wadhwani C, Chung KH. Effect of modifying the screw access channels of zirconia implant abutment on the cement flow pattern and retention of zirconia restorations. *J Prosthet Dent* 2014; **112**(1): 45–50.
67. Wadhwani C, Piñeyro A, Avots J. An esthetic solution to the screw-retained implant restoration: introduction to the implant crown adhesive plug: clinical report. *J Esthet Restor Dent* 2011; **23**(3): 138–143.
68. Linkevicius T. Restorative options that eliminate or reduce the potential for cement-induced peri-implant disease. In: Wadhwani C (ed). *Cementation in Dental Implantology: An Evidence-Based Guide.* Heidelberg: Springer Science 2015; 119–125.
69. Wadhwani CP. Restorative options that eliminate or reduce the potential for cement-induced peri-implant disease. In: Wadhwani C (ed). *Cementation in Dental Implantology: An Evidence-Based Guide.* Heidelberg: Springer Science 2015; 136–137.

CHAPTER 13
Implant Restoration of the Growing Patient

Clark M. Stanford
University of Illinois at Chicago College of Dentistry, Chicago, Illinois, USA

There is a number of reasons why teeth may be missing in the growing patient, including disease and its management, trauma, and/or congenital anomalies. Orofacial congenital anomalies occur in about 2–3% of newborns, with multiple environmental, genetic, and complex interactive etiologies being proposed.[1] There are multiple complex forms of craniofacial anomalies but for the purposes of this discussion, we will use the ectodermal dysplasias as an illustrative example of the complex management issues that arise in treating any of these conditions. The ectodermal dysplasias are not one disorder but a complex polyphenotype with more than 210 different forms being recognized.[2] The most common form is hypohidrotic ectodermal dysplasia (HED), which has an incidence rate of about 1 in 5000–10 000 live births.[3] Many of these conditions involve a loss or lack of formation of dentition, supportive skeletal and facial structures, and the need for a comprehensive, age appropriate orofacial care for the developing child and young adult.

One of the most common abnormalities affecting the dentition is congenital anomalies, followed by trauma or iatrogenic conditions caused by cancer management. In regard to congenital anomalies, the ectodermal dysplasias are defined as a diverse set of syndromic conditions derived from mutations affecting communication between the overlying ectoderm and the underlying mesoderm in embryonic development. The condition is seen throughout the animal kingdom. Conventionally, a clinical definition of this phenotype has been two or more ectodermally derived structures (hair, teeth, nails, sweat glands, etc.) being affected. Under some of these conditions, the structures either do not form (aplasia) or form an altered phenotype (dysplasia), such as conical-shaped or microdontic teeth.[4] Originally described in its current classification by Frieire-Maia and Pinheiro,[5] the most common form of ectodermal dysplasia syndrome is referred to as X-linked hypohidriotic ectodermal dysplasia or HED; note there is currently a significant effort to revise this system using molecular classification. The X-linked HED is defined by a combination of features including hypodontia (missing fewer than six teeth), oligodontia (missing six or more teeth) (Figure 13.1a, b), and, rarely, anodontia (complete loss of teeth), altered hair growth, distribution, and volume (trichodysplasia), reduced or altered sweating (dyshidrosis), altered mucosal sebaceous function (asteatosis) leading to dry mucosal surfaces and significant mucosal crusting, and altered keratin nail formation in some types (onychodyplasia).

In regard to the dental malformations, the issues are usually esthetics, self-perception, and awareness relative to unaffected peers, loss of perceived function, lack of alveolar ridge development, arch length/tooth size discrepancies, and hyposalivation. The latter can place the patient at a higher risk of dental caries (Figure 13.1c). Various groups have convened consensus conferences to develop expert experience-based guidelines for tooth replacement therapy, with or without oral implant options primarily for the skeletally immature adult.[6–11] Again, the data on outcomes are not strong and, as an evidence-based procedure, the clinician should proceed very carefully. A leading principle is to provide age-appropriate therapies holistically respecting the integrity of the patient and the caregiver's autonomy, cultural competence, and providing staged therapies allowing patients to adapt to each approach as they are undergoing what growth potential they have (Figure 13.1d–f).[12–14] Note, in this discussion, it is often better to use the medical term, "care plan" rather than "treatment plan", since the latter suggests something is needed (when it may not at this time) and indicates the long-term interests of the patient and their holistic outcomes of care are more important (family- and patient-centered care) than any clinical perception of care.[13–19]

In the young child (age 0–6 years), a care plan involving a removable prosthesis is usually considered, starting around the age of 3 years. A pediatric dentist is often the lead consultant and should see any patient starting around 1 year of age. In situations where there are multiple age-appropriate teeth, it may be useful to consult with a prosthodontist to assist in the staging of care. In this way, the affected individual builds a bond of trust

Evidence-based Implant Treatment Planning and Clinical Protocols, First Edition. Edited by Steven J. Sadowsky.

Companion website: www.wiley.com/go/sadowsky/implant

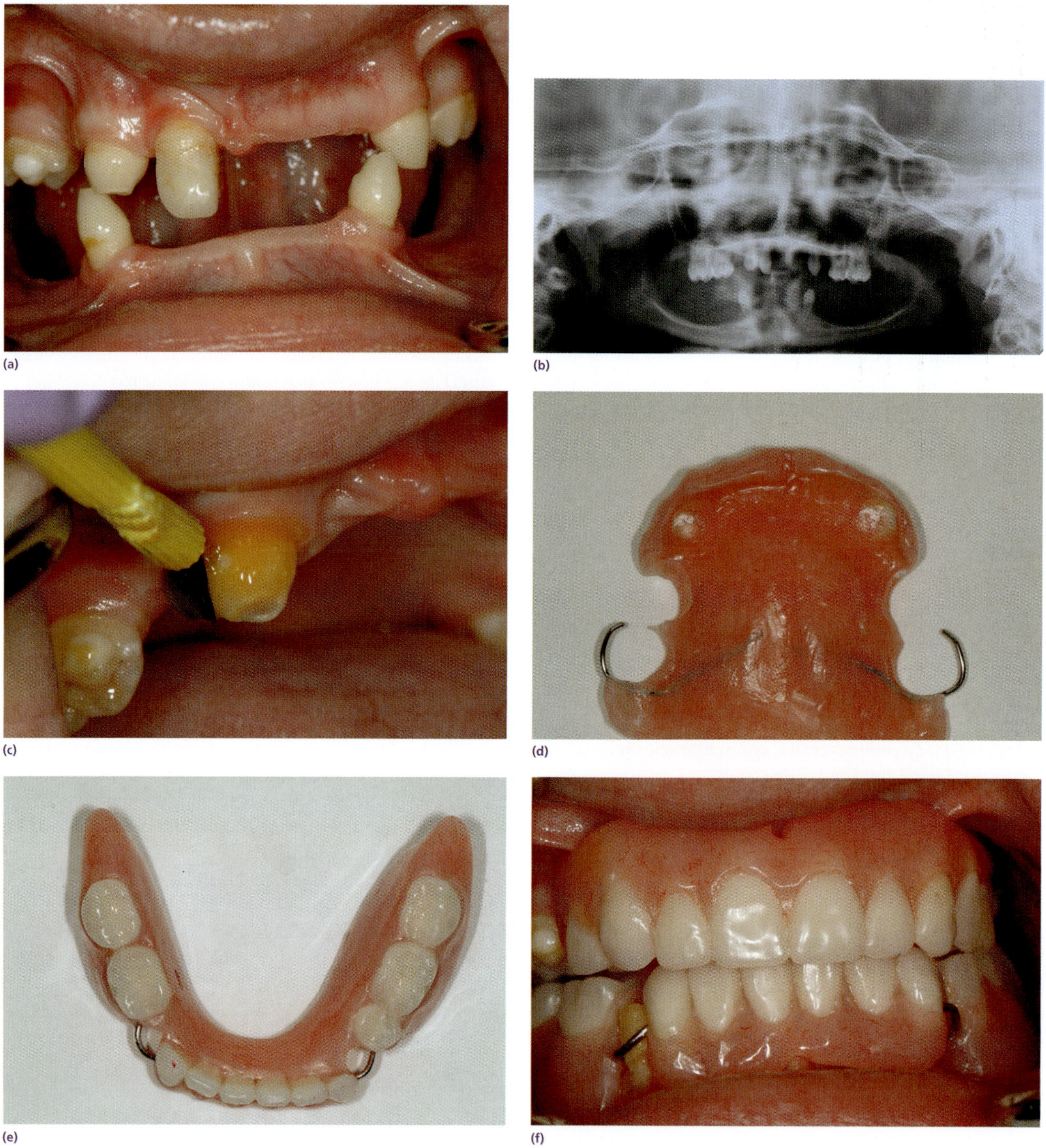

Figure 13.1 X-linked hypohidriotic ectodermal dysplasia. **(a)** Intraoral appearance shows the typical oligodontia, cone-shaped teeth, and retained primary teeth. The class III malocclusion, common in this population, is also evident in this image. **(b)** Radiographic appearance of the oligodontia. **(c)** Hyposalivation is common in this population since the salivary glands are derived in the same manner that sweat glands are formed. Use of frequent 5% NaF applications is recommended. **(d)** Provisional removable overdenture partial denture prosthesis for the maxilla. **(e)** Provisional removable partial denture for the mandible. **(f)** Prostheses in place at increased vertical dimension to match appropriate profile and need for interocclusal distance.

with the entire care team with enhanced communication between the members of the care team and enhanced transition of care as the patient reaches adulthood. In the young child, a removable or pediatric fixed prosthesis may be considered.[9] It is very helpful that the dentures and denture teeth be age appropriate in shape, size, and dimensions (Figure 13.2).[20,21]

In the young child, the prosthetic steps are often simplified relative to the adult complete or partial denture approaches, due

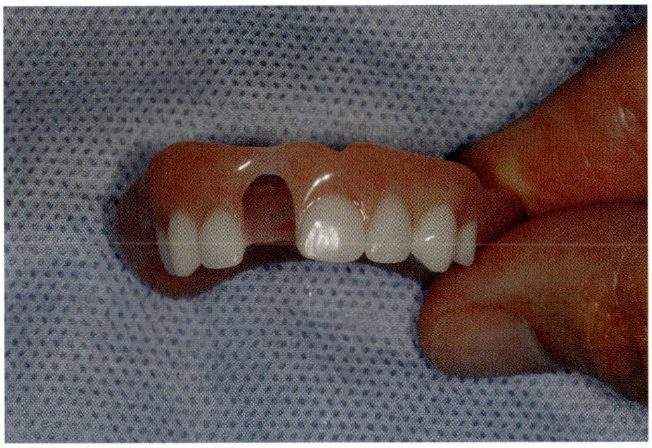
(a)

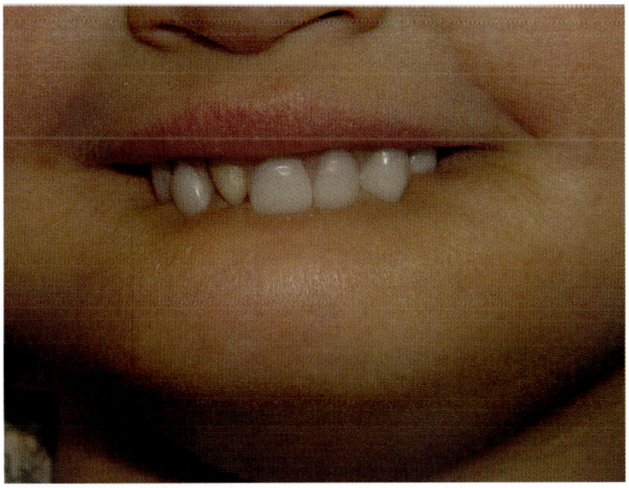
(b)

Figure 13.2 **(a, b)** Maxillary removable partial prosthesis. Age-appropriate sized replacement teeth used on the maxillary partial denture in a 5-year old.

to timing, need for frequent replacement, limited family resources, and patient and family tolerance. In a young patient presenting with multiple missing primary and permanent teeth, making a final impression, often with a well-fitting stock tray and a fast-setting impression material (e.g., occlusal registration material) may be sufficient. At the impression appointment, jaw relationships are made using a measure of the vertical dimension of rest in order to determine the vertical dimension of occlusion. A construct using about 2 mm of interocclusal distance is used with a measurement from the height of the posterior maxillary vestibule to the commissures of the lips (nodes of the orbicular oris) at approximately the vertical dimension of the anterior/posterior occlusion (canine and first and second primary molar). In a young child, this often translates to about 7 mm from the zygoma in the vestibule to the proposed posterior occlusal plane, coincident if possible with the corners of the mouth. This will develop in the laboratory phase of setting the prosthetic pediatric teeth (Milk Teeth, Nissin Dental Products, Japan, www.kilgoreinternational.com). If this approach is used, it is important to closely evaluate the patient at recall appointments and adjust the denture to allow eruption of any remaining teeth. This especially important since the growth of dento-alveolar bone creates about two-thirds of the vertical height of the mid- and lower face.[22] In the case of total anodontia, the mandibular region, from approximately the second primary molar to second primary molar, completes basilar growth around 5 years of age with ongoing growth at the condylar growth plates and on the distal aspect of the ramus (allowing the mandible to become more upright with growth and carrying the symphysis area passively forward). As such, in the congenitally edentulous mandible, after about the age of 5, the use of oral implant(s) may be considered. Do note if there are teeth in the arch and/or erupting permanent teeth, implant placement should be delayed until at least skeletal maturity. In females this is typically at least 18 years or older and, in males, 20 years or older. As discussed later, the most important aspect of premature implant placement is disruption of normal tooth eruption and changes in tooth position due to the ankylosed oral implant. For this application, it must be clearly determined from the patient, not the parents, the perceived functional, esthetic, phonetic, and emotional/social advantages of this invasive therapy. It is important to hear from the patient the request and desire for the perceived improved function, since the procedures will entail a general anesthesia protocol with the associated elevated risks in this population. With an understanding that one or two two-part or modular-style narrow-diameter implants can be used (e.g., 3 mm diameter), an overdenture-style approach can be considered in this age group. Obviously, implants should not be used in the partially edentulous jaw in the growing child since the implant will become more submerged as the teeth erupt around it and/or the implant can affect the eruption path (the so-called halo affect) of the adjacent teeth. Depending on the location and impact on eruption of adjacent teeth, ankylosed primary teeth may act as useful overdenture abutments and should be considered as a useful solution to prosthesis retention.

When the child reaches school age (7–12 years), the transition from primary to permanent dentition normally occurs. It is important to provide replacement teeth to allow for phonetics, mastication, and social/peer awareness.[20,23,24] Typically a more removable approach is used in this population allowing ongoing growth (Figure 13.1). This is often the time to consider an orthodontic evaluation, especially as permanent teeth erupt. Retained primary teeth that do not have a succedaneous replacement should be retained to preserve the alveolar bone. Evaluation for ankylosed primary teeth needs to be carried out, especially in bounded spaces with permanent teeth on both sides, commonly the canines and first molars. A key aspect is to evaluate if the ankylosed primary teeth are interfering with the eruption of the adjacent permanent teeth; if so, they should be surgically removed. If not, then they should be maintained until at least skeletal maturity.

In adolescents to young adults (13 years to skeletal maturity), orthodontic therapy should be considered if there are teeth in

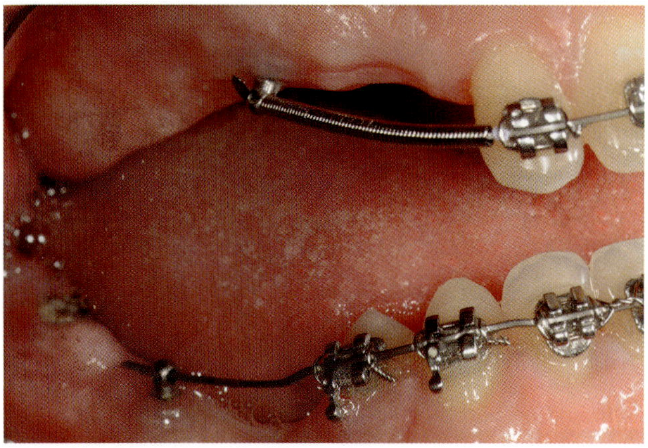

Figure 13.3 Use of TADs to assist in anchorage for orthodontic movement of the four anterior teeth that the patient formed.

the arch and space distribution is needed. Comprehensive care in this population should preferably be a team approach between pediatric dentists, prosthodontists, and orthodontists. Orthodontic care may be conventional full-banded appliances or assisted with temporary anchoring devices (TADs or non-integrated "temporary implants") to support anchorage for orthodontic care (Figure 13.3). In cases of minor hypodontia (e.g., missing maxillary lateral incisors), esthetic tooth replacement can be performed either with a removable partial denture, an orthodontic retainer, or with a unilateral bonded pontic. In the bonded pontic approach, this is typically made with a zirconia core, pressed with hydrofluoric acid etchable glass ceramic (e.g., EMaxPress, Ivoclar Vivadent, Amherst NY) and bonded to the mesial aspect of the canine with a veneer-based cement system (e.g., RelyX Veneer, 3M ESPE, St. Paul, MN).[25] An important goal for the transitional period is a stable, esthetic, and functional dentition without overtreatment or loss of retained primary teeth that are developing or maintaining alveolar bone. It is most important that the maximal potential of craniofacial growth be accomplished during this period.

If denture retention is insufficient, from the patient's perceptive, oral implant therapy can be considered in the edentulous anterior mandible during this period. It is best to plan for a definitive final prosthetic design in selecting the implant sites.[21] It is also preferable to avoid extensive bone grafting for site development in this age period.

Oral rehabilitation in the skeletally mature adult needs to be based on a comprehensive evaluation of systemic health and oral health risk factors, with a strong weighting on patient-oriented outcomes, desires, and values. In this population, a multidisciplinary team is critical with additional orthodontic and oral surgical phases of care (e.g., LeFort midface orthognathic procedures).[26] The prosthetic outcomes need to be carefully planned by the prosthodontist and strategic decisions made for retention of primary (or sometimes permanent) teeth, use of root canal therapy and removable partial overdentures for multiple missing contiguous teeth, and/or the need for extensive bone grafting for a multiple oral implant rehabilitation (Figure 13.4). The patient needs to understand that any prosthodontic intervention will have significant maintenance issues and will probably need to be replaced multiple times in the patient's lifetime.[15]

Regardless of the reasons for tooth loss, a careful systematic assessment of risk factors is always essential. A careful evaluation of keratinized mucosal tissue thickness and width and, where appropriate, the use of connective tissue grafting (alloplastic or autoplastic) should be considered. In a retrospective survey by Stanford *et al.*,[20] with 98 patients affected with ectodermal dysplasia (ED), treated with oral implants at the National Institutes of Health (NIH) in the 1980s, it was observed that a relatively high rate of implant maintenance complications occurred over time.[20] With 56 male and 46 female subjects having 73% of the implants in the lower jaw, it was observed 52% of the implants had maintenance or complications, such as infections, lost implants, loose dentures, remakes/relines, or a combination of complications. All of the oral implants were of one type (Brånemark System, NobelBiocare). Interestingly, in a later study by Bergendal *et al.*,[27] the authors reported on a retrospective study of Nordic regional treatment centers on ED-affected children treated with oral implants between 1985 and 2005. Twenty-one children, treated with 33 implants due to agenesis or trauma, with a subgroup of ED-affected children (five treated with 14 implants) at 5–12 years of age were reported. The authors reported nine of the 14 implants were lost prior to loading in the ED cohort, warranting caution with the approach and/or the implant system being used at that time.[27] In the Netherlands, a retrospective study following 129 subjects within the Dutch National Health Care System, having mostly hypodontia and some agenesis noted over an observation period of 3–79 months (mean of 46 months in function) that 36% of subjects had severe orthodontic root resorption, 12% had significant bone loss (more than 5 mm), and 57% had mucosal discoloration around the implant abutments.[28] The latter observation indicates the need to evaluate mucosal thickness and the critical need for rigorous long-term maintenance therapy.

As this population reaches adult maturity, the prosthetic treatment options become very diverse. Given that there is some debate as to when growth is completed, there is a general consensus to consider oral implant placement in the bounded edentulous space starting around the age of 18–20 years. Clinical assessments are needed, especially of post-orthodontic retention, tooth mobility, and the stability of the occlusion. As always, a part of the informed consent process is to outline the strengths and challenges of each procedure being proposed (within a health literacy perceptive and language the patient and caregivers can understand). Health literacy is an important aspect of this process and it is important to have the caregiver and patient reflect on what is being proposed and articulate back to the clinical team the elements of the conversation.[29,30] Supportive written, web, video, and related materials are also helpful, but are not a substitute for careful, health-literacy-appropriate conversations. Alteratives to the proposed care plan should be

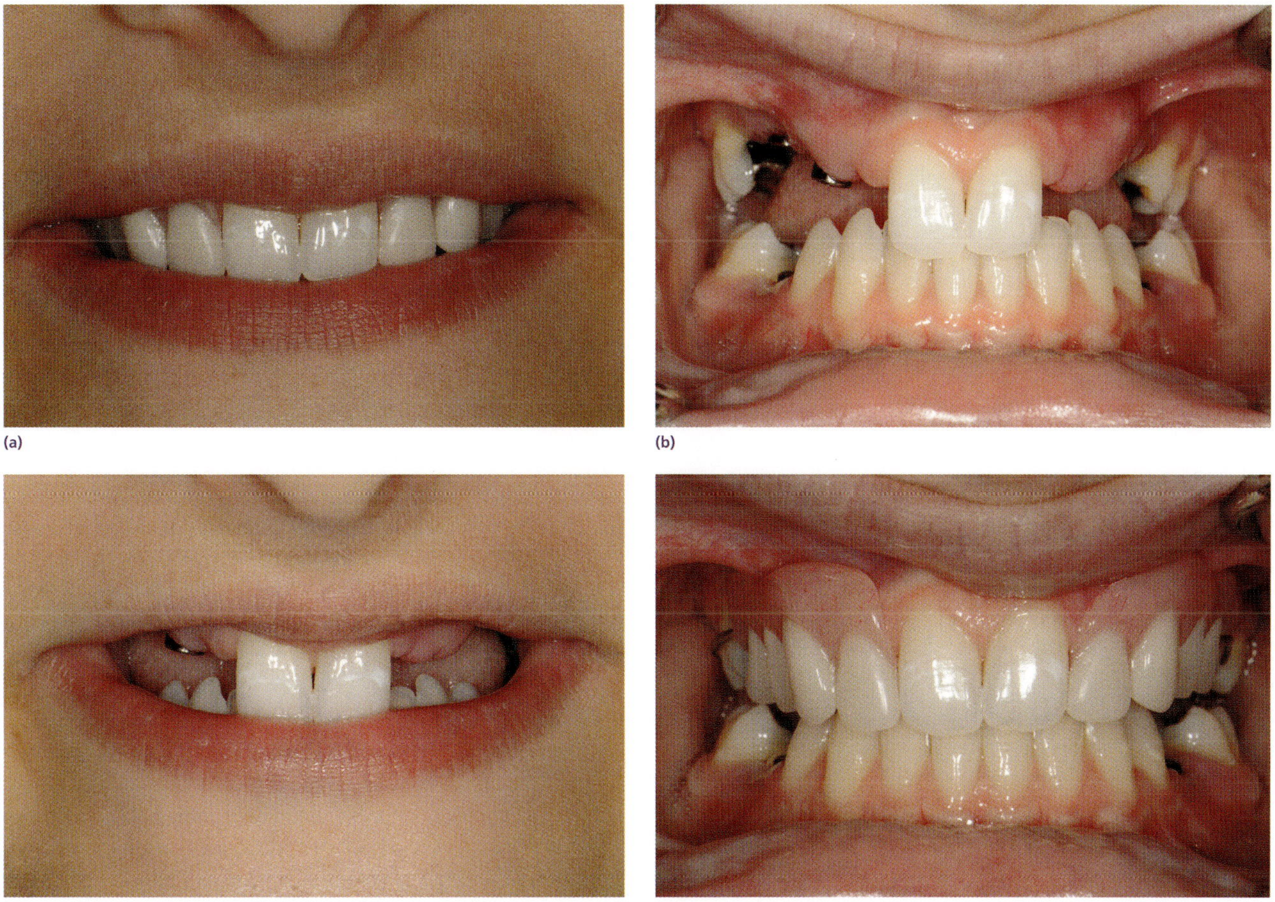

(a) (b) (c) (d)

Figure 13.4 (a–d) Interim restorations are useful as an expeditious approach to esthetics and phonetics in the growing child. This patient presented with healing implants that were placed in bone grafts; therefore, an interim removable partial denture was used during the healing period.

discussed (including risks, benefits, and alternatives) as well as reasonable expectations of outcomes if no intervention is done.[31]

As the care plan is developed, esthetic and functional outcomes of implant treatment require comprehensive diagnostic and care planning (Figure 13.5a, b). The initial assessment of the patient's medical and dental history is to determine the implant system and devices that will meet the patient's therapeutic and esthetic requirements. The assessment should determine a patient's risks for a surgical intervention, especially since some individuals who have congenital anomalies will have impaired wound healing.[32]

Steps to consider in the rehabilitation of the young adult patient

To create a predictable care plan, the prosthodontist should design the proposed prosthesis during the diagnostic phase. For implant-based rehabilitations, planning will dictate the number of implants, size, diameter, and their position and angulation (Figure 13.5c–f).[33,34] Based on this diagnostic information, a surgical guide or denture indicates the desired implant position, angulation, and need for hard or soft tissue augmentation before or during implant placement. During the clinical examination, the clinician should evaluate the residual ridge for its shape and contour. A careful evaluation of the patient's risk factors for soft and hard tissue changes, whatever final restoration is planned, should be made, to encourage realistic patient expectations.

Preoperative planning helps to achieve esthetic goals by ensuring the implant's three-dimensional position is restoratively driven. In some situations, implant fixed partial dentures (IFPD) are an excellent alternative to long edentulous spans conventionally restored with removable partial dentures (RPD). On the other hand, an RPD can be less expensive with fewer risks than a complex surgical intervention. During the informed consent process, care plan alternatives should include a discussion regarding the ability to control esthetics and function with the various methods of tooth replacement including conventional FPDs, adhesive resin restorations ("Maryland" bridges), implants, and/or removable partial dentures.

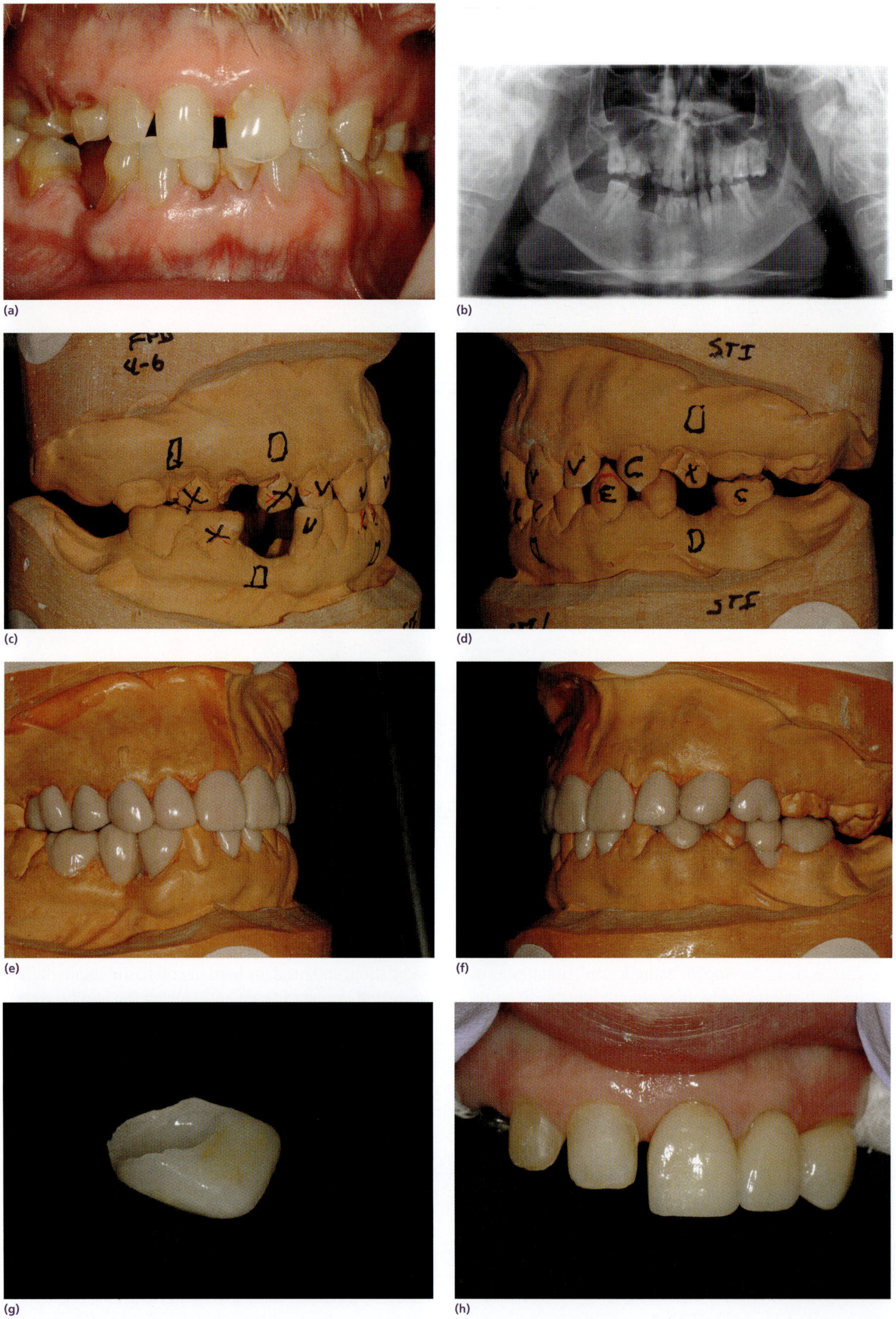

Figure 13.5 A 35-year-old male with Witkop's syndrome presents with multiple malformed permanent teeth and retained primary teeth. **(a)** Retained primary teeth in maxillary right quadrant have maintained the alveolar bone and soft tissue architecture in this area. The diastemas between the anterior teeth are created as part of the planning for ceramic veneers on these teeth. The mandibular right side has a significant facial bone atrophy in the premolar region. **(b)** Panoramic radiograph demonstrating the retained primary teeth. **(c)** Diagnostic casts showing planning for implant and veneers on the right side. **(d)** Diagnostic casts showing planning for implants and veneers on the left side. **(e, f)** Diagnostic wax-up performed to estimate contours.

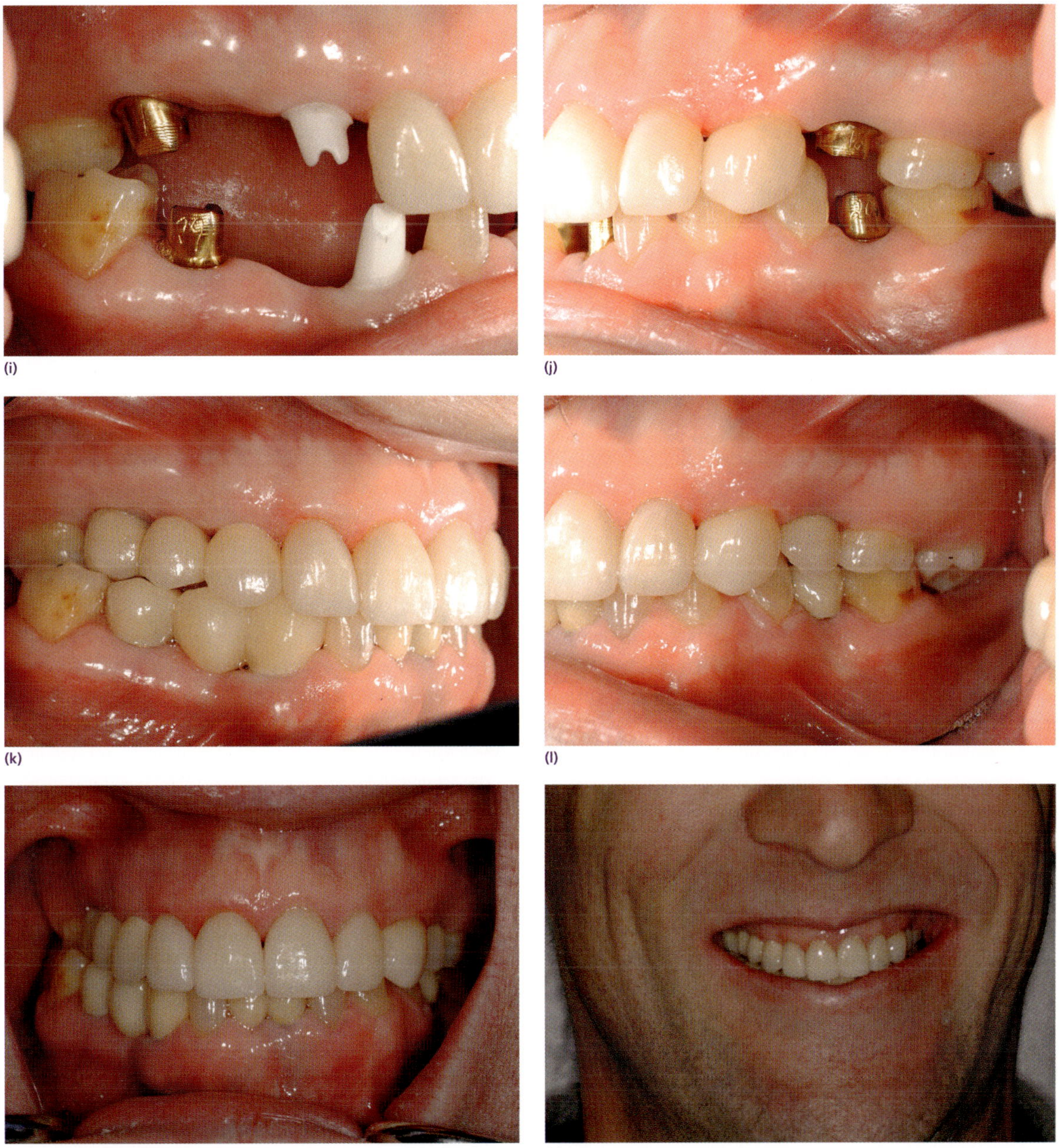

(i) (j) (k) (l) (m) (n)

Figure 13.5 (*Continued*) **(g)** Ceramic veneers (EMax lithium disilicate etchable glass) are very useful to establish contours and esthetics when teeth are malformed. Note the design is as full a wrap-around design as possible. **(h)** Clinical image showing change in incisal length and contours with the veneers. The veneers can be done either simultaneous with the implant restorations or the implants can be provisionalized, then the veneers placed, and then the final implant restorations made or the veneers can be completed as the implants are healing. In general, the second, three-step approach is most predictable. **(i, j)** Custom abutments are in place and final restorations are adjusted and the occlusion evaluated. **(k, l)** Lateral views of the completed restorations. **(m, n)** Final facial view of the completed restorations.

Mechanical considerations

The diagnostic phase should determine the number of endosseous-style implants to be placed. When replacing multiple adjacent teeth with dental implants, it is clinically useful to replace three teeth with a short-span FPD on two implants, utilizing the pontic to adjust for contours and final implant position. This approach is especially useful in the anterior maxilla involving multiple teeth, where the smallest tooth to be replaced is planned as a pontic with implants placed in the canine and central incisor region. It is also very useful to use ceramic veneers on the natural teeth to conservatively fill out contours and esthetics (Figure 13.5g, h).

When a tooth or teeth are missing in the anterior region, the dentition tends to be positioned more facially relative to the central axis of the alveolar ridge, resulting in a thin facial plate of bone over the teeth. Upon tooth loss, this facial plate is unevenly resorbed in a palatal and apical direction (e.g., an average of 3–4 mm of bone resorption) in the maxillae.[35–40] The position and stability of the facial/buccal plate of bone should be considered for any evidence of bone loss, which occurs in cases involving traumatic fracture or, potentially, during orthodontic therapy. In the mandible, the resorption pattern can occur at an uneven rate causing increased bone loss on the thin superior regions, producing a wider ridge with high muscle attachments. When determining the optimal tooth position for functional and esthetic purposes, a diagnostic set-up with denture teeth on a trial base with soft and hard tissue contours waxed out to full contour is useful. This can be duplicated as a radiographic guide for the CBCT planning study. Lower ionizing radiation with newer CBCT machines allows a less invasive diagnostic work-up for young patients. A vacuum-formed matrix of this diagnostic set-up can also assist the surgeon in determining the position, placement, and volume of site development (hard and soft tissue grafting) needed in a staged procedure with delayed implant placement.[22] In planning the occlusion one should consider tooth contacts in centric relation or maximum intercuspation, providing vertical loading down the long axis of the implant(s), if possible.[41,42] Large lateral sliding contacts may create elevated bending or torsional loads, leading to premature failure of abutments, fracture of crown or FDP mechanical components, mesial migration of anterior teeth away from posterior implants, and opening posterior contact points.[43–45] Further, it is important, especially in the premaxilla, to carefully consider the occlusion. If single-tooth implants are considered in the premaxilla, the occlusion on the adjacent natural teeth is very important. It is critical that there be definitive occlusal stops created either by the orthodontic phase or by the restorative dentist (using lingual composite stops). This is used to reduce the risk of ongoing passive eruption with time leading to changes in the position of the incisal edge of the natural teeth on either side of the restored oral implant.

Careful oral implant placement in the partially edentulous or single-tooth situation is critical for achieving a predictable esthetic outcome.[46] The initial evaluation considers factors associated with sufficient bone and soft tissue volume. Additionally, the prosthodontist should discuss these risk factors with the patient and members of the implant team. When evaluating any proposed site in all three dimensions for hard and soft tissue contours, the dentist should rely on clinical observations, mounted diagnostic casts, and a diagnostic wax-up. The evaluation of the soft-tissue contours for shape, quantity, texture, and color should include noting the parameters of the diagnostic wax-up for generation of radiographic and surgical guides. A thick periodontal tissue biotype typically has thick flattened osseous plates and offers a higher resistance to recession than a thin tissue biotype, especially on the mid-facial aspect. Long-term facial bone loss, especially in a thin tissue biotype, can be pronounced, regardless of whether an implant is placed or not. It may be useful to evaluate the gingiva on the contralateral tooth/teeth to consider size, shape, and color of the interdental papillae, the arcuate form of the free marginal gingiva, the relative root shape and size (i.e., transition contour of the abutment and restorative emergence profile), along with the width of attached gingiva and facial root prominence (Figure 13.5i–n).[47–50] Consideration should be given to using soft tissue augmentation procedures in sites of thin tissue biotype as previously discussed. In situations posing high risk of gingival recession, a screw-retained crown or prosthesis should be considered instead of a cemented prosthesis. This approach allows contours to be modified, especially if changes occur due to occlusion and/or growth.

The most uncomfortable aspect of implant dentistry is critically evaluating our outcomes. In conventional discussions of dental occlusion, there is often an emphasis on the static nature of occlusion (e.g., tripod occlusal schemes), implying that establishment of such approaches would protect the patient from long-term complications.[51] Implant dentistry, utilizing the common endosseous implant designs, has only existed in the US since the 1980s. As restored patients age, we are observing some old and new complications, which are worth discussing. Since oral implants act as a rigid anchorage to bone, their position allows for an accurate fiduciary marker for craniofacial growth.[52] In the "skeletally mature" adult, restored with oral implants, two common observations are made. One is that in certain patients with an orthognathic short facial height, as growth continues, an oral implant placed will tend to "drift" towards the palate, not because of the implant but due to mid-face growth directed from the mid-face growth plate.[53] Implants therefore become more palatally positioned as passive growth continues, especially those in the posterior maxilla.

Patients with a statistically "long" facial height present within a continuum in which there is a trend for more midface vertical growth. In this case, in some individuals there is the occlusal risk of managing passive eruption (common in every patient), along with a genetically defined risk for greater midface growth throughout life. The consequence of this has been explored in the orthodontic literature with measurements of midface growth for cohorts longitudinally followed for greater than 20 years. The underlying issue is the range of diversity in human response. Occlusion is inherently dynamic and the use of implants provides wonderful examples of this. The most significant issue is to provide patients with the current best evidence.

Conclusions

Providing tooth replacement therapy for missing teeth plays a strong role in the physiological, emotional, and physiological support of our patients. Understanding and conveying the strengths and challenges of the proposed care plan is a vital part of the health literacy process. Oral healthcare needs to start in the first year of life and interdisciplinary care is needed between all of the oral health specialties as the patient moves from childhood, though adolescence, and into adulthood. An important underlying feature is to provide care without being excessively aggressive and to allow the patient to continue to have as many options as possible throughout their life.

References

1. Craniofacial anomalies and associated birth defects. http://www.who.int/genomics/anomalies/en/Chapter02.pdf [accessed 16 May 2016].
2. Types of ectodermal dysplasias. http://nfed.org/index.php/about_ed/types_of_ectodermal_dysplasias [accessed 16 May 2016].
3. What is hypohidrotic ectodermal dysplasia? http://nfed.org/index.php/about_ed/hypohidrotic-ectodermal-dysplasia [accessed 16 May 2016].
4. Carmichael RP, Sandor GK. Use of dental implants in the management of syndromal oligodontia. *Atlas Oral Maxillofac Surg Clin North Am* 2008; **16**(1): 33–47.
5. Freire-Maia N, Pinheiro M. Ectodermal dysplasias – some recollections and a classification. *Birth Defects Orig Artic Ser* 1988; **24**(2): 3–14.
6. Paulus C, Martin P. Hypodontia due to ectodermal dysplasia: rehabilitation with very early dental implants. *Rev Stomatol Chir Maxillofac Chir Orale* 2013; **114**(3): e5–8.
7. Diz P, Scully C, Sanz M. Dental implants in the medically compromised patient. *J Dent* 2013; **41**(3): 195–206.
8. Al-Ibrahim HA, Al-Hadlaq SM, Abduljabbar TS, *et al.* Surgical and implant-supported fixed prosthetic treatment of a patient with ectodermal dysplasia: a case report. *Spec Care Dentist* 2012; **32**(1): 1–5.
9. Bidra AS, Martin JW, Feldman E. Complete denture prosthodontics in children with ectodermal dysplasia: review of principles and techniques. *Comp Cont Educ Dent* 2010; **31**(6): 426–433.
10. Van Sickels JE, Raybould TP, Hicks EP. Interdisciplinary management of patients with ectodermal dysplasia. *J Oral Implantol* 2010; **36**(3): 239–245.
11. Cronin RJ Jr, Oesterle LJ. Implant use in growing patients. Treatment planning concerns. *Dent Clin North Am* 1998; **42**(1): 1–34.
12. Yap AK, Klineberg I. Dental implants in patients with ectodermal dysplasia and tooth agenesis: a critical review of the literature. *Int J Prosthodont* 2009; **22**(3): 268–276.
13. Klineberg I, Cameron A, Hobkirk J, *et al.* Rehabilitation of children with ectodermal dysplasia. Part 2: an international consensus meeting. *Int J Oral Maxillofac Implants* 2013; **28**(4): 1101–1019.
14. Klineberg I, Cameron A, Whittle T, *et al.* Rehabilitation of children with ectodermal dysplasia. Part 1: an international Delphi study. *Int J Oral Maxillofac Implants* 2013; **28**(4): 1090–1100.
15. Bassi F, Carr AB, Chang TL, *et al.* Economic outcomes in prosthodontics. *Int J Prosthodont* 2013; **26**(5): 465–469.
16. Bassi F, Carr AB, Chang TL, *et al.* Psychologic outcomes in implant prosthodontics. *Int J Prosthodont* 2013; **26**(5): 429–434.
17. Bassi F, Carr AB, Chang TL, *et al.* Functional outcomes for clinical evaluation of implant restorations. *Int J Prosthodont* 2013; **26**(5): 411–418.
18. Bassi F, Carr AB, Chang TL, *et al.* Clinical outcomes measures for assessment of longevity in the dental implant literature: ORONet approach. *Int J Prosthodont* 2013; **26**(4): 323–330.
19. Bassi F, Carr AB, Chang TL, *et al.* Oral Rehabilitation Outcomes Network – ORONet. *Int J Prosthodont* 2013; **26**(4): 319–322.
20. Stanford CM, Guckes A, Fete M, *et al.* Perceptions of outcomes of implant therapy in patients with ectodermal dysplasia syndromes. *Int J Prosthodont* 2008; **21**(3): 195–200.
21. Stanford CM. Application of oral implants to the general dental practice. *J Am Dent Assoc* 2005; **136**(8): 1092–1100.
22. De Coster PJ, Marks LA, Martens LC, *et al.* Dental agenesis: genetic and clinical perspectives. *J Oral Pathol Med* 2009; **38**(1): 1–17.
23. Kohli R, Levy S, Kummet CM, *et al.* Comparison of perceptions of oral health-related quality of life in adolescents affected with ectodermal dysplasias relative to caregivers. *Spec Care Dentist* 2011; **31**(3): 88–94.
24. Stanford CM, Wagner W, Rodriguez YBR, *et al.* Evaluation of the effectiveness of dental implant therapy in a practice-based network (FOCUS). *Int J Oral Maxillofac Implants* 2010; **25**(2): 367–373.
25. Ozkurt Z, Kazazoglu E. Clinical success of zirconia in dental applications. *J Prosthodont* 2010; **19**(1): 64–68.
26. Le Fort fracture of skull. https://en.wikipedia.org/wiki/Le_Fort_fracture_of_skull [accessed 16 May 2016].
27. Bergendal B, Ekman A, Nilsson P. Implant failure in young children with ectodermal dysplasia: a retrospective evaluation of use and outcome of dental implant treatment in children in Sweden. *Int J Oral Maxillofac Implants* 2008; **23**(3): 520–524.
28. Dueled E, Gotfredsen K, Trab Damsgaard M, *et al.* Professional and patient-based evaluation of oral rehabilitation in patients with tooth agenesis. *Clin Oral Implants Res* 2009; **20**(7): 729–736.
29. Gong DA, Lee JY, Rozier RG, *et al.* Development and testing of the Test of Functional Health Literacy in Dentistry (TOFHLiD). *J Public Health Dent* 2007; **67**(2): 105–112.
30. Richman JA, Lee JY, Rozier RG, *et al.* Evaluation of a word recognition instrument to test health literacy in dentistry: the REALD-99. *J Public Health Dent* 2007; **67**(2): 99–104.
31. Chalmers I. Well informed uncertainties about the effects of treatments. *BMJ* 2004; **328**(7438): 475–476.
32. Monti P, Russo D, Bocciardi R, *et al.* EEC- and ADULT-associated TP63 mutations exhibit functional heterogeneity toward P63 responsive sequences. *Hum Mutat* 2013; **34**(6): 894–904.
33. Patzelt SB, Bahat O, Reynolds MA, *et al.* The all-on-four treatment concept: a systematic review. *Clin Implant Dent Relat Res* 2014; **16**(6): 836–855.
34. Cooper LF, Pin-Harry OC. "Rules of six" – diagnostic and therapeutic guidelines for single-tooth implant success. *Comp Cont Educ Dent* 2013; **34**(2): 94–101.
35. Sanz M, Cecchinato D, Ferrus J, *et al.* Implants placed in fresh extraction sockets in the maxilla: clinical and radiographic outcomes from a 3-year follow-up examination. *Clin Oral Implants Res* 2013; **25**(3): 321–327.
36. Lindhe J, Bressan E, Cecchinato D, *et al.* Bone tissue in different parts of the edentulous maxilla and mandible. *Clin Oral Implants Res* 2013; **24**(4): 372–377.

37. Januario AL, Duarte WR, Barriviera M, *et al.* Dimension of the facial bone wall in the anterior maxilla: a cone-beam computed tomography study. *Clin Oral Implants Res* 2011; **22**(10): 1168–1171.
38. Araujo MG, Lindhe J. Socket grafting with the use of autologous bone: an experimental study in the dog. *Clin Oral Implants Res* 2011; **22**(1): 9–13.
39. Huynh-Ba G, Pjetursson BE, Sanz M, *et al.* Analysis of the socket bone wall dimensions in the upper maxilla in relation to immediate implant placement. *Clin Oral Implants Res* 2010; **21**(1): 37–42.
40. Tomasi C, Sanz M, Cecchinato D, *et al.* Bone dimensional variations at implants placed in fresh extraction sockets: a multilevel multivariate analysis. *Clin Oral Implants Res* 2010; **21**(1): 30–36.
41. Stanford CM. Issues and considerations in dental implant occlusion: what do we know, and what do we need to find out? *J Calif Dent Assoc* 2005; **33**(4): 329–336.
42. Klineberg I, Murray G. Osseoperception: sensory function and proprioception. *Adv Dent Res* 1999; **13**: 120–129.
43. Goodacre CJ, Kan JY, Rungcharassaeng K. Clinical complications of osseointegrated implants. *J Prosthet Dent* 1999; **81**(5): 537–552.
44. Papaspyridakos P, Chen CJ, Chuang SK, *et al.* A systematic review of biologic and technical complications with fixed implant rehabilitations for edentulous patients. *Int J Oral Maxillofac Implants* 2012; **27**(1): 102–110.
45. Olsson M, Gunne J, Astrand P, *et al.* Bridges supported by free-standing implants versus bridges supported by tooth and implant. A five-year prospective study. *Clin Oral Implants Res* 1995; **6**(2): 114–121.
46. Stanford CM, Maze G. Prosthetic considerations for implant surgery. *Pract Proced Aesthet Dent* 2006; **18**(5): 8.
47. Bidra AS. Three-dimensional esthetic analysis in treatment planning for implant-supported fixed prosthesis in the edentulous maxilla: review of the esthetics literature. *J Esthetic Restorative Dent* 2011; **23**(4): 219–236.
48. Kan JY, Rungcharassaeng K, Liddelow G, *et al.* Periimplant tissue response following immediate provisional restoration of scalloped implants in the esthetic zone: a one-year pilot prospective multicenter study. *J Prosthet Dent* 2007; **97**(6 Suppl): S109–118.
49. Berglundh T, Lindhe J. Dimension of the periimplant mucosa. Biological width revisited. *J Clin Periodontol* 1996; **23**(10): 971–973.
50. Stanford CM. Achieving and maintaining predictable implant esthetics through the maintenance of bone around dental implants. *Comp Cont Educ Dent* 2002; **23**(9 Suppl 2): 13–20.
51. Stanford CM, Brand RA. Toward an understanding of implant occlusion and strain adaptive bone modeling and remodeling. *J Prosthet Dent* 1999; **81**(5): 553–561.
52. Garetto LP, Chen J, Parr JA, *et al.* Remodeling dynamics of bone supporting rigidly fixed titanium implants: a histomorphometric comparison in four species including humans. *Implant Dent* 1995; **4**(4): 235–243.
53. Carmichael RP, Sandor GK. Use of dental implants in the management of syndromal oligodontia. *Atlas Oral Maxillofac Surg Clin North Am* 2008; **16**(1): 33–47.

CHAPTER 14
Occlusion: The Role in Implant Prosthodontics

Avinash S. Bidra and Thomas D. Taylor
University of Connecticut School of Dental Medicine, Farmington, Connecticut, USA

Introduction

It is well recognized that occlusion is one of the most controversial aspects of implant prosthodontics.[1] This is because occlusion in implant prosthodontics has historically evolved through a combination of dogma, expert opinion, *in vitro* studies, animal studies, and extrapolation from concepts used on natural teeth. Interestingly, little scientific evidence exists in the field of occlusion to justify one concept over another. In an extensive review of the occlusion literature, Taylor *et al.*[1] concluded that there is minimal scientific evidence to support a direct cause–effect relationship between occlusal factors and deleterious biological outcomes for osseointegrated implants. The purpose of this chapter is to examine various occlusal considerations and disconsiderations for implant-borne restorations, scrutinize the available and applicable scientific evidence, and lend clarity on this topic to the reader. Recommendations on choice of occlusal schemes are also presented to the reader to simplify and aid in clinical practice.

Occlusal considerations for implant-borne restorations

Crown–implant ratio

The concept of crown–implant ratio has been directly derived from the concept of crown–root ratio described in natural teeth. In natural teeth, crown–root ratio is regarded as an important aspect of diagnosis, treatment planning, and predicting the prognosis of treatment.[2] A favorable crown–root ratio is 1:1.5, while the minimal accepted ratio is 1:1. While the scientific merits to this approach are debatable for natural teeth, it is important to understand that implants do not have the same characteristics as roots of natural teeth, nor can they be subjected to the same principles and rules.[3] A greater crown–implant ratio has been considered to be detrimental by previous authors.[4] However, a recent systematic review that investigated the influence of the crown–implant ratio on the success rate and marginal bone loss of dental implants showed that the higher the crown–implant ratio, the lesser the peri-implant marginal bone loss.[5] There was a significant negative association between the two variables, indicating that a higher crown–implant ratio had a beneficial effect on implants. In implant-borne restorations, crown–implant ratio is merely theoretical, as the height of a crown is dictated by esthetics and distance from the implant platform to the occlusal plane (Figure 14.1). The length of an implant is primarily dictated by the ability to gain primary stability and anatomic limitations (Figure 14.2). Multiple systematic reviews on short implants have shown high survival rates and marginal bone loss comparable to regular-length implants.[5–7] Therefore, once osseointegrated, a short implant is as efficacious as a long implant, and, within the scope of dental occlusion, clinicians may simply ignore the concept of crown–implant ratio as far as protecting the bone adjacent to an implant is concerned. However an increased crown–implant ratio may increase the risk of mechanical complications related to the implant components themselves. One method to reduce mechanical complications in such scenarios is to use an implant design that offers an internal connection for the abutment, whilst the restoration is supported by the implant pillar itself. This concept is similar to the ferrule effect concept used in restoring endodontically treated teeth with dowel and core restorations.

Progressive loading

Progressive loading has been defined as the "concept of gradually increasing the amount of functional load applied to a newly integrated dental implant or implants, by modifying the design and the material of the prosthesis."[8] Misch[3,9] has described that progressive loading can be attained by the practice of increasing occlusal load over a time period of 6 months, and thus provide the requisite time for bone to adapt to loading by a gradual enhancement of loading. Accompanying tenets to this philosophy include

Evidence-based Implant Treatment Planning and Clinical Protocols, First Edition. Edited by Steven J. Sadowsky.

Companion website: www.wiley.com/go/sadowsky/implant

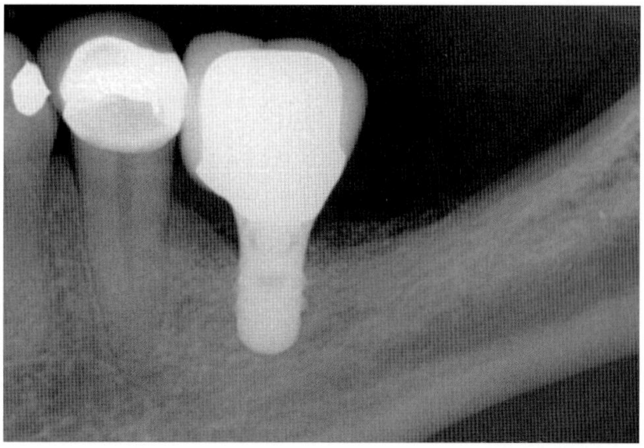

Figure 14.1 Periapical radiograph of a long-term successful outcome from a short implant supported single crown with excessive crown–implant ratio. Notice that the veneering porcelain on the occlusal surface is well supported by the metal coping.

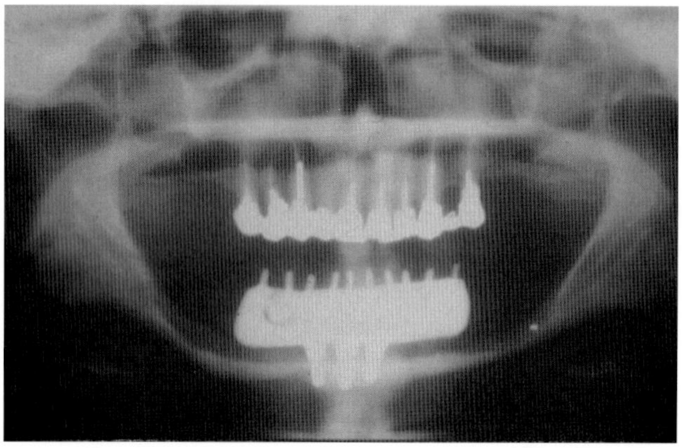

Figure 14.2 Panoramic radiograph of a long-term successful outcome of a mandibular fixed prosthesis with bilateral cantilevers, supported by only three short implants. The implant length was dictated by the height of the residual mandible that was severely resorbed.

using acrylic resin provisional restorations for an extended period of time during "bone adaptation", keeping the implant-borne restoration out of occlusion, and using shallower cusped teeth and a narrower occlusal table in the final restorations. While some of these tenets may be beneficial in patients with bruxism, or in immediate-loading situations, primarily due to risk management and the ease of adjustment, the scientific basis for progressive loading in osseointegrated implants is questionable.

Stegaroiu *et al.*[10] have shown that under static and nonimpact dynamic loading, three different types of superstructure materials tested (highly filled composite resin, acrylic resin, and gold alloy) had the same influence on the strain transmitted to a bone simulant that surrounded a single implant. Other authors have shown similar results, implying that keeping patients in provisional restorations solely for the purpose of progressive loading is a misconception.[11] The laws of physics state that one cannot make mechanical energy disappear simply by changing the material through which a force is applied. Stated another way, a pound applied to the occlusal surface of an implant-supported restoration is a pound transferred through the implant to the surrounding bone, regardless of the material the restoration is made of. With regards to using shallower cusps and reduced width of occlusal table, Morneburg *et al.*[12] have shown that cusp height had no effect in reducing the load on implants. However, severely reducing the occlusal table width by 30% (which is clinically not possible without compromising esthetics and function) did reduce bending forces. This again questions the theory behind progressive loading. Finally, keeping the provisional restorations out of occlusion (or in "progressively light occlusion") during maximum intercuspation is not advisable, because opposing natural teeth may supra-erupt to contact the provisional restoration and disrupt the occlusal plane. Additionally, it is well known that during natural chewing, the food itself acts as a force amplifier, negating the effect of "progressively light occlusion". Therefore, within the scope of dental occlusion, clinicians may ignore the concept of progressive loading in osseointegrated implants.

Occlusal overload

Occlusal overload has been defined as the "application of occlusal loading, through function or parafunction, in excess of what the prosthesis, implant component, or osseointegrated interface is capable of withstanding without structural or biologic damage."[8] To expound the implications of occlusal overload, it is important to first understand Wolff's Law. Wolff's law is defined as "principle of bone healing and/or remodeling based upon the understanding that bone remodels in response to physical stress by depositing bone in locations of increased stress and resorbing bone in areas of little or no stress."[8] It is named after German anatomist Julius Wolff, who first explained this concept. It is widely believed that occlusal overload can cause implant failure by failure of osseointegration, but interestingly the scientific evidence for this concept is lacking. Multiple animal studies have all demonstrated that osseointegrated implants are extremely resistant to occlusal overload.[13–17]

Contrarily, occlusal overload has been shown to promote new dense bone formation around the osseointegrated implants.[17,18] There are no clinical studies on occlusal overload that have demonstrated a cause-and-effect relationship between occlusal overload and loss of osseointegration. One animal study by Isidor *et al.*,[15] done on monkeys, demonstrated loss of implants when they were subjected to an unusually extreme loading environment, beyond what can be considered to be clinically relevant. In a recent systematic review by Chang *et al.*,[19] the authors concluded that there was no scientific evidence to clarify whether occlusal overload may cause marginal bone loss or complete loss of osseointegration when the applied load exceeds the biologically acceptable limit. The authors also stated that this biological limit is presently unknown.[19] Therefore, current scientific evidence does not demonstrate occlusal forces as being a substantial risk factor for the biological aspect of

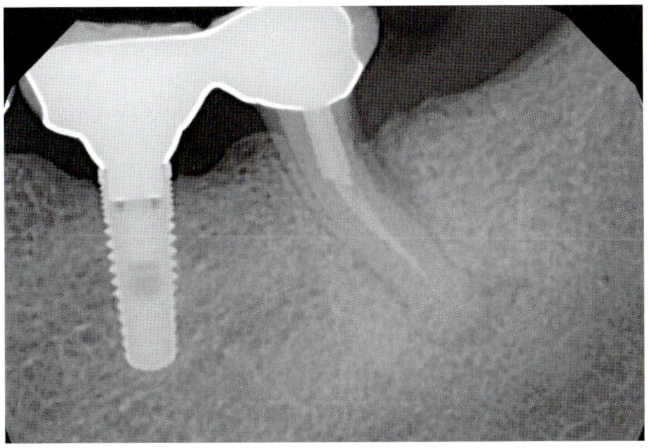

Figure 14.3 Periapical radiograph of a patient with an implant restoration splinted to natural tooth. This patient presented with pain and discomfort that was attributed to the failing natural tooth. *Source:* Reproduced with permission from Dr. Marie Falcone, DMD.

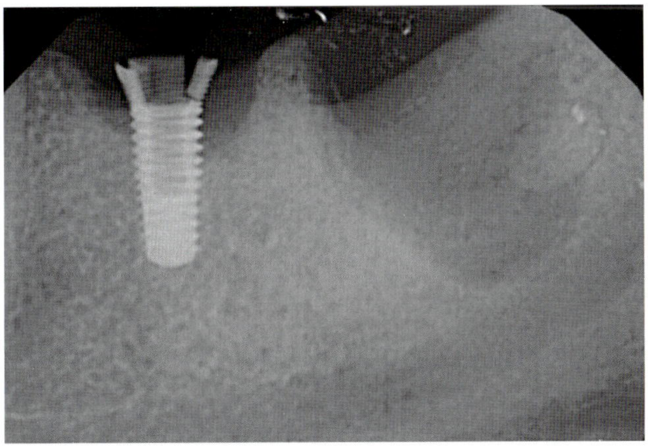

Figure 14.4 Periapical radiograph of patient in Figure 14.3 after removal of the restoration and extraction of the natural tooth indicates a fractured implant. This is a classic appearance of fracture of an internal-connection implant caused by hoop stress. *Source:* Reproduced with permission from Dr. Marie Falcone, DMD.

implant-borne restorations. However, it is important to consider the unfavorable outcomes of occlusal overload on the mechanical aspect of implant-borne restorations. The consequences of these detrimental effects may include fractured implants, fractured abutments, fractured occlusal screws, and, more commonly, fractured veneering resin or porcelain. Of these, fracture of the implant is obviously the most catastrophic complication (Figures 14.3 and 14.4). It is often difficult for clinicians to diagnose (before starting treatment) which patient may have higher occlusal loading and which patient may have parafunctional habits that are detrimental (Figures 14.5 and 14.6). Clinicians should recognize that the osseointegrated interface appears to be very strong and able to withstand occlusal overload within the limits of component structural integrity and appears to be the strongest link in the pillar of implant-borne restorations.

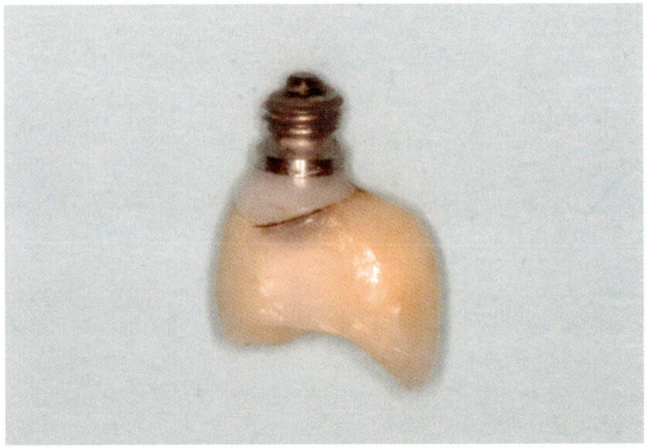

Figure 14.5 Clinical presentation of a fractured implant, which supported a single crown in the maxillary left second premolar region, from a bruxism patient.

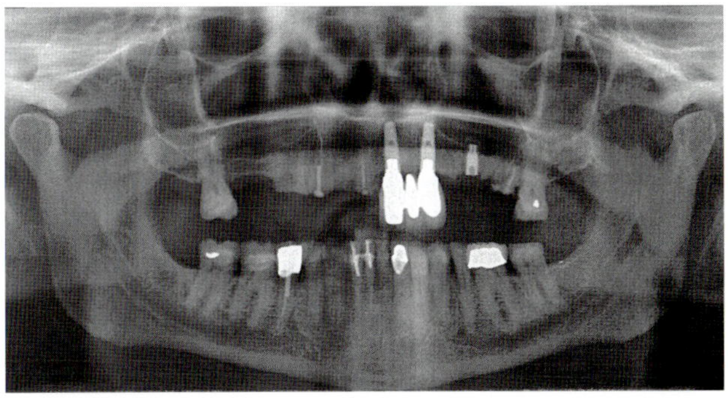

Figure 14.6 Panoramic radiograph of the bruxism patient from Figure 14.5 showing the extent of the fractured implant. Also notice multiple fractured teeth, fractured restorations, multiple missing teeth, as well as an acute gonial angle.

Nonaxial loading

Nonaxial loading refers to "loading of an implant body that is not along the long axis of an implant body,"[8] whereas axial loading refers to "application of load, usually by the forces of occlusion, in the direction of the long axis of an implant body or tooth."[8] It is important to recognize that axial loading is purely theoretical, and, by nature, occlusal forces in the human dentition are nonaxial. Therefore, all implant-borne restorations are subjected to nonaxial loading. A contemporary highly successful prosthodontic treatment that is based on nonaxial loading is the tilted implant concept, popularly known as the All-on-4® concept, which is a testimony to the lack of detrimental effects of nonaxial loading. Additional examples include successful usage of zygoma and pterygoid implants for maxillary rehabilitation (Figure 14.7). In natural teeth, occlusal load is transmitted to the surrounding bone through tensile loading of the periodontal ligament. With implants, the load is transferred directly from the implant to surrounding bone through an ankylotic connection. Previous animal studies have shown no adverse effects on bone surrounding implants, due to nonaxial loading.[20,21] At the same time, it is important to recognize that,

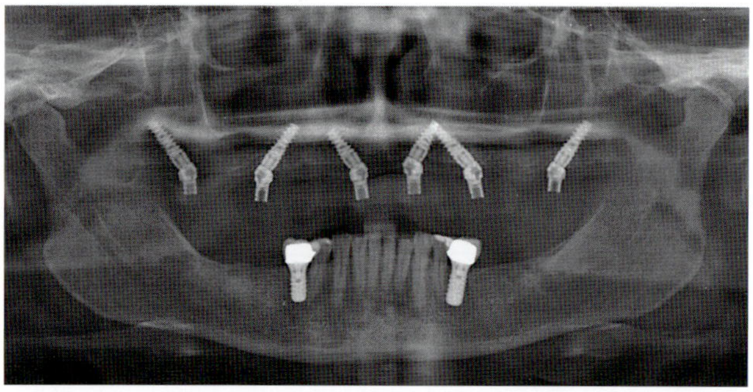

Figure 14.7 Panoramic radiograph showing all six maxillary implants being placed at a 30–45° tilt to overcome anatomic restrictions and allow a successful immediate load of the implants.

beyond a certain threshold, nonaxial loading may create strain through the implant–abutment connection and relative motion between components, and eventually result in prosthetic component flexure, fatigue, and eventual component failure. This may not be true in the presence of cross-arch splinting, as done in complete-arch fixed implant-supported prostheses.

Nature of implant–abutment connection

The nature of the implant–abutment connection can either be external (usually external hex) or internal (numerous designs and shapes). Within the scope of occlusion, it is important to note that load transfer in external hex connections is centripetal in nature, while load transfer in internal connections is usually centrifugal in nature (specifically termed "hoop stress").[22] Hoop stress is the stress in a cylindrical object, acting circumferentially in a plane perpendicular to the longitudinal axis.[22] Due to the higher clamping force (preload) required to secure the abutment in external hex connections, they are susceptible to abutment screw loosening, especially in single-crown restorations. A recent systematic review on clinical outcomes of implant abutments used exclusively in the anterior region (where forces are lower) showed that screw loosening was exclusively seen in external-hex implants and was entirely absent in internal-connection implants.[23] However, a recent study by Chae *et al.*, that compared post-loading complications on 2651 implants, concluded that implants with internal connection were more prone to technical complications, such as loosening or fracture of the abutment or screw, and the external connection was more vulnerable to biological complications, such as increased pocket depth, thread exposure, and soft tissue complications.[24] Whether the results of this large sample study are attributed to the specific implant systems studied should be verified by future clinical trials.

Internal-connection implants are known to offer good anti-rotational resistance, decreased dependence on clamping force, and good resistance to nonaxial loading. However, as these implants are hollow to accommodate the internal connection, they are susceptible to hoop stress, which requires the relatively thin walls of the implant to carry the load (Figure 14.8). Fortunately, the reported prevalence of implant fracture is very

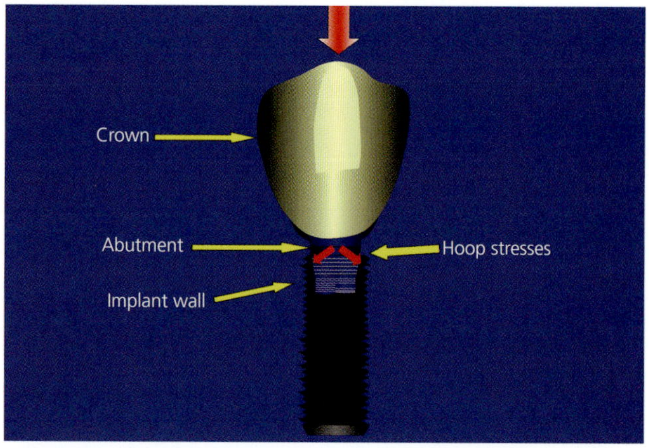

Figure 14.8 Illustration showing the susceptibility of an internal-connection implant to hoop stress, which requires the relatively thin walls of the implant to carry the load due to external-directed (centrifugal) forces.

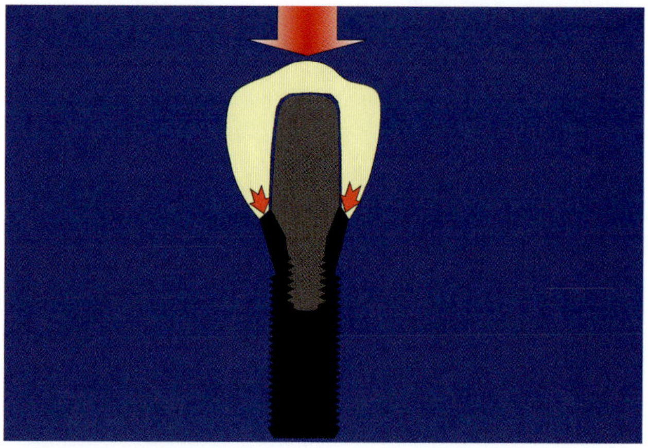

Figure 14.9 Illustration showing the advantage provided to an internal-connection implant when the restoration is supported by the implant pillar itself. In this situation, the implant is loaded by internally directed compressive (centripetal) forces.

low (1%) at the present time.[25] However, fatigue failure related to the implant material itself is an impending threat in the long term. One solution to mitigate this problem and still use an internal-connection implant, is to use an implant design that offers an internal connection for the abutment, whilst the restoration is supported by the implant pillar itself (e.g. Straumann Tissue Level Implant). Thus, the internal-connection implant is now loaded through internally directed compressive forces rather than externally directed hoop stresses (Figure 14.9). This concept is similar to the ferrule effect concept used in restoring endodontically treated teeth.

Passive fit

Passive fit has been defined as "the adaptation of one component to another in a manner that does not impart strain."[8] Achieving passively fitting prostheses is desirable in implant prosthodontics. Popular misconceptions about passive fit have stated that damage to the osseointegrated interface is much more likely to occur from a poorly adapted prosthesis than by the transient forces of occlusion.[3] Additionally, a popular thought has been that nonpassive adaptation creates permanent, unremitting strain between two or more implants. However, the scientific evidence (largely from animal studies) has shown no adverse effects on bone surrounding implants, due to misfit of prosthetic components.[26–31] One clinical study by Jemt *et al.*[27] on 14 patients also concluded that the marginal bone loss around implants was within normal limits when passive fit was absent. Therefore, it can be concluded that nonpassive prosthesis adaptation does not appear to be a major risk factor to the health of the osseointegrated interface.[32]

It is important for clinicians to acknowledge that some degree of passive fit may be important for the success and survival of prosthetic components, including porcelain fracture.[32] It is also important to recognize that some degree of misfit may be present amongst all prosthetic components. The threshold for misfit tolerance before failure of prosthetic components is yet to be defined. Use of computer-aided design and computer-aided manufacturing (CAD/CAM) technology and laser welding technology has certainly improved the passive fit of components compared to the conventional casting and soldering techniques. Currently available tools for the clinician and laboratory technician to verify passive fit of prosthetic components over the implants include: 1) plain visual examination; 2) use of a disclosing medium to aid in visual examination (Figures 14.10 and 14.11); 3) tactile feedback from palpation; 4) tactile feedback from a one-screw test; 5) tactile feedback from a dental plastic explorer; 6) tactile feedback from screw-clamping force; and 7) radiographs. It is obvious that none of these methods appear scientifically sound nor accurately measurable and reproducible. Moreover, passive fit between an abutment and implant is more difficult to verify in implants with internal connection using the above techniques, and this does not provide confidence of passive fit to the clinician. Finally, it is important to recognize that passive fit in cement-retained restorations can result in less strain between implants, compared to screw-retained restorations.[33,34] This is perhaps due to the cement behaving as the "slop factor" or as a gasket and ameliorating the adverse effects of increased preload of the abutment screw or occlusal screw.

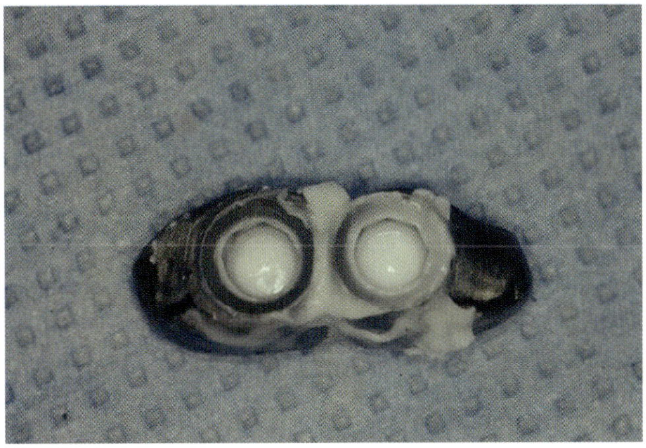

Figure 14.10 Image showing initial attempt at obtaining a complete and passive seating of a splinted implant-supported restoration using a silicone disclosing medium.

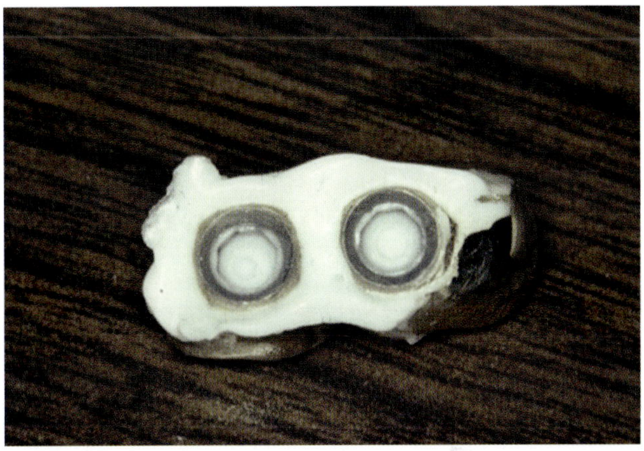

Figure 14.11 Image of the same restoration as Figure 14.10, after adjustments of internal aspect, and proximal contacts show complete seating as revealed by the silicone disclosing medium.

Splinting

The concept of splinting implants to decrease the force magnification around osseointegrated implants is debatable. Scientific evidence is lacking on the beneficial effects of splinting for the osseointegrated interface itself. A recent 10-year follow-up randomized controlled trial (RCT) study on 44 patients by Vigolo *et al.* reported that there was no difference in crestal bone loss with splinted or nonsplinted designs.[35] As discussed in the topic of occlusal overload, once osseointegration has been achieved, occlusal overload may only play a role in component failure rather than osseointegration failure. The advantages of splinting two or three adjacent implants is primarily a clinical decision, which provides the advantage of minimizing the number of adjustable proximal contacts at the time of insertion. However, the disadvantages to this approach include potential for compromised patient's oral hygiene performance, as well as the need for remake of the entire prosthesis should the veneering ceramic fracture. Splinting multiple restorations is an obvious choice when a distal or mesial cantilever is necessary. Splinting across the arch (or commonly called cross-arch splinting), as done in complete-arch fixed implant-supported prostheses, provides the opportunity for simplicity of the prosthetic design and may avoid remaking the prosthesis if there is a future failure of one of the implants. However, cross-arch splinting does compromise the patient's oral hygiene performance as well as repair of the prosthesis. Therefore, screw-retained prosthesis is the obvious choice in such situations.

Splinting of implants to natural teeth should be avoided because of risk of intrusion of the natural tooth or teeth, and risk of secondary caries and periodontal disease resulting in failure of the entire prosthesis. Finally, the opportunity to obtain an adequately fitting prosthesis on the implant abutments and with closed margins on the natural teeth is challenging. In a recent systematic review on splinting natural teeth to implants for fixed prosthesis, intrusion of the abutment teeth occurred in about 5% of cases (all were nonrigid connectors), and about 10% of natural teeth were lost after 10 years. Loss of implants or implant fractures was 15.6% after 10 years, resulting in the survival rate of splinted tooth and implant-supported restorations at 77.8% after 10 years.[36] Another systematic review showed a survival rate of 77.7% in the fixed prostheses connected to natural teeth and implants.[37] These data are compelling enough to suggest clinicians should avoid splinting implants to natural teeth.

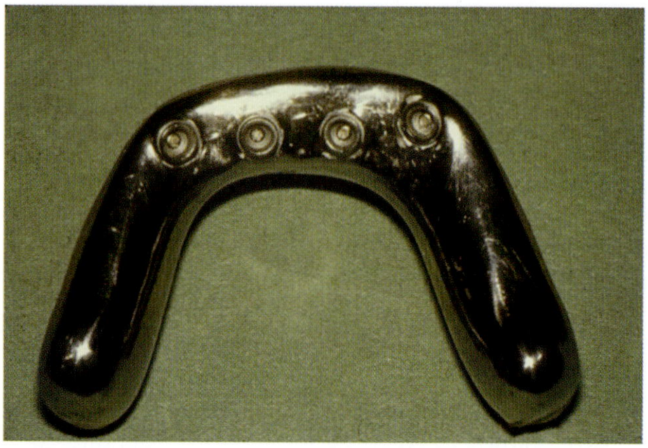

Figure 14.12 Image of a cast metal–resin mandibular fixed prosthesis showing excessive cantilever. This type of cantilever is detrimental to the prosthetic components but not necessarily detrimental to the osseointegration surface itself.

Cantilevers

Cantilevers in completely edentulous patients treated with implant-supported fixed prostheses have been used in since the evolution of osseointegration.[38] They have a long track record of successful usage for complete-arch fixed implant-supported prostheses in the edentulous jaw.[39] This is perhaps due to the cross-arch splinting and the load-distribution mechanism (Figure 14.12). However, the data are largely restricted to the edentulous mandible, while there are minimal data for the edentulous maxilla. Based on the theoretical models of anterior–posterior (AP) spread, *in vitro* studies, and empiricism, a cantilever length of 1.5 times the AP spread has been adopted for the mandible by clinicians worldwide.[40] This model is not applicable for the maxilla, where reduced cantilever length is usually favored due the biomechanical considerations of the moving mandible that occludes against it. The scientific evidence indicates no adverse effects to bone adjacent to implants due to cantilevers, as discussed in the section of occlusal overload.[41] A clinical retrospective study by Shakleton *et al.*[42] on 28 edentulous jaws with fixed prostheses (24 mandibles and four maxillae) compared patients with cantilevers less than 15 mm, to patients with cantilevers greater than 15 mm. They also subdivided cantilevers as right and left sides. The authors showed that prostheses with cantilevers less than or equal to 15 mm had significantly higher prosthetic survival rate (and reduced mechanical complications) than prostheses with cantilevers greater than 15 mm. It is well known that 15 mm is the average width of two premolars, implying that these posterior teeth could be cantilevered if implants are placed in the anterior region of the edentulous jaw. However, the type of prosthesis in the opposing jaw, nature of the prosthetic biomaterial, and amount of prosthetic space should be carefully considered. Gallucci *et al.*[43] showed that, in 45 mandibular edentulous patients with average cantilever length of 15 mm, there were more mechanical complications related to the prosthesis, and the implants themselves had a 100% survival rate.

Cantilevers in partially edentulous patients have been widely used in the maxilla and mandible, primarily to overcome anatomic restrictions.[44–46] Based on short-term and medium-term studies on cantilevered FDP, it is clear that there are no differences in marginal bone levels between partial FDPs, with or without cantilevers. However, mechanical complications are frequently observed in prostheses with cantilevers.[46] This may be sufficient to warrant careful consideration and not to opt for cantilever restorations as a first choice in treatment planning. A systematic review by Aglietta *et al.* identified multiple mechanical complications in cantilever restorations and lack of evidence on the influence of mesial or distal cantilevers on mechanical complications.[47] However, as forces are much higher in the posterior regions of the jaw, it can be suggested that mesial cantilevers may be preferable to distal cantilevers in partial FDPs. Within the scope of dental occlusion, clinicians should be prepared to deal with future technical complications when cantilevers are chosen. The difference in cost and long-term patient satisfaction between use of a cantilevered prosthesis versus preprosthetic surgery and placement of an additional implant, versus avoidance of cantilever with a shortened dental arch is an area that needs further exploration.

Bruxism

Bruxism has been defined by the glossary of prosthodontics terms as: "an oral habit consisting of involuntary rhythmic or spasmodic nonfunctional gnashing, grinding, or clenching of teeth, in other than chewing movements of the mandible, which may lead to occlusal trauma."[48] In the glossary of oral and maxillofacial terms, it has been defined as the "involuntary grinding, clenching, or gnashing of teeth."[8] This parafunctional activity may occur either diurnally and/or nocturnally and commonly results in excessive occlusal wear, periodontal trauma, pain, and neuromuscular problems. It is a complex condition of multifactorial etiologies that is not well understood and is linked to a central nervous system disorder.[49] Irrespective of the etiology, treatment of bruxism patients will require in-depth education of the patient, risk management, clinical precautions, and lifelong dental professional maintenance. Recent findings have

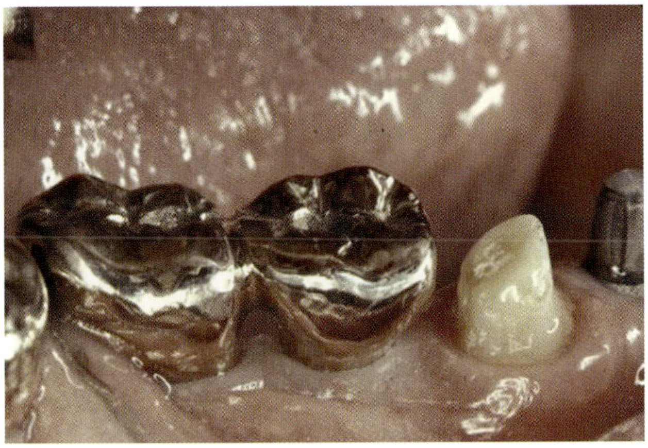

Figure 14.13 Use of implant-supported cast gold restorations in a patient with severe bruxism.

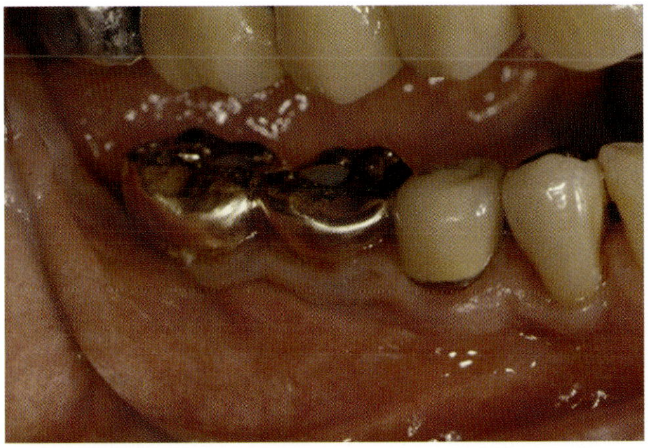

Figure 14.14 Image of the same patient from Figure 14.13, at a 10-year follow-up showing wear facets and changes in soft tissue but absence of restoration failure.

suggested that in patients with natural dentition, bruxism cannot cause periodontal damage *per se*.[50] With respect to dental implants, multiple systematic reviews have suggested that it is unlikely that it has any effect on the osseointegration interface.[51,52]

Bruxism does, however, pose a high risk for mechanical complications related to prosthetic components. Therefore, it is necessary to take prophylactic steps in the management of dental occlusion in the bruxism patient. Some suggestions include: 1) mutually protected articulation scheme with canine disclusion; 2) use of monolithic restorative materials with a long track record on at least the occlusal surface (Figures 14.13 and 14.14); 3) limiting or avoidance of cantilevers; 4) choosing an implant design that minimizes or eliminates hoop stresses; 5) fixed prosthetic design that is easily retrievable for the likely necessity of repairs and maintenance; 6) fabrication of a protective occlusal device; and 7) patient education and institution of a lifelong professional maintenance regimen. The need for occlusal devices in bruxism patients undergoing implant therapy was recently questioned in a systematic review which showed that presently there is no scientific evidence to support the use of occlusal devices.[53] However, the risk-to-benefit ratio and the minimal invasiveness of fabricating an occlusal device is quite low, so they can be recommended as a safeguard to protect the expensive restorations in these patients. An empirical suggestion, based on the author's experience, for successful management of repeated prosthesis fractures in a complete-arch fixed implant-supported prosthesis, is to revert to an implant-supported overdenture. This will allow simplified and inexpensive repair or remake procedures, allows the patient to function with a spare prosthesis, and allows the patient to remove the prosthesis during sleep (in cases of nocturnal bruxism). It would be helpful to provide patients with two overdentures in such situations, so that in the likely event of a fracture/prosthetic complication, the patient can wear the second overdenture while the first overdenture is being repaired.

Absence of proprioception

Proprioception is the perception of movement and spatial orientation of the body or parts of the body.[54] It is defined as the "the reception of stimulation of sensory nerve terminals within the tissues of the body that give information concerning movements and the position of the body; perception mediated by proprioceptors."[48] The scientific evidence is clear that loss of the periodontal ligament affects sensory perception and that implants are not as discriminating as natural teeth.[55–58] However, the difference in sensory perception in implant restorations may not be clinically significant, since proprioceptive nerve endings are still present in the mucosa, periosteum, muscles of mastication, and temporomandibular joint and capsule. Jacobs and van Steenberghe[54] have described the term "osseoperception" as the specialized sensory perception that patients with implants may develop within a few months following implant placement. A peripheral feedback pathway may be reestablished allowing physiologic integration of the implant in the human body and more natural function. The validity and testimony of all of these concepts is provided by the consistently high patient satisfaction rates after implant therapy across the world.

It is well recognized that the threshold for passive tactile sensitivity perceived for dental implants is significantly higher than for natural teeth.[53,55] Jacobs and van Steenberghe[59] showed that the threshold level of implants is 50 times higher than that of natural teeth when tapping was avoided, which might otherwise trigger distant receptors. Similarly Hammerle *et al.*[57] showed that the mean threshold values for implants were 8.75 times higher than for teeth. It is not known if the difference in the threshold for passive tactile sensitivity is of clinical consequence. One possible clinical implication is that it behooves clinicians to accurately confirm for uniform occlusal contacts, especially around existing natural teeth, during insertion of implant-borne restorations (Figure 14.15). Absence of proprioception has often incorrectly been attributed as the main cause for mechanical complications (including fractured porcelain or other prosthetic

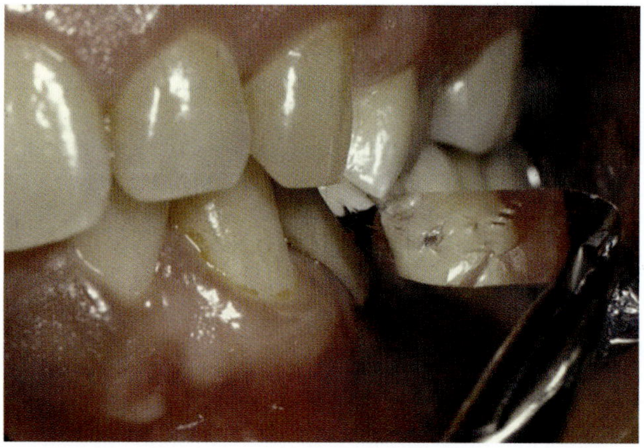

Figure 14.15 Image showing use of an 8 μm shim stock to confirm occlusal contacts of natural teeth while inserting a posterior implant-supported restoration.

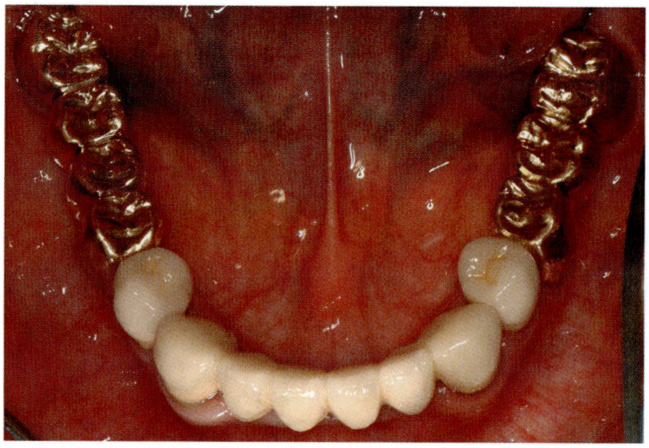

Figure 14.16 Occlusal view of a patient with severe bruxism being restored with cast gold restorations in the second premolar and molar regions (where forces are significantly higher) and restored with metal–ceramic restorations in the remaining natural teeth.

components) in implant-borne restorations. These complications are a result of a myriad of factors that have been discussed thus far, including the simple laboratory error of providing unsupported veneering porcelain for restorations. However, when edentulous patients have both jaws restored with fixed implant-supported prostheses, it is likely that these patients may have more mechanical complications as they are more proprioceptively challenged.[60,61]

Occlusal materials

A large number of biomaterials have evolved in implant prosthodontics with many having little or no long-term scientific evidence. The most common occlusal materials used currently in implant dentistry are: 1) resin (acrylic resin, composite resin); 2) metal alloy (high noble, noble, base metal, milled titanium); and 3) ceramic (feldspathic supported by metal coping, lithium disilicate, zirconia). Some of these materials can be used in a monolithic form and some are required to be blended, for use in a bi-layered form. Historically, resin occlusal surfaces were advocated by Branemark in order to provide a "cushioning effect" over the implants to compensate for the resilience of the periodontium and allow the occlusal surface to be the weakest link in an implant-borne restoration.[38] With improved understanding of the osseointegration interface, and increased application of implants for replacing single and multiple missing teeth in partially edentulous spaces, the use of metal alloys and ceramic as an occlusal surface became popular. Presently, there is no scientific evidence for breakdown of osseointegration due to differences in occlusal material. Additionally, there appears to be no difference in the strain transmitted to the bone by different occlusal materials.[10]

Despite this, fracture of the occlusal material is one of the most common complications that have been reported in the literature.[25,46] Historically, denture teeth were designed for use in complete dentures, and they were conveniently adopted by clinicians and laboratory technicians for fixed implant-supported prostheses, primarily due to their decreased cost. However, there is minimal evidence to show that these denture teeth can withstand the long-term load in an increased masticatory load environment in patients with fixed implant-supported prostheses. Significant wear and fracture of the resin denture teeth in complete-arch fixed implant-supported prostheses is now widely recognized as a consequence (rather than as a complication) of prosthodontic treatment. Purcell *et al.* noted that patients were 52.5 times more likely to need posterior tooth replacement at over 5 years than at less than 2 years in mandibular metal–resin fixed prostheses.[62] At the same time, ceramic fracture in SCs and FDPs is reported to be as high as 20.3%.[63] This is obviously unfavorable to both clinicians and patients and renders the true endpoint of implant therapy (patient satisfaction) discouraging. To mitigate ceramic fracture problem (especially in bruxism patients), occlusal materials with a long-term track record could be used. Complete-coverage gold (cast or milled) is a simple monolithic restoration that has a long track record that may be an acceptable material especially in bruxism patients (Figure 14.16). If the color of gold is objectionable to patients, then conventional metal–ceramic restorations with metal on the occlusal surface and porcelain on the facial surface can satisfy both purposes (Figure 14.17). However, patients should be cautioned that depending upon their physical height, there could be display of metal during speech or laughter. Bruxism patients objecting to this metal display should be offered the option of monolithic ceramic materials, but educated about the lack of long-term data on monolithic zirconia and lithium disilicate, especially for implant-supported restorations.

Reasons for ceramic fracture have been traditionally assigned to previously discussed factors such as occlusal overload, and absence of proprioception. However, an important factor may be found in the design and construction of implant-supported restorations by the dental laboratory. Metal–ceramic restorations

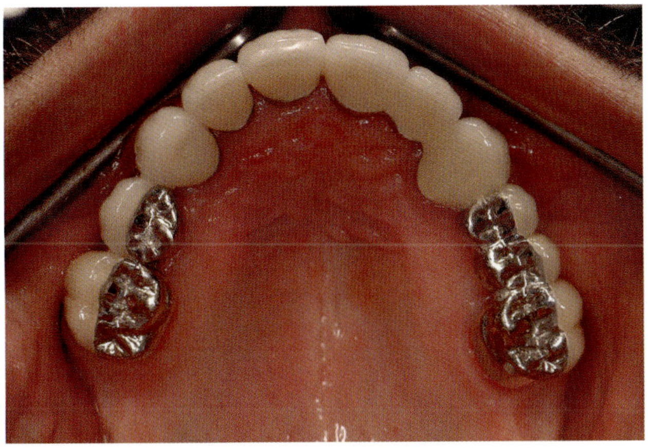

Figure 14.17 Occlusal view of a patient with severe bruxism who declined cast gold restorations. Metal occlusion can prevent porcelain fracture, which is a common implant occlusion complication. Monolithic zirconia or lithium disilicate restorations are alternatives to a metal occlusal surface.

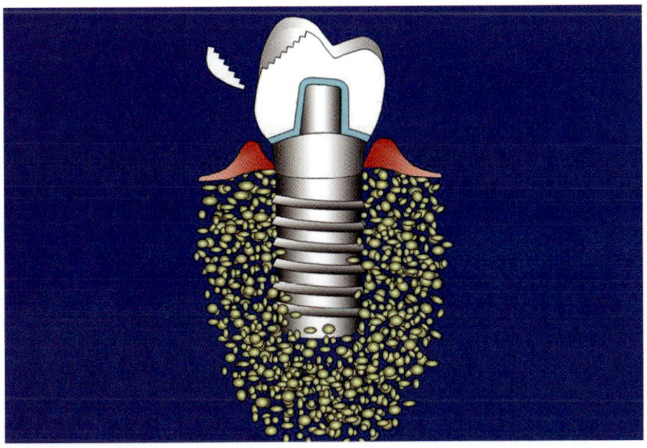

Figure 14.18 Illustration showing the common reason for fracture of porcelain in an implant- supported restoration. The inner metal/ceramic coping lacks normal tooth preparation contours and the final restoration results in the build-up of excess veneering porcelain that has a high risk of fracture. *Source:* Figure courtesy of Dr. Reza Kazemi, DDS.

are still popular for implant-supported single crowns (SCs) and fixed dental prosheses (FDPs) due to their long track record, strength, and acceptable esthetics. In a natural tooth situation, the tooth is prepared for a crown by relatively uniform reduction of normal tooth contours to create space for the restoration. When an implant-supported restoration is fabricated, it is frequently created from a prefabricated coping provided by the implant manufacturer. The coping lacks normal tooth preparation contours and the final restoration may result in the build-up of excess veneering porcelain. The resulting unsupported porcelain is more susceptible to fracture (Figure 14.18). One solution for this problem is to use custom abutments (manually or digitally fabricated) that allow for uniform thickness of the substructure coping and occlusal porcelain (Figure 14.19). A second solution is to fabricate a coping (manually or digitally) to

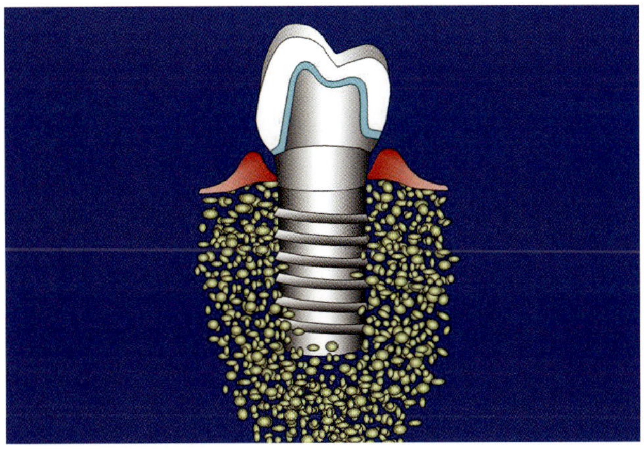

Figure 14.19 Illustration showing that custom abutment can more closely reflect the shape of the final restoration and minimize porcelain fracture. *Source:* Figure courtesy of Dr. Reza Kazemi, DDS.

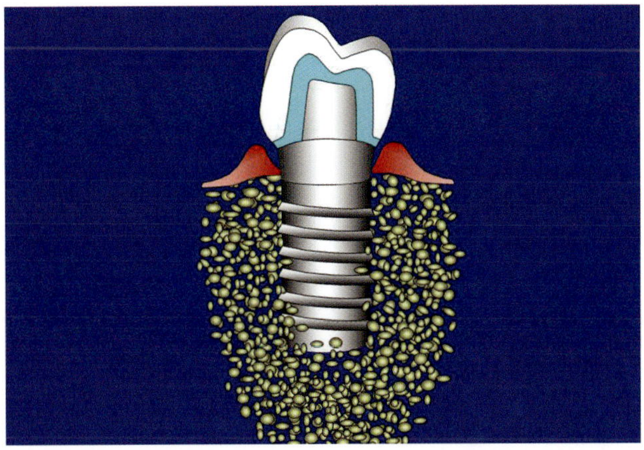

Figure 14.20 By requesting that the dental laboratory technician generate a full contour wax-up of the final restoration and then manually trimming back by 1.5–2 mm to make space for veneering porcelain of even thickness, the risk for porcelain fracture is minimized. *Source:* Figure courtesy of Dr. Reza Kazemi, DDS.

closely reflect the final contour of the anticipated implant-supported restoration (Figure 14.20). This can be accomplished by waxing (manual or digital) to full contour, and then manually trimming back by 1.5–2 mm before casting in metal, to make space for a 1.5–2 mm veneering porcelain of even thickness. Many dentists and dental laboratories around the world use base metal alloys (usually cobalt–chromium) in order to reduce metal alloy costs, compared to noble and high noble alloys. From classic fixed prosthodontics, it is well known that base metal alloys form thicker oxides and are detrimental to porcelain bonding.[64,65] While high noble alloys (containing gold) are the ideal alloys to cast and minimize porcelain fracture, their high cost precludes most clinicians from using them. It is advisable to use noble alloys as they offer similar advantages at a reduced cost. Clinicians should request the alloy certificate for each implant restoration and store it as a permanent part of the patient's treatment record.

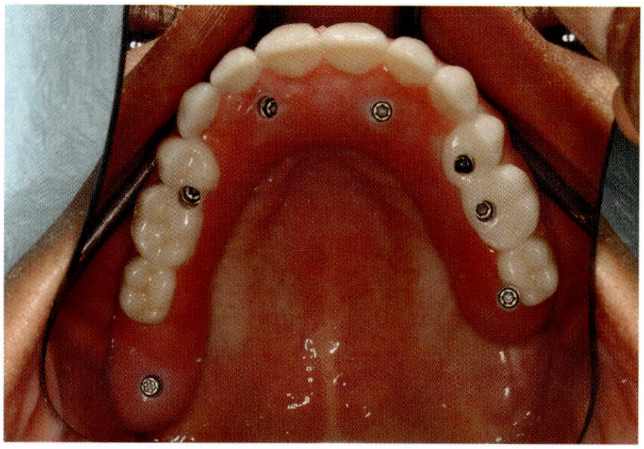

Figure 14.21 Occlusal view of a maxillary complete-arch implant-supported fixed prosthesis fabricated with monolithic zirconia with minimal veneering of porcelain only in the gingival region. Monolithic zirconia is an emerging material that is highly esthetic compared to resin and has promising potential to decrease occlusal material complications.

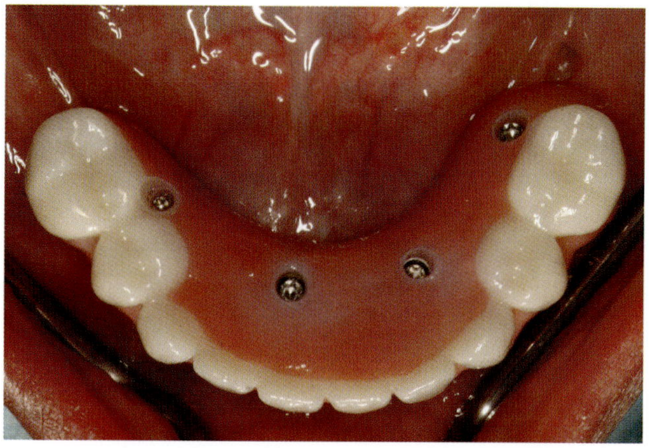

Figure 14.22 Occlusal view of a mandibular complete-arch implant-supported fixed prosthesis in the same patient shown in Figure 14.21, fabricated with monolithic zirconia with minimal veneering of porcelain only in the gingival region.

All-ceramic restorations have an emerging popularity in implant prosthodontics, primarily due to improved esthetics, relatively lower cost, and manufacturer's warranty. However, long-term data on clinical outcomes for materials like zirconia and lithium disilicate (in monolithic or bilayered form) for implant restorations are presently lacking for implants as well as for natural teeth restorations.[66,67] Therefore, clinicians should follow the same precautions of avoiding unsupported veneering porcelain. Additionally, for implant-supported FDPs, it is advisable to use metal–ceramic materials given their long-term successful track record for several decades. Presently, there is a lack of evidence for using popular all-ceramic materials, such as lithium disilicate, for FDPs, especially in the posterior region, and caution is advised for their use in the clinical setting.[66]

With the confluence of advancements of digital dentistry and all-ceramic materials, an emerging trend is the use of monolithic occlusal materials such as zirconia and lithium disilicate for implant-supported crowns and FDPs. They are especially useful in patients with bruxism and other parafunctional habits. One recognized disadvantage of these materials is their difficulty in occlusal adjustment and polishing after adjustment, which may cause increased wear of opposing dentition. Additionally, it is difficult to add minor interproximal contacts and missing occlusal contacts to a monolithic designed restoration. However, they offer a significant advantage over gold-colored or metal-colored occlusal surfaces that are often considered objectionable to patients. For complete-arch fixed implant-supported prostheses, an emerging material is monolithic zirconia, with either stained or minimally veneered gingival porcelain (Figures 14.21 and 14.22). This prosthesis eliminates the possibility of veneering occlusal material fracture that is common with resin or porcelain, and offers superior esthetics and high strength. Moreover, this prosthesis is relatively inexpensive and backed by manufacturer's warranty or dental laboratory warranty, ranging from 5 to 7 years. Until further scientific evidence is available, it is suggested that clinicians should monitor their outcomes with emerging materials and have a clear understanding of manufacturer's warranty and their dental laboratory's service warranty before universally embracing these modern materials.

Screw retention versus cement retention of restorations

The debate between screw-retained restorations and cement-retained restorations has spanned at least two decades, resulting in multiple clinical studies and multiple systematic reviews, all of which have offered minimal conclusive evidence.[68–73] It is obvious from this debate that there are advantages and disadvantages to each method of retention. However, the literature is not clear on elucidating screw-retention outcomes with external-connection implants versus internal-connection implants. Additionally, screw-retention outcomes at implant level (which uses the longer abutment screw) versus screw-retention outcomes at abutment level (which uses the smaller occlusal/prosthetic screw) have not been clarified and compared. It is also important for clinicians to avoid grouping the advantages and disadvantages of each type of restoration in general, but rather to examine them distinctly for each region of the mouth (anterior versus posterior versus complete arch) and type of restoration (SC, FDP, or complete-arch fixed implant-supported prostheses).

In complete-arch fixed implant-supported prostheses, screw retention is an obvious choice due to easier retrievability and opportunity for future revisions. In the anterior region, where masticatory forces and mechanical complications are lower, it may be preferable for both SCs and FDPs to be screw-retained, due to numerous biological and restorative advantages, such as: 1) improved soft tissue outcomes;[74] 2) increased buccal bone thickness and gingival esthetics due to palatal positioning of the implant; 3) improved dental ceramic esthetics of the restoration due to increased availability of facial restorative space for technician; 4) easier retrievability and adjustments to accommodate for long-term changes in growth, color, and contours with respect to adjacent teeth; and 5) elimination of the catastrophic biological and esthetic failure related to potential residual excess cement. In a recent systematic review, screw loosening in the maxillary anterior region was minimal (1%) and was exclusively seen in implants with an external connection, indicating that perhaps abutment screw loosening in implants with internal connection is virtually nonexistent.[23] At the same time, it is important for clinicians to recognize that due to anatomic constraints related to decreased buccal–lingual thickness of bone, implant angulations may prohibit screw retention, and cement retention may outweigh the alternative option of additional bone grafting and soft tissue grafting surgeries. Newer solutions have emerged to mitigate this problem and allow screw-retained restorations to be fabricated. Presently, there are a few manufacturers offering an angle correction up to 25° using both a screw and a screwdriver with a unique tip. However, no clinical studies presently exist, to determine the short-term or long-term outcomes of this solution.

In the posterior region, where the masticatory forces are known to be higher, the choice of screw versus cement retention should be considered from two perspectives. One is the type of restoration (SC versus FDP) and the other is the need to minimize mechanical complications. For posterior single crowns, screw retention or cement retention are acceptable options, but screw retention may still be preferable to allow for easier retrievability for future revisions, or to allow utilization of the implant as an FDP for a future change in treatment plan. Within the scope of dental implant occlusion, the authors suggest cement retention for all posterior FDPs, except when it is occluding against a similar prosthesis in the opposing jaw. This is because of the higher risk for ceramic fracture or other mechanical complications, as observed in completely edentulous patients rehabilitated with implant-supported fixed prostheses in both jaws.[60,61] In all other scenarios, cement retention in posterior FDPs offers distinct advantages such as: 1) optimal occlusal contacts due to absence of a large screw-access channel; 2) reduced need for ideal implant placement, bone augmentation, or site development compared to screw-retained restorations; 3) potential for reduced ceramic fracture due to absence of screw-access channel; 4) easier to obtain passive fit of the substructure and potential for indemnity to passive fit due to the luting cement; 5) easier to obtain and correct implant parallelism compared to screw-retention scenario; and 6) inexpensive due to simplicity in fabrication of the restorations.

Some of the disadvantages related to use of cement retention in these situations could be mitigated by systematic execution of a few additional steps before insertion of the restorations. Firstly, the authors advocate use of a definitive ("permanent") cement as opposed to provisional cement. This is to ensure adequate control of the restoration in the patient's mouth and eliminate inadvertent debonding of the restoration. The second step is to ensure easy retrievability of the restoration in the future. This is done by fabrication of a clear vacuum-formed matrix (termed as the "screw-access matrix") over the restorations as a routine practice, before cementation in the mouth (Figure 14.23). Once the clear matrix is fabricated, access holes are then drilled and black lines can be drawn on the buccal and lingual surfaces of the matrix, using a permanent ink marker to indicate the direction of the screw channel (Figure 14.24). This matrix should be preserved in the dentist's office as a permanent part of the patient's treatment record. In the event of a future implant occlusal complication, such as porcelain fracture, screw loosening or screw fracture, the clear matrix can simply be placed in the patient's mouth and the exact site of screw access can be drilled to access the screw channel for a quick and easy retrieval

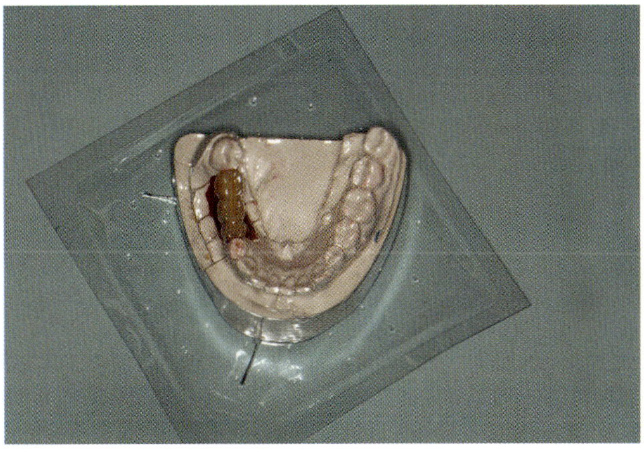

Figure 14.23 Image showing fabrication of a thin clear vacuum-formed matrix (screw-access matrix) for cement-retained implant restorations. The vacuum-formed matrix is fabricated directly over the master cast encompassing all remaining teeth.

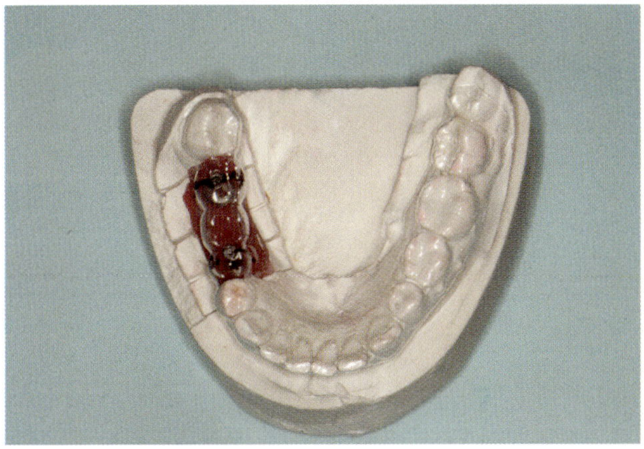

Figure 14.24 The implant restoration is removed from the master cast and the screw-access matrix is replaced on the master cast and the screw-access holes are then drilled, and black lines can be drawn on the buccal and lingual surfaces of the matrix, indicating the direction of the screw channel.

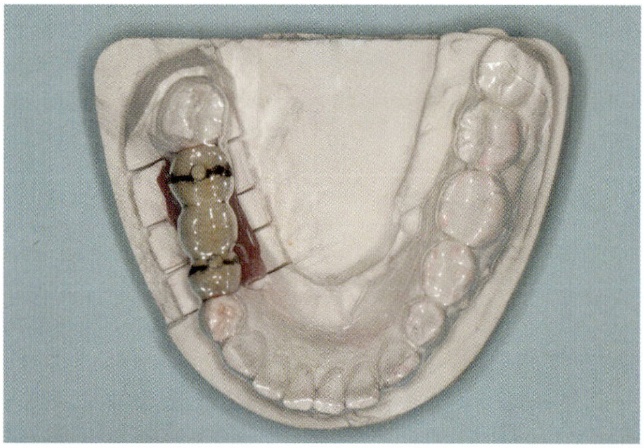

Figure 14.25 Image illustrating the occlusal view of the screw-access matrix in place with the screw-access holes marked. This matrix should be preserved in the dentist's office as a permanent part of the patient's treatment record.

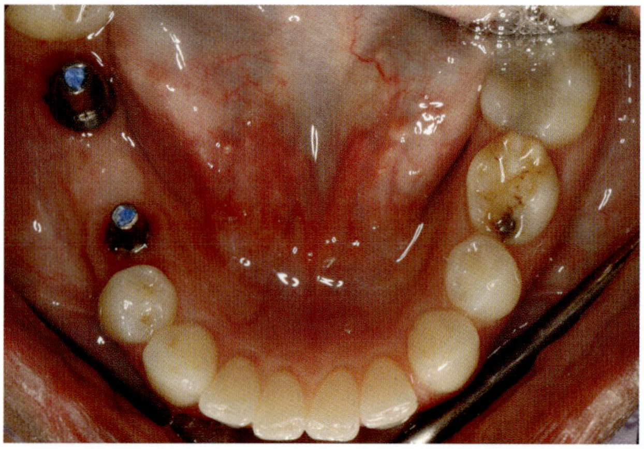

Figure 14.26 Image illustrating the use of nonwhite colored polytetrafluoroethylene (PTFE) tape to fill the screw-access channel. Using a colored tape allows easier visibility and access to the screw, if the screw-access site is drilled through the restoration.

of the restoration (Figure 14.25). The cemented abutment–crown complex can then be returned to the dental laboratory where the abutment can be retrieved by simply placing it in a ceramic furnace and following appropriate protocols for firing and cooling.[75] It is advisable to protect the abutment screw by filling the screw-access channel with a nonwhite colored polytetrafluorethylene (Teflon) tape to ensure easy visibility when the screw access site is drilled (Figure 14.26). The third step is the utilization of a trial cementation technique immediately before cementation of the restoration in the mouth. Trial cementation can be accomplished by cementing the restoration over an implant analog or a copy abutment fabricated from a silicone material (Figure 14.27). This will allow extrusion of all excess cement extraorally and ensure minimal residual cement that can be removed easily.

In summary, given the weak evidence regarding which method of prosthesis anchorage is best from the standpoint of occlusion and future mechanical complications, clinicians may use both screw-retained and cement-retained restorations, to utilize the unique advantages of each mode of anchorage.

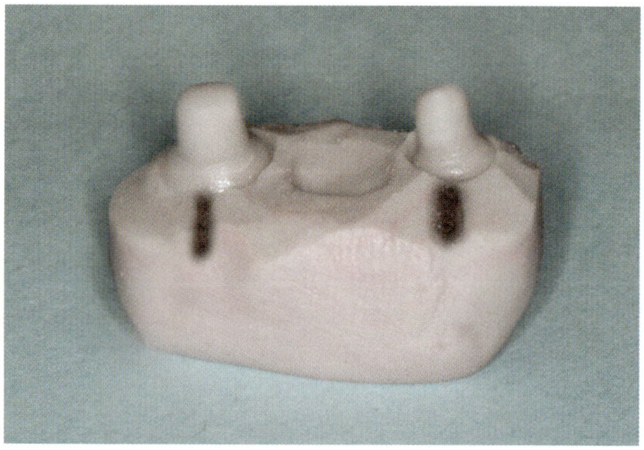

Figure 14.27 Image showing copy abutments of a three-unit fixed dental prosthesis fabricated from a silicone material. The copy abutments aid in trial cementation and clean-up of excess cement extruding from the restoration, which allows easier clean-up in the mouth and minimal residual cement.

Occlusal schemes

In the absence of scientific evidence, it is difficult to justify recommendation of one occlusal scheme over another.[1] However, due to the fact that implants are not, and do not behave like, natural teeth, it is essential to choose the simplest possible occlusal scheme, that can minimize mechanical complications and provide longer durability of the restorations for the patient. For all single crowns and fixed dental prostheses, the authors suggest restoring to the existing occlusal scheme of the patient, without any nonworking interferences on the implant restoration(s) itself. A mutually protected articulation scheme with canine guidance is the suggested occlusal scheme for all other implant-supported restorations (including complete-arch fixed implant-supported prostheses and implant-supported overdentures), whenever possible. When canine guidance in a patient's clinical situation is not an option, the premolar tooth should be used for guidance. The rationale for this is to use the most anteriorly located posterior tooth, far enough from the mandibular condyles, and minimize the discluding forces. When guidance from a single first premolar tooth is not an option, then it is suggested to use both premolars for guidance, in a partial group function occlusal scheme.[76] Utilizing a complete group function occlusal scheme where guidance is provided by one or both molars (in addition to the premolars) is undesirable, due to their distal location where higher forces may be detrimental to the occlusal material as well as prosthetic components, and there is a risk of a higher incidence of mechanical complications.

Summary

Implants are not, and do not behave like natural teeth. Therefore, many of the theories that may be applicable to natural teeth are neither valid nor clinically useful for implants. Current scientific evidence indicates that the osseointegrated interface is very strong and able to withstand occlusal forces within the limits of component structural integrity, and appears to be the strongest link in the pillar of implant-borne restorations. Therefore, it is necessary to maintain a simple approach to occlusion in implant prosthodontics and yet be meticulous about the technical steps in the execution of treatment.

References

1. Taylor TD, Wiens J, Carr A. Evidence-based considerations for removable prosthodontic and dental implant occlusion: a literature review. *J Prosthet Dent* 2005; **94**(6): 555–560.
2. Ante JH. The fundamental principles, design and construction of crown and bridge prosthesis. *Dental Item Int* 1928; **50**(5): 215–232.
3. Misch CE. *Dental Implant Prosthetics*. St. Louis: Mosby 2004; 511–530.
4. Garaicoa-Pazmiño C, Suárez-López del Amo F, Monje A, *et al.* Influence of crown/implant ratio on marginal bone loss: a systematic review. *J Periodontol* 2014; **85**(9): 1214–1221.
5. Lee SA, Lee CT, Fu MM, *et al.* Systematic review and meta-analysis of randomized controlled trials for the management of limited vertical height in the posterior region: short implants (5 to 8 mm) vs longer implants (>8 mm) in vertically augmented sites. *Int J Oral Maxillofac Implants* 2014; **29**(5): 1085–1097.
6. Srinivasan M, Vazquez L, Rieder P, *et al.* Survival rates of short (6 mm) micro-rough surface implants: a review of literature and meta-analysis. *Clin Oral Implants Res* 2014; **25**(5): 539–545.
7. Atieh MA, Zadeh H, Stanford CM, *et al.* Survival of short dental implants for treatment of posterior partial edentulism: a systematic review. *Int J Oral Maxillofac Implants* 2012; **27**(6): 1323–1331.
8. Laney WR. *Glossary of Oral and Maxillofacial Implants*. Chicago: Quintessence Publishing Co 2007; 40, 102, 113, 133.
9. Misch CE. Endosteal implants for posterior single tooth replacement: alternatives, indications, contraindications, and limitations. *J Oral Implantol* 1999; **25**(2): 80–94.
10. Stegaroiu R, Khraisat A, Nomura S, *et al.* Influence of superstructure materials on strain around an implant under 2 loading conditions: a technical investigation. *Int J Oral Maxillofac Implants* 2004; **19**(5): 735–742.
11. Juodzbalys G, Kubilius R, Eidukynas V, *et al.* Stress distribution in bone: single-unit implant prostheses veneered with porcelain or a new composite material. *Implant Dent* 2005; **14**(2): 166–175.
12. Morneburg TR, Pröschel PA. In vivo forces on implants influenced by occlusal scheme and food consistency. *Int J Prosthodont* 2003; **16**(5): 481–486.
13. Heitz-Mayfield L, Schmid B, Weigel C, *et al.* Does excessive occlusal load affect osseointegration? An experimental study in the dog. *Clin Oral Implants Res* 2004; **15**(3): 259–268.
14. Hurzeler M, Quinones C, Kohal R, *et al.* Changes in peri-implant tissues subjected to orthodontic forces and ligature breakdown in monkeys. *J Periodontol* 1998; **69**(3): 396-404.
15. Isidor F. Loss of osseointegration caused by occlusal load of oral implants. A clinical and radiographic study in monkeys. *Clin Oral Implants Res* 1996; **7**(2): 143–152.
16. Miyata T, Kobayashi Y, Araki H, *et al.* The influence of controlled occlusal overload on peri-implant tissue: a histologic study in monkeys. *Int J Oral Maxillofac Implants* 1998; **13**(5): 677–683.
17. Ogiso M, Tabata T, Kuo P, *et al.* A histologic comparison of the functional loading capacity of an occluded dense apatite implant and the natural dentition. *J Prosthet Dent* 1994; **71**(6): 581–588.
18. Taylor TD. Osteogenesis of the mandible associated with implant reconstruction: a patient report. *Int J Oral Maxillofac Implants* 1989; **4**(3): 227–231.
19. Chang M, Chronopoulos V, Mattheos N. Impact of excessive occlusal load on successfully-osseointegrated dental implants: a literature review. *J Investig Clin Dent* 2013; **4**(3): 142–150.
20. Celletti R, Pameijer CH, Bracchetti G, *et al.* Histologic evaluation of osseointegrated implants restored in nonaxial functional occlusion with preangled abutments. *Int J Periodontics Restorative Dent* 1995; **15**(6): 562–573.
21. Asikainen P, Klemetti E, Vuillemin T, *et al.* Titanium implants and lateral forces. An experimental study with sheep. *Clin Oral Implants Res* 1997; **8**(6): 465–468.
22. Flanagan D, Phillips J, Connor M, *et al.* Hoop stress and the conical connection. *J Oral Implantol* 2015; **41**(1): 37–44.
23. Bidra AS, Rungruanganunt P. Clinical outcomes of implant abutments in the anterior region: a systematic review. *J Esthet Restor Dent* 2013; **25**(3): 159–176.
24. Chae SW, Kim YS, Lee YM, *et al.* Complication incidence of two implant systems up to six years: a comparison between internal and external connection implants. *J Periodontal Implant Sci* 2015; **45**(1): 23–29.
25. Goodacre CJ, Bernal G, Rungcharassaeng K, *et al.* Clinical complications with implants and implant prostheses. *J Prosthet Dent* 2003; **90**(2): 121–132.
26. Carr AB, Gerard DA, Larsen PE. The response of bone in primates around unloaded dental implants supporting prostheses with different levels of fit. *J Prosthet Dent* 1996; **76**(5): 500–509.
27. Jemt T, Book K. Prosthesis misfit and marginal bone loss in edentulous implant patients. *Int J Oral Maxillofac Implants* 1996; **11**(5): 620–625.
28. Gotfredsen K, Berglundh T, Lindhe J. Bone reactions adjacent to titanium implants subjected to static load. A study in the dog (I). *Clin Oral Implants Res* 2001; **12**(1): 1–8.
29. Duyck J, Rønold HJ, Van Oosterwyck H, *et al.* The influence of static and dynamic loading on marginal bone reactions around osseointegrated implants: an animal experimental study. *Clin Oral Implants Res* 2001; **12**(3): 207–218.
30. De Pauw GA, Dermaut LR, Johansson CB, *et al.* A histomorphometric analysis of heavily loaded and non-loaded implants. *Int J Oral Maxillofac Implants* 2002; **17**(3): 405–412.
31. Miyamoto Y, Koretake K, Hirata M, *et al.* Influence of static overload on the bony interface around implants in dogs. *Int J Prosthodont* 2008; **21**(5): 437–444.
32. Taylor TD. Prosthodontic problems and limitations associated with osseointegration. *J Prosthet Dent* 1998; **79**(1): 74–78.

33. Karl M, Taylor TD, Wichmann MG, *et al.* In vivo stress behavior in cemented and screw-retained five-unit implant FPDs. *J Prosthodont* 2006; **15**(1): 20–24.
34. Guichet DL, Caputo AA, Choi H, *et al.* Passivity of fit and marginal opening in screw- or cement-retained implant fixed partial denture designs. *Int J Oral Maxillofac Implants* 2000; **15**(2): 239–246.
35. Vigolo P, Mutinelli S, Zaccaria M, *et al.* Clinical evaluation of marginal bone level change around multiple adjacent implants restored with splinted and nonsplinted restorations: a 10-year randomized controlled trial. *Int J Oral Maxillofac Implants* 2015; **30**(2): 411–418.
36. Lang NP, Pjetursson BE, Tan K, *et al.* A systematic review of the survival and complication rates of fixed partial dentures (FPDs) after an observation period of at least 5 years. II. Combined tooth–implant-supported FPDs. *Clin Oral Implants Res* 2004; **15**(6): 643–653.
37. Mamalis A, Markopoulou K, Kaloumenos K, *et al.* Splinting osseointegrated implants and natural teeth in partially edentulous patients: a systematic review of the literature. *J Oral Implantol* 2012; **38**(4): 424–434.
38. Brånemark PI. Osseointegration and its experimental background. *J Prosthet Dent* 1983; **50**(3): 399–410.
39. Adell R, Lekholm U, Rockler B, *et al.* A 15-year study of osseointegrated implants in the treatment of the edentulous jaw. *Int J Oral Surg* 1981; **10**(6): 387–416.
40. English CE. Critical A-P spread. *Implant Soc* 1990; **1**(1): 2–3.
41. Hälg GA, Schmid J, Hämmerle CH. Bone level changes at implants supporting crowns or fixed partial dentures with or without cantilevers. *Clin Oral Implants Res* 2008; **19**(10): 983–990.
42. Shackleton JL, Carr L, Slabbert JC, *et al.* Survival of fixed implant-supported prostheses related to cantilever lengths. *J Prosthet Dent* 1994; **71**(1): 23–26.
43. Gallucci GO, Doughtie CB, Hwang JW, *et al.* Five-year results of fixed implant-supported rehabilitations with distal cantilevers for the edentulous mandible. *Clin Oral Implants Res* 2009; **20**(6): 601–607.
44. Wennström J, Zurdo J, Karlsson S, *et al.* Bone level change at implant-supported fixed partial dentures with and without cantilever extension after 5 years in function. *J Clin Periodontol* 2004; **31**(12): 1077–1083.
45. Romeo E, Tomasi C, Finini I, *et al.* Implant-supported fixed cantilever prosthesis in partially edentulous jaws: a cohort prospective study. *Clin Oral Implants Res* 2009; **20**(11): 1278–1285.
46. Brägger U, Karoussis I, Persson R, *et al.* Technical and biological complications/failures with single crowns and fixed partial dentures on implants: a 10-year prospective cohort study. *Clin Oral Implants Res* 2005; **16**(3): 326–334.
47. Aglietta M, Siciliano VI, Zwahlen M, *et al.* A systematic review of the survival and complication rates of implant supported fixed dental prostheses with cantilever extensions after an observation period of at least 5 years. *Clin Oral Implants Res* 2009; **20**(5): 441–451.
48. The glossary of prosthodontic terms. *J Prosthet Dent* 2005; **94**(1): 10–92.
49. Feu D, Catharino F, Quintão CC, *et al.* A systematic review of etiological and risk factors associated with bruxism. *J Orthod* 2013; **40**(2): 163–171.
50. Manfredini D, Ahlberg J, Mura R, *et al.* Bruxism is unlikely to cause damage to the periodontium: findings from a systematic literature assessment. *J Periodontol* 2015; **86**(4): 546–555.
51. Chrcanovic BR, Albrektsson T, Wennerberg A. Bruxism and dental implants: a meta-analysis. *Implant Dent* 2015; **24**(5): 505–516.
52. Manfredini D1, Poggio CE, Lobbezoo F. Is bruxism a risk factor for dental implants? A systematic review of the literature. *Clin Implant Dent Relat Res* 2014; **16**(3): 460–469.
53. Mesko ME, Almeida RC, Porto JA, *et al.* Should occlusal splints be a routine prescription for diagnosed bruxers undergoing implant therapy? *Int J Prosthodont* 2014; **27**(3): 201–203.
54. Jacobs R, Van Steenberghe D. From osseoperception to implant-mediated sensory-motor interactions and related clinical implications. *J Oral Rehabil* 2006; **33**(4): 282–292.
55. Jacobs R, van Steenberghe D. Role of periodontal ligament receptors in the tactile function of teeth: a review. *J Periodontal Res* 1994; **29**(3): 153–167.
56. Mericske-Stern R, Hofmann J, Wedig A, *et al.* In vivo measurements of maximal occlusal force and minimal pressure threshold on overdentures supported by implants or natural roots: a comparative study, Part 1. *Int J Oral Maxillofac Implants* 1993; **8**(6): 641–649.
57. Hämmerle CH, Wagner D, Brägger U, *et al.* Threshold of tactile sensitivity perceived with dental endosseous implants and natural teeth. *Clin Oral Implants Res* 1995; **6**(2): 83–90.
58. El-Sheikh AM, Hobkirk JA, Howell PG, *et al.* Passive tactile sensibility in edentulous subjects treated with dental implants: a pilot study. *J Prosthet Dent* 2004; **91**(1): 26–32.
59. Jacobs R, van Steenberghe D. Comparison between implant-supported prostheses and teeth regarding passive threshold level. *Int J Oral Maxillofac Implants* 1993; **8**(5): 549–554.
60. Eliasson A, Palmqvist S, Svenson B, *et al.* Five-year results with fixed complete-arch mandibular prostheses supported by 4 implants. *Int J Oral Maxillofac Implants* 2000; **15**(4): 505–510.
61. Maló P, Araújo Nobre MD, Lopes A, *et al.* Double full-arch versus single full-arch, four implant-supported rehabilitations: a retrospective, 5-year cohort study. *J Prosthodont* 2015; **24**(4): 263–570.
62. Purcell BA, McGlumphy EA, Holloway JA, *et al.* Prosthetic complications in mandibular metal-resin implant-fixed complete dental prostheses: a 5- to 9-year analysis. *Int J Oral Maxillofac Implants* 2008; **23**(5): 847–857.
63. Wittneben JG, Buser D, Salvi GE, *et al.* Complication and failure rates with implant-supported fixed dental prostheses and single crowns: a 10-year retrospective study. *Clin Implant Dent Relat Res* 2014; **16**(3): 356–364.
64. Wataha JC. Alloys for prosthodontic restorations. *J Prosthet Dent* 2002; **87**(4): 351–363.
65. Wataha JC, Messer RL. Casting alloys. *Dent Clin North Am* 2004; **48**(2): 499–512.
66. Pieger S, Salman A, Bidra AS. Clinical outcomes of lithium disilicate single crowns and partial fixed dental prostheses: a systematic review. *J Prosthet Dent* 2014; **112**(1): 22–30.
67. Raigrodski AJ, Hillstead MB, Meng GK, *et al.* Survival and complications of zirconia-based fixed dental prostheses: a systematic review. *J Prosthet Dent* 2012; **107**(3): 170–177.
68. Michalakis KX, Hirayama H, Garefis PD. Cement-retained versus screw-retained implant restorations: a critical review. *Int J Oral Maxillofac Implants* 2003; **18**(5): 719–728.
69. Nissan J, Narobai D, Gross O, *et al.* Long-term outcome of cemented versus screw-retained implant-supported partial restorations. *Int J Oral Maxillofac Implants* 2011; **26**(5): 1102–1107.

70. Sherif S, Susarla SM, Hwang JW, *et al.* Clinician- and patient-reported long-term evaluation of screw- and cement-retained implant restorations: a 5-year prospective study. *Clin Oral Investig* 2011; **15**(6): 993–999.
71. Vigolo P, Mutinelli S, Givani A, *et al.* Cemented versus screw-retained implant-supported single-tooth crowns: a 10-year randomised controlled trial. *Eur J Oral Implantol* 2012; **5**(4): 355–364.
72. Sailer I, Mühlemann S, Zwahlen M, *et al.* Cemented and screw-retained implant reconstructions: a systematic review of the survival and complication rates. *Clin Oral Implants Res* 2012; **23**(Suppl 6): 163–201.
73. Wittneben JG, Millen C, Brägger U. Clinical performance of screw-versus cement-retained fixed implant-supported reconstructions – a systematic review. *Int J Oral Maxillofac Implants* 2014; **29**(Suppl): 84–98.
74. Weber HP, Kim DM, Ng MW, *et al.* Peri-implant soft-tissue health surrounding cement- and screw-retained implant restorations: a multi-center, 3-year prospective study. *Clin Oral Implants Res* 2006; **17**(4): 375–379.
75. Alsiyabi AS, Felton DA. Technique for removing cement between a fixed prosthesis and its substructure. *J Prosthodont* 2009; **18**(3): 279–282.
76. Fox CW, Doukoudakis A, Fox SW, *et al.* A method for occlusal reshaping. *J Prosthodont* 1992; **1**(2): 101–105.

CHAPTER 15

Evolving Technologies in Implant Prosthodontics

David G. Gratton
University of Iowa College of Dentistry, Iowa City, Iowa, USA

Along the pathway of prosthodontics, a plethora of evolving technologies is available to the practitioner at each of the crucial intersections of treatment. These technologies are offered for diagnosis and treatment planning, mouth and tooth preparation, interim prostheses, impressions, jaw-relationship records, prostheses fabrication, prostheses delivery, and patient maintenance. Yet, the clinician may be conflicted in determining if these evolving technologies provide a better patient experience and overall better treatment outcome compared with the conventional methods of prosthodontic treatment delivery. If one does not embrace these evolving technologies, is he or she practicing inferior dentistry? Asked another way, "What is wrong with the way I have always done it?" There are extrinsic factors, such as industry trends and patient perceptions, along with intrinsic factors, such as clinical efficiencies and clinical precision and accuracy, that must be analyzed when considering embracing these evolving technologies for everyday practice. An assessment of these various technologies will aid the clinician in the decision process of whether or not to disrupt current workflows to incorporate a few or many of these evolving technologies.

The flow of patient data in digital implant prosthodontics (the language of digital prosthodontics)

In consideration of the "virtualization" of the prosthodontic implant patient, there are three basic phases that comprise the digital workflow: data acquisition, data processing and manipulation, computer-aided prosthesis fabrication. The success of the digital workflow is predicated upon the successful integration of the data at each of these phases (Figure 15.1). Multiple "languages" are spoken throughout the process; every instance in which translation is necessary may result in the loss of data trueness and precision. Digital dental systems are classified as open architecture or closed architecture, with some systems being a hybrid of the two. In a closed-architecture system the data is locked with proprietary file extensions. The clinician is restricted to transferring the data among the three phases, using only the particular hardware and software supplied by the manufacturer. This may limit the clinical indications available to the clinician but should ensure a certain level of robustness of the workflow. In contrast, an open-architecture system gives the clinician full access to the data, thereby providing unlimited possibilities to transfer the data among the three phases of the workflow. At this point the maximum clinical indications are realized, and there is literally global access to various design and manufacturing platforms. However, the clinician should be cautioned, as has been previously stated with the limited standardization of data language, that a process of workflow validation is required to ensure the clinically desired outcome is realized.

For the data-acquisition phase there is standardization of the digital radiographic data through the Digital Imaging and Communications in Medicine (DICOM). DICOM is a standard developed by American College of Radiology (ACR) and National Electrical Manufacturers Association (NEMA) for the handling, storing, printing, and transfer of information in medical imaging. However, for dental CAD/CAM systems, there is no equivalent standard. The industry has gravitated to using an STL (stereolithography) file format as a *de facto* standard. STL is a file format created by 3D Systems (3D Systems, Rock Hill, SC) in the 1970s; today it is also referred to as "Standard Triangulation Language" or "Standard Tessellation Language," both misnomers, as it is not a true standard. Using this file format, the surface of a three-dimensional (3-D) object is defined by a series of triangles. A limitation of this file format in dentistry is that it has no representation of color or texture. The accuracy of representation of a curved surface is determined by the size and density of the triangles (Figure 15.2). In recognition of these limitations, other standard file formats are under development

Evidence-based Implant Treatment Planning and Clinical Protocols, First Edition. Edited by Steven J. Sadowsky.

Companion website: www.wiley.com/go/sadowsky/implant

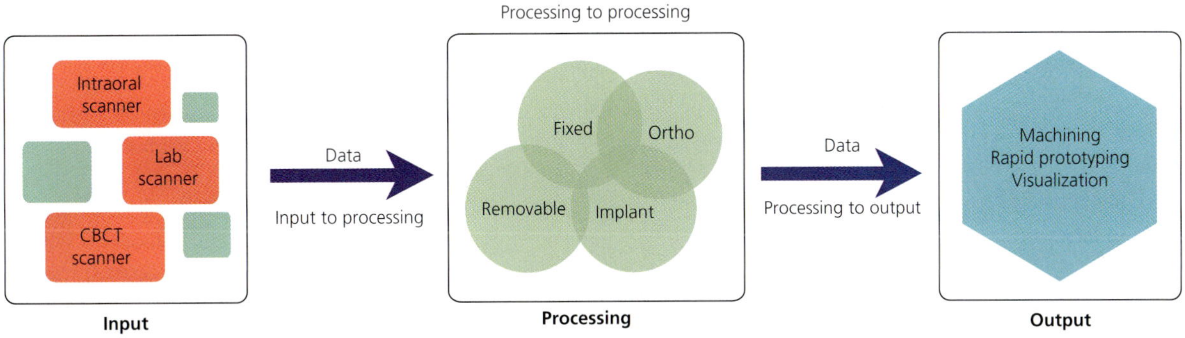

Figure 15.1 Digital prosthodontics platform flow of data.

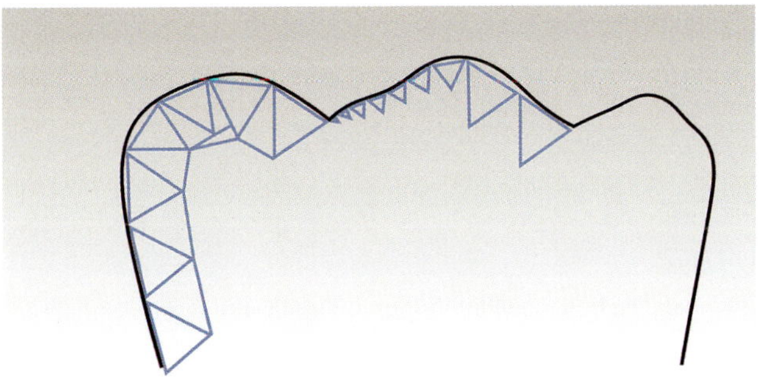

Figure 15.2 Three-dimensional surface geometry as described by an STL (stereolithography) file. Black line is original tooth contour, blue line is STL model. Note how the size and density of the triangles will affect the trueness of the model to the original anatomy.

but as of yet have not been adopted. One such example is Additive Manufacturing File Format (AMF). This open source ISO/ASTM Standard 52915:2013 supports color, materials, lattices, and constellations.

Technologies for implant diagnosis and treatment planning

The success of any prosthodontic treatment is predicated upon a sound diagnosis and treatment plan. Radiographic survey and mounted diagnostic casts form the foundation. Paramount to the evolving digital workflow for implant prosthodontics is the use of digital radiographs, whether planar films or three-dimensionally reconstructed images (Figure 15.3). Digital radiography has been shown to result in decreased time and radiation dose for an equivalent diagnostic accuracy[1–3] and image analysis time savings.[4,5] Cone-beam computed tomography (CBCT) allows for linear measurement, analysis of the 3-D topography of potential implant sites, and determinations of proximity to critical anatomical structures (Figure 15.4). Ultimately, CBCT assists in the fabrication of implant surgical guides;[6–9] however, deviations between planned and actual implant location have been noted, emphasizing the need for clinical care.[6]

Can the use of an intraoral scanner replace alginate and dental stone? Casts from an intraoral scanner can be produced through either a subtractive milling process or an additive 3D printing process (Figure 15.5). The Cadent iTero scanner (Align Technology, Inc., San Jose, CA) uses milled casts. Linear measurements of the mesial–distal, buccal–lingual, and occlusal–gingival dimensions of the digital models resulted in near-perfect agreement (interclass correlation, 0.91–0.99) with caliper measurements on 60 dry skulls.[10,11]

The use of digital technologies has shown comparable results of pretreatment diagnostic wax-up casts completed in a conventional wax-up technique to those of a digital wax-up in regard to axial tooth morphology (Figure 15.6).[12]

A third source of diagnostic data, not yet fully realized in implant prosthodontics, is the use of an extraoral 3-D scanner (Figure 15.7). Not only are these devices able to capture static images but they can also be used to capture four-dimensional images – the incorporation of real-time motion of facial expression and features.[13–15] The application of these four-dimensional data sets in the diagnostic planning for the complex implant patient will allow for the virtual assessment of changes in vertical dimension of occlusion and facial esthetics as a result of prosthesis/tooth position. As of yet there is no software readily available to the clinician that incorporates the volumetric radiographic data, the intraoral scan data, and the extraoral four-dimensional data.

Technologies for implant placement

Although the use of surgical robotics is becoming more common in medicine, no such protocol exists for the routine use of surgical robotics for the placement of dental implants. The work on this in the dental arena is decidedly preliminary; however, initial studies have commenced with system validation and actual placement of implants.[16,17]

The more common approach is to use implant planning software such as NobelClinician® (Nobel Biocare, Yorba Linda, CA), SimPlant® (DENTSPLY Implants, Molndal, Sweden), coDiagnostiX™ (Dental Wings, Montreal, Canada), or Implant Studio™ (3Shape A/S, Copenhagen, Denmark). These software

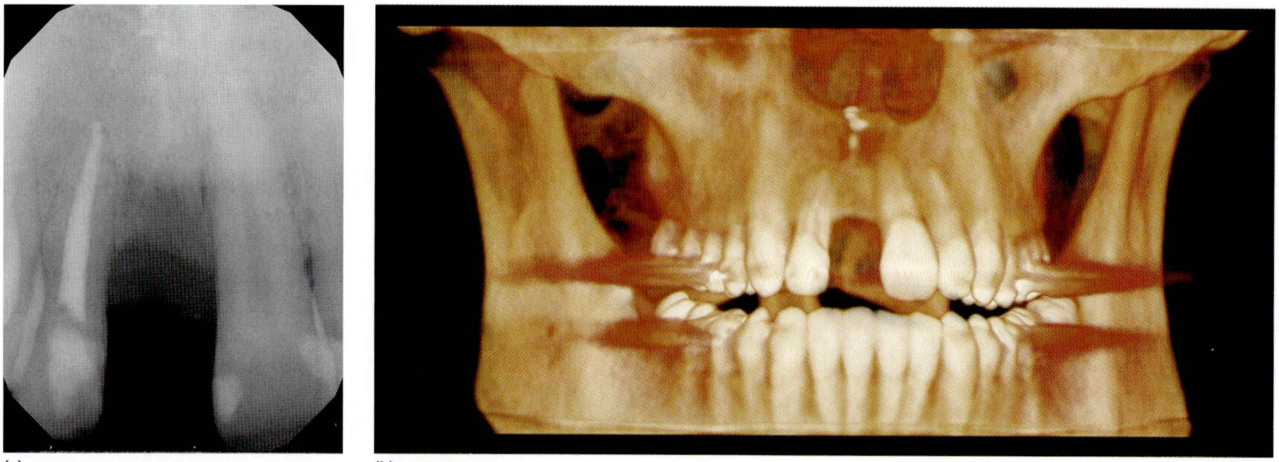

(a) (b)

Figure 15.3 **(a)** Digital periapical radiograph of potential implant site. **(b)** Three-dimensionally reconstructed CBCT image.

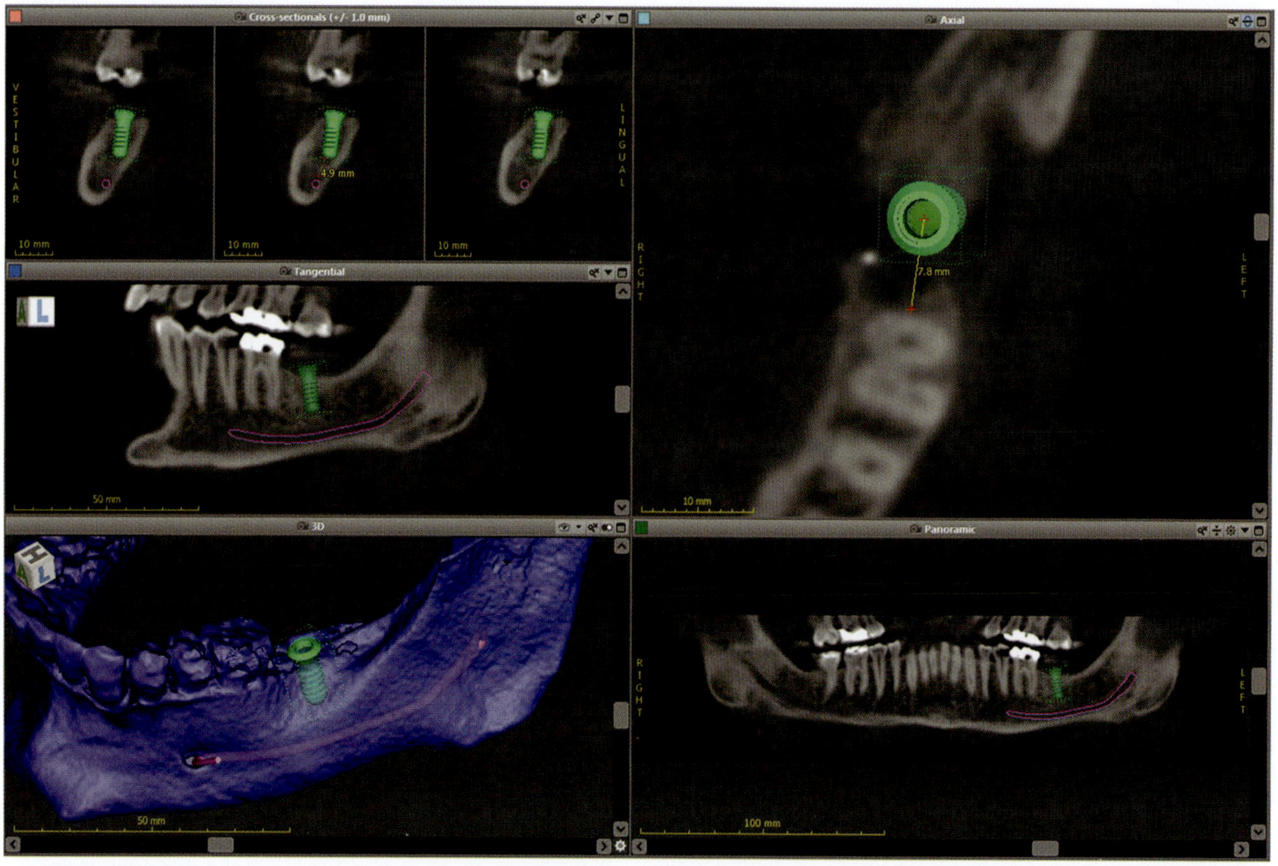

Figure 15.4 Implant-planning software showing linear measurements, proximity to vital structures, and 3-D surface topography.

platforms allow the superimposition of CBCT data, intraoral scanner (or lab-based cast scanner) data, and digital diagnostic plans of the final prosthesis for the planning of implant placement and the production of surgical guides.[18–21] These guides can be produced using a subtractive process such as milling (Figure 15.8),[22] or an additive process such as stereolithography or selective laser sintering.[23,24] Recently, workflows have been developed for chairside dental CAD/CAM systems for milling of surgical guides in-office.[25–27] *In vitro* investigation has revealed an accuracy range of 0.17–1.3 mm for pilot drill preparation on stone casts for chairside-milled CAD/CAM guides.[28]

The use of CAD/CAM surgical guides is more accurate than a freehand approach for implant placement,[29,30] and implants

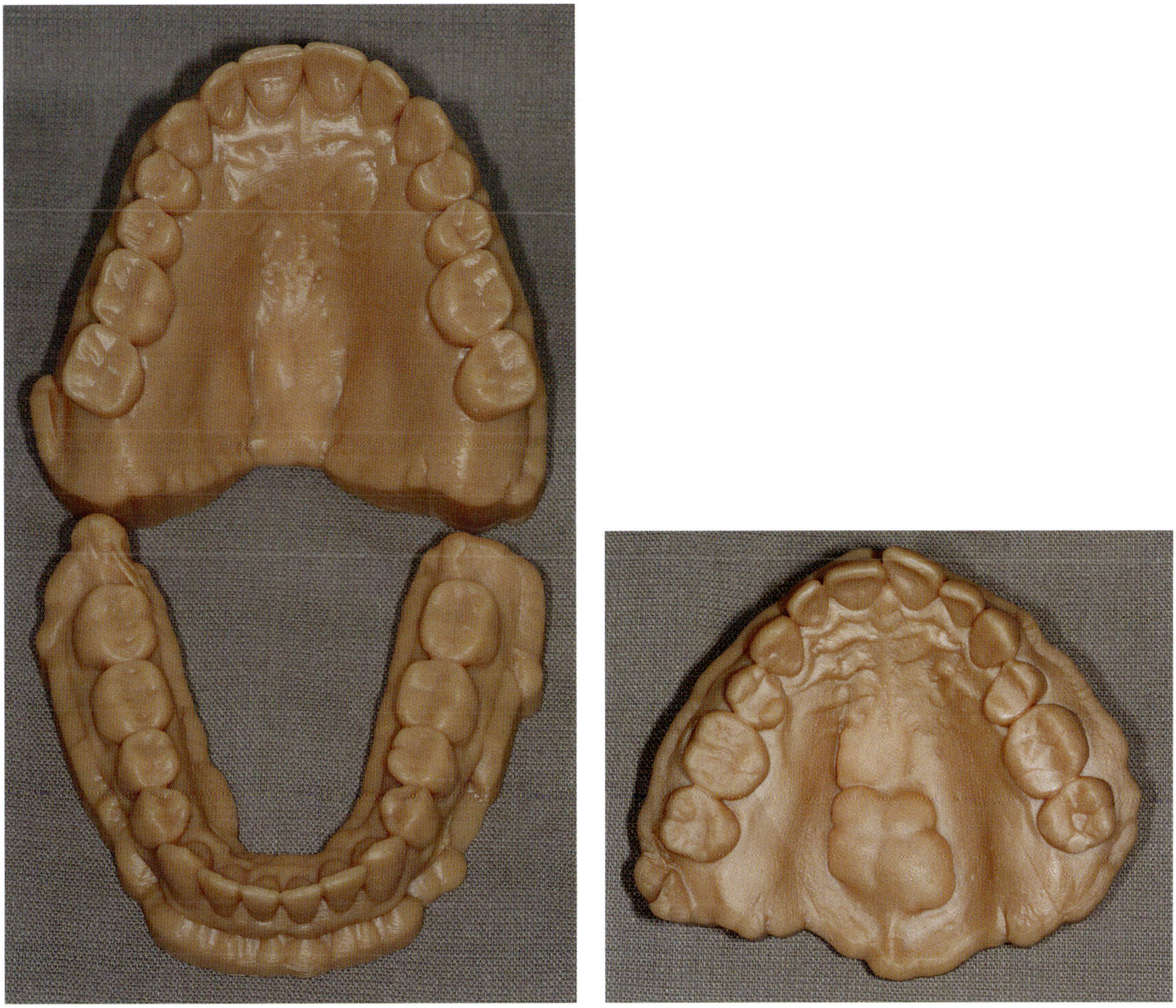

(a) (b)

Figure 15.5 **(a)** An example of three-dimensionally printed casts. **(b)** An example of three-dimensionally printed maxillary cast with reproduction of maxillary torus.

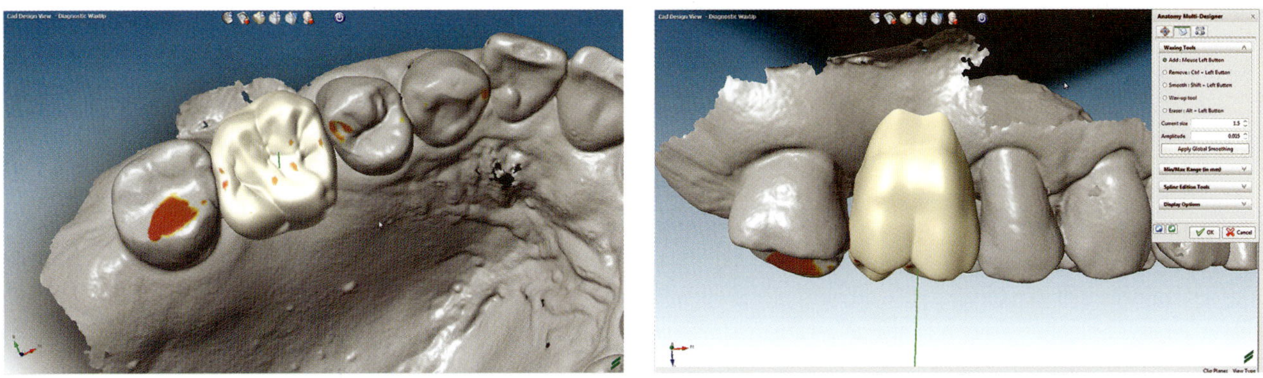

(a) (b)

Figure 15.6 **(a)** A digital diagnostic wax-up for a maxillary right first molar, occlusal view. **(b)** A digital diagnostic wax-up for a maxillary right first molar, buccal view.

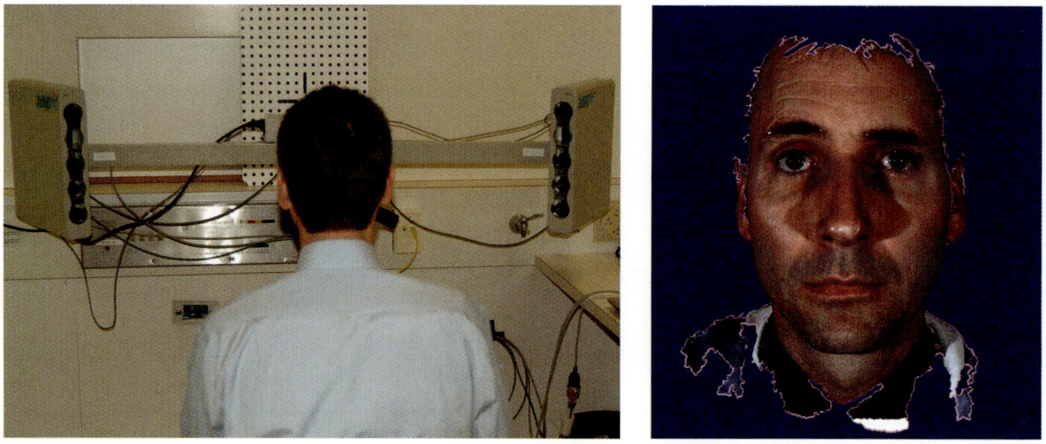
(a) (b)

Figure 15.7 (a) Extraoral 3-D camera set-up. (b) Extraoral 3-D facial image.

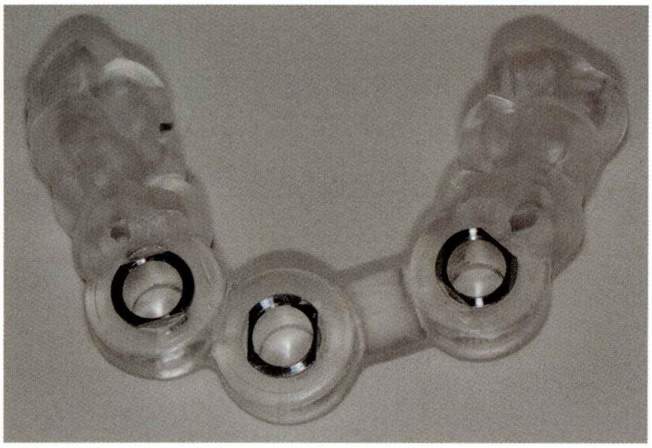

Figure 15.8 Milled implant surgical guide for a guided surgery protocol.

placed with the aid of a CAD/CAM surgical guide are positioned more accurately and with more consistent deviation from the planned location compared with those placed with conventional surgical guides.[31] Comparing planned versus actual implant placement based on postoperative CT scans, the trend is toward tooth-supported guides being more accurate with less deviation of implant position than mucosa-supported guides.[29,32–34] *In vivo* analysis of 111 implants placed in 24 patients revealed mean angular deviations of $1.72 \pm 1.67°$ and $2.71 \pm 2.58°$, mean deviations in position of the implant neck of 0.27 ± 0.24 mm and 0.69 ± 0.66 mm, mean deviations in position at the implant apex of 0.37 ± 0.35 mm and 0.94 ± 0.75 mm, and mean depth deviations of 0.32 ± 0.32 mm and 0.51 ± 0.48 mm, for tooth- and mucosa-supported stereolithographic guides, respectively ($P < .05$ for all).[32] For mucosa-supported guides, findings confirm that maximizing the supporting surface area and using rigid fixation improves the accuracy of implant placement. Additionally the reduced mucosal thickness of nonsmokers allows for less coronal and apical deviation of implant position as compared with smokers, and reduced bone density may affect accuracy negatively.[35,36]

In a study comparing implant surgical guides fabricated conventionally with acrylic resin, based on CBCT scan data only, or based on optical scan data, the fit of the conventional guides and those fabricated from the optical scan data had greater accuracy of fit than the guides fabricated from the CBCT scan.[37] This is not unexpected due to the artifact scatter caused by metallic restorations, but also points to the potential for inaccuracies in the superimposition of intraoral scan data onto the CBCT data during implant planning. If such a malalignment has occurred, the planned implant placement will not be represented intraorally as the CAD/CAM guide is now positioned in a different 3-D position than in the software. The clinician may still consider the value of a surgical guide try-in with radiographs to confirm implant position and angulation, or, at a minimum, an initial scout radiograph at the time of implant surgery (Figure 15.9). The mean survival rate of implants placed using computer-guided surgery with a follow-up period of at least 12 months was 97.3% (n = 1941), which is comparable to implants placed following conventional procedures.[38]

Technologies for implant interim prostheses

The rehabilitation of the implant patient may involve a period of time in which interim prostheses may be indicated. The use of the interim prosthesis is valuable in the validation of the diagnostic design,[39–41] occlusal function,[41] esthetics,[39–42] contours,[39–44] and patient phonetics[41] that are ultimately duplicated in the definitive prosthesis.[45–47] The interim prosthesis also allows for the monitoring of gingival tissue response and development of appropriate emergence profiles,[44–46,48] allowing the gingival tissue to mature to the planned definitive prosthesis contours,[42,49–51] all the while confirming osseointegration of the implant.[51] This interim phase of treatment could be a relatively short period of time or could be quite lengthy, at which point the physical properties of the material become important (Figure 15.10).[52]

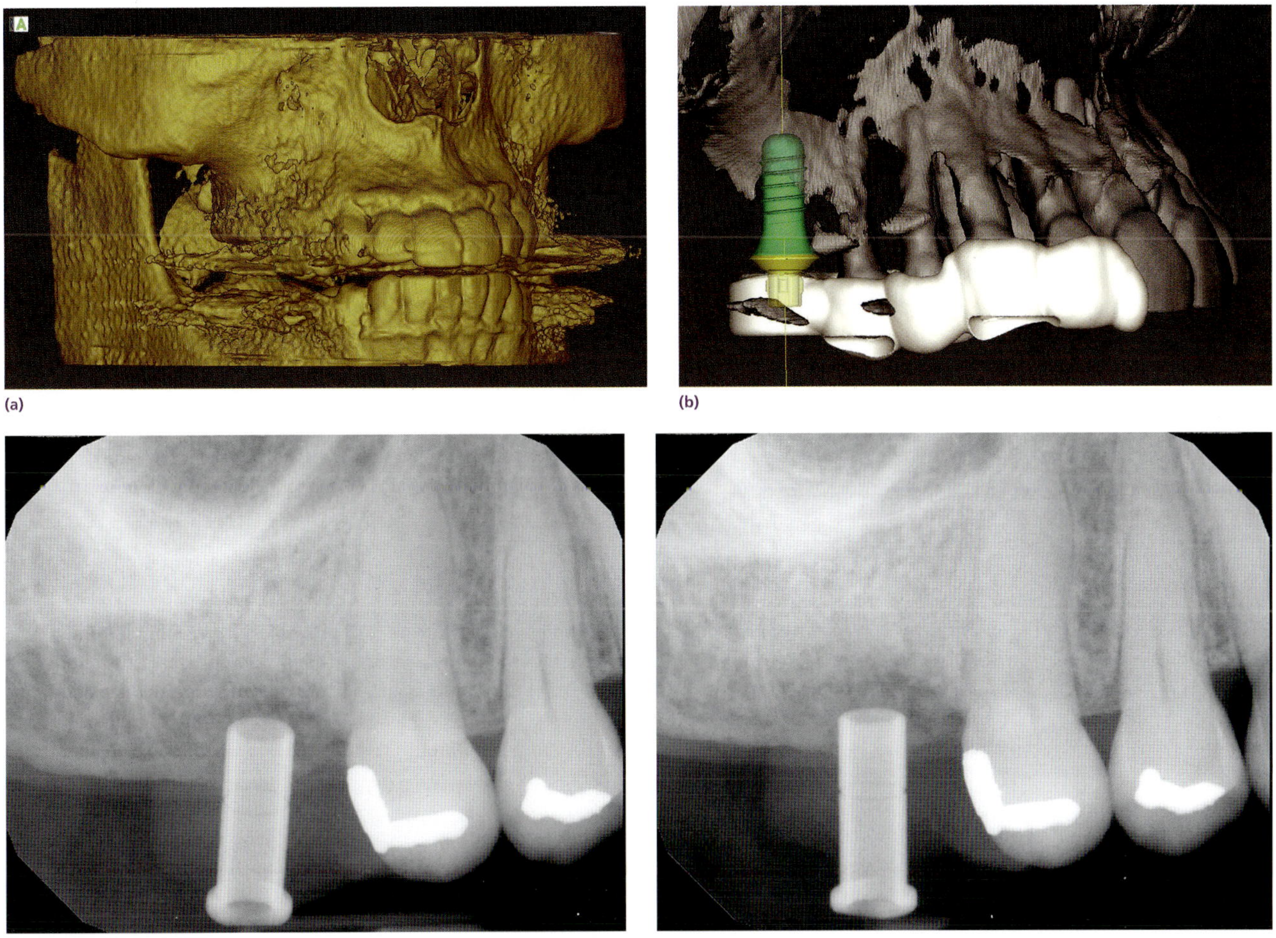

Figure 15.9 **(a)** Example of metallic artifact in CBCT data set. **(b)** Planned implant position for maxillary right first molar site. **(c)** Radiographic try-in of milled surgical guide from digital implant plan showing angle deviation from original plan. This is most likely due to metallic artifact causing an inaccurate registration of the CBCT data set and the intraoral scan data set. **(d)** Corrected implant position and angulation after manual correction of surgical guide.

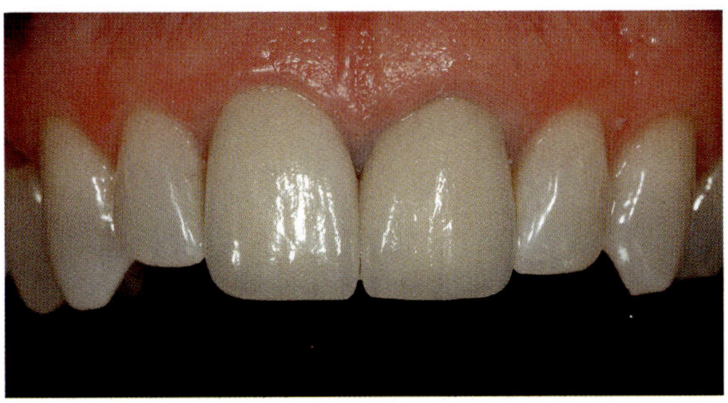

Figure 15.10 Long-term milled CAD/CAM interim crowns for central incisor implants at the time of prosthesis delivery. Surface characterization and staining completed by hand.

An *in vitro* study of interim prosthesis materials for single-unit interim premolar crowns demonstrated that CAD/CAM milled interim crowns from a polymethylmethacrylate material (Cercon Base PMMA blocks, DENTSPLY, York, PA) demonstrated enhanced color stability, higher mechanical properties, and better fit than the crowns made from a direct technique using autopolymerizing polymethylmethacrylate, automixing bis-acryl compound, and thermoplastic highly crystalline acetal copolymer resins.[53] Similar findings were reported for a study involving molar crowns, in which the two CAD/CAM materials, Vita Cad-Temp (VITA North America, Yorba Linda, CA) and Telio CAD (Ivoclar Vivadent, Inc., Amherst, NY), demonstrated significantly less mean marginal gaps than the two direct-fabrication materials, ProTemp 4 (3M ESPE, St. Paul, MN) and Structure 2 SC/QM (VOCO GmbH, Cuxhaven, Germany), both before and after thermal cycling.[54] The authors also produced 25 × 2 × 2 mm bars from the four materials and subjected the specimens to three-point bend tests both with and without thermal cycling. All groups exhibited significantly decreased flexural strength after thermal cycling, with the Telio CAD possessing the highest flexural strength. The authors concluded that CAD/CAM interim prostheses should be used for long-term and long-span clinical situations.[54] In an investigation of interim fixed dental prostheses (FDPs), three-unit FDPs milled from Telio CAD exhibited similar flexural strength to directly fabricated interim FDPs that were reinforced with a resin-impregnated light-polymerized glass fiber (GrandTEC, VOCO GmbH, Cuxhaven, Germany), which were significantly stronger than those fabricated without the reinforcing fiber.[55]

The digital implant workflow allows for the fabrication of interim abutments and prostheses prior to implant surgery.[56] Through the use of CAD/CAM technologies, the cement margin can be optimally positioned in the sulcus to reduce soft tissue complications and maintain long-term peri-implant health.[57,58] The role of crown contours, namely overcontouring, which could lead to bacterial biofilm accumulation and limits the patient and dental professional hygiene access, has been postulated as a potential cause of peri-implant mucositis and peri-implantitis.[59] The authors go on to suggest that use of available 3-D computer technology for implant prosthesis planning and design, along with enhanced communication among all members of the implant team, especially the dental technologists, may allow for a decreased incidence of peri-implant disease.[59]

Technologies for definitive impressions

Although the focus of this chapter is on evolving technologies for implant prosthodontics, when it comes to the discussion of intraoral scanning for implants, much of the foundational data pertains to the use of intraoral scanners with natural teeth. It will be instructive to briefly review the natural tooth data that have established a baseline of accuracy and precision, allowing the expansion of scanning indications to include implant scanning. However, there are limitations unique to intraoral scanning of implants, especially with regard to large-span edentulous regions.

Intraoral scanning for single-tooth indications

In a unique clinical study involving three intraoral scanners and one lab-based scanner that measured marginal gap using the established replica technique,[60–65] the authors found the following marginal gaps: 88 μm (68–136 μm) [median/inter-quartile range] for the True Definition (3 M ESPE, St. Paul, MN), 112 μm (94–149 μm) for the Heraeus Cara TRIOS (3Shape A/S, Copenhagen, Denmark), 113 μm (81–157 μm) for the laboratory scanner (3Shape D700, 3Shape A/S, Copenhagen, Denmark), and 149 μm (114–218 μm) for the CEREC AC Omnicam (Sirona Dental, Inc., Charlotte, NC). A statistically significant difference between the OmniCam group and all other groups ($p < 0.05$) was realized. The authors concluded that except for the one group, zirconia copings for single-tooth restorations fabricated from intraoral scans and analog impressions combined with laboratory scans had comparable marginal fit.[66]

In summary, it has been demonstrated that intraoral scanning can produce single-unit and multi-unit dentate or implant prostheses of equal or better accuracy and precision of fit compared with prostheses fabricated from analog techniques.

Intraoral scanning for complete-arch indications

Having earned a certain level of validity for single-tooth intraoral scanning, the clinical indications may be expanded for impressions with the intraoral scanner. It is with these more complex clinical situations that differentiation between hardware and software may be realized. In an *in vitro* investigation that focused on the trueness and precision of four intraoral scanners used to scan a model arch with 14 units, the Lava COS (3M ESPE, St. Paul, MN) produced the most accurate results (trueness 38.0 ± 14.3 μm; precision 37.9 ± 19.1 μm) compared with the CEREC AC Bluecam (Sirona Dental, Inc., Charlotte, NC), which produced the least accurate results (trueness 332.9 ± 64.8 μm; precision 99.1 ± 37.4 μm). It was concluded that three of the tested systems – Lava COS, iTero, and Zfx IntraScan (Zfx GmbH, Dachau, Germany) – exhibited comparable results.[67] The iTero datasets were converted to 3Shape (3Shape A/S, Copenhagen, Denmark) and Dental Wings (Dental Wings, Inc., Montreal, Canada) STL files. No differences were noted for the trueness of precision between the two software platforms (Figure 15.11).[67]

Intraoral scanning for implant indications

To employ an intraoral scanner for the capture of an implant level impression, a surrogate means of registering the spatial 3-D position of the implant and its rotational timing must be used. Currently, two fundamental approaches are applied. First is the use of a special healing abutment that is placed at the time of implant surgery; the second is the use of a scan body that is interfaced with the implant after the healing abutment has been removed.

The BellaTek® Encode® System (Zimmer Biomet, Warsaw, IN), launched in 2007[68] for conventional impressioning techniques, is one such system that uses unique patterns milled into the occlusal surface of the healing abutment that are used downstream to indicate the depth, rotational timing, platform diameter, and external versus internal connection type (Figure 15.12).[69] Provided that there is no gingival overgrowth of the healing, this is a simplified clinical approach, as no removal of the healing abutment and placement of a unique scan body is required.[70–72] However, it seems that the use of a coded healing abutment produces implant-definitive casts that are less accurate than those produced from conventional open and closed tray techniques.[73–75] More recently the coded healing abutment has been advocated with the use of intraoral scanners;[76,77] however, no *in vitro* or *in vivo* data have been reported.

The more common and rapidly evolving method for intraoral scanning involves the use of unique scan bodies (Figure 15.13). These scan bodies can be procured from the original implant manufacturer or from a third party manufacturer. Through the application of the digital workflow, analog casts can be fabricated through either a milling or printing

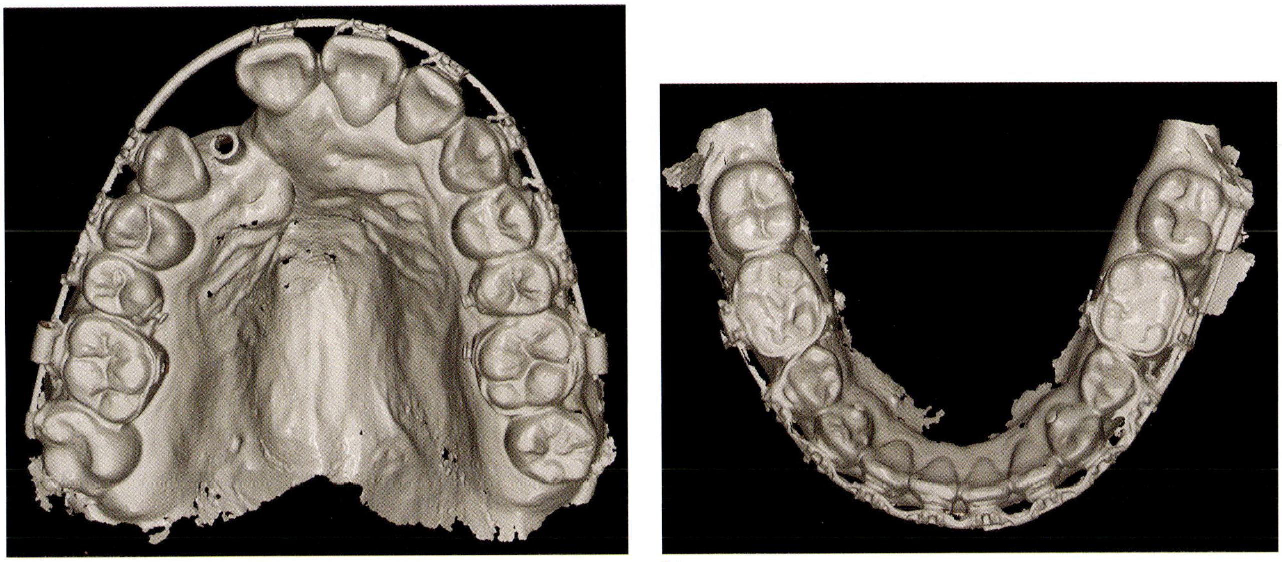

(a) (b)

Figure 15.11 (a) Maxillary full-arch digital diagnostic impression from an intraoral scanner. (b) Mandibular full-arch digital diagnostic impression from an intraoral scanner.

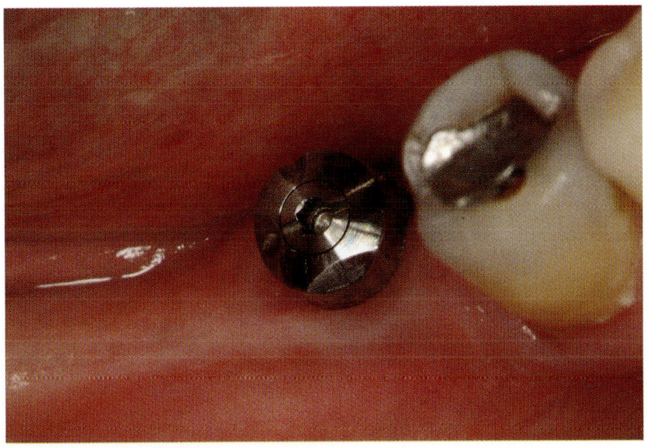

Figure 15.12 Specialized healing abutment with milled patterns to indicate implant depth, rotational timing, platform diameter, and external versus internal connection type. *Source:* Reproduced with permission from Dr. Abraham Stein, DMD, MS.

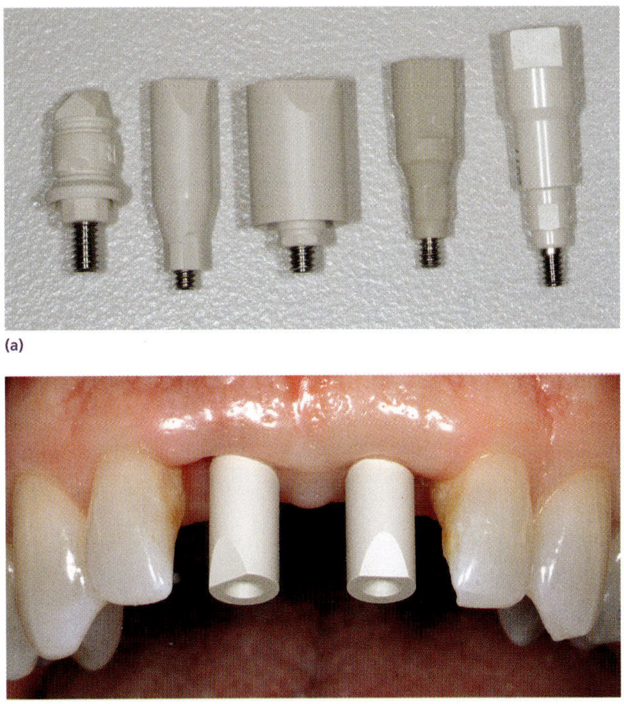

Figure 15.13 (a) Various scanbody geometries from different manufacturers. (b) Intraoral implant scanbodies for digital impressioning systems. Note the incisal bevel that must be oriented to the facial for proper CAD software registration.

process (Figure 15.14). It has been shown that milled casts from data sets obtained from the iTero intraoral scanner are comparable to gypsum casts obtained from conventional impression materials. Variation was noted in the secondary anatomy features of grooves and fossae, with gypsum casts exhibiting more detail and prominent anatomy.[78] It was noted that both gypsum and milled casts had a significant ($P = 0.020$) discrepancy in the vertical axis of the implant position as compared with the master model, with the gypsum casts having an apical position (-0.088 ± 0.044 mm) of the implant analog whereas the milled casts from the intraoral scanner had an occlusal position (0.093 ± 0.061 mm) of the implant analog compared with the master model.[78] The clinical implication one might derive from this study is that implant crowns fabricated from either cast will have occlusal inaccuracies; those from gypsum casts would be in hyperocclusion and those fabricated from the milled cast in hypoocclusion clinically. Crowns in hypoocclusion would require a laboratory procedure to achieve occlusal harmony.

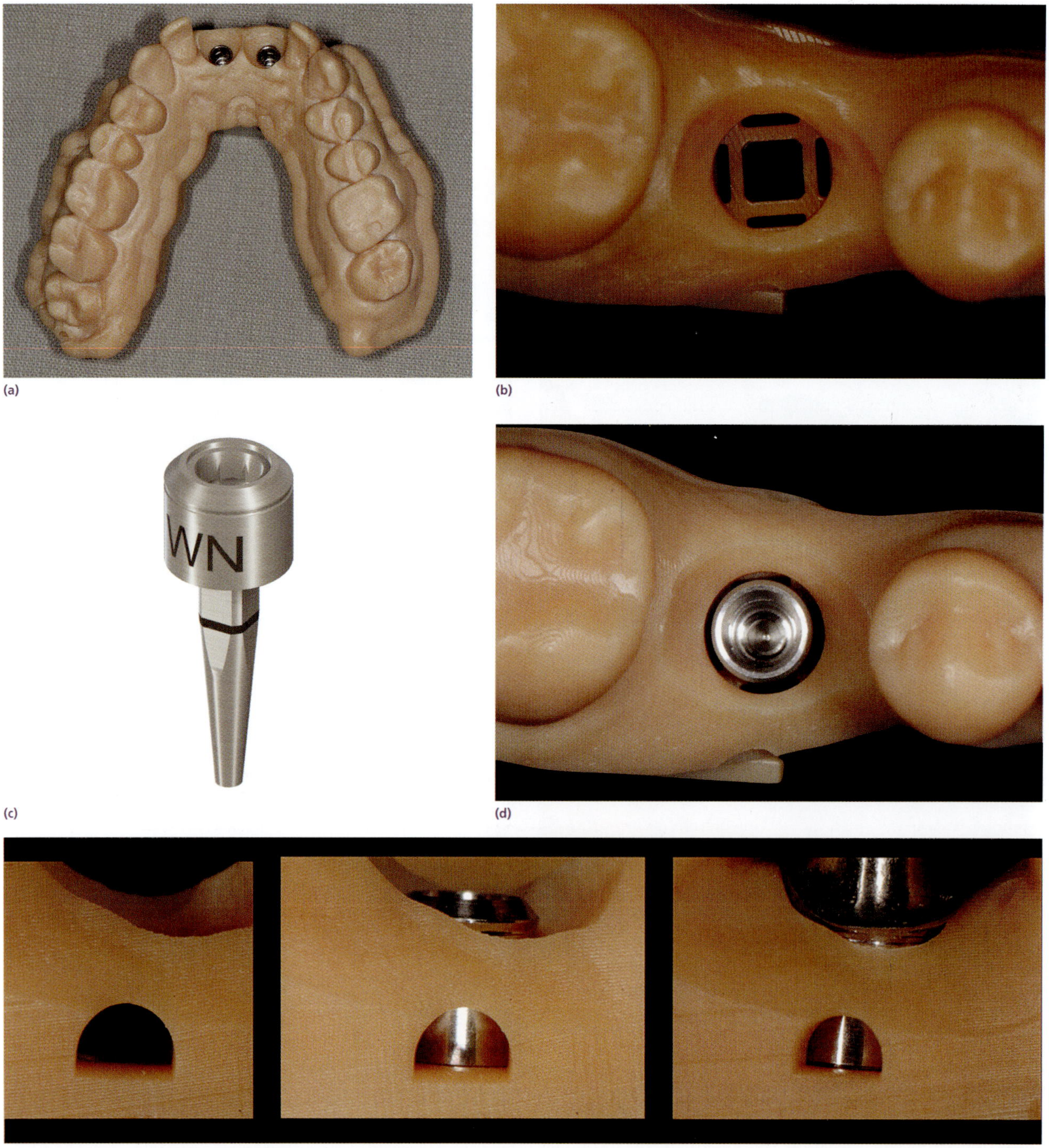

(a) (b) (c) (d) (e)

Figure 15.14 (a) Three-dimensionally printed implant definitive cast. (b) Close-up of the printed detail of the socket to receive the implant analog. (c) Implant analog for milled or printed casts. (d) Implant analog inserted into printed cast. (e) Verification window in printed casts to confirm complete seating of implant analog and/or abutment.

The accuracy of implant impressions generated from the use of intraoral scanners may be hardware/software dependent as well as clinical-indication dependent. An investigation that involved complete-arch scanning of a dentate model that had three reference scan bodies positioned in the mandibular first molar positions and right central incisor position realized differences in mean distance and angular errors among the three scanners tested. The scanner that used video capture technology and a high-accuracy scanning protocol had smaller and more consistent errors compared with the two point-and-click scanners in regard to mean distance errors.[79]

Intraoral scanning for edentulous indications

Limited data exist pertaining to the use of intraoral scanners for edentulous arches. One *in vitro* study of four intraoral scanners (iTero, Lava COS, CEREC AC Bluecam, and Zfx IntraScan) used to digitize maxillary and mandibular edentulous reference models found mean trueness values ranging from 44.1–591.8 μm and mean precision values ranging from 21.6–698.0 μm. The greatest visual deviations of the superimposed data sets occurred in the maxillary arch, with digital mismatches in the palatal region.[80] Although the Lava COS scanner achieved the highest level of accuracy in the study, the authors concluded that, because of the high degree of inaccuracy found in the study, the expectation was that even less accuracy would be realized due to saliva and mobile tissue intraorally. Therefore further enhancements were required before a clinical recommendation could be given to use these scanners for clinical edentulous arch scanning.[80] New hardware and software have been released, but this study has not been replicated to validate manufacturer claims of the ability to scan soft tissues.

A unique *in vivo* study evaluated 25 patients who had mandibular bar overdentures fabricated previously. The original definitive master casts for each patient were digitized and served as the reference comparison for the intraoral scan data sets obtained with an iTero scanner.[81] The authors concluded that the distance errors and the mean angular errors were too large to fabricate a well-fitting superstructure for the two implants in the edentulous mandible. In fact, for four of the 25 patients, no clinically acceptable scan could be achieved. This was discussed as a limitation of the scanner technology and hardware. The intraoral scanner captures a maximum area of 14 × 18 mm.[82] Stitching of the photographs was not possible if there was a large distance between the implants and a lack of definitive mucosal landmarks to function as reference points.[81] However, some patients with large inter-implant distances could be scanned because of the presence of stable mucosa that had adequately variable tissue height, allowing for appropriate reference for the software calculations.[81] The authors demonstrated stitching errors in 10 of the 21 patients, four of the 21 patient scans exhibited deformation of the scan abutments, and one patient had both stitching and deformation errors. Five scans appeared to be optically correct; however, only one of those scans had acceptable errors (distance error of 60 μm and angle error of 0.342°).[81] As discouraging as these results may seem, one must consider that at the time of the study this particular scanner was not indicated for this type of clinical situation; it has since gone through multiple software and, more recently, hardware updates. Highlighting the evolving nature of technology related to implant prosthodontics is important to assess the impact of new developments on the comparative accuracy with conventional techniques.

Intraoral scanning systems can be differentiated on the basis of whether or not an agent is required on the tissues to be scanned. The use of powder or other contrast media is required for different purposes, but in general is used to combat the challenges faced while scanning intraorally,[83–85] and could prove beneficial in assisting the scanning of edentulous arches. The optical properties of the target surface, such as the translucency and reflectivity, vary between enamel, dentin, restorative materials, gingiva, and mucosa, and influence the accuracy of the scan. The geometry of the target surface, sharp line angles, and presence or lack of a supragingival margin are challenges for intraoral scanners, as are the moisture and humidity present in the oral cavity. Random relative motion can create artifacts in the dataset. The development of scan spray application has resulted in thinner coatings, enhanced image acquisition, and improvement in marginal fidelity of milled prostheses over conventional powdering techniques.[85] The original CEREC Redcam and Bluecam (Sirona Dental, Inc., Charlotte, NC) required essentially a complete surface coating of the tissue in question, so that the projected striped light pattern could be reflected off the tissue surface and captured by the optical sensor. The 3M ESPE Lava COS and, more recently, True Definition scanners rely on the distinct macro-features of the powder in the various images captured to allow aligning of the images in creating the 3-D image (Figure 15.15). These contrast media typically consist of some combination of titanium dioxide, zirconium dioxide, and zinc stearate. The powder is used to reflect light and to minimize the scattering of the light off the target surface.[86] These compounds are commonly found in food coloring and dyes. It has been shown that the neither the optical properties, composition, nor form of titanium and alumina oxides found in various contrast media had an impact on the marginal gaps of zirconia crowns fabricated using a lab-based scanner.[86] Similar results have been realized with infrared laser CEREC 3/RedCam and LED CEREC AC/BlueCam (Sirona Dental, Inc., Charlotte, NC) and different powdering techniques, as no differences were found on internal adaptation and marginal precision.[87,88]

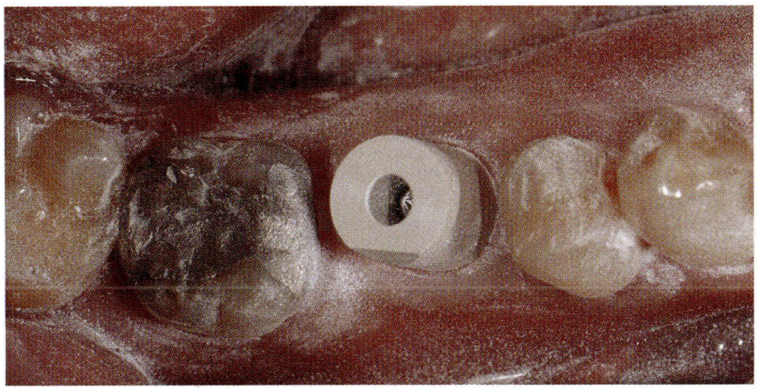

Figure 15.15 Proper isolation, field control, and contrast medium application for intraoral scanning of implant scanbodies.

The consistency of application of the contrast media has been shown to be operator dependent. An *in vitro* investigation determined that experienced dentists generated more homogeneous ($p < .001$) and thinner ($p < .007$) applications of the scan spray than did inexperienced dentists.[89] The experienced group consisted of three dentists with over 10 years of experience with prosthodontics and daily use of CAD/CAM systems, whereas the inexperienced group consisted of postgraduate dentists with no clinical experience with a CAD/CAM system. The thickness of the coating for the experienced group was 43.1 ± 14.09 μm and 70.19 ± 31.26 μm for the inexperienced group for all crown surfaces.[89] It has been suggested that inconsistent surface coating could result in poor marginal adaptation of prostheses.[84] The extension of this suggestion to implant prosthodontics would imply that inconsistency in surface coating may result in ill-fitting surgical guides, and inaccuracies of implant scanbody registration (or even complete lack of registration) downstream in the computer-aided design software. However, anecdotal clinical experience with multiple "powder-free" scanners has revealed that scanning progresses more efficiently when a contrast medium has been applied.

The use of Pressure Indicator Paste (Mizzy, Inc., Cherry Hill, NJ) applied with a toothbrush has been suggested as an alternative to scan sprays to decrease the reflectivity of cast restorations and avoid any issues with the inhalation of fine dust particles.[90]

The clinician looking to become an adopter of intraoral scanning should be cautious to not place too much emphasis on whether a particular device uses a contrast medium or not. It may seem that a device that does not "require" the use of a contrast medium would be simpler to use and would be recommended for a novice user; however, the base tenet of intraoral scanning is maintaining a dry and isolated work field. It is plausible that, through the extra effort of applying a contrast medium, proper retraction and moisture control will be precisely maintained, resulting in consistently accurate scans. An informal survey of the currently available intraoral scanners reveals that, in general terms, the intraoral scanners that require a contrast medium are less expensive, incorporate simpler and possibly more robust technology, and are as accurate (or more accurate) than the intraoral scanners that do not require a contrast medium. Other considerations must be factored into the decision process before acquiring an intraoral scanner: clinical indications, especially an implant workflow with the implant manufacturer currently using clinically, company reputation, product life cycle (first generation or later iteration?), initial cost, ongoing costs such as service contracts and data plans, open architecture or closed architecture, how readily it interfaces with local or at-distance dental laboratories, size, weight, balance of scanner, user interface, local or cloud storage (short term and long term) of patient data, data encryption and HIPAA compliant, speed and efficiency of clinical workflow, etc.

Technologies for jaw-relation records

It has been demonstrated that the use of a digital pretreatment wax-up can result in increased contact numbers as compared with the pretreatment casts ($p = 0.00$); however, no difference in contact numbers existed between the conventional wax-up casts and digital wax-up casts ($p = 0.07$).[91] With respect to contact area, the conventional and digital wax-up casts had similar contact area ($p = 0.11$), with the conventional wax-up cast having greater contact area than the pretreatment casts ($p = 0.01$). The contact accuracy for pretreatment casts exhibited greater contact precision than the two wax-up casts ($p = 0.00$). Overall the conventional and digital wax-up casts exhibited similar contact accuracy ($p = 0.07$).[91] The authors concluded that the digital wax-up was comparable to a conventional wax-up, but noted that physical casts from each should be subjected to further investigation.[91] In a study evaluating the lateral occlusal scheme developed from both a conventional wax-up and a digitally developed wax-up, minimal difference in the number and pattern of the excursive contacts was noted between the two methods, suggesting that, although early in its development, the digital method is a clinically relevant method of developing a lateral occlusal scheme.[92]

It has been demonstrated that for virtual prosthodontics, patient occlusal contacts computed using a "three-point alignment" method from aligned virtual casts accurately reproduce the contacts on the analog articulator.[93] Limitations of this approach include the lack of verification if this truly represents the best possible maximum intercuspation position and the reliance on establishing the occlusion on dental stone casts initially.[94] Expanding on this methodology, a rigid motion engine is enabled to prevent the virtual penetration of maxillary and mandibular dental models when aligning casts with a freehand movement tool. Additionally, a guided movement tool allows the operator to direct the final occlusion from an idealized initial position, and, after three such positions have been selected, a "spring connection" is assigned. Once the forces applied by the springs equal the contact reaction forces as defined by the rigid motion engine, a stable occlusal position is realized.[95] Using this method in a validation study, it was determined that due to the small variations between a manually and virtually defined occlusion, this system could be used clinically.[95] Again, it has been suggested that without first seeing physical casts, it may be difficult to digitize the corresponding points on the maxillary and mandibular models.[94] To that end, an automated method of articulation of digital dental models into maximum intercuspation position has been developed and demonstrated to produce accurate and effective articulation.[94] This method employs an initial alignment based on the dental curve and point matching algorithms, and the final maximum intercuspation position achieved through an iterative surface-based minimal-distance-mapping algorithm that includes collision constraints.[94] There is a learning curve to digitally derived occlusions; as with the analog method, the individual can "feel" the casts intercuspate, whereas, with the digital, the individual only "sees" the resultant occlusion on the screen (Figure 15.16).[95]

Technologies used in the fabrication of prostheses

The dental laboratory industry has embraced digital technologies for the fabrication of virtually any type of dental prosthesis. For implant prostheses, this typically is in the form of a subtractive process to mill patient-specific abutments, custom implant bars or substructure frameworks, and the definitive

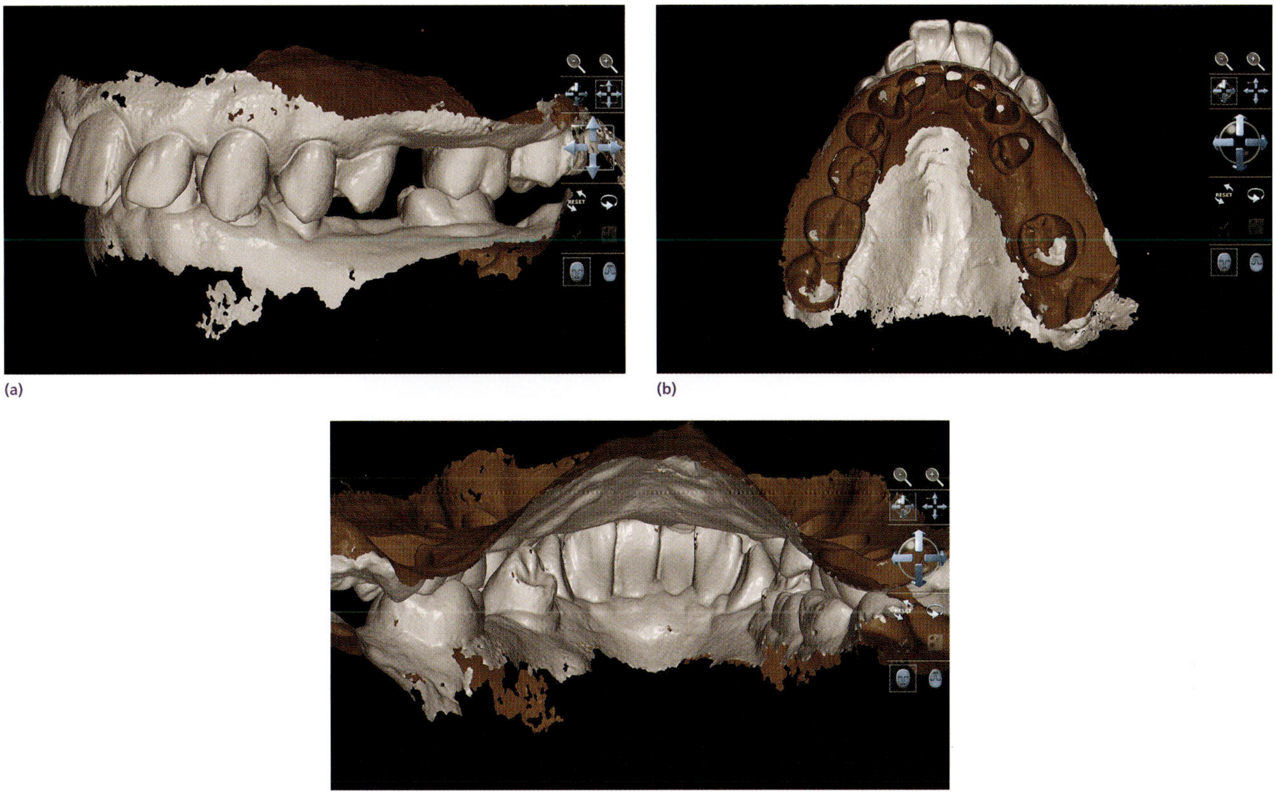

(a) (b) (c)

Figure 15.16 (a) A maximum intercuspation position acquired with an intraoral scanner. Instructing the patient to close with even pressure bilaterally is helpful in obtaining an accurate registration. (b) Occlusal registration as verified from "underneath". Even distribution of white "burn through" would be indicative of appropriate occlusal registration. Use of shim stock to verify key occlusal stops is a good practice. (c) The unique lingual perspective of the occlusion.

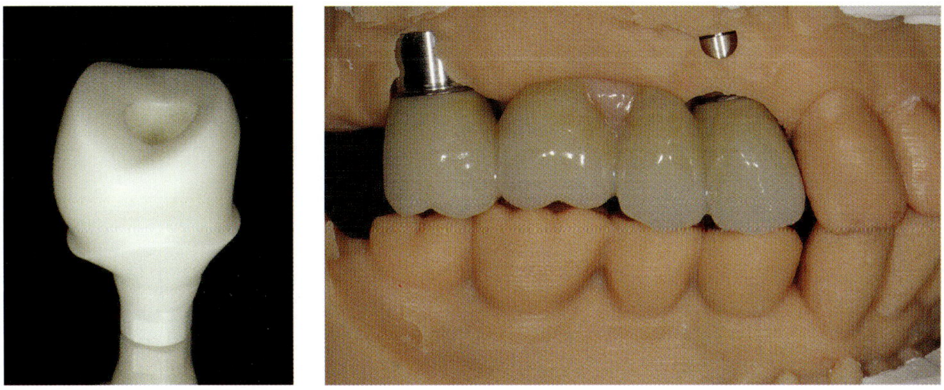

(a) (b)

Figure 15.17 (a) Custom-milled zirconia abutment from manufacturer blank that has premachined implant interface. (b) Custom-milled monolithic zirconia screw-retained implant fixed dental prosthesis.

prosthetic suprastructure.[96–98] Much attention has been devoted to zirconium dioxide as a material for custom implant abutments and implant prosthesis frameworks (Figure 15.17). It has been shown that the strength of the custom-milled zirconia abutments is equal to or superior to that of prefabricated custom abutments; however, the implant/abutment interface fit is less accurate.[99] Similar findings were reported for copy-milled zirconia abutments having a less accurate fit than prefabricated titanium abutments; however, this decrease in fit did not compromise their ability to maintain the applied preload torque.[100] Investigation of multiple implant–abutment interface configurations revealed micromotion at the interface ranging from 1.52 to 94.00 μm. CAD/CAM zirconia abutments exhibited less micromotion than did CAD/CAM titanium abutments. If micromotion can be used as a surrogate measure for the fit at the implant–abutment interface, this would suggest a better fit of the CAD/CAM zirconia abutments.

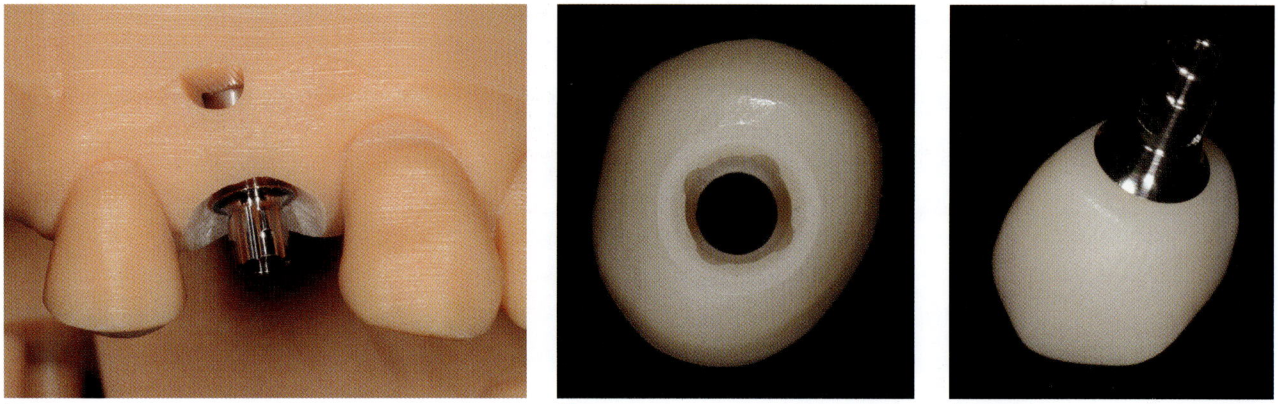

(a) (b) (c)

Figure 15.18 (a) Titanium base for a hybrid abutment. (b) Milled custom zirconia crown. Note the milled anti-rotational features on the intaglio surface. (c) Hybrid abutment components assembled and bonded together.

The long-term clinical significance is unknown. CAD/CAM abutments interfaced to proprietary and competing implant systems exhibited inconsistent levels of micromotion. Pronounced variations in interface micromotion were realized with clone abutments and clone implant systems.[101] Given the degree of implant–abutment interface micromotion, concern for wear at the interface, resulting in loss of preload and/or component fracture, and ultimately the release of titanium debris, has been raised.[102] Clinical findings of titanium tattooing associated with zirconia abutments has been reported and should now be considered a potential complication for use of zirconia abutments in clinical situations of high esthetic demand,[103] precisely one of the primary indications for the use of custom zirconia abutments!

The recent addition of hybrid abutments, consisting of a titanium base that interfaces with the titanium implant and a custom CAD/CAM zirconia meso- or suprastructure, may become more routine in practice. The advantage of this system is the mating of like materials at the implant–abutment interface along with the esthetics and soft tissue benefits of zirconia placed into the gingival sulcus (Figure 15.18). However, concern exists about the durability of the bonded interface between the titanium base and the zirconia structure. An *in vitro* study evaluating the integrity of the bonded interface between titanium and zirconia has shown that air abrasion of the titanium as well as the zirconia coping, along with a 30 μm luting gap resulted in significantly greater retention of the copings than copings bonded with a 60 μm gap.[104] The use of air abrasion on both the titanium and zirconia, along with alcohol cleaning of the components prior to bonding results in stable retention;[105,106] more recently, the use of a phosphate-based primer to further enhance the retention has been recommended.[106] The load-bearing capacity of a bonded zirconia abutment to a titanium base has been shown to be greater than that of a friction fit interface between the titanium and zirconia as well as an all zirconia abutment.[107] Based on the limited, yet positive, *in vitro* findings, further *in vivo* investigations are required to confirm the clinical acceptability of the hybrid abutment concept. Chairside CAD/CAM systems now have the workflows that allow the milling of custom zirconia abutment structures in-office that can then be bonded to the corresponding titanium base.

The precision of fit of short-span (five units) and long-span (10 units) implant-supported screw-retained FDPs manufactured from CAD/CAM titanium and ceramic veneer have shown clinically acceptable values, with five-unit FDPs being statistically more precise than the 10-unit FDPs. Total median vertical microgaps were 23 μm (range 2–38 μm) for the long-span group and 7 μm (4–24 μm) for short-span group.[108] The porcelain firing process has been shown to have no effect on the precision of fit of 10-unit CAD/CAM titanium FDPs.[109] A study evaluating the accuracy of fit of three-unit implant-supported, screw-retained frameworks fabricated from CAD/CAM zirconia and cobalt–chromium compared with cast cobalt–chromium frameworks, with either premachined cast to abutments or castable abutments, concluded that the CAD/CAM frameworks had better fit accuracy than the cast frameworks. The mean vertical misfit values were 5.9 ± 3.6 μm for CAD/CAM-fabricated zirconia, 1.2 ± 2.2 μm for CAD/CAM-fabricated cobalt–chromium frameworks, 11.8 ± 9.8 μm for conventionally fabricated cobalt–chromium frameworks with premachined abutments, and 12.9 ± 11.0 μm for conventionally fabricated frameworks with castable abutments.[110]

Further advances of additive manufacturing techniques, such as selective laser sintering (SLS) and selective laser melting (SLM), may allow these technologies that are conducive to the rapid fabrication of high-precision parts with complex geometries to replace the current mainstay subtractive process of milling.[111]

Technologies for implant prosthesis delivery

As aspirational as it may be to hire a humanoid robot for the dental office to assist in the delivery of prosthodontic care, no such entity exists today. However, the development of artificial limb prostheses for amputee patients with sensory feedback

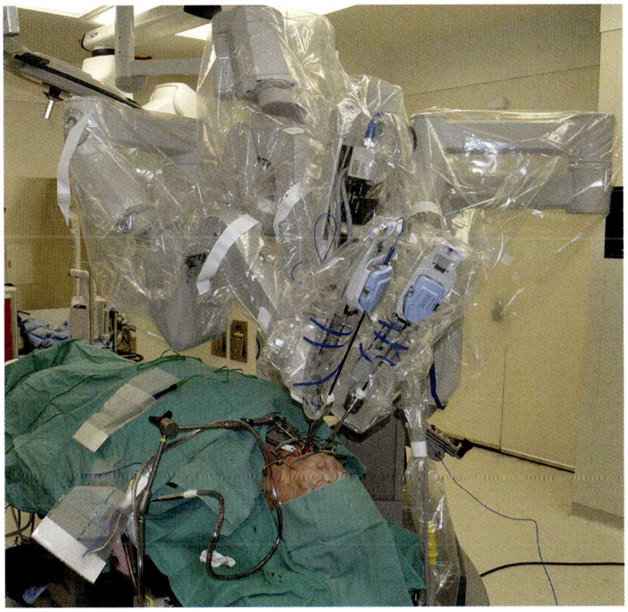

(a)

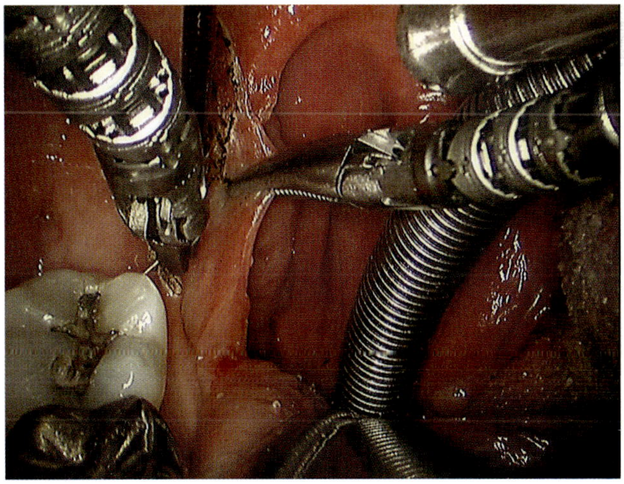

(b)

Figure 15.19 (a) daVinci surgical robot in position for transoral-robotic assisted radical tonsillectomy (Intuitive Surgical, Inc., Sunnyvale, CA). (b) Intraoperative view during radical tonsillectomy for T1 tonsillar cancer. *Source:* Reproduced with permission from Dr. Rodrigo Bayon.

from the artificial hand[112] and tactile sense rivaling the touch of a human finger[113] may be precursors to the prosthodontic robot. Our surgical colleagues in medicine have adapted surgical robots for the treatment of head and neck cancers.[114–117] Transoral robotic surgery (TORS) has been advocated for the following anatomical subsets: oropharynx, hypopharynx, supraglottic larynx, larynx, parapharyngeal space, and skull base (Figure 15.19).[115,117] TORS has been shown to decrease the number of tracheotomies required, facilitate more rapid swallowing rehabilitation, and decrease the time of in-patient hospital stays.[115] As these technologies continue to evolve, their adaption to implant surgical procedures and operative/prosthodontics procedures are closer to being realized. In the interim, the clinician can employ existing digital technologies to decrease the number of procedures rendered, improve clinical outcomes, and enhance the patient experiences as well as those of the clinician.

Time efficiencies

An *in vitro* investigation looked at time efficiencies of analog versus digital impression making for three different scenarios: a single right maxillary first molar crown abutment, a maxillary right second molar and second premolar for a two-abutment three-unit FDP, and a complete arch of 14 prepared crown abutments.[118] The scanners investigated consisted of the CEREC AC with Bluecam, Lava COS, and iTero. The results were that for the single-abutment scenario, the digital impressions were up to 23 minutes faster, for the three-unit FDP scenario the digital impressions were up to 22 minutes faster, and for the full arch scenario the digital impressions were up to 13 minutes faster.[118] The authors suggest that computer-aided impression methods create a more time-efficient work flow than can be achieved with conventional impression techniques.[118] In comparing a conventional and a digital impression work flow, the only steps eliminated by the digital workflow is the disinfection of the impression and pouring of the impression.[118]

Similar time efficiencies were realized in a study that compared the digital versus conventional impression techniques for a single-unit implant prosthesis. The mean total time for the conventional impression was 24 minutes and 42 seconds compared with only 12 minutes and 29 seconds for the digital impression, a significant difference of over 12 minutes ($p < .001$).[119] It should be noted this study involved novice clinicians, second-year dental students, and that the times also included retakes or rescans.[119] More recently, an *in vivo* study involved 50 patients who had both a conventional and a digital full-arch implant impression for a single-unit premolar implant prosthesis. The mean time for the digital impression was 6 minutes and 39 seconds, whereas the time for the analog impression was 12 minutes and 13 seconds. The difference was significant at $p < .001$ and large effect size (d) of 2.7.[120]

In a study comparing time requirements for alginate and intraoral scans of complete arches for orthodontic purposes, the mean chairside time for the alginate impressions was 7 minutes and 35 seconds compared with 20 minutes and 27 seconds for the Lava COS intraoral scans, and the difference was significant ($p < 0.05$).[121] However, when the procedure processing time was factored in there was no difference ($p < 0.05$) between the conventional and digital impressions, 22 minutes and 12 seconds versus 20 minutes and 47 seconds respectively.[121] The authors go on to discuss how in an office with only one scanner, only about 16 to 20 scans can be performed in an 8-hour workday, in contrast to alginates that could be made simultaneously by several staff throughout the same time period, suggesting that conventional impressions are more practical when considering time requirements and performing multiple procedures simultaneously.[121] A clinician must critically assess office and patient flow as part of the decision process regarding the incorporation of digital techniques into everyday dentistry.

Patient preferences

The patient experience surrounding the impression-making process is of utmost importance. A documented trend of patient preference for digital impressions over conventional impression techniques has been established.[120,122,123] Patient-reported reasons for favoring digital impressions include: less inconvenience, shortness of breath, and fear of repeating the impression; fewer feelings of helplessness during the procedure,[120] preparatory activities, and taste effects;[122] decreased queasiness, time mouth opened, TMJ discomfort, smell, heat, and overall discomfort.[123] In one study, patients perceived the length of time of the intraoral scan to be negative compared with the analog impression technique,[122] which conflicts with positive perception of the overall time of impression for the digital impression in a separate study.[123] Intraoral scanners on the market today come in a variety of sizes and shapes. In considering an intraoral scanner, not only is the overall size and weight important, but also size and geometry of the specific intraoral portion of the scanner. This will have significant influence on ease of access to various areas of the oral cavity and the overall patient comfort during scanning (Figure 15.20). Of interest is the clinicians' perception of the use of the intraoral scanner; as one would expect, with proper training and increased experience, their views toward the use of the intraoral scanner may be changed in a positive direction.[124]

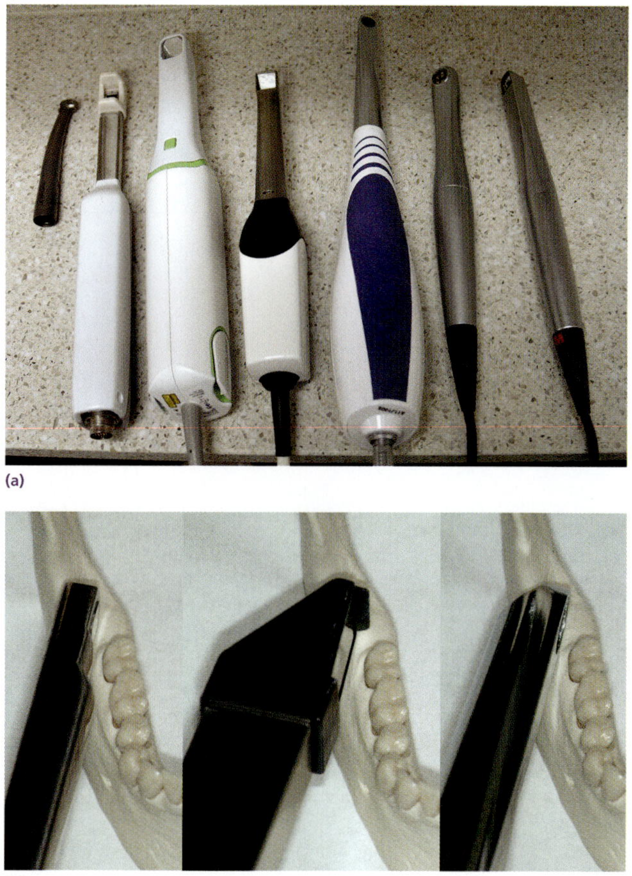

(a)

(b)

Figure 15.20 **(a)** Example of various sizes and shapes of intraoral scanners. **(b)** Impact of the physical geometry on oral access of intraoral scanners.

Technologies for implant prosthodontic patient maintenance

As the technologies for intraoral scanning and extraoral scanning continue to evolve, data acquisition and accuracy will no doubt continue to improve, and this will lead to new diagnostic and patient monitoring modalities over the standard indications of today's scanners. Superimposition of serial partial or complete-arch intraoral scan 3-D data sets will allow for the monitoring of volumetric changes of hard and soft tissues,[125–127] restorative materials, 3-D tooth positional changes, and postural changes in jaw position at various points in time (Figure 15.21). Diagnoses and rendered treatment can now be analyzed over time.[128,129] This will ultimately lead to the development of more robust, evidenced-based treatment protocols.

We have come to appreciate that with implant patients there are craniofacial growth/atrophy changes that can occur over the life of the adult patient, resulting in positional changes of the implant prosthesis relative to adjacent teeth for the partially edentulous patient (Figure 15.22).[130–135] The effect of these craniofacial changes for the patient restored with an implant-supported complete denture on multiple implants is unknown and should give pause. Additionally, an instrument such as the Tekscan (Tekscan, Inc., South Boston, MA) may be beneficial in establishing a baseline occlusion record post-delivery of an implant prosthesis that can be compared against future dynamic occlusal registrations at subsequent recall appointments, to analyze any changes to the location, timing, and force magnitude of the occlusal contacts.[136–138] Through the use of CBCT and 3-D analysis, the hard and soft tissue changes after implant site augmentation and implant placement can be monitored, spectrophotometry can be employed to analyze the color of gingival tissues around implants and natural teeth, nonionizing modalities, such as magnetic resonance imaging and ultrasonography, hold promise for future application in the evaluation of hard and soft tissues defects, and optical scanning and optical coherence tomography may assist in the evaluation of implant prosthesis misfit.[127]

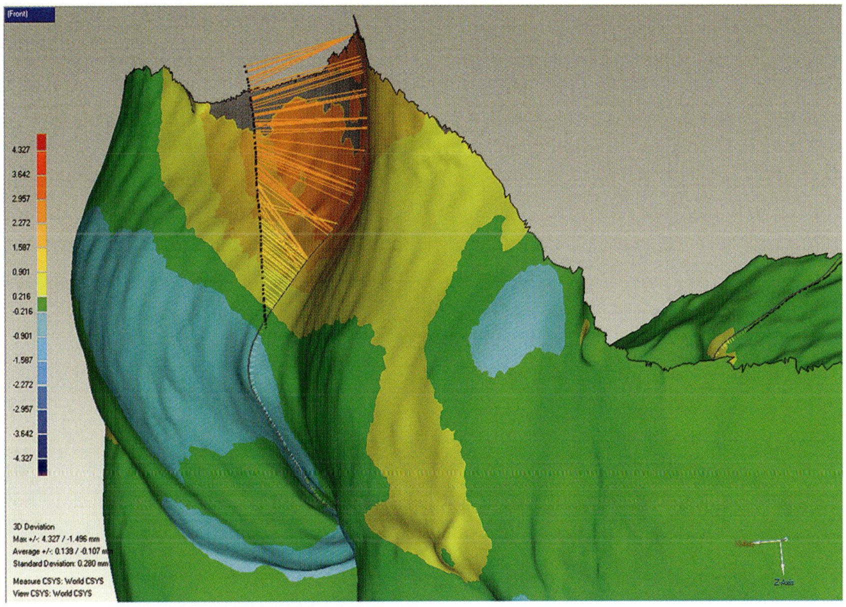

Figure 15.21 Overlay of intraoral scans to monitor the volumetric change of a bone graft in a potential implant site.

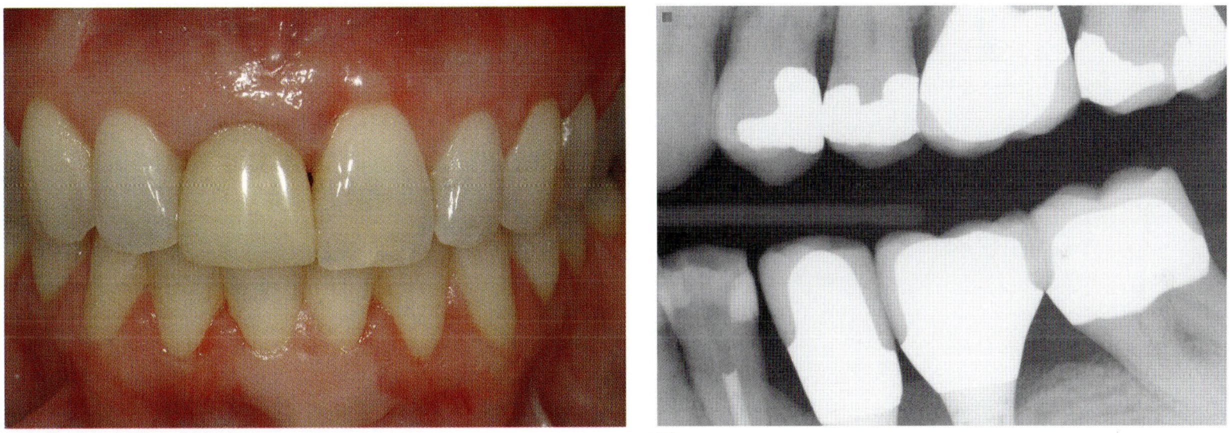

(a) (b)

Figure 15.22 **(a)** Incisal edge positional change of natural teeth relative to implant in right central incisor. **(b)** Opening up of mesial contact between implant crown and natural tooth.

Evolving technologies in implant maxillofacial prosthodontics

For the treatment of the complex maxillofacial patient, dental implants have been most beneficial in the restoration of form and function. The delivery of maxillofacial prosthodontic care today is benefiting from an extensive application of the complete digital workflow, as has been presented above.[139,140] The diagnostic work-up is based on the medical computed tomography (CT) data sets of the primary surgical site and the donor graft site. From these medical CTs, a process of virtual surgical planning is completed using sophisticated software (VSP, Medical Modeling, Boulder, CO), in which the tumor resection is completed, donor graft is manipulated to reconstruct the defect, implants are placed in the graft, and all of it is based on the definitive prosthesis, designed not only to restore form but also functional occlusion. Once the surgical and prosthetic plan has been approved by the treating team, the virtual plan is converted into a series of models, cutting guides, implant placement guides, and reconstruction plates that will be used at the time of surgery. If desired, the surgery and reconstruction can be practiced using these physical models (Figure 15.23). The use of this technique has resulted in a decrease in operative times and increased rates of dental rehabilitation,[141] and in some instances allows complete reconstruction in a single stage.[142,143] In a retrospective *in vivo* study of 10 patients who underwent a VSP protocol, preoperative planning and postoperative CT scans revealed no difference in the dimensions of

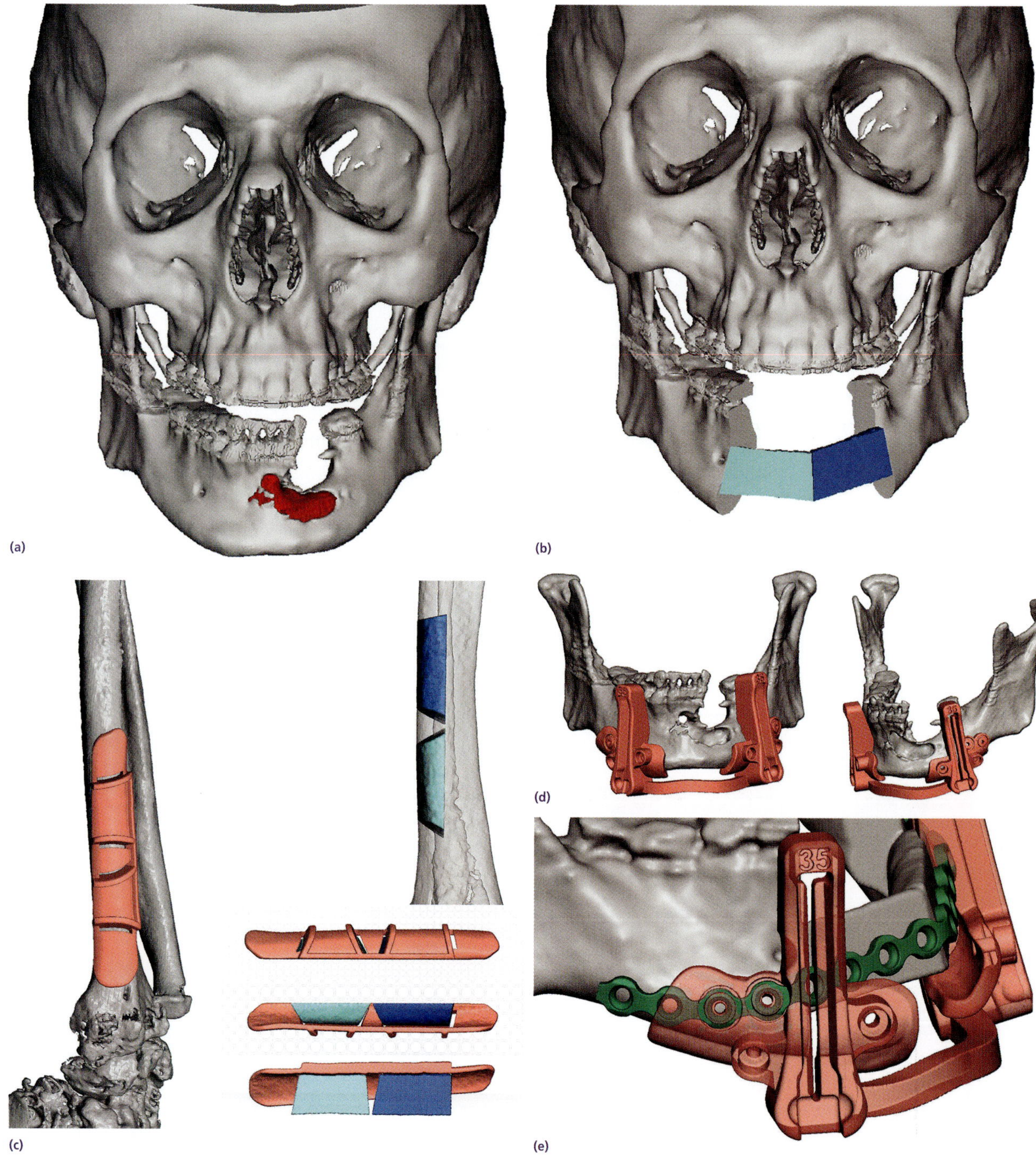

Figure 15.23 **(a)** Three-dimensional reconstruction of tumor. **(b)** Proposed mandibular reconstruction with radial forearm free flap graft. **(c)** Cutting guides on radius for mitered cuts. **(d)** Cutting guides on mandible for precise resection. **(e)** Close-up of guide on mandible indicating shared holes for guide and reconstruction plate, and right mandible cut guide.

the fibula osteotomies. A 12.4° and −12.5° difference of the anterior and posterior mandibular angles was noted postoperatively as compared to the preoperative plan, respectively. A 1.7 mm and 4.6° difference was noted for the condylar distance and inclination, respectively, postoperatively as compared with the preoperative VSP plan. The authors concluded that this virtual surgical approach delivered reproducible accuracy and precision when used for mandibular fibula free flap reconstructions, especially the reconstructions requiring multiple fibula sections.[144]

Future trends in implant prosthodontics

With the current debate between cement-retained and screw-retained implant prostheses[145–150] and the possible pendulum swing back to predominately screw-retained prostheses, the application of a digital workflow from diagnosis, implant planning, surgical guide fabrication, and implant surgery will be critical for locating screw-access holes in clinically appropriate locations and also working with systems that incorporate abutments that allow for angulated screw channels (ASC, NobelBiocare, Yorba Linda, CA).

As the field of additive manufacturing continues to expand and evolve in medicine and dentistry, new health technologies – defined as any equipment, materials, drugs, or procedures used by healthcare professionals, and the systems within which they are used – will be realized. An example is the incorporation of antimicrobial agents into 3-D printed polymers, allowing for implant prosthetic materials that may be effective against implant mucositis and peri-implantitis. Recent work has demonstrated that adding positively charged quaternary ammonium groups to diurethanedimethacrylate/glycerol dimethacrylate photocurable resins, as part of the stereolithographic workflow, produced composite resins that were bactericidal upon contact, without loss of the mechanical properties.[151]

Much intriguing investigation is ongoing in the development of patient-specific bioprinting of biologic structures and tissues.[152] Osteoconductive calcium phosphate scaffolds have been successfully fabricated using low-temperature thermal inkjet printing for proposed synthetic bone graft materials,[153] as have osteoinductive resorbable materials from brushite and monetite.[154] In a study comparing monolithic monetite versus autografts for vertical onlay grafts in a rabbit model, it was found that osseous tissue within the autograft occupied 60% of volume, whereas the monetite graft had new bone formation in 43% of its volume.[155] Further investigation has demonstrated the successful osseointegration of dental implants into sites augmented with 3-D printed monolithic microporous monetite bioresorbable synthetic onlay grafts in the rabbit model.[156] To further enhance the biologic activity of these printed synthetic scaffolds, it has been shown that the application of a cell-laid extracellular matrix to the scaffold results in osteoblastic differentiation due to an upregulation of osteoblastic genes (RUNX2, alkaline phosphatase, osteocalcin, and osteopontin), along with an increase in calcium deposition.[157] More effort is required in the development of these printing methodologies, that not only produce the customized scaffold for cells to adhere to, proliferate, and migrate on, but also incorporate growth factors, pharmaceuticals, and living cells.[152,158] In a 1-year follow-up of a prospective study on 10 patients who received patient-specific scaffolds milled from porous hydroxyapatite blocks for maxillary ridge augmentation, the authors concluded the scaffolds were clinically acceptable in regard to size, shape, and appearance, and they matched the residual defect. This allowed for a reduction in surgical time and produced acceptable healing of the defects.[159] The obvious benefit of synthetic graft materials for the implant patient with deficient alveolar bone in the proposed implant site is the lack of a donor site surgery and the associated morbidity and avoidance of off-axis implant placement. In the future these patient-specific synthetic bone graft substitutes may be used in the repair of periodontal defects,[160] or ultimately in the reconstruction of more complex congenital or acquired craniofacial defects.[158]

Summary

With the advent of osseointegrated dental implants, our ability to restore stomatognathic form and function has been greatly enhanced. A once predominantly analog process now has succumbed to the digital era, with current and evolving technologies for each phase of the treatment of the implant patient. As is common with any health technology, there is a lag in adoption from the time of introduction, in part due to the rapid development of technologies, concurrent with limited clinical documentation. However, as this body of literature continues to mature, additional enhanced and validated digital treatment algorithms will evolve, enabling a more efficient and effective delivery of care for our implant patients.

References

1. Ashwinirani SR, Suragimath G, Jaishankar HP, *et al.* Comparison of diagnostic accuracy of conventional intraoral periapical and direct digital radiographs in detecting interdental bone loss. *J Clin Diagn Res* 2015; **9**(2): ZC35–38.
2. Morner-Svalling AC, Tronje G, Andersson LG, *et al.* Comparison of the diagnostic potential of direct digital and conventional intraoral radiography in the evaluation of peri-implant conditions. *Clin Oral Implants Res* 2003; **14**(6): 714–719.
3. Dias da Silva PR, Martins Marques M, Steagall W Jr, *et al.* Accuracy of direct digital radiography for detecting occlusal caries in primary teeth compared with conventional radiography and visual inspection: an in vitro study. *Dentomaxillofac Radiol* 2010; **39**(6): 362–367.
4. Celik E, Polat-Ozsoy O, Toygar Memikoglu TU. Comparison of cephalometric measurements with digital versus conventional cephalometric analysis. *Eur J Orthod* 2009; **31**(3): 241–246.
5. Uysal T, Baysal A, Yagci A. Evaluation of speed, repeatability, and reproducibility of digital radiography with manual versus computer-assisted cephalometric analyses. *Eur J Orthod* 2009; **31**(5): 523–528.
6. D'Haese J, Van De Velde T, Komiyama A, *et al.* Accuracy and complications using computer-designed stereolithographic surgical guides for oral rehabilitation by means of dental implants: a review of the literature. *Clin Implant Dent Relat Res* 2012; **14**(3): 321–335.
7. Kalra M, Aparna IN, Dhanasekar B. Evolution of surgical guidance in implant dentistry. *Dent Update* 2013; **40**(7): 577–582.
8. Nickenig HJ, Eitner S, Rothamel D, *et al.* Possibilities and limitations of implant placement by virtual planning data and surgical guide templates. *Int J Comput Dent* 2012; **15**(1): 9–21.

9. Benavides E, Rios HF, Ganz SD, *et al.* Use of cone beam computed tomography in implant dentistry: the International Congress of Oral Implantologists consensus report. *Implant Dent* 2012; **21**(2): 78–86.
10. Akyalcin S, Cozad BE, English JD, *et al.* Diagnostic accuracy of impression-free digital models. *Am J Orthod Dentofacial Orthop* 2013; **144**(6): 916–922.
11. Anadioti E, Aquilino SA, Gratton DG, *et al.* 3D and 2D marginal fit of pressed and CAD/CAM lithium disilicate crowns made from digital and conventional impressions. *J Prosthodont* 2014; **23**(8): 610–617.
12. Abduo J, Bennamoun M, Tennant M. Influence of conventional and digital wax-ups on axial tooth contour. *Int J Periodontics Restorative Dent* 2015; **35**(4): e50–59.
13. Shujaat S, Khambay BS, Ju X, *et al.* The clinical application of three-dimensional motion capture (4D): a novel approach to quantify the dynamics of facial animations. *Int J Oral Maxillofac Surg* 2014; **43**(7): 907–916.
14. Ju X, O'Leary E, Peng M, *et al.* Evaluation of the reproducibility of nonverbal facial expressions using a 3D motion capture system. *Cleft Palate Craniofac J* 2016; **53**(1): 22–29.
15. Lee JG, Jung SJ, Lee HJ, *et al.* Quantitative anatomical analysis of facial expression using a 3D motion capture system: application to cosmetic surgery and facial recognition technology. *Clin Anat* 2015; **28**(6): 735–744.
16. Sun X, McKenzie FD, Bawab S, *et al.* Automated dental implantation using image-guided robotics: registration results. *Int J Comput Assist Radiol Surg* 2011; **6**(5): 627–634.
17. Sun X, Yoon Y, Li J, *et al.* Automated image-guided surgery for common and complex dental implants. *J Med Eng Technol* 2014; **38**(5): 251–259.
18. Jabero M, Sarment DP. Advanced surgical guidance technology: a review. *Implant Dent* 2006; **15**(2): 135–142.
19. Scherer MD, Kattadiyil MT, Parciak E, *et al.* CAD/CAM guided surgery in implant dentistry. A review of software packages and step-by-step protocols for planning surgical guides. *Alpha Omegan* 2014; **107**(1): 32–38.
20. Guichet D. Digitally enhanced dentistry: the power of digital design. *J Calif Dent Assoc* 2015; **43**(3): 135–141.
21. Ganz SD. Techniques for the use of CT imaging for the fabrication of surgical guides. *Atlas Oral Maxillofac Surg Clin North Am* 2006; **14**(1): 75–97.
22. Park JM, Yi TK, Koak JY, *et al.* Comparison of five-axis milling and rapid prototyping for implant surgical templates. *Int J Oral Maxillofac Implants* 2014; **29**(2): 374–383.
23. Di Giacomo GA, da Silva JV, da Silva AM, *et al.* Accuracy and complications of computer-designed selective laser sintering surgical guides for flapless dental implant placement and immediate definitive prosthesis installation. *J Periodontol* 2012; **83**(4): 410–419.
24. Di Giacomo GA, Cury PR, de Araujo NS, *et al.* Clinical application of stereolithographic surgical guides for implant placement: preliminary results. *J Periodontol* 2005; **76**(4): 503–507.
25. Bindl A, Ritter L, Mehl A. Cerec guide: rapid and streamlined manufacture of surgical guides in dental practice. *Int J Comput Dent* 2012; **15**(1): 45–54.
26. Bindl A. Clinical application of fully digital Cerec surgical guides made in-house. *Int J Comput Dent* 2015; **18**(2): 163–175.
27. Neugebauer J, Kistler F, Kistler S, *et al.* CAD/CAM-produced surgical guides: optimizing the treatment workflow. *Int J Comput Dent* 2011; **14**(2): 93–103.
28. Ritter L, Palmer J, Bindl A, *et al.* Accuracy of chairside-milled CAD/CAM drill guides for dental implants. *Int J Comput Dent* 2014; **17**(2): 115–124.
29. Noharet R, Pettersson A, Bourgeois D. Accuracy of implant placement in the posterior maxilla as related to 2 types of surgical guides: a pilot study in the human cadaver. *J Prosthet Dent* 2014; **112**(3): 526–532.
30. Arisan V, Karabuda CZ, Mumcu E, *et al.* Implant positioning errors in freehand and computer-aided placement methods: a single-blind clinical comparative study. *Int J Oral Maxillofac Implants* 2013; **28**(1): 190–204.
31. Farley NE, Kennedy K, McGlumphy EA, *et al.* Split-mouth comparison of the accuracy of computer-generated and conventional surgical guides. *Int J Oral Maxillofac Implants* 2013; **28**(2): 563–572.
32. Geng W, Liu C, Su Y, *et al.* Accuracy of different types of computer-aided design/computer-aided manufacturing surgical guides for dental implant placement. *Int J Clin Exp Med* 2015; **8**(6): 8442–8449.
33. Cassetta M, Giansanti M, Di Mambro A, *et al.* Accuracy of two stereolithographic surgical templates: a retrospective study. *Clin Implant Dent Relat Res* 2013; **15**(3): 448–459.
34. Verhamme LM, Meijer GJ, Berge SJ, *et al.* An accuracy study of computer-planned implant placement in the augmented maxilla using mucosa-supported surgical templates. *Clin Implant Dent Relat Res* 2015; **17**(6): 1154–1163.
35. Cassetta M, Giansanti M, Di Mambro A, *et al.* Accuracy of positioning of implants inserted using a mucosa-supported stereolithographic surgical guide in the edentulous maxilla and mandible. *Int J Oral Maxillofac Implants* 2014; **29**(5): 1071–1078.
36. Ochi M, Kanazawa M, Sato D, *et al.* Factors affecting accuracy of implant placement with mucosa-supported stereolithographic surgical guides in edentulous mandibles. *Comput Biol Med* 2013; **43**(11): 1653–1660.
37. Reyes A, Turkyilmaz I, Prihoda TJ. Accuracy of surgical guides made from conventional and a combination of digital scanning and rapid prototyping techniques. *J Prosthet Dent* 2015; **113**(4): 295–303.
38. Bornstein MM, Al-Nawas B, Kuchler U, *et al.* Consensus statements and recommended clinical procedures regarding contemporary surgical and radiographic techniques in implant dentistry. *Int J Oral Maxillofac Implants* 2014; **29**(Suppl): 78–82.
39. Capp NJ. The diagnostic use of provisional restorations. *Restorative Dent* 1985; **1**(4): 92–98.
40. Moscovitch MS, Saba S. The use of a provisional restoration in implant dentistry: a clinical report. *Int J Oral Maxillofac Implants* 1996; **11**(3): 395–399.
41. Gratton DG, Aquilino SA. Interim restorations. *Dent Clin North Am* 2004; **48**(2): vii, 487–497.
42. Neale D, Chee WW. Development of implant soft tissue emergence profile: a technique. *J Prosthet Dent* 1994; **71**(4): 364–368.
43. Breeding LC, Dixon DL. Transfer of gingival contours to a master cast. *J Prosthet Dent* 1996; **75**(3): 341–343.
44. Saba S. Anatomically correct soft tissue profiles using fixed detachable provisional implant restorations. *J Can Dent Assoc* 1997; **63**(10): 767–770.
45. Biggs WF, Litvak AL Jr. Immediate provisional restorations to aid in gingival healing and optimal contours for implant patients. *J Prosthet Dent* 2001; **86**(2): 177–180.

46. Proussaefs P. The use of healing abutments for the fabrication of cement-retained, implant-supported provisional prostheses. *J Prosthet Dent* 2002; **87**(3): 333–335.
47. Sze AJ. Duplication of anterior provisional fixed partial dentures for the final restoration. *J Prosthet Dent* 1992; **68**(2): 220–223.
48. Listgarten MA, Lang NP, Schroeder HE, *et al.* Periodontal tissues and their counterparts around endosseous implants [corrected and republished with original paging, article orginally printed in *Clin Oral Implants Res* 1991; **2**(1): 1–19]. *Clin Oral Implants Res* 1991; **2**(3): 1–19.
49. Biggs WF. Placement of a custom implant provisional restoration at the second-stage surgery for improved gingival management: a clinical report. *J Prosthet Dent* 1996; **75**(3): 231–233.
50. Daftary F, Bahat O. Prosthetically formulated natural aesthetics in implant prostheses. *Pract Periodontics Aesthet Dent* 1994; **6**(9): 75–83.
51. Lewis S. Anterior single-tooth implant restorations. *Int J Periodontics Restorative Dent* 1995; **15**(1): 30–41.
52. Lin WS, Harris BT, Ozdemir E, *et al.* Maxillary rehabilitation with a CAD/CAM-fabricated, long-term interim and anatomic contour definitive prosthesis with a digital workflow: a clinical report. *J Prosthet Dent* 2013; **110**(1): 1–7.
53. Rayyan MM, Aboushelib M, Sayed NM, *et al.* Comparison of interim restorations fabricated by CAD/CAM with those fabricated manually. *J Prosthet Dent* 2015; **114**(3): 414–419.
54. Yao J, Li J, Wang Y, *et al.* Comparison of the flexural strength and marginal accuracy of traditional and CAD/CAM interim materials before and after thermal cycling. *J Prosthet Dent* 2014; **112**(3): 649–657.
55. Penate L, Basilio J, Roig M, *et al.* Comparative study of interim materials for direct fixed dental prostheses and their fabrication with CAD/CAM technique. *J Prosthet Dent* 2015; **114**(2): 248–253.
56. Proussaefs P, Proussaefs P. Use of CAD/CAM healing abutment immediately after dental implant placement for the non-esthetic zone. A guided soft tissue healing technique. *J Oral Implantol* 2015; **42**(2): 189–193.
57. Galindo-Moreno P, Leon-Cano A, Monje A, *et al.* Abutment height influences the effect of platform switching on peri-implant marginal bone loss. *Clin Oral Implants Res* 2016; **27**(2): 167–173.
58. Galindo-Moreno P, Leon-Cano A, Ortega-Oller I, *et al.* Prosthetic abutment height is a key factor in peri-implant marginal bone loss. *J Dent Res* 2014; **93**(7 Suppl): 80S–85S.
59. Chaves ES, Lovell JS, Tahmasebi S. Implant-supported crown design and the risk for peri-implantitis. *Clin Adv Periodontics* 2013; **4**(2): 118–126.
60. Boening KW, Wolf BH, Schmidt AE, *et al.* Clinical fit of Procera AllCeram crowns. *J Prosthet Dent* 2000; **84**(4): 419–424.
61. Laurent M, Scheer P, Dejou J, *et al.* Clinical evaluation of the marginal fit of cast crowns – validation of the silicone replica method. *J Oral Rehabil* 2008; **35**(2): 116–122.
62. Reich S, Uhlen S, Gozdowski S, *et al.* Measurement of cement thickness under lithium disilicate crowns using an impression material technique. *Clin Oral Investig* 2011; **15**(4): 521–526.
63. Fransson B, Oilo G, Gjeitanger R. The fit of metal-ceramic crowns, a clinical study. *Dent Mater* 1985; **1**(5): 197–199.
64. Renne W, McGill ST, Forshee KV, *et al.* Predicting marginal fit of CAD/CAM crowns based on the presence or absence of common preparation errors. *J Prosthet Dent* 2012; **108**(5): 310–315.
65. Karlsson S. The fit of Procera titanium crowns. An in vitro and clinical study. *Acta Odontol Scand* 1993; **51**(3): 129–134.
66. Boeddinghaus M, Breloer ES, Rehmann P, *et al.* Accuracy of single-tooth restorations based on intraoral digital and conventional impressions in patients. *Clin Oral Investig* 2015; **19**(8): 2027–2034.
67. Patzelt SB, Emmanouilidi A, Stampf S, *et al.* Accuracy of full-arch scans using intraoral scanners. *Clin Oral Investig* 2014; **18**(6): 1687–1694.
68. Eliasson A, Ortorp A. The accuracy of an implant impression technique using digitally coded healing abutments. *Clin Implant Dent Relat Res* 2012; **14**(Suppl 1): e30–38.
69. Mahn DH, Prestipino T. CAD/CAM implant abutments using coded healing abutments: a detailed description of the restorative process. *Compend Contin Educ Dent* 2013; **34**(8): 612–615.
70. Grossmann Y, Pasciuta M, Finger IM. A novel technique using a coded healing abutment for the fabrication of a CAD/CAM titanium abutment for an implant-supported restoration. *J Prosthet Dent* 2006; **95**(3): 258–261.
71. Carpentieri JR, Lazzara RJ. A simplified impression protocol for fabrication of anatomical, cement-retained CAD/CAM abutments. *Int J Periodontics Restorative Dent* 2014; **34**(Suppl 3): s19–25.
72. Telleman G, Raghoebar GM, Vissink A, *et al.* The use of a coded healing abutment as an impression coping to design and mill an individualized anatomic abutment: a clinical report. *J Prosthet Dent* 2011; **105**(5): 282–285.
73. Howell KJ, McGlumphy EA, Drago C, *et al.* Comparison of the accuracy of Biomet 3i Encode Robocast Technology and conventional implant impression techniques. *Int J Oral Maxillofac Implants* 2013; **28**(1): 228–240.
74. Ng SD, Tan KB, Teoh KH, *et al.* Three-dimensional accuracy of a digitally coded healing abutment implant impression system. *Int J Oral Maxillofac Implants* 2014; **29**(4): 927–936.
75. Al-Abdullah K, Zandparsa R, Finkelman M, *et al.* An in vitro comparison of the accuracy of implant impressions with coded healing abutments and different implant angulations. *J Prosthet Dent* 2013; **110**(2): 90–100.
76. Ramsey CD, Ritter RG. Utilization of digital technologies for fabrication of definitive implant-supported restorations. *J Esthet Restor Dent* 2012; **24**(5): 299–308.
77. Nayyar N, Yilmaz B, McGlumphy E. Using digitally coded healing abutments and an intraoral scanner to fabricate implant-supported, cement-retained restorations. *J Prosthet Dent* 2013; **109**(4): 210–215.
78. Lee SJ, Betensky RA, Gianneschi GE, *et al.* Accuracy of digital versus conventional implant impressions. *Clin Oral Implants Res* 2015; **26**(6): 715–719.
79. van der Meer WJ, Andriessen FS, Wismeijer D, *et al.* Application of intra-oral dental scanners in the digital workflow of implantology. *PLoS One* 2012; **7**(8): e43312.
80. Patzelt SB, Vonau S, Stampf S, *et al.* Assessing the feasibility and accuracy of digitizing edentulous jaws. *J Am Dent Assoc* 2013; **144**(8): 914–920.
81. Andriessen FS, Rijkens DR, van der Meer WJ, *et al.* Applicability and accuracy of an intraoral scanner for scanning multiple implants in edentulous mandibles: a pilot study. *J Prosthet Dent* 2014; **111**(3): 186–194.
82. Fasbinder DJ. Digital dentistry: innovation for restorative treatment. *Compend Contin Educ Dent* 2010; **31**(Spec No 4): 2–11.

83. Dehurtevent M, Robberecht L, Behin P. Influence of dentist experience with scan spray systems used in direct CAD/CAM impressions. *J Prosthet Dent* 2015; **113**(1): 17–21.
84. Kurbad A. The optical conditioning of Cerec preparations with scan spray. *Int J Comput Dent* 2000; **3**(4): 269–279.
85. Willershausen I, Lehmann KM, Robeta A, *et al.* Influence of three scan spray systems on human gingival fibroblasts. *Quintessence Int* 2012; **43**(6): e67–72.
86. Alghazzawi TF, Al-Samadani KH, Lemons J, *et al.* Effect of imaging powder and CAD/CAM stone types on the marginal gap of zirconia crowns. *J Am Dent Assoc* 2015; **146**(2): 111–120.
87. da Costa JB, Pelogia F, Hagedorn B, *et al.* Evaluation of different methods of optical impression making on the marginal gap of onlays created with CEREC 3D. *Oper Dent* 2010; **35**(3): 324–329.
88. Cook KT, Fasbinder DJ. Accuracy of CAD/CAM crown fit with infrared and LED cameras. *Int J Comput Dent* 2012; **15**(4): 315–326.
89. Dehurtevent M, Robberecht L, Behin P. Influence of dentist experience with scan spray systems used in direct CAD/CAM impressions. *J Prosthet Dent* 2015; **113**(1): 17–21.
90. Lee JH, Lee KB. Alternative antireflection substance for a digital impression. *J Prosthet Dent* 2015; **114**(3): 460–461.
91. Abduo J, Bennamoun M, Tennant M, *et al.* Effect of prosthodontic planning on intercuspal occlusal contacts: comparison of digital and conventional planning. *Comput Biol Med* 2015; **60**: 143–150.
92. Abduo J, Bennamoun M, Tennant M, *et al.* Effect of prosthodontic planning on lateral occlusion scheme: a comparison between conventional and digital planning. *J Appl Oral Sci* 2015; **23**(2): 196–205.
93. Delong R, Ko CC, Anderson GC, *et al.* Comparing maximum intercuspal contacts of virtual dental patients and mounted dental casts. *J Prosthet Dent* 2002; **88**(6): 622–630.
94. Chang YB, Xia JJ, Gateno J, *et al.* In vitro evaluation of new approach to digital dental model articulation. *J Oral Maxillofac Surg* 2012; **70**(4): 952–962.
95. Nadjmi N, Mollemans W, Daelemans A, *et al.* Virtual occlusion in planning orthognathic surgical procedures. *Int J Oral Maxillofac Surg* 2010; **39**(5): 457–462.
96. Fuster-Torres MA, Albalat-Estela S, Alcaniz-Raya M, *et al.* CAD/CAM dental systems in implant dentistry: update. *Med Oral Patol Oral Cir Bucal* 2009; **14**(3): E141–145.
97. Kapos T, Evans C. CAD/CAM technology for implant abutments, crowns, and superstructures. *Int J Oral Maxillofac Implants* 2014; **29**(Suppl): 117–136.
98. Abduo J, Lyons K. Rationale for the use of CAD/CAM technology in implant prosthodontics. *Int J Dent* 2013; 768121.
99. Park JI, Lee Y, Lee JH, *et al.* Comparison of fracture resistance and fit accuracy of customized zirconia abutments with prefabricated zirconia abutments in internal hexagonal implants. *Clin Implant Dent Relat Res* 2013; **15**(5): 769–778.
100. Alikhasi M, Monzavi A, Bassir SH, *et al.* A comparison of precision of fit, rotational freedom, and torque loss with copy-milled zirconia and prefabricated titanium abutments. *Int J Oral Maxillofac Implants* 2013; **28**(4): 996–1002.
101. Karl M, Taylor TD. Parameters determining micromotion at the implant–abutment interface. *Int J Oral Maxillofac Implants* 2014; **29**(6): 1338–1147.
102. Klotz MW, Taylor TD, Goldberg AJ. Wear at the titanium-zirconia implant–abutment interface: a pilot study. *Int J Oral Maxillofac Implants* 2011; **26**(5): 970–975.
103. Taylor TD, Klotz MW, Lawton RA. Titanium tattooing associated with zirconia implant abutments: a clinical report of two cases. *Int J Oral Maxillofac Implants* 2014; **29**(4): 958–960.
104. Ebert A, Hedderich J, Kern M. Retention of zirconia ceramic copings bonded to titanium abutments. *Int J Oral Maxillofac Implants* 2007; **22**(6): 921–927.
105. Gehrke P, Alius J, Fischer C, *et al.* Retentive strength of two-piece CAD/CAM zirconia implant abutments. *Clin Implant Dent Relat Res* 2014; **16**(6): 920–925.
106. von Maltzahn NF, Holstermann J, Kohorst P. Retention forces between titanium and zirconia components of two-part implant abutments with different techniques of surface modification. *Clin Implant Dent Relat Res* 2015; doi: 0.1111/cid.12352. [Epub ahead of print].
107. Kim JS, Raigrodski AJ, Flinn BD, *et al.* In vitro assessment of three types of zirconia implant abutments under static load. *J Prosthet Dent* 2013; **109**(4): 255–263.
108. Katsoulis J, Muller P, Mericske-Stern R, *et al.* CAD/CAM fabrication accuracy of long- vs. short-span implant-supported FDPs. *Clin Oral Implants Res* 2015; **26**(3): 245–249.
109. Katsoulis J, Mericske-Stern R, Enkling N, *et al.* In vitro precision of fit of computer-aided designed and computer-aided manufactured titanium screw-retained fixed dental prostheses before and after ceramic veneering. *Clin Oral Implants Res* 2015; **26**(1): 44–49.
110. de Franca DG, Morais MH, das Neves FD, *et al.* Influence of CAD/CAM on the fit accuracy of implant-supported zirconia and cobalt-chromium fixed dental prostheses. *J Prosthet Dent* 2015; **113**(1): 22–28.
111. Torabi K, Farjood E, Hamedani S. Rapid prototyping technologies and their applications in prosthodontics, a review of literature. *J Dent (Shiraz)* 2015; **16**(1): 1–9.
112. Rosen B, Ehrsson HH, Antfolk C, *et al.* Referral of sensation to an advanced humanoid robotic hand prosthesis. *Scand J Plast Reconstr Surg Hand Surg* 2009; **43**(5): 260–266.
113. Maheshwari V, Saraf R. Tactile devices to sense touch on a par with a human finger. *Angew Chem Int Ed Engl* 2008; **47**(41): 7808–7826.
114. Byeon HK, Holsinger FC, Kim DH, *et al.* Feasibility of robot-assisted neck dissection followed by transoral robotic surgery. *Br J Oral Maxillofac Surg* 2015; **53**(1): 68–73.
115. Hans S, Delas B, Gorphe P, *et al.* Transoral robotic surgery in head and neck cancer. *Eur Ann Otorhinolaryngol Head Neck Dis* 2012; **129**(1): 32–37.
116. Park YM, Kim WS, Byeon HK, *et al.* Clinical outcomes of transoral robotic surgery for head and neck tumors. *Ann Otol Rhinol Laryngol* 2013; **122**(2): 73–84.
117. Rinaldi V, Pagani D, Torretta S, *et al.* Transoral robotic surgery in the management of head and neck tumours. *Ecancermedicalscience* 2013; **7**: 359.
118. Patzelt SB, Lamprinos C, Stampf S, *et al.* The time efficiency of intraoral scanners: an in vitro comparative study. *J Am Dent Assoc* 2014; **145**(6): 542–551.
119. Lee SJ, Gallucci GO. Digital vs. conventional implant impressions: efficiency outcomes. *Clin Oral Implants Res* 2013; **24**(1): 111–115.
120. Schepke U, Meijer HJ, Kerdijk W, *et al.* Digital versus analog complete-arch impressions for single-unit premolar implant crowns: operating time and patient preference. *J Prosthet Dent* 2015; **114**(3): 403–406 e1.

121. Grunheid T, McCarthy SD, Larson BE. Clinical use of a direct chairside oral scanner: an assessment of accuracy, time, and patient acceptance. *Am J Orthod Dentofacial Orthop* 2014; **146**(5): 673–682.
122. Wismeijer D, Mans R, van Genuchten M, *et al.* Patients' preferences when comparing analogue implant impressions using a polyether impression material versus digital impressions (Intraoral Scan) of dental implants. *Clin Oral Implants Res* 2014; **25**(10): 1113–1138.
123. Yuzbasioglu E, Kurt H, Turunc R, *et al.* Comparison of digital and conventional impression techniques: evaluation of patients' perception, treatment comfort, effectiveness and clinical outcomes. *BMC Oral Health* 2014; **14**: 10.
124. Park HR, Park JM, Chun YS, *et al.* Changes in views on digital intraoral scanners among dental hygienists after training in digital impression taking. *BMC Oral Health* 2015; **15**(1): 151.
125. Chappuis V, Engel O, Reyes M, *et al.* Ridge alterations post-extraction in the esthetic zone: a 3D analysis with CBCT. *J Dent Res* 2013; **92**(12Suppl): 195S–201S.
126. Chappuis V, Engel O, Shahim K, *et al.* Soft tissue alterations in esthetic postextraction sites: a 3-dimensional analysis. *J Dent Res* 2015; **94**(9 Suppl): 187S–193S.
127. Benic GI, Elmasry M, Hammerle CH. Novel digital imaging techniques to assess the outcome in oral rehabilitation with dental implants: a narrative review. *Clin Oral Implants Res* 2015; **26**(Suppl 1): 86–96.
128. Mehl A, Koch R, Zaruba M, *et al.* 3D monitoring and quality control using intraoral optical camera systems. *Int J Comput Dent* 2013; **16**(1): 23–36.
129. Zaruba M, Ender A, Mehl A. New applications for three-dimensional follow-up and quality control using optical impression systems and OraCheck. *Int J Comput Dent* 2014; **17**(1): 53–64.
130. Lammie GA, Posselt U. Progressive changes in the dentition of adults. *J Periodontol* 1965; **36**(6): 443–454.
131. Oesterle LJ, Cronin RJ Jr. Adult growth, aging, and the single-tooth implant. *Int J Oral Maxillofac Implants* 2000; **15**(2): 252–260.
132. Heij DG, Opdebeeck H, van Steenberghe D, *et al.* Facial development, continuous tooth eruption, and mesial drift as compromising factors for implant placement. *Int J Oral Maxillofac Implants* 2006; **21**(6): 867–878.
133. Jemt T, Ahlberg G, Henriksson K, *et al.* Tooth movements adjacent to single-implant restorations after more than 15 years of follow-up. *Int J Prosthodont* 2007; **20**(6): 626–632.
134. Daftary F, Mahallati R, Bahat O, *et al.* Lifelong craniofacial growth and the implications for osseointegrated implants. *Int J Oral Maxillofac Implants* 2013; **28**(1): 163–169.
135. Greenstein G, Carpentieri J, Cavallaro J. Open contacts adjacent to dental implant restorations: etiology, incidence, consequences, and correction. *J Am Dent Assoc* 2016; **147**(1): 28–34.
136. Baba K, Tsukiyama Y, Clark GT. Reliability, validity, and utility of various occlusal measurement methods and techniques. *J Prosthet Dent* 2000; **83**(1): 83–89.
137. Saracoglu A, Ozpinar B. In vivo and in vitro evaluation of occlusal indicator sensitivity. *J Prosthet Dent* 2002; **88**(5): 522–526.
138. Koos B, Godt A, Schille C, *et al.* Precision of an instrumentation-based method of analyzing occlusion and its resulting distribution of forces in the dental arch. *J Orofac Orthop* 2010; **71**(6): 403–410.
139. Guth JF, Edelhoff D, Ihloff H, *et al.* Complete mouth rehabilitation after transposition osteotomy based on intraoral scanning: an experimental approach. *J Prosthet Dent* 2014; **112**(2): 89–93.
140. Patel A, Levine J, Brecht L, *et al.* Digital technologies in mandibular pathology and reconstruction. *Atlas Oral Maxillofac Surg Clin North Am* 2012; **20**(1): 95–106.
141. Avraham T, Franco P, Brecht LE, *et al.* Functional outcomes of virtually planned free fibula flap reconstruction of the mandible. *Plast Reconstr Surg* 2014; **134**(4): 628e–634e.
142. Levine JP, Bae JS, Soares M, *et al.* Jaw in a day: total maxillofacial reconstruction using digital technology. *Plast Reconstr Surg* 2013; **131**(6): 1386–1391.
143. Schepers RH, Raghoebar GM, Vissink A, *et al.* Fully 3-dimensional digitally planned reconstruction of a mandible with a free vascularized fibula and immediate placement of an implant-supported prosthetic construction. *Head Neck* 2013; **35**(4): E109–114.
144. Metzler P, Geiger EJ, Alcon A, *et al.* Three-dimensional virtual surgery accuracy for free fibula mandibular reconstruction: planned versus actual results. *J Oral Maxillofac Surg* 2014; **72**(12): 2601–2612.
145. Wilson TG Jr. The positive relationship between excess cement and peri-implant disease: a prospective clinical endoscopic study. *J Periodontol* 2009; **80**(9): 1388–1392.
146. Anchieta RB, Machado LS, Hirata R, *et al.* Platform-switching for cemented versus screwed fixed dental prostheses: reliability and failure modes: an in vitro study. *Clin Implant Dent Relat Res* 2015; doi: 10.1111/cid.12363. [Epub ahead of print].
147. Kotsakis G, Zhang L, Gaillard P, *et al.* Investigation of the association between cement retention and prevalent peri-implant diseases: a cross-sectional study. *J Periodontol* 2016; **87**(3): 212–220.
148. Lemos CA, de Souza Batista VE, Almeida DA, *et al.* Evaluation of cement-retained versus screw-retained implant-supported restorations for marginal bone loss: a systematic review and meta-analysis. *J Prosthet Dent* 2016; **115**(4): 419–427.
149. Ma S, Fenton A. Screw- versus cement-retained implant prostheses: a systematic review of prosthodontic maintenance and complications. *Int J Prosthodont* 2015; **28**(2): 127–145.
150. Millen C, Bragger U, Wittneben JG. Influence of prosthesis type and retention mechanism on complications with fixed implant-supported prostheses: a systematic review applying multivariate analyses. *Int J Oral Maxillofac Implants* 2015; **30**(1): 110–124.
151. Yue J, Zhao P, Gerasimov JY, *et al.* 3D-printable antimicrobial composite resins. *Adv Funct Mater* 2015; **25**(43): 6756–6767.
152. Obregon F, Vaquette C, Ivanovski S, *et al.* Three-dimensional bioprinting for regenerative dentistry and craniofacial tissue engineering. *J Dent Res* 2015; **94**(9 Suppl): 143S–152S.
153. Inzana JA, Olvera D, Fuller SM, *et al.* 3D printing of composite calcium phosphate and collagen scaffolds for bone regeneration. *Biomaterials* 2014; **35**(13): 4026–4034.
154. Habibovic P, Gbureck U, Doillon CJ, *et al.* Osteoconduction and osteoinduction of low-temperature 3D printed bioceramic implants. *Biomaterials* 2008; **29**(7): 944–953.
155. Tamimi F, Torres J, Gbureck U, *et al.* Craniofacial vertical bone augmentation: a comparison between 3D printed monolithic monetite blocks and autologous onlay grafts in the rabbit. *Biomaterials* 2009; **30**(31): 6318–6326.
156. Tamimi F, Torres J, Al-Abedalla K, *et al.* Osseointegration of dental implants in 3D-printed synthetic onlay grafts customized according to bone metabolic activity in recipient site. *Biomaterials* 2014; **35**(21): 5436–5445.

157. Pati F, Song TH, Rijal G, *et al.* Ornamenting 3D printed scaffolds with cell-laid extracellular matrix for bone tissue regeneration. *Biomaterials* 2015; **37**: 230–241.
158. Ricci JL, Clark EA, Murriky A, *et al.* Three-dimensional printing of bone repair and replacement materials: impact on craniofacial surgery. *J Craniofac Surg* 2012; **23**(1): 304–308.
159. Mangano F, Macchi A, Shibli JA, *et al.* Maxillary ridge augmentation with custom-made CAD/CAM scaffolds. A 1-year prospective study on 10 patients. *J Oral Implantol* 2014; **40**(5): 561–569.
160. Rasperini G, Pilipchuk SP, Flanagan CL, *et al.* 3D-printed bioresorbable scaffold for periodontal repair. *J Dent Res* 2015; **94**(9 Suppl): 153S–157S.

CHAPTER 16

Implant Dentistry: Challenges in the Treatment of the Edentulous Patient

Steven J. Sadowsky[1], Howard M. Landesman[2], and W. Peter Hansen[1]
[1] University of the Pacific Arthur A. Dugoni School of Dentistry, San Francisco, California, USA
[2] Encino, California, USA

When considering the impact of innovation, it is noteworthy that only 1 per 1000 articles has studied undesirable consequences from new discoveries, a proportion that has not changed since the 1960s, as reported in a position paper by the Hanken School of Economics in 2009. This is explained by pro-innovation bias or the fundamental value that innovation is good. However, this widespread attitude may limit decision makers and change agents to anticipate and respond to unforeseen outcomes. Perhaps, as a result of the salvation that dental implants have offered edentulous patients, such an analysis would be sacrosanct. However, enhanced patient-centered care may hinge on it. As clinicians and academicians, we are in an opportune position to identify and address these trends.

Since the introduction of the osseointegration concept to North America in 1982, there has been a number of unexpected discoveries that have changed the therapeutic model for treatment of the edentulous patient. The advent of affordable and low-dose radiation three-dimensional (3-D) imaging, using cone-beam computed tomography (CBCT) with attendant software programs, has enabled virtual treatment planning from surgical placement to prosthetic design.[1] Further developments have included a digital implant workflow, allowing for fabrication of surgical guides,[2,3] interim abutments and provisional prostheses prior to implant surgery,[4] intraoral scanning for complete arch impressions,[5] and ultimately CAD/CAM production of the definitive restoration.[6,7] The developing science of surface topography of dental implants has focused on enhanced formation of osteoblastic proliferation on titanium implants.[8–10] Data now have demonstrated an upregulation of genes associated with signaling osteogenic differentiation following early exposure of osteoprogenitor cells to moderately roughened surfaces.[11,12] These investigations have influenced original clinical guidelines for the time span necessary between implant placement and loading the prosthetic rehabilitation.[13–15] Coupled with the evidence from systematic reviews on the similar fate of tilted and orthogonally placed implants for edentulous arches,[16,17] the "All-on-4" concept has gained immense traction in the prosthodontic community. Anatomic limitations, including pneumatized maxillary sinus, proximity of the inferior alveolar nerve, and lack of available native bone, usually requiring invasive and costly grafting procedures prior to implant placement, have been circumvented. In line with reducing surgical morbidity, cost, and failure rates, augmentation procedures have been replaced with the use of four zygomatic implants when addressing severe atrophy of the maxilla.[18,19] Considering oral health-related quality-of-life indices and patient preferences for minimally invasive procedures, graftless implant rehabilitation of complete edentulism has become more mainstream. It is notable that patient satisfaction averaged 94% with tilted implant placement, 91% with flapless implant placement, 90% with a reduced number of implants, 89% with short implants, 87% with narrow-diameter implants, and 83% with zygomatic fixtures.[20] Another example of this "less is more" direction is the evolution from the original *ad modum* Branemark prototype with six implants for the rescue of the mandibular denture cripple to a solitary symphyseal implant-retained overdenture for a selected cohort of patients.[21–23]

The aforementioned advancements have the potential to improve our diagnostic acumen, render care in an expeditious time period, circumvent extensive and costly preprosthetic surgery, and offer patients more cost-effective outcomes. With that in mind, one would think that the discipline of implant prosthodontics is moving swiftly down the highway of customized treatment planning with an emphasis on minimally invasive procedures. However, the elephant in the room is the burgeoning reputation that implants are the *deus ex machina* for all patients requiring minimal surveillance for life. This myth, in conjunction with six prevailing trends, has, on the contrary, resulted in a diminished ability to conservatively treat edentulous patients and an increased likelihood of implant prosthodontic mishaps.

Evidence-based Implant Treatment Planning and Clinical Protocols, First Edition. Edited by Steven J. Sadowsky.

Companion website: www.wiley.com/go/sadowsky/implant

Education

The teaching of complete denture prosthodontics has been marginalized in dental school curricula.

Due to crowded curricula, because of advances in technology[24] and implant rehabilitation,[25] along with decreasing edentulism,[26] there has been a progressive diminution of didactic, laboratory, and clinical training in complete denture prosthodontics.[27,28] New graduates are now less well equipped to practice complete denture prosthodontics than in the 1990s.[29] Dental schools have low expectations for their undergraduate students to be practically trained in the production and insertion of complete dentures, with lead teachers reporting that course work did not ensure competence on graduation.[30,31] Despite that fact 63% of graduates felt complete dentures were an important aspect of dentistry, only 5% expressed confidence in removable prosthodontics.[32] A decreased load of core coursework and clinical reinforcement in complete denture principles, incorporating the sphere of troubleshooting denture complications, diagnostic criteria for edentulism, vertical dimension of occlusion (VDO), occlusal harmony, and esthetic arrangement of teeth, has spawned poor management of both conventional and implant prosthodontics.

Troubleshooting denture complications

A typical patient presents with a nonretentive maxillary denture. Instead of assessing the peripheral seal, width of the flange, the allowance for muscle attachments, intimacy of fit of the intaglio surface, and occlusal harmony, a reline is recommended. When this fails, the discussion migrates to implant prosthetic options. For example, if the vibrating line (junction between the movable and immovable soft palate) is up to 8 mm anterior to the distal limit of the denture (Figure 16.1) and there is space in the retrozygomatic vestibular region between the flange and fornix (Figure 16.2), a reline that does not address these deficiencies is destined for failure. When this occurs, the patient considers the "evidence" that a tissue-borne prosthesis offers little benefit for dependable retention and stability. On the other hand, if the distal limit is adjusted, the flanges are developed by functional border molding, and a thin wash is placed in the relieved intaglio of the denture (Figure 16.3),[33] followed by occlusal equilibration, the clinician and patient have the opportunity to assess the prospect of conservative conventional treatment. However, the edentulous mandible has routinely offered more challenges to patients to adapt to a tissue-borne prosthesis, which especially has been predicated on systemic,[34,35] local,[36,37]

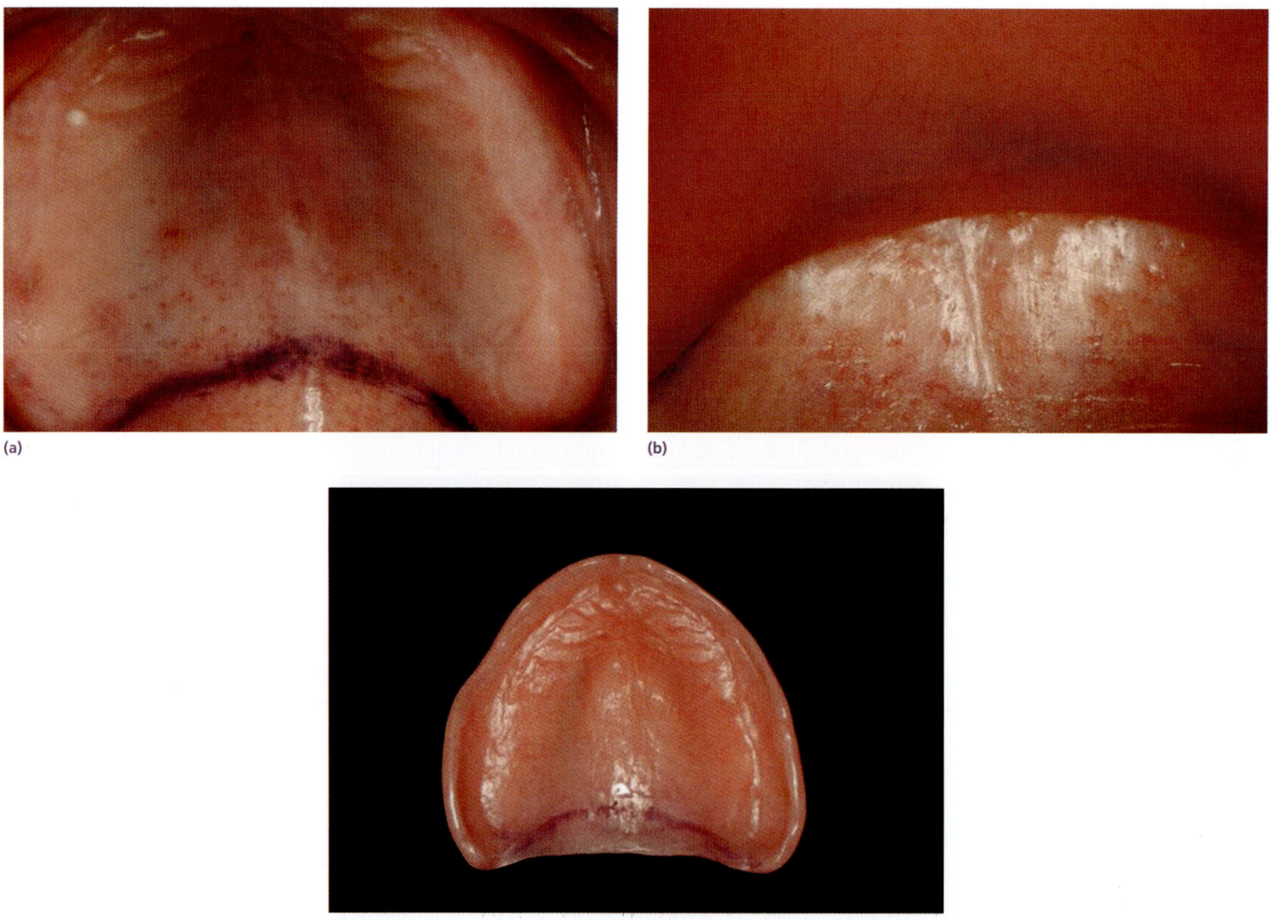

(a) (b) (c)

Figure 16.1 (a) Vibrating line established with indelible marker. (b) Denture in place, demonstrating distal limit engaging the movable soft palate beyond the vibrating line. (c) Vibrating line visible on intaglio surface of denture.

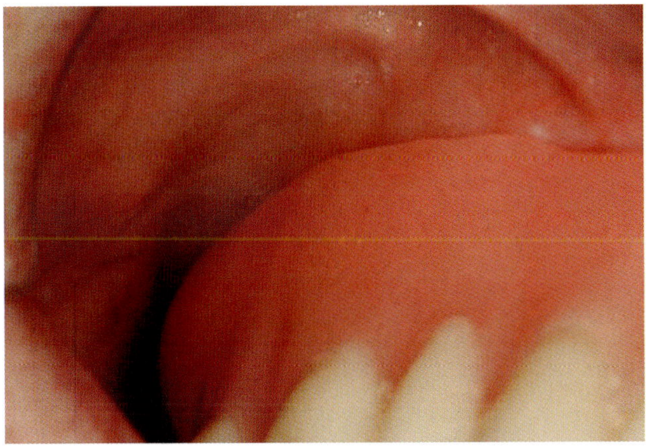

Figure 16.2 Peripheral seal lacking with short flange in the retrozygomatic region.

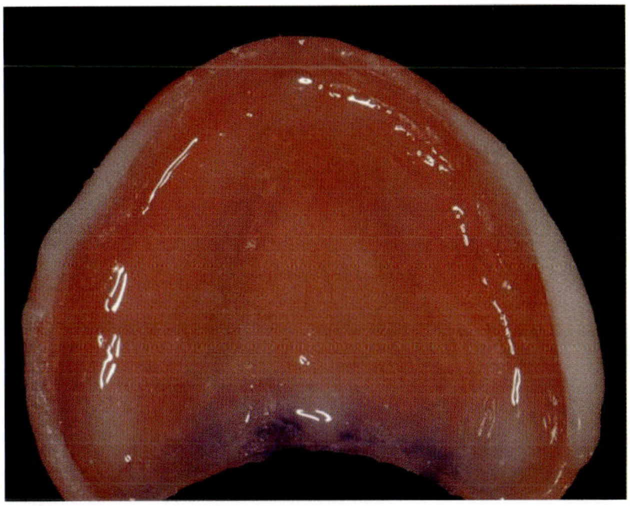

Figure 16.3 Tissue conditioner used first to develop the periphery with a higher viscosity powder/liquid ratio and then a very thin wash for the intaglio surface.

and psychosocial factors.[38–40] Ironically, the introduction of implants for the restoration of the edentulous mandible has facilitated a progressive erosion of the education in complete denture prosthodontics.

Diagnostic criteria for complete edentulism

In 2002, the McGill Consensus concluded that the minimum standard of care for the edentulous mandible was a two-implant overdenture.[41] This statement did not differentiate among different classes of edentulism, patients' prognosis for success with complete dentures, or their limitations in embracing an implant therapy. To address the question posed by the edentulous patient, "Do I need implants?", the focus is generally directed to the mandibular arch. In an attempt to organize the diagnostic criteria for complete edentulism, McGarry *et al.*[42] introduced a classification system for pretreatment evaluation of patients considered for complete dentures (Table 16.1). The Prosthodontic Diagnostic Index identified two classifications (class III and IV) which were in need of implant/surgical intervention. These included patients with residual ridge deficiencies, muscle attachments challenging retention (Figure 16.4a), history of parethesia/dysesthesia, incoordination, retracted tongue position (Figure 16.4b), hyperactive gag reflex, and, most importantly, a high maladaptive quotient. Since 10–15% of patients receiving new and technically well-made dentures, and 25–35% with older dentures, are generally not satisfied with the treatment because of maladaptive tendencies,[43] Friedman *et al.*[44] offered a classification system to assist the clinician in identifying a spectrum of physical and psychological maladaptive responses of patients who are made edentulous. Therefore, despite the advent of implants, for a class of patients that physically, anatomically, and psychosocially present with favorable conditions, a tissue-borne prosthesis is a viable option, especially for the patient with financial limitations. On the other hand, there has been a presumption that implants not only can overcome anatomic deficiencies but also maladaptation. In this regard, it is notable to consider that implant patients have higher expectations than those treated with conventional prostheses.[45] Over 60 years ago, M.M. House delineated four different personality profiles influencing the prognosis of complete denture therapy (philosophical, exacting, hysterical and indifferent). His classification still has relevance in the decision to rehabilitate the patient conventionally, with implants or not at all. In the final resolve, adding implants to the arsenal of therapeutic options for patients should not minimize the effective application of tissue-supported prostheses for selected patients or underestimate the role that psychosocial issues have in accommodating to implant prostheses.

Vertical dimension of occlusion

The ability to assess the appropriate vertical dimension of occlusion (VDO) is paramount in predictable prosthodontics for the edentate as well as for the dentulous patient who has lost adequate vertical stops. Historically, predoctoral training in complete denture fabrication offered students multiple opportunities to practice calibrating this measurement. Errors in establishing the correct VDO could be seen as causing contact of teeth when speaking or a collapsed edentulous appearance. As complete denture education waned, more sophisticated implant rehabilitations requiring this skill were at risk of being mismanaged, often with irreversible consequences. Various prosthetic modalities, such as implant overdentures (with diverse anchorage systems and dimensional requirements), implant-fixed complete dentures, and metal–ceramic designs, all require different interarch spatial allowance.[46,47] Specific guidelines are discussed in Chapters 17 and 18. Errors in this calculation not only may handcuff accurate surgical planning for alveoplasty, but once the implants are placed, the intended design may not be able to be executed. Insufficient space afforded for the prosthetic components often leads to material fatigue and/or fracture.[48]

There are several techniques for determining the correct VDO. These methods include the use of physiologic rest position, swallowing, phonetic, esthetic, and facial measurements. Today these techniques seem difficult for students to grasp

Table 16.1 Checklist for prognostic classification of complete edentulism. *Source:* Reproduced with permission from the American College of Prosthodontists.

		Class I	Class II	Class III	Class IV
Bone height – mandibular					
	21 mm or greater				
	16–20 mm				
	11–15 mm				
	10 mm or less				
Ridge morphology – maxilla					
	Type A – resists vertical and horizontal movement, hamular notch, no tori				
	Type B – no buccal vestibule, poor hamular notch, no tori				
	Type C – no anterior vestibule, min support, mobile anterior ridge				
	Type D – no anterior/posterior vestibules, tori, redundant tissue				
Muscle attachments – mandibular					
	Type A – adequate attached mucosa				
	Type B – no buccal attached mucosa (22–27), + mentalis m				
	Type C – no anterior buccal and lingual vestibule (22–27), + genioglossus & mentalis m				
	Type D – attached mucosa in posterior only				
	Type E – no attached mucosa, cheek/lip moves tongue				
Maxillomandibular relationships					
	Class I				
	Class II				
	Class III				
Conditions requiring preprosthetic surgery					
	Minor soft tissue procedures				
	Minor hard tissue procedures				
	Implants – simple				
	Implants with bone graft – complex				
	Correction of dentofacial deformities				
	Hard tissue augmentation				
	Major soft tissue revisions				
Limited interarch space					
	18–20 mm				
	Surgical correction needed				
Tongue anatomy					
	Large (occludes interdental space)				
	Hyperactive – with retracted position				
Modifiers					
	Oral manifestation of systemic disease				
	Mild				
	Moderate				
	Severe				
	Psychosocial				
	Moderate				
	Severe				
	Temporomandibular joint disorder symptoms				
	History of paresthesia or dysesthesia				
	Maxillofacial defects				
	Ataxia				
	Refractory patient				
ICD-9-CM diagnostic codes		525.41	525.42	525.43	525.44

Guidelines for use of the worksheet

1. Any single criterion of a more complex class places the patient into the more complex class
2. Initial preprosthetic treatment and/or adjunctive therapy can change the initial classification level
3. In the situation where the patient presents with an edentulous maxilla opposing a partially edentulous mandible, each arch is diagnosed with the appropriate classification system

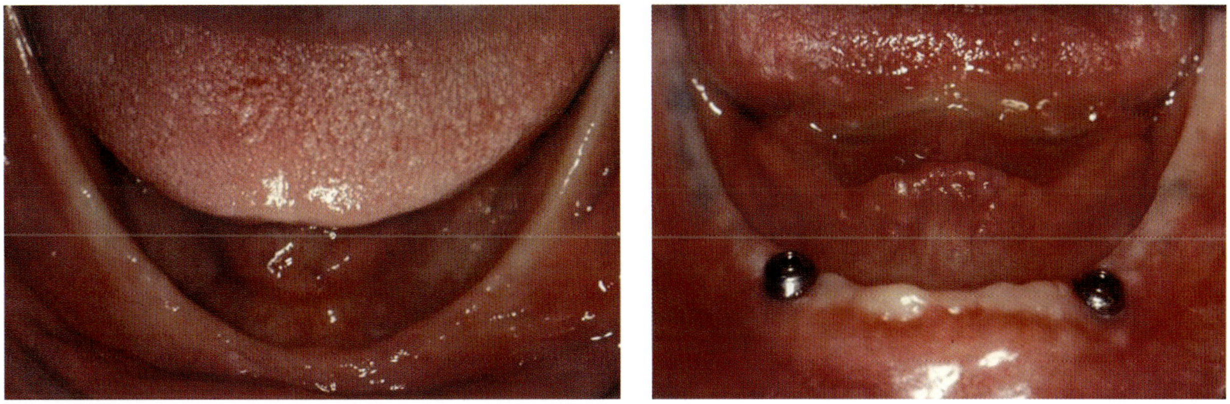

(a) (b)

Figure 16.4 (a) High muscle attachment which negatively affects the prognosis of a complete denture. (b) Retruded tongue compromising prognosis of complete denture leading to appropriate implant treatment.

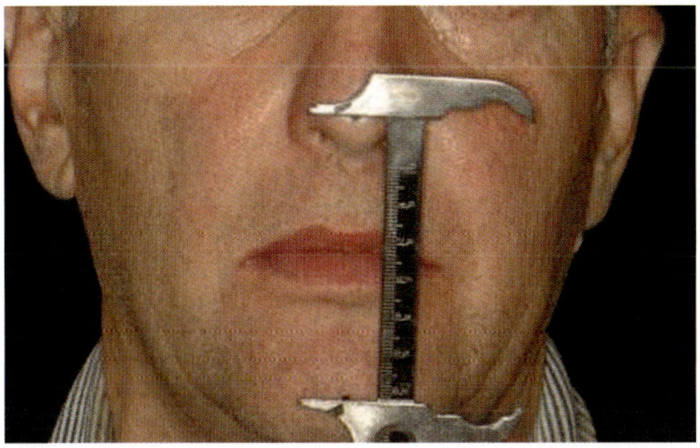

(a)

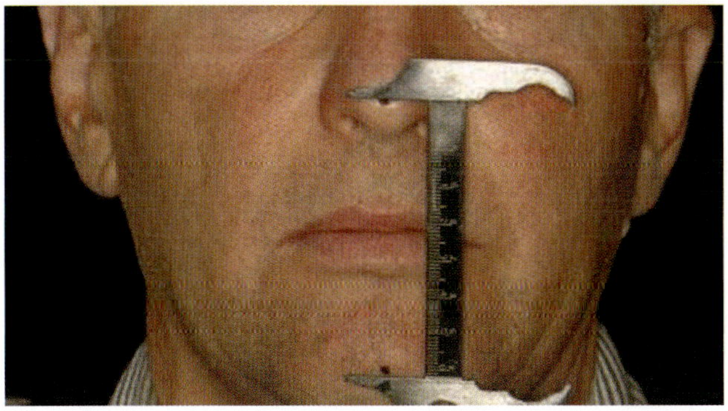

(b)

Figure 16.5 (a) Vertical dimension of rest (VDR) recorded with a boley gauge. (b) Vertical dimension of occlusion (VDO) registered with less than 1 mm difference between VDR and VDO. This demonstrates insufficient interocclusal distance for a class I patient.

without focused training. There is consensus that the use of multiple determinants is helpful in establishing VDO.[49–51] One measurement used is the vertical dimension of rest (VDR),[52,53] which is the mandibular position assumed when the head is in an upright position[54] and the involved muscles, particularly the elevator and depressor groups, are in equilibrium in tonic contraction and the condyles are in a neutral and unstrained position. The interocclusal distance (IOD) is the space between VDR and VDO (Figure 16.5). A weak correlation has been documented between speaking /s/ space and IOD.[55] For class I patients there is approximately 3 mm of IOD, class II patients more than 3 mm and class III patients less than 3 mm.[56] A 15-year longitudinal study using lateral cephalometric radiographs to record the VDO of patients after assessment of VDR, the "m"[57] and swallowing[58] technique, confirmed a small range of stability in all subjects throughout the follow-up.[59] Esthetic and facial analyses have also been recommended to verify VDO.[60–62]

Occlusal harmony

It has been said that there is no better discipline to learn occlusal concepts and equilibration than complete denture prosthodontics (Figure 16.6). Identifying the interrelationship of the occlusal plane, curve of Spee, curve of Wilson, condylar inclination, and incisal guidance is facilitated when balanced set-ups are generated. There is little debate that a harmonious occlusion in various forms improves the stability and comfort of a tissue-borne prosthesis.[63,64] The clinical remount allows for a recording of guided ligamentous centric relation position, a verifiable occlusal record, and the opportunity to identify disruptive occlusal interferences (Figure 16.7). However, the teaching of complete denture occlusion has been marginalized in the dental school curriculum.[56] While there is controversy over the optimal occlusal scheme for various implant prosthetic designs (canine guidance, group function, balanced occlusion), the goal is to develop an absence of deflective contacts in centric and excursive positions, providing disseminated load distribution and chewing efficiency. Interceptive contacts encourage mechanical complications because of the diminution of proprioception, especially in double-arch reconstructions.[65,66] Furthermore, material fractures, as a result of preferential forces in fixed implant reconstructions, mean that fixed implant reconstructions carry a greater time/economic burden than do removable prosthetic designs.

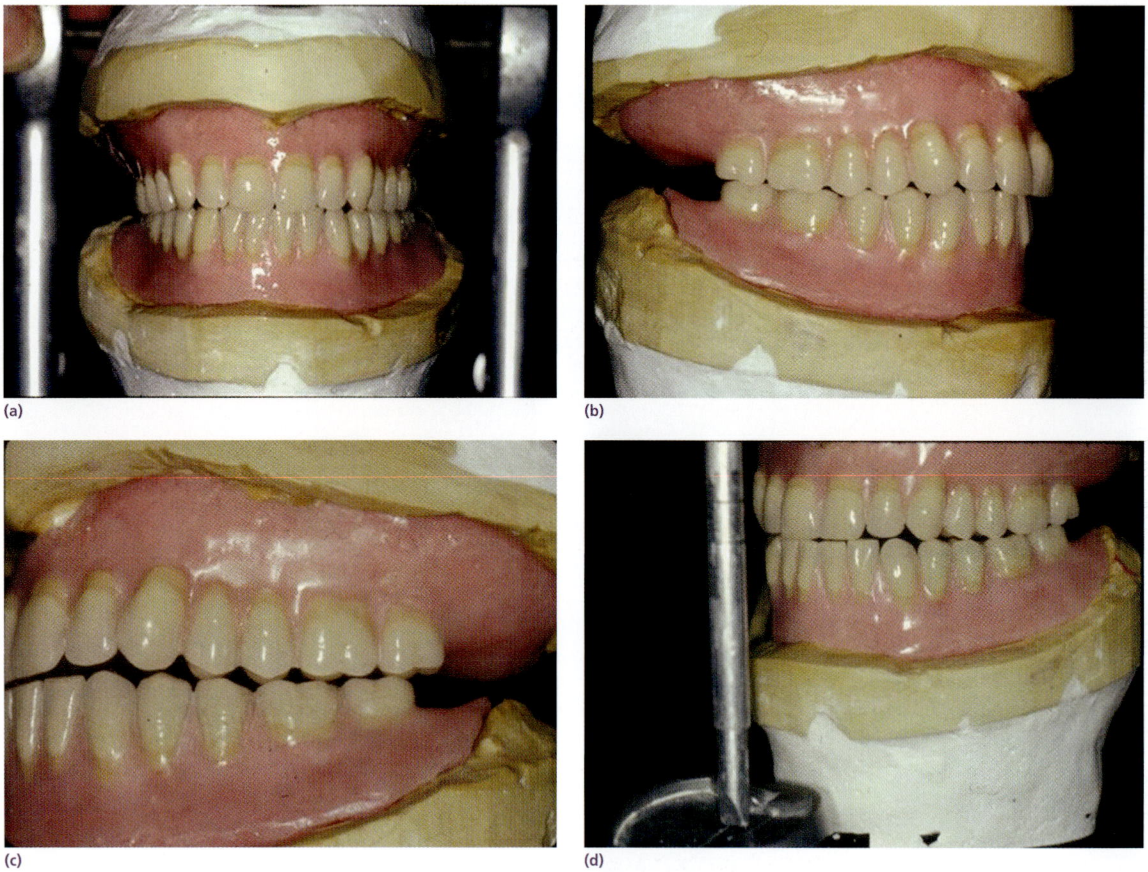

Figure 16.6 (**a**) Balanced complete denture wax-up (centric relation position). (**b**) Balanced complete denture wax-up (right working excursion). (**c**) Balanced complete denture wax-up (right balancing excursion). (**d**) Balanced complete denture wax-up (protrusive excursion).

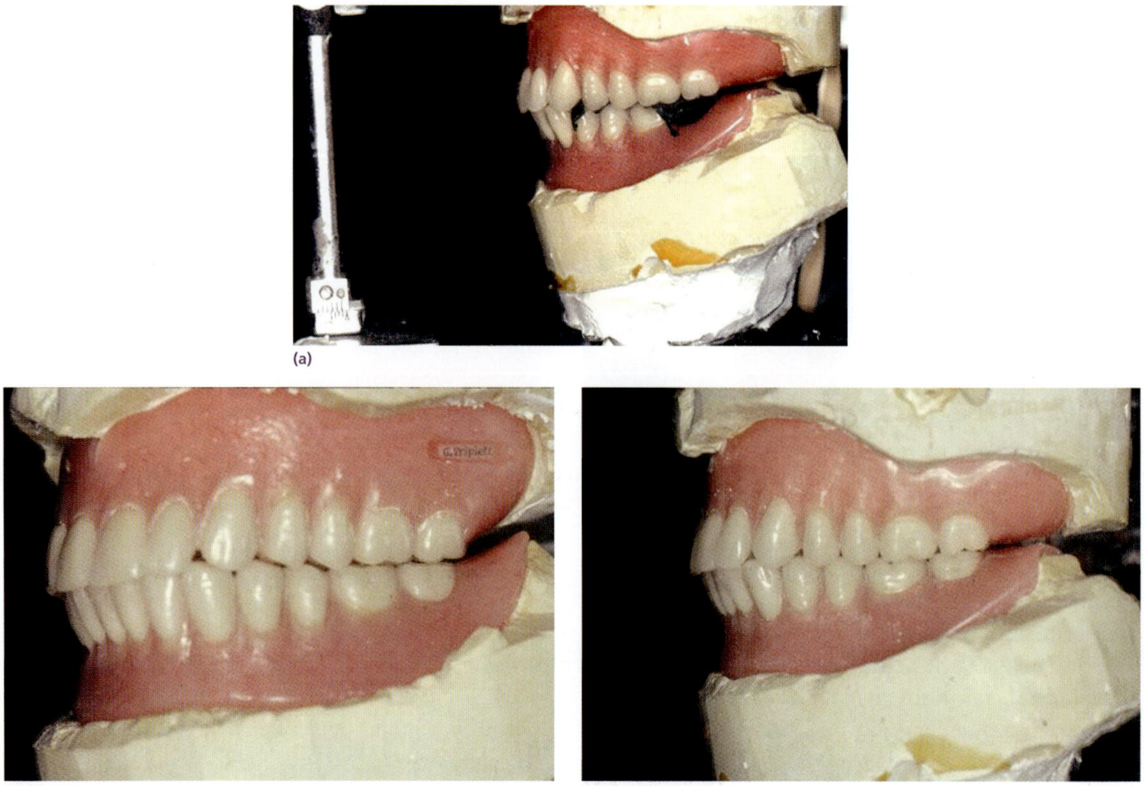

Figure 16.7 (**a**) Articulator mounting with remount record in place. (**b**) Lack of posterior bilateral contacts demonstrated on the articulator but not visualized intraorally because of resilient and like effect (REALEFF) of the soft tissue foundation. (**c**) Equilibrated dentures.

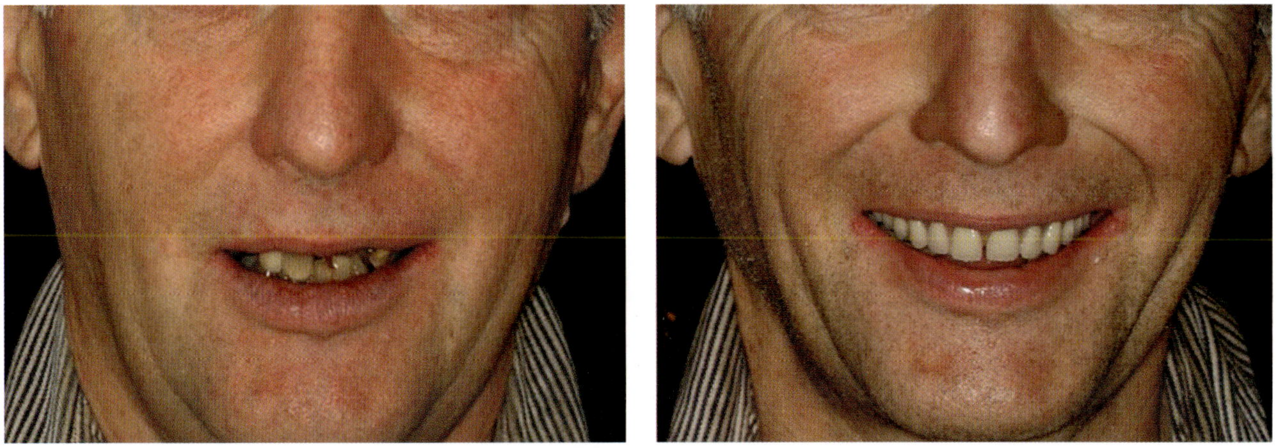

(a) (b)

Figure 16.8 (a) Patient presenting with terminal dentition with a loss of dental landmarks. (b) Patient restored with complete denture following facial references to create an authentic appearance.

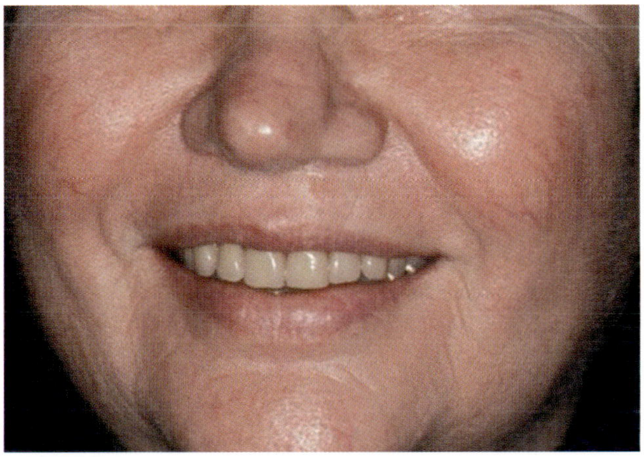

Figure 16.9 Smile line serving as an envelope for the incisal edges of maxillary anterior teeth.

Esthetic arrangement of teeth

The esthetic zeitgeist that we have all experienced may have been promulgated by the baby boomer generation who became invested in delaying the passages of life to retard the sense of aging.[67] Medical, pharmaceutical, and dental solutions have been pursued by increasing numbers of patients to "regain" their youthful vigor and appearance. As a result, the ability to develop an authentic and customized anterior arrangement of teeth, when there has been an abject loss of dental landmarks, is even more critical for patients today (Figure 16.8). The art and biometric science of complete denture esthetics have identified general guidelines. These include the bisection of the face for midline,[68] envelope of the lower lip for maxillary incisal line (Figure 16.9),[56] averages for width and length of maxillary central incisors in white male (9 mm, 10.5 mm),[69] phonetic sounds for incisal position of maxillary incisors (Figure 16.10a),[70,71] and lip support and sibilant sounds for labial placement of anterior teeth (Figure 16.10b).[57] The dynesthetic and dentogenic concept has been advanced for practitioners to restore edentulous patients' dignity and unique individuality with asymmetrical, but balanced, set-ups, considering age, gender, and personality (Figure 16.11a–d).[72] Incorporating variety in axial inclination of the teeth will open up the incisal embrasures accentuating a figure/ground contrast, adding a dynamic interplay (Figure 16.11e). The anterior try-in procedure is invaluable for practitioners to practice these principles. It is ironic that given implant patients are concerned about esthetics only second to function,[73] curriculum hours dedicated to complete denture principles have declined significantly.[29,74,75]

Economic burden

New graduates face a heavier economic burden than their predecessors.

Escalating postsecondary educational costs in the US have elevated student loan debt second only to mortgages.[76] The direct cost of obtaining a dental education has had an upward turn over the last 10 years. New clinical technologies, technology costs, and main campus taxes have been reported to be the main source of rising tuitions.[77] Reduced state appropriations to public schools and decreases in private giving to all schools have also had a significant influence.[78] The average debt load of new dental graduates has grown to $247,097 (based on the American Dental Education Association, Survey of Dental School Seniors, 2014 Graduating Class). This trend, in combination with a continued decline in the real income that has occurred since 2000, has had a negative impact on the return of investment (ROI). The prospect of lower dental insurance reimbursement, increased market share of dental service organizations, and rising interest rates could influence the financial viability of the practice of dentistry. Future estimates of the growth in number of new dental schools, expansion of existing schools, and associated increment of new graduates could exert further downward pressure to the ROI.[76] This economic forecast for new graduates may have a subtle effect on treatment planning decision making, providing a

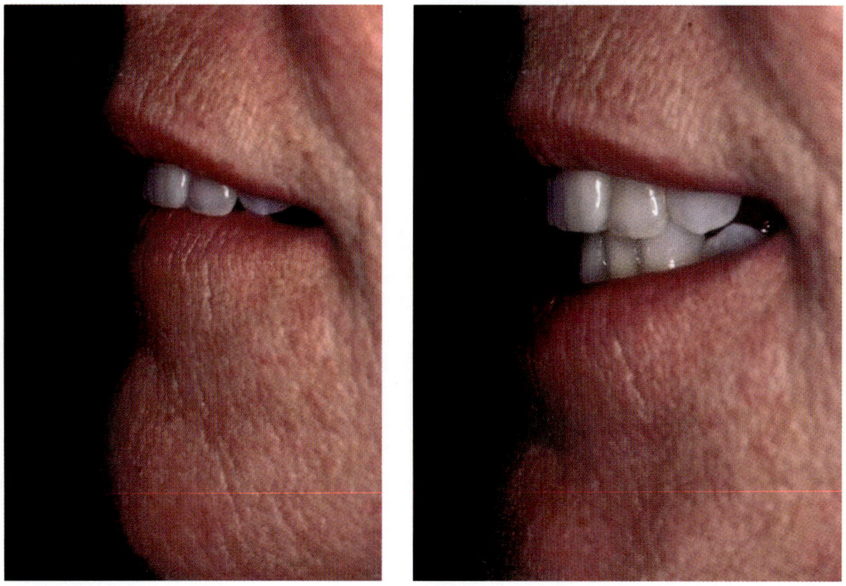

Figure 16.10 **(a)** Fricative /f/ sound aiding the practitioner in assessing the coronoapical position of the maxillary central incisors. The incisal edge should lightly touch the vermillion border of the lower lip. **(b)** Sibilant /s/ sound aiding the practitioner in assessing the horizontal overlap of the anterior teeth. Typically the teeth should be 1 mm apart with the /s/ sound.

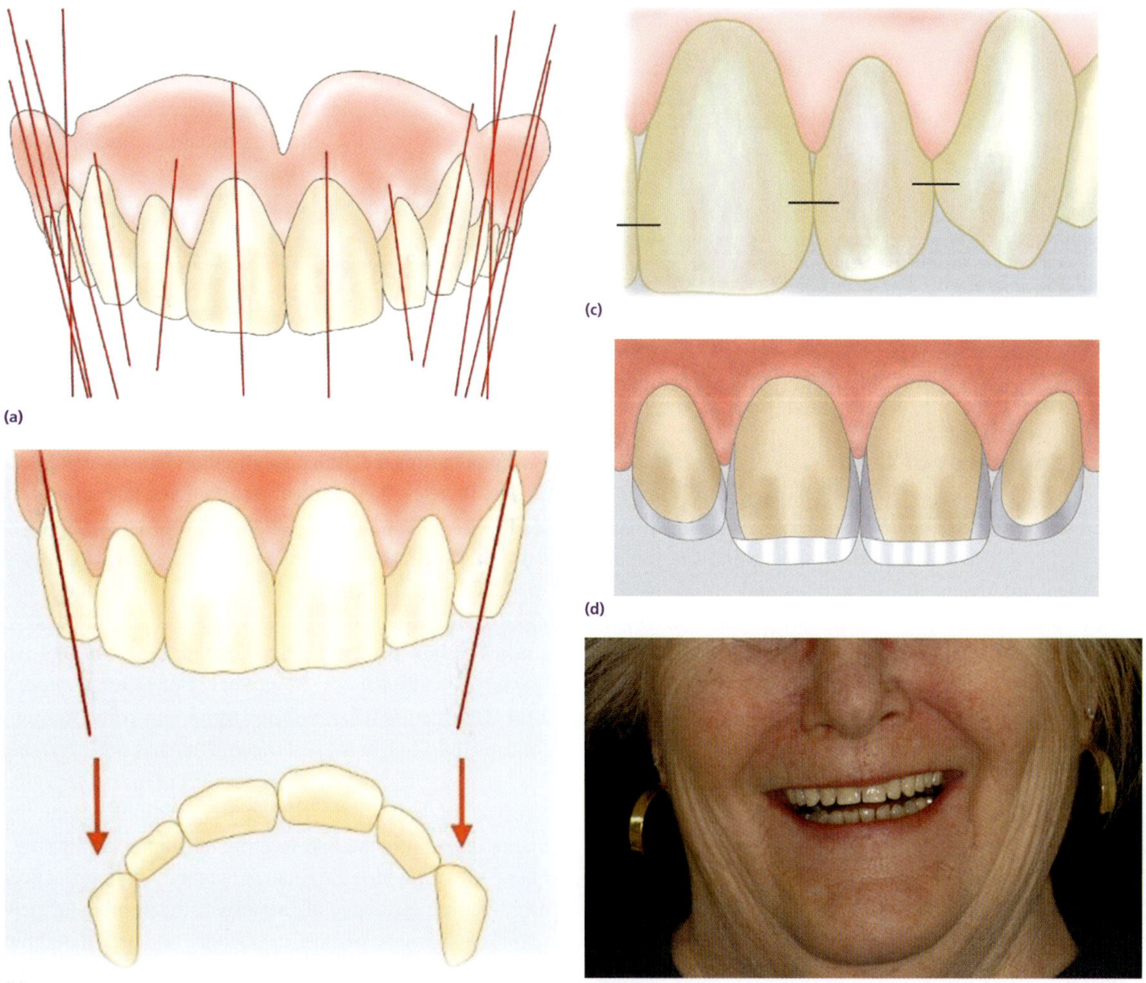

Figure 16.11 **(a)** Variation in axial inclination but the asymmetries do not disrupt a visual balance. **(b)** Horizontal plane view demonstrating bodily displacement of the teeth from a single arc. Note the facial view does not reveal the stark asymmetries but the teeth will appear more individualized and break up the light in a nonuniform fashion. **(c)** Important differences in contact points to guard againt a "denture look". The incisal embrasures are distinctive. **(d)** Age-relevant selective grinding of the incisal edges is important to create a natural appearance. *Source for* **(a–d)**: Courtesy of Jeff Miles. **(e)** Patient with a maxillary complete denture fabricated with these principles in mind.

potential conflict of interest. Brennan and Spencer[79] have identified provider-based factors impacting the provision of dental services, such as desire for income, desire for style of practice, and personal characteristics. The pressure to meet financial obligations may prompt practitioners to pursue a more extensive implant rehabilitation than is absolutely necessary. It is of note that individuals edentulous in one or both jaws have a lower probability to desire implant treatment than those with all teeth remaining, or with missing teeth replaced by fixed partial dentures.[80]

New technologies

The allure of new technologies has lulled initiates into the belief that implant restorations can be managed predictably and easily with the assistance of a digital workflow.

From the surgical domain to the restorative province, evolving technologies have offered the promise of accuracy and efficiency, even for the less experienced clinician. However, when evaluating the effect of surgical guide design and surgeon's experience on accuracy of implant placement, there was a difference in accuracy based on experience level. In an *in vitro* study, four operators placed a total of 100 implants on 20 photopolymer resin edentulous mandibles scanned with CBCT to generate a stereolithographic surgical template. Specifically, the inexperienced group had a mean error of angular deviation of 3.96° ± 1.64° and the experienced group had an angular deviation of 2.60° ± 1.25°. In the same vein, the advent of digital dentures offers the practitioner a time saving by reducing the number of appointments usually required for denture fabrication from five to two. Fifteen predoctoral students fabricated two sets of complete dentures, one digital and one conventional. Both students and patients preferred the digital denture and noted enhanced retention.[81] A telling outcome of the study, however, was the reliance on faculty supervision and the fact that students reported their clinical concerns with proceeding with the digital denture workflow without the expertise of an accomplished practitioner. For example, accurate functional impressions, determination of vertical and horizontal records, customized esthetic set-up of the teeth, assessment of occlusal plane, and execution of occlusal harmony will be even more rigorous for the clinician because of the reduction of the number of visits and reversible checks. It is therefore understandable that the learning curve for new technologies has been reported to be challenging and the dental team must rely on traditional skills to capitalize on the benefits of these advances.[82]

Marketing

Implants have been marketed in mainstream advertising propelling patients to seek implant restorations.

Patients who want to be informed consult websites to gather information about dental implants. However, online information regarding implant treatment is generally low in quality and data on longitudinal outcomes and complications are overlooked.[83] Advertising in sundry media promoting implant treatment modalities, such as the All-on-4®, produced in a day, appeals to a growing cohort of patients. However, this treatment regimen is not a "one-size fits all". Parel and Phillips[84] addressed the associated risk factors in the protocol of immediately loading four implants on the maxilla. They recommended patient profiling with respect to factors that contribute to implant failure. Such characteristics as opposing natural dentition (due to inability to manage the occlusal scheme well), lack of bone density, and parafunction were significant enough to warrant a delayed approach or the addition of more implants. However, the prevailing theme in the media is that this regimen can be universally applied with high implant survival, giving rise to patient enthusiasm. The role of individual perception of potential reasons for treatment selection should not be underestimated as a force controlling the decision-making process for patients.[85] The clinician may be highly influenced to comply with the patient's wishes, notwithstanding the limitations of the patient, clinician, or procedure.

Assumptions

There is an assumption by clinicians that implant-fixed restorations are preferred by edentulous patients and have a higher survival/success rate with lower maintenance incidence in comparison with removable designs.

Most practitioners believe that a fixed prosthesis is the treatment of choice for the edentulous patient.[86] However, there are a number of studies that do not support this view. For example, in a within-subject clinical cross-over trial, functional and psychometric outcomes were evaluated after edentulous patients utilized mandibular long-bar overdentures and implant fixed complete dentures (IFCD) opposing complete dentures.[87] While the subjects found the fixed alternative to be superior for chewing hard foods, there was no difference in general satisfaction. In the maxilla, a similar crossover study was conducted comparing IFCDs and implant supported overdentures opposing mandibular implant-supported overdentures.[88] Patients selected the long-bar overdentures (>2:1) in preference to the fixed prosthesis because of ease of speaking and cleaning the restoration. In another study, 20 patients were evenly distributed with either a fixed or removable implant prosthetic treatment and queried after 6 months of function.[89] While treatment costs were significantly higher with the fixed prosthetic design, no differences were found between the two groups in how the implant therapy was assessed or patients' level of well-being, using a visual analog scale. Finally, in a cross-over investigation, one group received a maxillary long-bar overdenture with palatal coverage and a second group received the same design without palatal coverage, with both groups opposing an implant-fixed prosthesis. No differences were noted in patient satisfaction, but what was even more compelling was the fact that the ratings for the maxillary implant prostheses were not significantly higher than the maxillary conventional prostheses. This underscores the importance maximizing the comfort, retention, stability, and esthetics of the patient's denture before consideration of an implant prosthetic replacement, requiring complete denture skills. Patients that truly are candidates for a maxillary implant rehabilitation have anatomic deficiencies that limit retention, psychogenic barriers to palatal coverage, or intransigent gagging.[90]

When considering implant survival, a number of researchers compared mandibular fixed and removable implant prostheses with follow-up of at least 5 years.[91–93] Fixed and removable prosthetic designs were reported to have clinically similar levels of overall implant survival in the mandible and maxilla.[94] In addition, similar levels of crestal bone loss were recorded after the first year of prosthetic function for the two designs on both arches. Zitzmann and Marinello[95] explored comparative maintenance occurrences with implant-fixed and removable prostheses on the edentulous maxilla. No differences in prosthodontic outcome were noted with more than 2 years of follow-up. While other reports of prosthetic success have ranged widely across prosthetic types, heterogeneity has been notable in defining events. One additional confounding variable when comparing prosthetic stability of fixed and removable prostheses is the design of the removable anchorage system. Investigations have shown that a rigid milled bar versus resilient attachments results in a much reduced maintenance burden.[96,97] Given the level of evidence, it is reasonable to assume that continued prosthetic maintenance should be anticipated for all implant-supported prostheses in the edentulous arch. Fixed restorations often involve more implants, morbidity, and economic investment than removable designs and, therefore, this burden should be carefully weighed based on clinician- and patient-mediated factors.[89,98,99] Clinical factors may rule out a fixed solution because of bone or soft tissue deficiencies. If the resorptive process has led to inadequate facial scaffolding, speech incompetence, or prognathism, or if there are esthetic problems related to exposure of the tissue/prosthetic junction, a removable design is preferable.[89] One of the most important patient-mediated factors requiring discussion is the difficulty with hygiene access attendant to fixed restorations, which is amplified in the elderly.

Periodontal compromise

When the remaining dentition is compromised periodontally, a terminal diagnosis has been fueled by high implant-survival outcomes, in spite of the fact that compromised teeth can be maintained successfully in compliant patients.

Moderate generalized periodontal attachment loss has prompted some to consider extraction of the remaining teeth and placing implants in order to preserve the bone before more precipitous loss ensues. However, Raspirini *et al.*[100] conducted a longitudinal study on 120 patients to evaluate the survival and success of periodontally compromised teeth and implants, using standardized serial radiographs taken at the time of implant placement and 10 years later. Natural teeth yielded superior results with respect to both survival and crestal bone loss compared to implants. Given that adequate periodontal treatment and maintenance have been performed, implant replacement of teeth with moderate attachment loss should be considered with caution.

A most discerning question relates to the management of patients with aggressive periodontitis, a destructive malady characterized by a high rate of progression and early onset without concomitant systemic disease. Graetz *et al.*[101] conducted a paired study of 34 patients with one arm chronic periodontitis and the other arm aggressive periodontitis. He evaluated survival rates and marginal bone loss of both questionable (≥50 to <70% bone loss) and hopeless teeth (≥70% bone loss), after 15 years of regular supportive periodontal therapy. There was no difference in the outcome of the two arms and 88.2% of the 237 questionable teeth and 59.5% of the 37 hopeless teeth survived. Despite continued supportive care, there may be reason to extract. The decision to extract has been predicated on residual 6 mm periodontal pocketing, bleeding on probing at least 30% of the time on recall, and multi-unit teeth with furcal involvement of class II–III.[102,103]

When considering salvaging a patient's compromised dentition, compliance with a consistent supportive periodontal maintenance program is critical for long-term survival of the natural dentition.[104,105] However, complete-arch implant prosthetic rehabilitation also requires assiduous aftercare and is not a solace for patients who are refractory to accept post-insertion protocols. It has been documented that 32% of complete-arch implant rehabilitations sustain a biologic complication, which increases with more than five implants.[106] Furthermore, mechanical aftercare burden in this scenario has been reported to be 3.8 times the incidence of biologic problems.[48] Additionally, mechanical maintenance was significantly higher for patients with double-arch implant reconstructions.[65] Therefore patients seeking implant restorative therapy must also be committed to a recall program a minimum of every 5–6 months.[107]

Future trends

The combination of reduced curriculum time allocation for complete denture theory and practice, scarcity of skilled faculty knowledgeable in removable prosthodontics, and paucity of edentulous patients appointing at dental schools has created a formidable challenge to dental schools to promote this discipline. One approach, that has been conceived and executed by Drs. Landesman, Hansen, and LaBarre at the University of the Pacific Arthur A. Dugoni School of Dentistry (Pacific), has been the Denture Block. It has capitalized on attracting outside prosthodontists to the school to supervise dental students in a hands-on supervision of the fabrication of a conventional complete denture during five to six clinic sessions. This has facilitated a 4:1 student to instructor ratio. It has also enabled faculty cross-training between specialists and faculty generalists to improve their knowledge base in complete dentures. The dearth of available patients has been remedied by contacting social services (Project Homeless Connect) and they have supplied a source for the required number of patients. Outside donations to offset school costs have been relatively easy to attract, providing a zero-based budget. The feedback from the students and patients has been universally positive.

Another approach at Pacific to tackle the battle over curriculum time is the strategy of overlapping disciplines to teach core courses. For example, teaching occlusal equilibration in fixed prosthodontics has been reinforced with clinical remounts of duplicated processed dentures. Likewise, the fundamentals of esthetics for the dentate patient can be reinforced by anterior arrangement of teeth in wax for the edentulous patient. Technological advances using a 3-D extraoral scanner and facility for virtual anterior set-ups is the next natural step to engage students and link facial references to tooth position. Abduo *et al.*[108] has shown comparable results of analog wax-up casts completed and those of a digital wax-up in regard to axial tooth morphology. These enhanced skills will foster a more patient-centered approach to conventional and implant removable prosthodontic care.

For dental schools, new revenue strategies have to be explored to find alternatives to tuition increases and mounting student debt. To remain viable, the dental education system will require a transformational change.[109] Donations for capital projects, educational grants, endowed professorships, and research funding all are becoming more commonplace and are primary in providing income to offset rising costs passed on to the students.[110] The incorporation of sound business-management principles also could offset clinic operation costs. A private practice model was implemented to increase senior dental student production, which resulted in a 63% increase in revenue.[111] Another approach to reducing clinic operations cost is to integrate community-based rotations into the senior dental curriculum. The University of Colorado was the first to implement this program (Advanced Clinical Training Service).[112] Outcomes related to community-based education predicted a net saving per school of $2.7 million or 8.1% of total school expenses.[113] Collaboration with private industry which once was considered best at arm's length, has evolved into a mutually beneficial partnership. Having commercial companies offer technological equipment at reduced costs and supplement the teaching of their clinical application will provide a practical service to the students and faculty. Another novel approach is to enlist private industry to offer support of dental schools in exchange for promoting their services. For example, Nara Bank and UCLA Dental School have partnered to offer low-income patients special loan programs to receive dental treatment, and have extended lines of credit to help graduates buy practices in underserved areas.[114] There are also a number of programs that are offsetting the tuition inflation in dental schools. The state of Mexico is offering a loan to enroll in selected out-of-state dental schools with the entire loan forgiven if the graduate returns to New Mexico to practice for a minimum number of years. The US Department of Health & Human Services offers repayment assistance in exchange for working and also teaching in urban and rural underserved areas. This is duplicated by many states who have a formal loan-repayment program for graduates who commit to practicing in these areas.

Finally, the excitement generated in the scientific community for implants has been seismic and sustained. However, the pendulum is rightly beginning to swing back to the center. Implant survival is no longer the most important outcome measurement. Success speaks to the biologic and technical integrity of the restoration tested over time. It is now apparent that natural teeth, even with compromised attachment levels, outperform implants in motivated patients. Peri-implant disease has been shown to be more prevalent and challenging to treat than formally considered. The disease process appears to be different than the periodontal model and future etiological analyses will undoubtedly uncover new risk factors for patient profiling. The emphasis is turning to diagnosis rather than treatment. This is fitting because, as George Bernard Shaw rightly observed, one of the most common diseases is diagnosis.

Summary

P-I Branemark's concept of osseointegration has arguably changed treatment-planning algorithms more than any other discovery in the last 50 years. But the immensity of this advancement has yet to be revealed. It has germinated a cascade of innovations in surgical and restorative permutations for implant treatment. It has fostered a nondental model for understanding implant biomechanical and biological processes. But perhaps even more compelling is the fact that such conundrums as dental school curriculum limitations, spiraling student debt, unrealistic implant treatment claims, and biases are the doorways to the next level of innovation.

References

1. Jansen CE. CBCT technology for diagnosis and treatment planning: what general practitioners should consider. *Compend Contin Educ Dent* 2014; **35**(10): 749–753.
2. Benavides E, Rios HF, Ganz SD, *et al.* Use of cone beam computed tomography in implant dentistry: the International Congress of Oral Implantologists consensus report. *Implant Dent* 2012; **21**(2): 78–86.
3. Nickenig HJ, Eitner S, Rothamel D, *et al.* Possibilities and limitations of implant placement by virtual planning data and surgical guide templates. *Int J Comput Dent* 2012; **15**(1): 9–21.
4. Lin WS, Harris BT, Ozdemir E, *et al.* Maxillary rehabilitation with a CAD/CAM-fabricated, long-term interim and anatomic contour definitive prosthesis with a digital workflow: a clinical report. *J Prosthet Dent* 2013; **110**(1): 1–7.

5. Papaspyridakos P, Gallucci GO, Chen CJ, *et al.* Digital versus conventional implant impressions for edentulous patients: accuracy outcomes. *Clin Oral Implants Res* 2016; **27**(4): 465–472.
6. Limmer B, Sanders AE, Reside G, *et al.* Complications and patient-centered outcomes with an implant-supported monolithic zirconia fixed dental prosthesis: 1 year results. *J Prosthodont* 2014; **23**(4): 267–275.
7. Altarawneh S, Limmer B, Reside GJ, *et al.* Dual jaw treatment of edentulism using implant-supported monolithic zirconia fixed prostheses. *J Esthet Restor Dent* 2015; **27**(2): 63–70.
8. Qu Z, Rausch-Fan X, Wieland M, *et al.* The initial attachment and subsequent behavior regulation of osteoblasts by dental implant surface modification. *J Biomed Mater Res A* 2007; **82**(3): 658–668.
9. Masaki C, Schneider GB, Zaharias R, *et al.* Effects of implant surface microtopography on osteoblast gene expression. *Clin Oral Implants Res* 2005; **16**(6): 650–656.
10. Schneider GB, Perinpanayagam H, Clegg M, *et al.* Implant surface roughness affects osteoblast gene expression. *J Dent Res* 2003; **82**(5): 372–376.
11. Vlacic-Zischke J, Hamlet SM, Friis T, *et al.* The influence of surface microroughness and hydrophilicity of titanium on the up-regulation of TGFbeta/BMP signalling in osteoblasts. *Biomaterials* 2011; **32**(3): 665–671.
12. Chakravorty N, Ivanovski S, Prasadam I, *et al.* The microRNA expression signature on modified titanium implant surfaces influences genetic mechanisms leading to osteogenic differentiation. *Acta Biomater* 2012; **8**(9): 3516–3523.
13. De Bruyn H, Raes S, Ostman PO, *et al.* Immediate loading in partially and completely edentulous jaws: a review of the literature with clinical guidelines. *Periodontol 2000* 2014; **66**(1): 153–187.
14. Bergkvist G. Immediate loading of implants in the edentulous maxilla. *Swed Dent J Suppl* 2008; **196**: 10–75.
15. Afrashtehfar KI, Cardenas-Bahena JT, Afrashtehfar CD. Predictable immediate loading of mandibular implants. *Tex Dent J* 2013; **130**(7): 596–607.
16. Monje A, Chan HL, Suarez F, *et al.* Marginal bone loss around tilted implants in comparison to straight implants: a meta-analysis. *Int J Oral Maxillofac Implants* 2012; **27**(6): 1576–1583.
17. Del Fabbro M, Ceresoli V. The fate of marginal bone around axial vs. tilted implants: a systematic review. *Eur J Oral Implantol* 2014; 7(Suppl2): S171–189.
18. Wang F, Monje A, Lin GH, *et al.* Reliability of four zygomatic implant-supported prostheses for the rehabilitation of the atrophic maxilla: a systematic review. *Int J Oral Maxillofac Implants* 2015; **30**(2): 293–298.
19. Davo R, Pons O. 5-year outcome of cross-arch prostheses supported by four immediately loaded zygomatic implants: a prospective case series. *Eur J Oral Implantol* 2015; **8**(2): 169–174.
20. Pommer B, Mailath-Pokorny G, Haas R, *et al.* Patients' preferences towards minimally invasive treatment alternatives for implant rehabilitation of edentulous jaws. *Eur J Oral Implantol* 2014; 7(Suppl 2): S91–109.
21. Ismail HA, Mahrous AI, Banasr FH, *et al.* Two years retrospective evaluation of overdenture retained by symphyseal single implant using two types of attachments. *J Int Oral Health* 2015; **7**(6): 4–8.
22. Cordioli G, Majzoub Z, Castagna S. Mandibular overdentures anchored to single implants: a five-year prospective study. *J Prosthet Dent* 1997; **78**(2): 159–165.
23. Krennmair G, Ulm C. The symphyseal single-tooth implant for anchorage of a mandibular complete denture in geriatric patients: a clinical report. *Int J Oral Maxillofac Implants* 2001; **16**(1): 98–104.
24. Brownstein SA, Murad A, Hunt RJ. Implementation of new technologies in U.S. dental school curricula. *J Dent Educ* 2015; **79**(3): 259–264.
25. Barwacz CA, Avila-Ortiz G, Allareddy V, *et al.* An overview of U.S. predoctoral dental implant programs and their directors. *J Dent Educ* 2015; **79**(3): 265–277.
26. Ong CT, Pan N, Tiang R, *et al.* General dental practitioners' perceptions of removable prosthodontics in the undergraduate curriculum. *N Z Dent J* 1999; **95**(421): 80–83.
27. McCord F. Understanding prosthodontics – where did it all go wrong? *Int Dent J* 2003; **53**(5Suppl): 335–339.
28. Clark RK. The future of teaching of complete denture construction to undergraduates. *Br Dent J* 2002; **193**(1): 13–14.
29. Ettinger RL. Who is going to treat our edentulous older adults? *Spec Care Dentist* 2004; **24**(6): 281–282.
30. Wieder M, Faigenblum M, Eder A, *et al.* An investigation of complete denture teaching in the UK: part 1. A survey of undergraduate teaching. *Br Dent J* 2013; **215**(4): 177–181.
31. Clark RK, Radford DR, Juszczyk AS. Current trends in complete denture teaching in British dental schools. *Br Dent J* 2010; **208**(5): E10; discussion 214–215.
32. Wieder M, Faigenblum M, Eder A, *et al.* An investigation of complete denture teaching in the UK: part 2. The DF1 experience. *Br Dent J* 2013; **215**(5): 229–236.
33. Landesman HM. A technique for the delivery of complete dentures. *J Prosthet Dent* 1980; **43**(3): 348–351.
34. Carlsson GE. Clinical morbidity and sequelae of treatment with complete dentures. *J Prosthet Dent* 1998; **79**(1): 17–23.
35. Al-Dwairi Z, Lynch E. Xerostomia in complete denture wearers: prevalence, clinical findings and impact on oral functions. *Gerodontology* 2014; **31**(1): 49–55.
36. Martori E, Ayuso-Montero R, Martinez-Gomis J, *et al.* Risk factors for denture-related oral mucosal lesions in a geriatric population. *J Prosthet Dent* 2014; **111**(4): 273–279.
37. Anil S, Vellappally S, Hashem M, *et al.* Xerostomia in geriatric patients: a burgeoning global concern. *J Investig Clin Dent* 2016; **7**(1): 5–12.
38. Cooper LF. The current and future treatment of edentulism. *J Prosthodont* 2009; **18**(2): 116–122.
39. Fenlon MR, Sherriff M. An investigation of factors influencing patients' satisfaction with new complete dentures using structural equation modelling. *J Dent* 2008; **36**(6): 427–434.
40. Koper A. Human factors in prosthodontic treatment. *J Prosthet Dent* 1973; **30**(4Pt2): 678–679.
41. Feine JS, Carlsson GE, Awad MA, *et al.* The McGill consensus statement on overdentures. Mandibular two-implant overdentures as first choice standard of care for edentulous patients. Montreal, Quebec, May 24–25, 2002. *Int J Oral Maxillofac Implants* 2002; **17**(4): 601–602.
42. McGarry TJ, Nimmo A, Skiba JF, *et al.* Classification system for complete edentulism. The American College of Prosthodontics. *J Prosthodont* 1999; **8**(1): 27–39.
43. Berg E. Acceptance of full dentures. *Int Dent J* 1993; **43**(3 Suppl 1): 299–306.

44. Friedman N, Landesman HM, Wexler M. The influences of fear, anxiety, and depression on the patient's adaptive responses to complete dentures. Part I. *J Prosthet Dent* 1987; **58**(6): 687–689.
45. Allen PF, McMillan AS, Walshaw D. Patient expectations of oral implant-retained prostheses in a UK dental hospital. *Br Dent J* 1999; **186**(2): 80–84.
46. Phillips K, Wong KM. Vertical space requirement for the fixed-detachable, implant-supported prosthesis. *Compend Contin Educ Dent* 2002; **23**(8): 750–756.
47. Phillips K, Wong KM. Space requirements for implant-retained bar-and-clip overdentures. *Compend Contin Educ Dent* 2001; **22**(6): 516–522.
48. Dhima M, Paulusova V, Lohse C, *et al.* Practice-based evidence from 29-year outcome analysis of management of the edentulous jaw using osseointegrated dental implants. *J Prosthodont* 2014; **23**(3): 173–181.
49. Koller MM, Merlini L, Spandre G, *et al.* A comparative study of two methods for the orientation of the occlusal plane and the determination of the vertical dimension of occlusion in edentulous patients. *J Oral Rehabil* 1992; **19**(4): 413–425.
50. Millet C, Jeannin C, Vincent B, *et al.* Report on the determination of occlusal vertical dimension and centric relation using swallowing in edentulous patients. *J Oral Rehabil* 2003; **30**(11): 1118–1122.
51. Miralles R, Dodds C, Palazzi C, *et al.* Vertical dimension. Part 1: comparison of clinical freeway space. *Cranio* 2001; **19**(4): 230–236.
52. Wagner AG. Comparison of four methods to determine rest position of the mandible. *J Prosthet Dent* 1971; **25**(5): 506–514.
53. Geerts GA, Stuhlinger ME, Nel DG. A comparison of the accuracy of two methods used by pre-doctoral students to measure vertical dimension. *J Prosthet Dent* 2004; **91**(1): 59–66.
54. Makzoume JE. Variations in rest vertical dimension: effects of headrest in edentulous patients. *Gen Dent* 2007; **55**(4): 316–319.
55. de Souza RF, Compagnoni MA. Relation between speaking space of the /s/ sound and freeway space in dentate and edentate subjects. *Braz Oral Res* 2004; **18**(4): 333–337.
56. Sadowsky SJ. The role of complete denture principles in implant prosthodontics. *J Calif Dent Assoc* 2003; **31**(12): 905–909.
57. Pound E. Recapturing esthetic tooth position in the edentulous patient. *J Am Dent Assoc* 1957; **55**(2): 181–191.
58. Shanahan TE. Physiologic vertical dimension and centric relation. 1956. *J Prosthet Dent* 2004; **91**(3): 206–209.
59. Williamson EH, Woelfel JB, Williams BH. A longitudinal study of rest position and centric occlusion. *Angle Orthod* 1975; **45**(2): 130–136.
60. Mack MR. Facially generated occlusal vertical dimension. *Compend Contin Educ Dent* 1997; **18**(12): 1183–1190.
61. Mack MR. Perspective of facial esthetics in dental treatment planning. *J Prosthet Dent* 1996; **75**(2): 169–176.
62. Sarver D, Jacobson RS. The aesthetic dentofacial analysis. *Clin Plast Surg* 2007; **34**(3): 369–394.
63. Zhao K, Mai QQ, Wang XD, *et al.* Occlusal designs on masticatory ability and patient satisfaction with complete denture: a systematic review. *J Dent* 2013; **41**(11): 1036–1042.
64. Rehmann P, Balkenhol M, Ferger P, *et al.* Influence of the occlusal concept of complete dentures on patient satisfaction in the initial phase after fitting: bilateral balanced occlusion vs canine guidance. *Int J Prosthodont* 2008; **21**(1): 60–61.
65. Malo P, Araujo Nobre MD, Lopes A, *et al.* Double full-arch versus single full-arch, four implant-supported rehabilitations: a retrospective, 5-year cohort study. *J Prosthodont* 2015; **24**(4): 263–270.
66. Eliasson A, Palmqvist S, Svenson B, *et al.* Five-year results with fixed complete-arch mandibular prostheses supported by 4 implants. *Int J Oral Maxillofac Implants* 2000; **15**(4): 505–510.
67. Dychtwald K. 'Age power': how the new-old will transform medicine in the 21st century. Interview by Alice V. Luddington. *Geriatrics* 1999; **54**(12): 22–27.
68. Lombardi RE. The principles of visual perception and their clinical application to denture esthetics. *J Prosthet Dent* 1973; **29**(4): 358–382.
69. McArthur DR. Determination of approximate size of maxillary anterior denture teeth when mandibular anterior teeth are present. Part III: relationship of maxillary to mandibular central incisor widths. *J Prosthet Dent* 1985; **53**(4): 540–542.
70. Small BW. Location of incisal edge position for esthetic restorative dentistry. *Gen Dent* 2000; **48**(4): 396–367.
71. Zitzmann NU, Marinello CP. Treatment plan for restoring the edentulous maxilla with implant-supported restorations: removable overdenture versus fixed partial denture design. *J Prosthet Dent* 1999; **82**(2): 188–196.
72. Jameson WS. Dynesthetic and dentogenic concept revisited. *J Esthet Restor Dent* 2002; **14**(3): 139–148.
73. Simensen AN, Boe OE, Berg E, *et al.* Patient knowledge and expectations prior to receiving implant-supported restorations. *Int J Oral Maxillofac Implants* 2015; **30**(1): 41–47.
74. Christensen GJ. Removable prosthodontics: a forgotten part of dentistry. *Alpha Omegan* 2006; **99**(1): 26–28.
75. Graser GN. Predoctoral removable prosthodontics education. *J Prosthet Dent* 1990; **64**(3): 326–333.
76. Stafford GL, Nourzad F, Lobb WK, *et al.* The economic costs and benefits of dental education: an empirical analysis. *J Dent Educ* 2014; **78**(11): 1497–1507.
77. McAllister DE, Garrison GE, Feldman CA, *et al.* U.S. dental school deans' perceptions of the rising cost of dental education and borrowing pressures on dental students: report of survey results. *J Dent Educ* 2015; **79**(6): 719–727.
78. Stafford GL. Dental student indebtedness: where did it come from and where will it lead? *J Am Coll Dent* 2013; **80**(4): 38–48.
79. Brennan DS, Spencer AJ. The role of dentist, practice and patient factors in the provision of dental services. *Community Dent Oral Epidemiol* 2005; **33**(3): 181–195.
80. Narby B. Factors shaping demand for prosthetic dentistry treatment with special focus on implant dentistry. *Swed Dent J Suppl* 2011; **218**: 3–65.
81. Lundgren D, Rylander H, Laurell L. To save or to extract, that is the question. Natural teeth or dental implants in periodontitis-susceptible patients: clinical decision-making and treatment strategies exemplified with patient case presentations. *Periodontol 2000* 2008; **47**: 27–50.
82. Fasbinder D. Using digital technology to enhance restorative dentistry. *Compend Contin Educ Dent* 2012; **33**(9): 666–672.
83. Ali S, Woodmason K, Patel N. The quality of online information regarding dental implants. *Br Dent J* 2014; **217**(9): E16.
84. Parel SM, Phillips WR. A risk assessment treatment planning protocol for the four implant immediately loaded maxilla: preliminary findings. *J Prosthet Dent* 2011; **106**(6): 359–366.

85. Leles CR, Martins RR, Silva ET, *et al.* Discriminant analysis of patients' reasons for choosing or refusing treatments for partial edentulism. *J Oral Rehabil* 2009; **36**(12): 909–915.
86. DeBoer J. Edentulous implants: overdenture versus fixed. *J Prosthet Dent* 1993; **69**(4): 386–390.
87. de Grandmont P, Feine JS, Tache R, *et al.* Within-subject comparisons of implant-supported mandibular prostheses: psychometric evaluation. *J Dent Res* 1994; **73**(5): 1096–1104.
88. Heydecke G, Boudrias P, Awad MA, *et al.* Within-subject comparisons of maxillary fixed and removable implant prostheses: patient satisfaction and choice of prosthesis. *Clin Oral Implants Res* 2003; **14**(1): 125–130.
89. Zitzmann NU, Marinello CP. Treatment outcomes of fixed or removable implant-supported prostheses in the edentulous maxilla. Part I: patients' assessments. *J Prosthet Dent* 2000; **83**(4): 424–433.
90. Sadowsky SJ, Fitzpatrick B, Curtis DA. Evidence-based criteria for differential treatment planning of implant restorations for the maxillary edentulous patient. *J Prosthodont* 2015; **24**(6): 433–446.
91. Tinsley D, Watson CJ, Russell JL. A comparison of hydroxylapatite coated implant retained fixed and removable mandibular prostheses over 4 to 6 years. *Clin Oral Implants Res* 2001; **12**(2): 159–166.
92. Watson RM, Davis DM. Follow up and maintenance of implant supported prostheses: a comparison of 20 complete mandibular overdentures and 20 complete mandibular fixed cantilever prostheses. *Br Dent J* 1996; **181**(9): 321–327.
93. Makkonen TA, Holmberg S, Niemi L, *et al.* A 5-year prospective clinical study of Astra Tech dental implants supporting fixed bridges or overdentures in the edentulous mandible. *Clin Oral Implants Res* 1997; **8**(6): 469–475.
94. Bryant SR, MacDonald-Jankowski D, Kim K. Does the type of implant prosthesis affect outcomes for the completely edentulous arch? *Int J Oral Maxillofac Implants* 2007; **22**(Suppl): 117–139.
95. Zitzmann NU, Marinello CP. Treatment outcomes of fixed or removable implant-supported prostheses in the edentulous maxilla. Part II: clinical findings. *J Prosthet Dent* 2000; **83**(4): 434–442.
96. Krennmair G, Krainhofner M, Piehslinger E. The influence of bar design (round versus milled bar) on prosthodontic maintenance of mandibular overdentures supported by 4 implants: a 5-year prospective study. *Int J Prosthodont* 2008; **21**(6): 514–520.
97. Weinlander M, Piehslinger E, Krennmair G. Removable implant-prosthodontic rehabilitation of the edentulous mandible: five-year results of different prosthetic anchorage concepts. *Int J Oral Maxillofac Implants* 2010; **25**(3): 589–597.
98. Locker D. Patient-based assessment of the outcomes of implant therapy: a review of the literature. *Int J Prosthodont* 1998; **11**(5): 453–461.
99. Lewis DW. Optimized therapy for the edentulous predicament: cost-effectiveness considerations. *J Prosthet Dent* 1998; **79**(1): 93–99.
100. Rasperini G, Siciliano VI, Cafiero C, *et al.* Crestal bone changes at teeth and implants in periodontally healthy and periodontally compromised patients. A 10-year comparative case-series study. *J Periodontol* 2014; **85**(6): e152–159.
101. Graetz C, Dorfer CE, Kahl M, *et al.* Retention of questionable and hopeless teeth in compliant patients treated for aggressive periodontitis. *J Clin Periodontol* 2011; **38**(8): 707–714.
102. Salvi GE, Mischler DC, Schmidlin K, *et al.* Risk factors associated with the longevity of multi-rooted teeth. Long-term outcomes after active and supportive periodontal therapy. *J Clin Periodontol* 2014; **41**(7): 701–707.
103. Matuliene G, Pjetursson BE, Salvi GE, *et al.* Influence of residual pockets on progression of periodontitis and tooth loss: results after 11 years of maintenance. *J Clin Periodontol* 2008; **35**(8): 685–695.
104. Klokkevold PR, Han TJ. How do smoking, diabetes, and periodontitis affect outcomes of implant treatment? *Int J Oral Maxillofac Implants* 2007; **22**(Suppl): 173–202.
105. Garcia-Bellosta S, Bravo M, Subira C, *et al.* Retrospective study of the long-term survival of 980 implants placed in a periodontal practice. *Int J Oral Maxillofac Implants* 2010; **25**(3): 613–619.
106. Passoni BB, Dalago HR, Schuldt Filho G, *et al.* Does the number of implants have any relation with peri-implant disease? *J Appl Oral Sci* 2014; **22**(5): 403–408.
107. Monje A, Aranda L, Diaz KT, *et al.* Impact of maintenance therapy for the prevention of peri-implant diseases: a systematic review and meta-analysis. *J Dent Res* 2016; **95**(4): 372–379.
108. Abduo J, Bennamoun M, Tennant M, *et al.* Impact of digital prosthodontic planning on dental esthetics: Biometric analysis of esthetic parameters. *J Prosthet Dent* 2016; **115**(1): 57–64.
109. Walker MP, Duley SI, Beach MM, *et al.* Dental education economics: challenges and innovative strategies. *J Dent Educ* 2008; **72**(12): 1440–1449.
110. Spalding PM, Bradley RE. Commercialization of dental education: have we gone too far? *J Am Coll Dent* 2006; **73**(3): 30–35.
111. Pousson RG, McDonald GT. A model for increasing senior dental student production using private practice principles. *J Dent Educ* 2004; **68**(12): 1272–1277.
112. Berg R, Berkey DB. University of Colorado School of Dentistry's Advanced Clinical Training and Service Program. *J Dent Educ* 1999; **63**(12): 938–943.
113. Bailit HL, Beazoglou TJ, Formicola AJ, *et al.* Financing clinical dental education. *J Dent Educ* 2007; **71**(3): 322–330.
114. Mitchell T, Mito R, Hong B, *et al.* A dental school and a bank: partnership for community service. *J Calif Dent Assoc* 2005; **33**(7): 562–564.

CHAPTER 17

Implant Restoration of the Maxillary Edentulous Patient

Nicola U. Zitzmann
School of Dental Medicine, University of Basel, Switzerland

Implant restorations in the maxillary edentulous patient are one of the most daunting challenges in dentistry, due to high patient expectations, complex diagnosis, difficult initial morphological situations, and compound surgical and restorative requirements. This chapter will examine the current knowledge on patient selection and risk factors for fixed and removable implant prostheses for the edentulous maxilla through the lens of a methodical diagnostic regimen. Guidelines will be offered for specific design considerations of implant prostheses. While long-term treatment success has been an elusive achievement, a discussion of patient-reported outcome measurements will assist the clinician in prognosis as part of a comprehensive informed consent.

Morphology of the edentulous maxilla

Tooth loss generally occurs earlier in the maxilla than in the mandible, which is most likely related to early damage from anterior trauma and vulnerability to periodontal disease, particularly with furcation involvement in the first premolars and molar teeth. Further, periodontal and endodontic treatment of maxillary molars is very demanding, due to contorted root canal anatomy, which complicates treatment and tooth preservation. As a consequence edentulism in the maxilla is more frequent, affecting approximately 40% of the population 65 years and older; in this age group 27% are edentulous in the mandible and these patients are almost invariably edentulous in both jaws.[1,2]

The scaffold of the maxillary bone is susceptible to severe alveolar ridge resorption following tooth loss, particularly in the anterior region, with thin cortical bone plates on the buccal aspect. In the posterior region, an increase in the pneumatization of the maxillary sinus reduces the bone volume (Figure 17.1a). Due to normal tooth inclination in the maxilla, the arch circumference of the maxillary dentition is larger than its bony foundation and normally overlaps the mandibular dentition. The faciolingual axial inclination of the central incisors, described as the angle between the long axis of the tooth and a line drawn perpendicular to a horizontal plane, measures 28°, it is on average 26° for lateral incisors, and 16° for canines.[3] This tooth angulation, particularly in the anterior region, contributes to the resorptive pattern of the edentulous maxilla, which is superiorly and medially directed, resulting in a reduced arch circumference (Figure 17.2).[4,5] For implant placement, the edentulous maxilla frequently has limited bone height and width, with a bone foundation displaced cranially and medially when compared to the ideal position of the clinical crowns. Depending on the progression of the bone resorption, this initial morphological situation frequently leads to a wide, unparalleled, fanned implant position, unless buccal augmentation has been anticipated. These morphological changes following tooth loss, accompanied by difficult implant procedures, require a thorough initial diagnosis by the clinician to visualize the three-dimensional (3-D) relationship between the ideal tooth position and the underlying soft and hard tissues. When there are high esthetic demands in addition to full display of the maxillary sextant, the margin for error is minimal. For this diagnostic sequence extra- and intraoral factors should be assessed systematically (Table 17.1), so that a reasoned treatment recommendation can be given and explained to the patient.

Diagnostic phase

An adequate existing complete denture (CD) can be used for diagnostics, and the thickness of the buccal flange can be indicative of the necessary lip and cheek support (Figure 17.1b, c).[6,7] A resilient cast can be produced, which is mounted in the

Evidence-based Implant Treatment Planning and Clinical Protocols, First Edition. Edited by Steven J. Sadowsky.

Companion website: www.wiley.com/go/sadowsky/implant

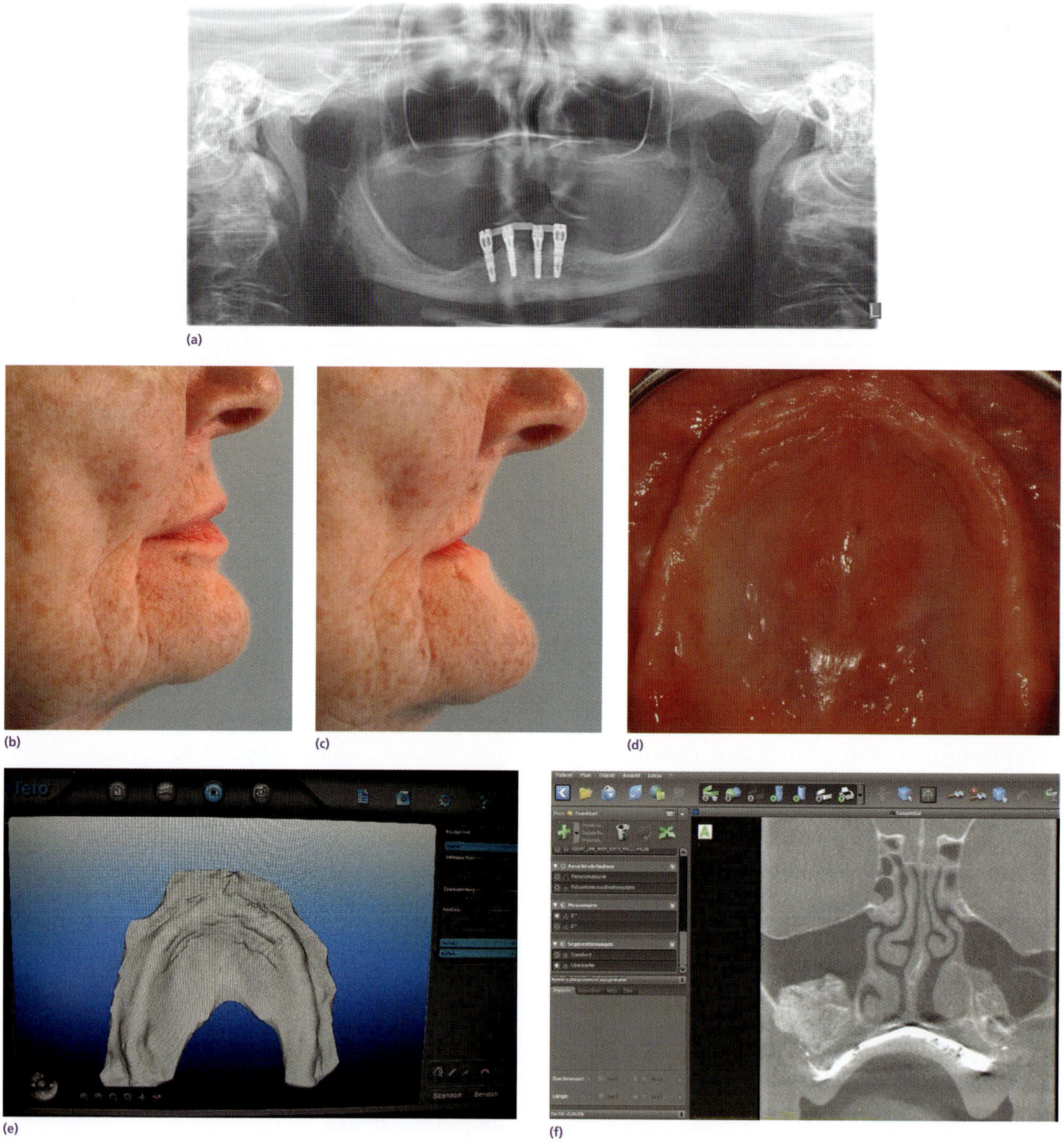

Figure 17.1 **(a)** Panoramic radiograph showing advanced bone resorption in both jaws with increased pneumatization of the maxillary sinuses and alveolar ridge resorption in the anterior maxilla. **(b, c)** Patient's profile with and without complete dentures in place with obvious need for facial support by prosthesis flanges. **(d)** Clinical situation of the patient with advanced bone resorption following bilateral maxillary sinus augmentation. **(e)** Intraoral surface scan of the mucosal tissues (iTero, San Jose, California). **(f)** CBCT scan with mucosal contour displayed by using jodoform paste applied onto the prosthesis base. **(g)** Image created with coDiagnostiX-software superimposing the CBCT data with the iTero-surface-scan (black line) and an additional surface scan of the prosthesis (Projektor MPT, Breuckmann GmbH, Meersburg, Germany; red line). **(h)** Prosthetically-driven implant planning for an implant overdenture with bar retention (black line illustrates mucosal contour, red line indicates prosthesis contour). **(i)** Six implants planned. **(j)** Virtual template designed according to the determined implant positions including blueprint for the sleeves. **(k)** Printed template based on exported iTero data transferred as stl.-file to a 3D-Printer (Objet Eden, Stratasys; right). **(l)** Postoperative panoramic radiograph after implant placement, using the template for guided preparation of implant beds. **(m)** Prefabricated round Dolder bar (soldered gold bar). **(n)** IOD with cast framework and clips inserted (Galak, Cendres & Métaux). (Technician: Clemens Gessner, Basel.) *Source:* Reproduced with permission from Dr. Sebastian Kühl.

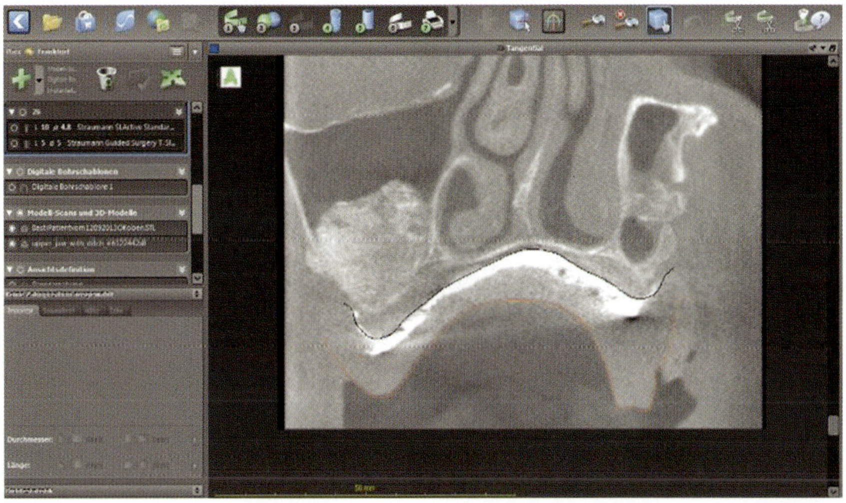

(g)

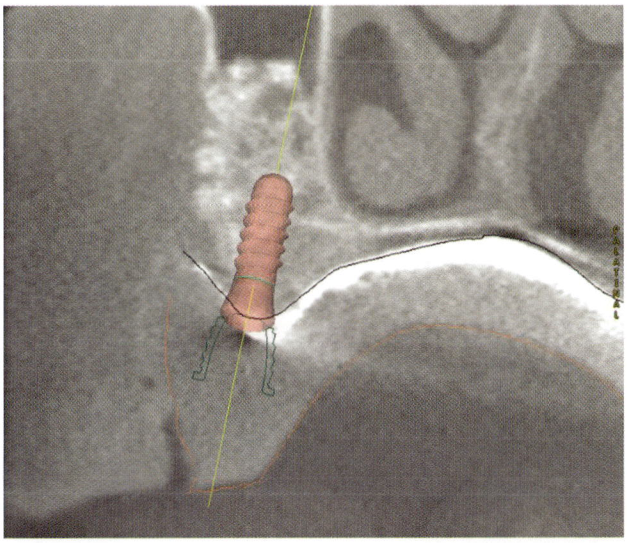

(h)

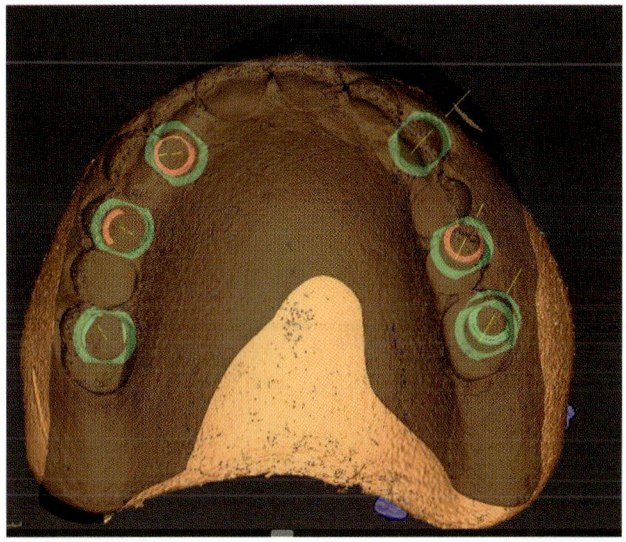

(i)

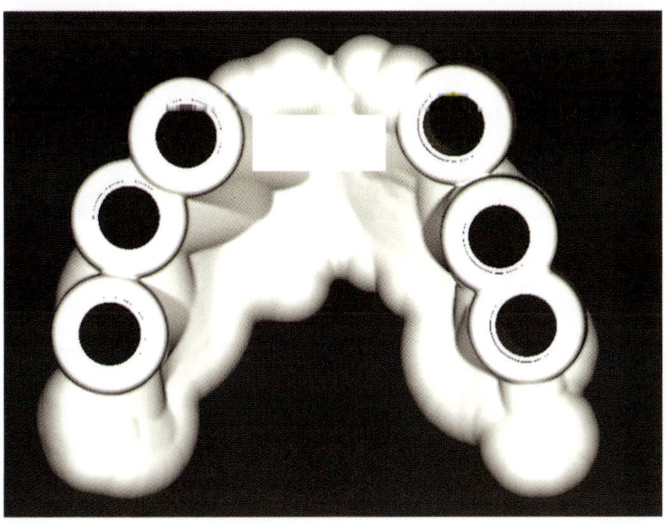

(j)

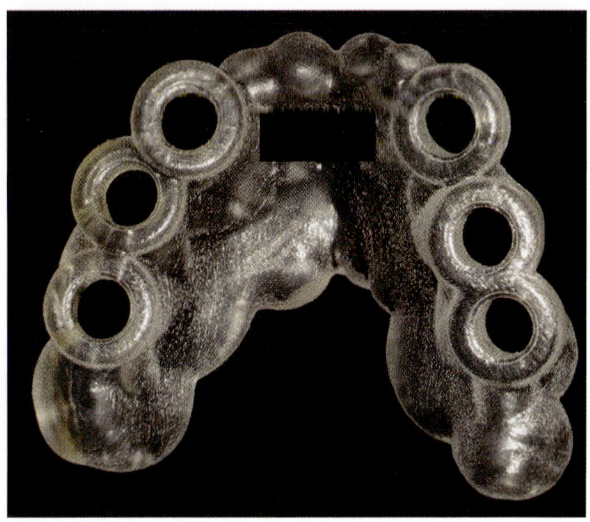

(k)

Figure 17.1 (*Continued*)

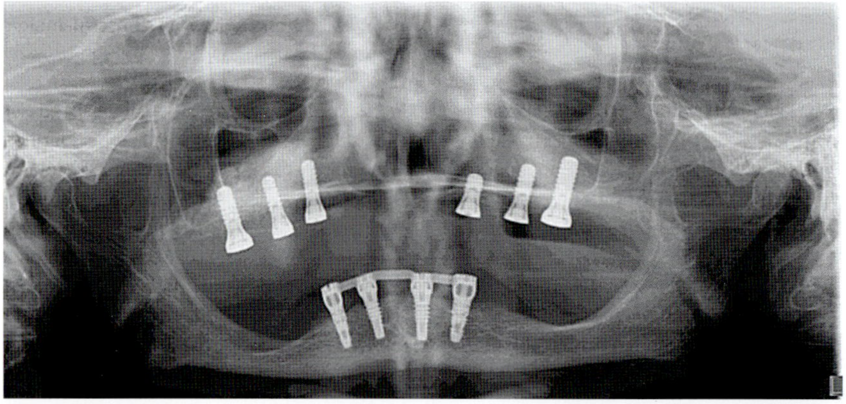

(l)

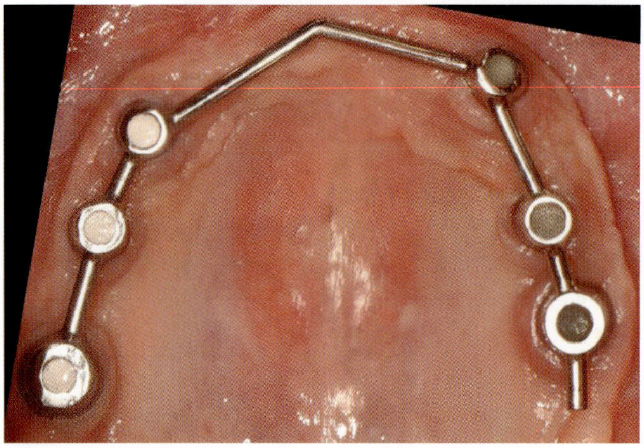

(m)

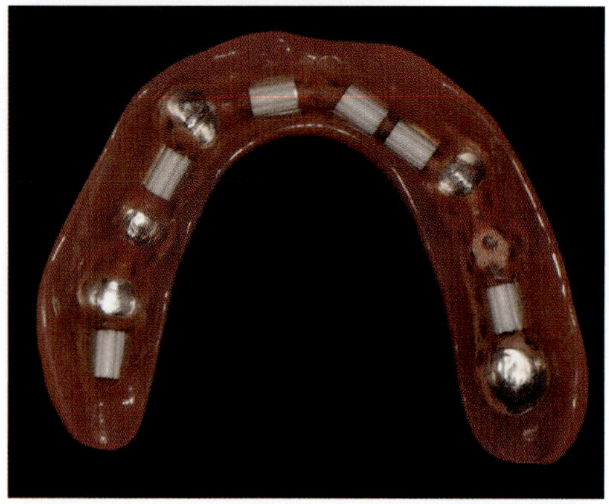

(n)

Figure 17.1 (*Continued*)

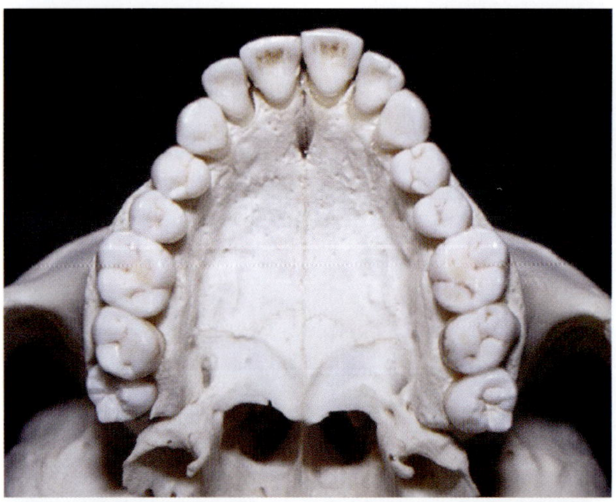

(a)

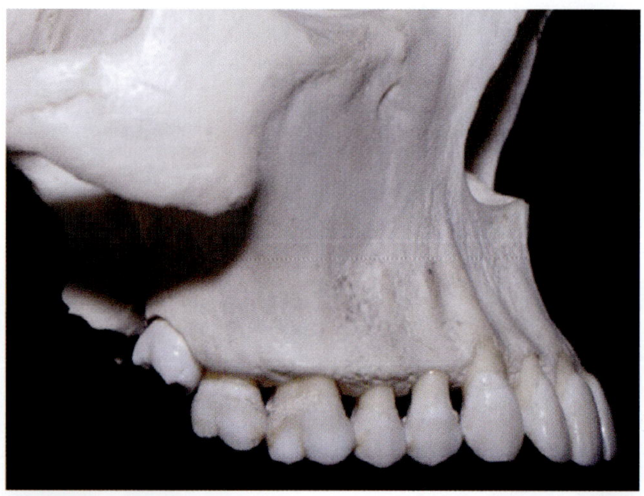

(b)

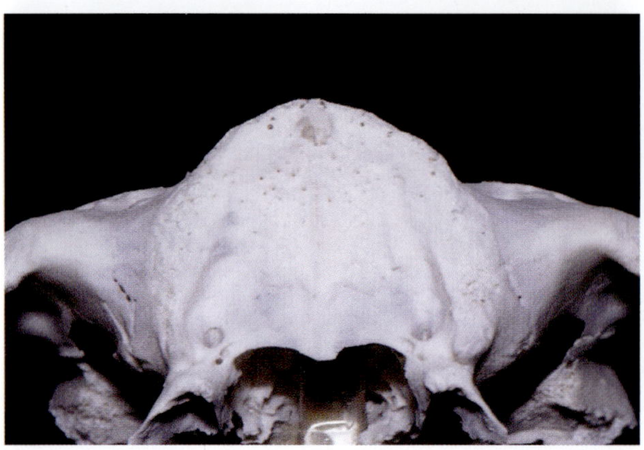

(c)

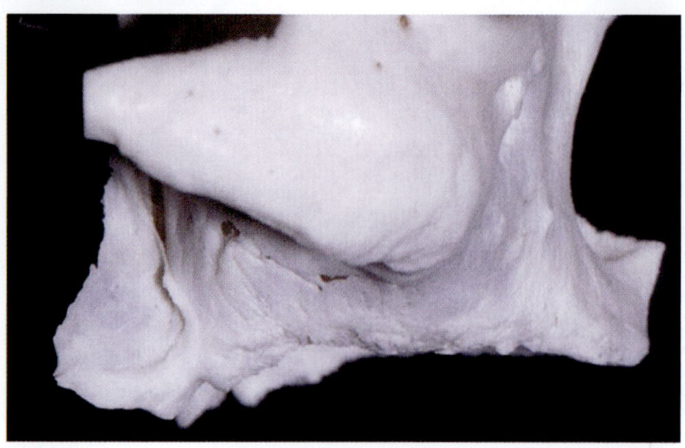

(d)

Figure 17.2 Dentate (**a, b**) and edentulous (**c, d**) maxillae (occlusal and lateral views).

Table 17.1 Diagnostic form for the edentulous maxilla (distribution of crosses indicate recommended prosthesis design).

a) Patient factors. General risk factors for implant treatment and bone augmentation: smoking, history of aggressive periodontal disease, residual probing pocket depth of ≥5 mm at implant placement					
Patient's request	Fixed ☐		Removable ☐		
			No palatal coverage ☐	Palatal coverage accepted ☐	
Reason for request	Psychological impairment ☐		Poor stability and retention of CD (no CD improvement feasible) ☐		
Finances	Acceptance ☐		Acceptance ☐	Limitations ☐	
Oral hygiene dexterity	Excellent ☐	Excellent ☐	Good ☐	Limitations ☐	
b) Extraoral factors					
Smile line	Low ☐		Average ☐	High ☐	
Lip and facial support	Not required ☐			Needed ☐	
Intermaxillary relation/ skeletal class	Class I (congruent) ☐ Class II (retrognathic mandible) ☐			Class III (prognathic appearance), small max. arch circumference, and/or concave profile ☐	
c) Intraoral factors					
Degree of alveolar ridge resorption	Moderate ☐		Advanced ☐	Advanced to severe ☐	
Ridge defects	None ☐		Only vertical ☐	Horizontal or combined ☐	
Intermaxillary space (max. mucosa to mand. incisal edges)	8–10 mm ☐ for PFM design		≥12 mm ☐ for IFCD design	≥12 mm ☐ for bar design	≥8 mm ☐ for single attachments
d) Recommended implant restoration					
Description	Implant-supported fixed dental prosthesis (metal–ceramic, PFM) ☐	Implant-supported fixed complete denture ☐	Implant overdenture (IOD) ☐		
Anchorage	Preferably screw-retained ☐		Bar splint ☐		Single attachments/ solitary anchors ☐
Number of implants	6–8 ☐	4–6 ☐	4–6 ☐		4 ☐
Implant position and angulation	In accordance with clinical crown position ☐	Approximately at crown positions ☐	Compensation of divergent implant angulations ☐ Varying implant positions requiring milled bar with overcast ☐	Every 2nd tooth position for approx. 8 mm clip length of prefabricated bar ☐	Limited options for divergent implant angulation ☐

articulator at the appropriate occlusal vertical dimension.[8] The anterior dentition is then keyed with silicone to visualize the available intermaxillary space and the thickness of the buccal prosthesis flange, which will indicate facial and lip support needs and further dictate a fixed or removable prosthesis (Figure 17.3a–c).

If the existing dentition and restoration deviate from an ideal vertical dimension of occlusion or tooth position, a new set-up (similar to the wax trial for a complete denture) should be made to establish the occlusal plane with a correct maxillary incisal edge position and to evaluate the tooth display during smiling.[9,10] This set-up can be prepared without a buccal flange to simplify the clinical analysis of a potential need for facial and lip support during try-in, especially when a fixed restoration is desired by the patient (Figure 17.3d). The major factors for establishing the correct anterior tooth arrangement and the occlusal plane are based on complete denture principles and are specifically elucidated in the following protocols.[10,11]

- Determine the incisal edge position of the central incisors, which overlap the occlusal plane about 2 mm (normal vertical overlap) and contact the vermillion border of the lower lip when an F-sound is produced. Depending on the upper lip length (see below), 1–2 mm of the incisal edge should be displayed in repose in the average patient, while more is visible during smiling. The length of the central incisor is 10.5 mm on average,[3] but may be more in elderly patients, in whom some gingival recession can be expected.
- The length of the upper lip, measured from the base of the columnella (subnasal) to the philtrum location, is related to the amount of the maxillary anterior dentition being exposed

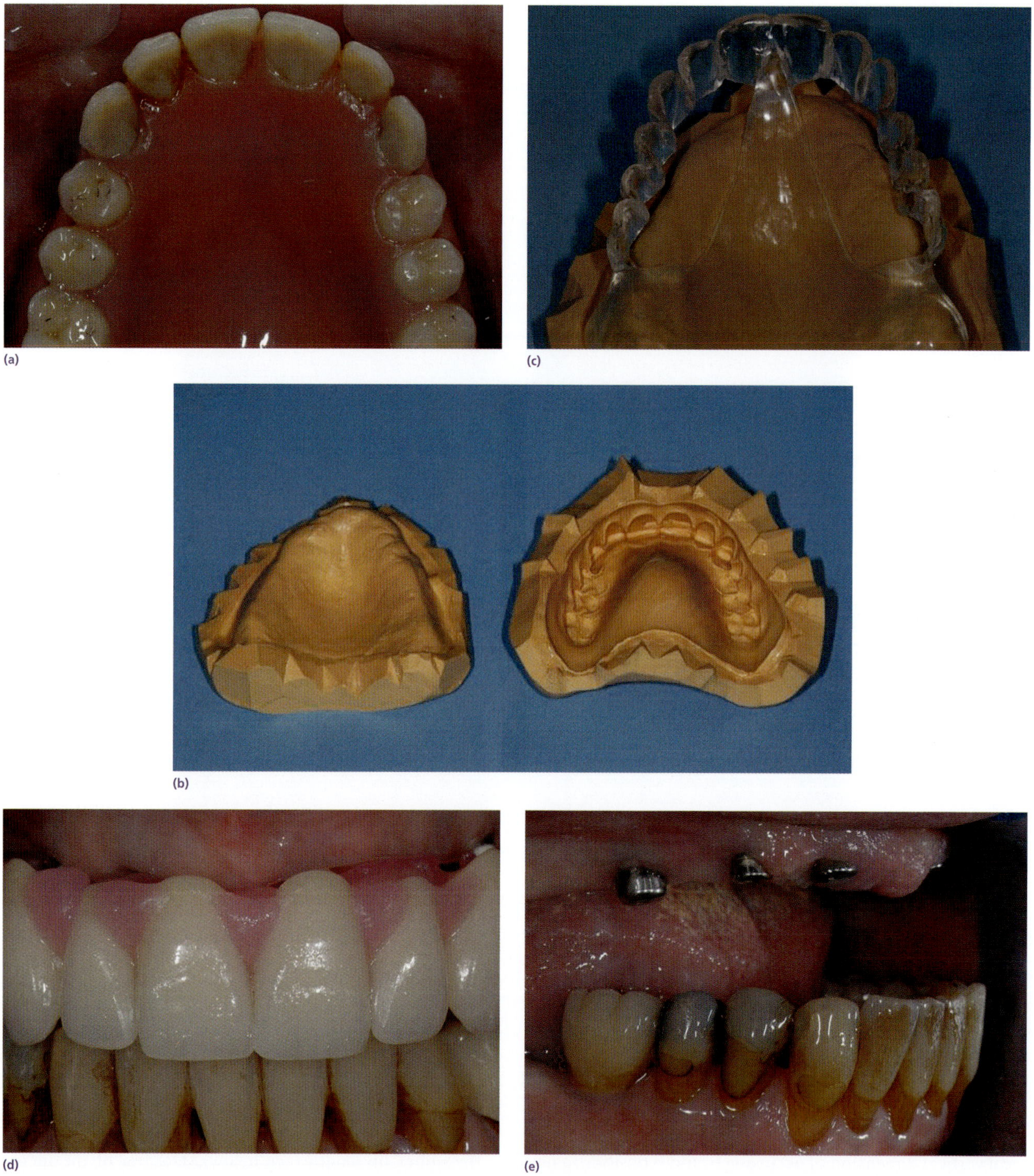

Figure 17.3 **(a)** Clinical situation of existing denture with adequate tooth position. **(b)** Denture is used to fabricate a resilient cast, which is keyed to visualize the relationship between ideal tooth position and underlying tissues. **(c)** Cast is used to fabricate a surgical template. **(d)** Set-up made without buccal flange, clearly illustrating that soft tissue support can only be provided by an implant overdenture. **(e)** Clinical situation with six implants placed. **(f)** IOD retained at stud abutments (locators) and an anterior bar (Bredent Vario Soft) with an overcast. **(g, h)** Clinical situation with reduced palatal coverage and buccal flange extension. (Technician: Alwin Schönenberger, Vision Dental Chiasso.)

in repose and also influences the incisal edge position and the occlusal plane (Figure 17.4a, b).[12]

- The smile line is determined by the tonus of the orofacial muscles influencing the movement of the upper lip during speech and smiling (Table 17.1b).[13] Tjan *et al.* described the average smile as having the position of the upper lip such that 75–100% of the upper incisors and the interproximal gingiva are displayed during smiling. This position was distinguished from the high smile line,

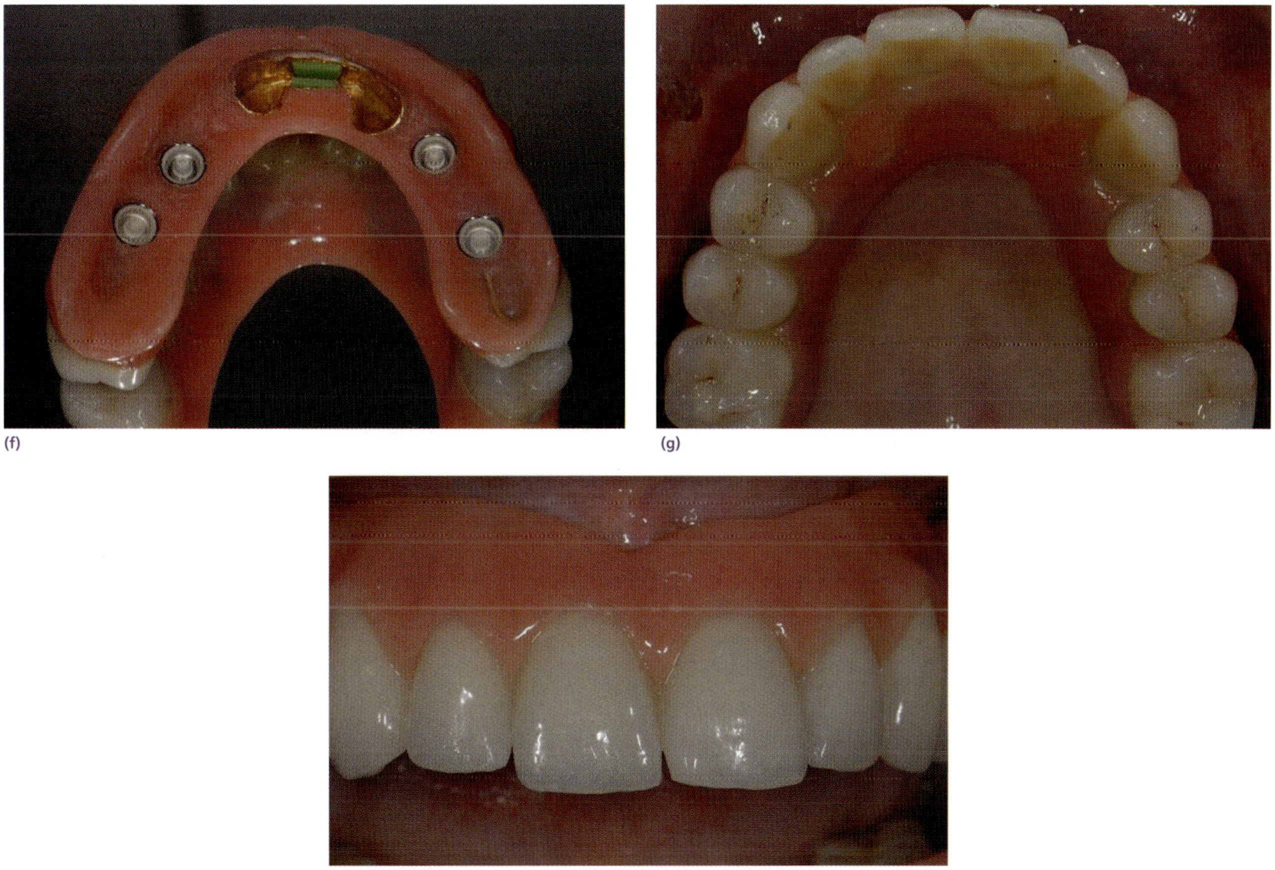

(f) (g) (h)

Figure 17.3 (*Continued*)

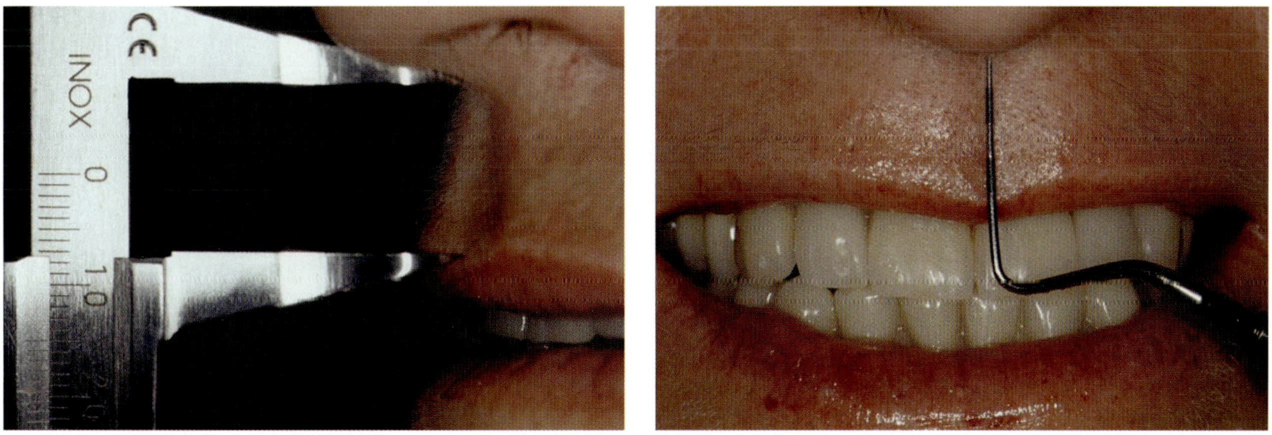

(a) (b)

Figure 17.4 (**a, b**) Initial examination in a patient with a short lip line (15 mm measured from subnasal to philtrum in repose) with adequate denture or diagnostic set-up in place. The full length of a periodontal probe serves as a reference for the average length of maxillary incisors (23.5 mm), which have to fit below the subnasal point, and helps to determine the adequate incisal edge position.

where there is additional exposure of part of the gingiva, and from the low smile line, where less than 75% of the maxillary anterior teeth is displayed.[14] In patients designated for implant treatment in the maxilla, evaluation of the smile line should be performed without the denture in place. When even the alveolar ridge is displayed during smiling, the use of a buccal flange in a removable prosthesis may be advisable to prevent esthetic problems with exposure of the prosthesis–tissue junction.[15] Alternatively, a reduction of the alveolar ridge can be considered, provided that sufficient bone height exists for implant placement.[16]

- Vertical dimension of occlusion: for the diagnostic set-up, the height of the lower face, ensuring harmony of the three thirds of the face, and an adequate interocclusal space for correct phonation, must be taken into account.
- Once the incisal edge position, crown length, and angulation have been determined, the relationship to the underlying soft and hard tissues is assessed for implant treatment planning (Figure 17.3c). In the dentate maxilla, lip support is primarily derived from the alveolar ridge shape and the cervical crown contour of the maxillary incisors, but in the edentulous maxilla, the alveolar ridge is frequently located posterior and cranially to the incisors. For an implant fixed dental prosthesis (implant FDP) with a porcelain-fused-to-metal design (PFM), the cervical aspect of the clinical crown should ideally end at the soft tissue level of the alveolar ridge (Table 17.1c, d). In this case, only minimal bone resorption and a limited interarch space with an optimal tooth–lip relationship is present. If a large vertical distance results between the ideally positioned artificial teeth and the underlying tissues, moderate to severe resorption of the maxilla may have occurred (Table 17.1c). Depending on this discrepancy in the bucco-oral dimension, the practitioner must assess if compensation is feasible with a gingival base of an implant FDP or with an implant fixed complete denture (IFCD) design, without causing oral hygiene constraints. If these requirements cannot be ensured, an implant overdenture (IOD) with a denture base is preferable, which also allows individual contouring on the palate to enable adequate tooth–tongue contact for T- and D-sounds, and to avoid any speech disruption and S-sound deficiencies (e.g., sigmatism, lisping). This is even more important in patients with a retrognathic appearance of the maxilla with a concave profile, or for compensation of prognathism (Table 17.1b, d; Figure 17.3e–h).[10]

Radiologic diagnosis and treatment planning

The panoramic radiograph provides a good two-dimensional overview of the anatomic structures and the available bone in the vertical dimension (Figure 17.1a). Due to the challenges related to the described resorption pattern in the maxilla and the need for implant positioning according to the planned prosthetic restoration, three-dimensional (3-D) imaging (e.g., cone beam computed tomography (CBCT) scan) is frequently indicated for thorough diagnostics. Attempts should be made to perform the 3-D imaging in conjunction with a scan of the diagnostic set-up (or the adequate existing denture) that allows identification of the tooth position, digital implant planning according to the clinical crown position, and subsequent transfer into a surgical template (Fig. 17.1d–g).[17] In former years, radiopaque markers (e.g., titanium pins) were incorporated into a template (Figure 17.5a), depicting the ideal implant position and angulation for a screw-retained fixed complete denture and were arranged parallel in a surveyor with a similar path of insertion (Figure 17.5b). The horizontal slices of the computed tomography were oriented perpendicular to these titanium pins and perpendicular cross-sectional reformations were processed, which served for the detailed implant planning and identification of augmentation needs (Figure 17.5c).[10] Today, selection of the implant length and diameter in an adequate position and angulation can be performed digitally with specialized software programs, and a surgical template is then printed and designed for support on the mucosa or the bone (Figure 17.1h–k).[18]

The transverse cross-sections from the 3-D radiographs are analyzed to determine if the available bone allows for implant placement at an ideal angulation.[19] For fixed implant restorations with a PFM design, it must be feasible to place implants meticulously with respect to the correct position and angulation for the prosthesis (Figure 17.6a–n). If any buccal concavities in the anterior are present notwithstanding grafting, the implant angulation may have to be altered to some degree, which means that the use of angulated or individualized abutments is inevitable. When an ideal selection of implant sites and positioning is not feasible, the PFM-design is ruled out and a IFCD design can be considered or, if clinical diagnosis indicates the need for facial support, an IOD should be recommended. In patients with more advanced bone resorption and larger vertical distances but no need for facial support, a screw-retained IFCD with a gingival base allows more flexibility with implants not exactly congruent with the clinical crown position (Figure 17.7a–e). Even with buccal screw access in a temporary, these can be covered using composite resin. When an IOD is planned, the space requirements of the preferred retention system (bar or single attachments) have to be taken into account when planning implant position and angulation (Figure 17.5d–k). In particular, a milled bar design allows more latitude in inter-implant distance (Table 17.1d).

Restoration design options and implant numbers

Implant fixed complete denture

In the early reports on maxillary implant prostheses, the established method for restoring the edentulous mandible was adopted for the edentulous maxilla.[20,21] Thus, screw-retained, implant fixed prostheses with cantilever pontics were installed, regardless of the degree of bone resorption that had occurred.[21] In patients with advanced or severe bone resorption, the large vertical distance associated with bone atrophy was dealt with by installing long standard abutments ("high water design"), but open interproximal spaces compromised esthetics and function. To avoid such a "high water design" or extended tooth lengths, gingiva-colored prosthetic material (porcelain, zirconium, or acrylics) can be used in contact with the alveolar ridge to compensate for the vertical discrepancy.[9] With this design of an implant fixed complete denture, the soft tissue

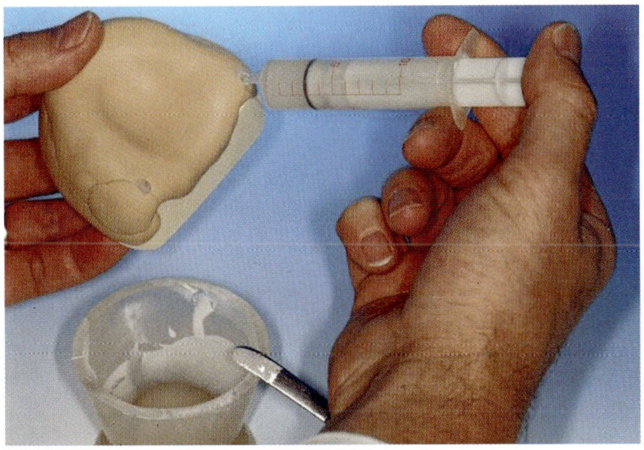

(a)

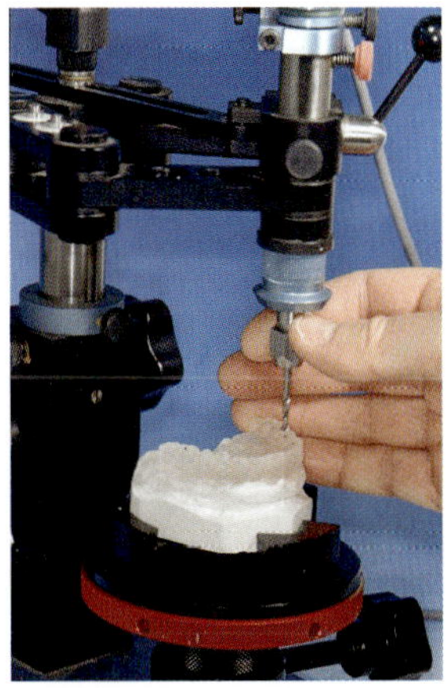

(b)

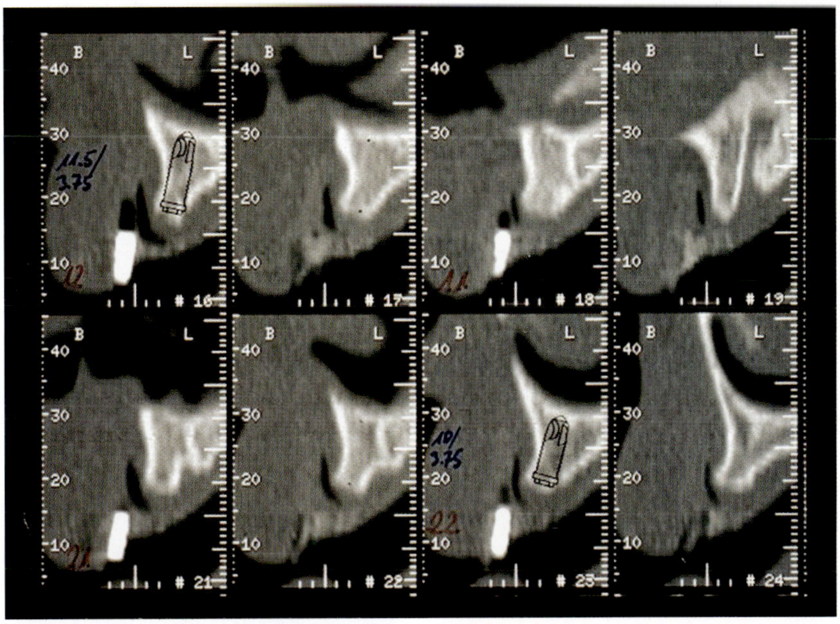

(c)

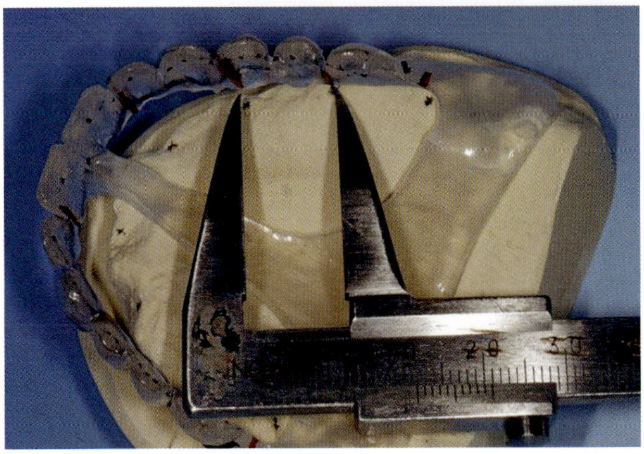

(d)

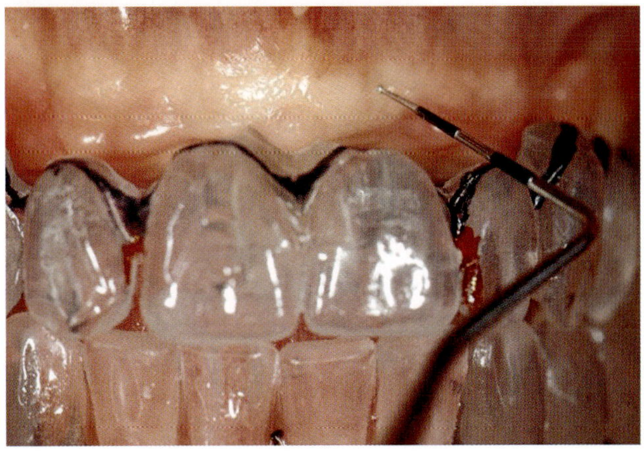

(e)

Figure 17.5 **(a)** Set-up keyed to produce a transparent template. **(b)** Template mounted in a surveyor to determine a similar path of insertion and to mill the holes for titanium markers. **(c)** Reformatted CT scan illustrates large discrepancy between ideal tooth position (indicated by titanium markers) and underlying maxillary bone. **(d)** Radiographic template modified for application during implant placement. **(e)** Template try-in illustrating discrepancy between alveolar ridge and diagnostic tooth position in the horizontal dimension. **(f)** IOD retention with casted gold bar with Bredent Vario soft elements. **(g)** IOD in place. **(h)** Anterior view with buccal flange. **(i)** Matrix exchange in the metal reinforcement. **(j)** Anterior view. **(k)** Side view. **(j)** and **(k)** illustrate adequate soft tissue support. (Technician: Fernando Pasamontes, Zug.)

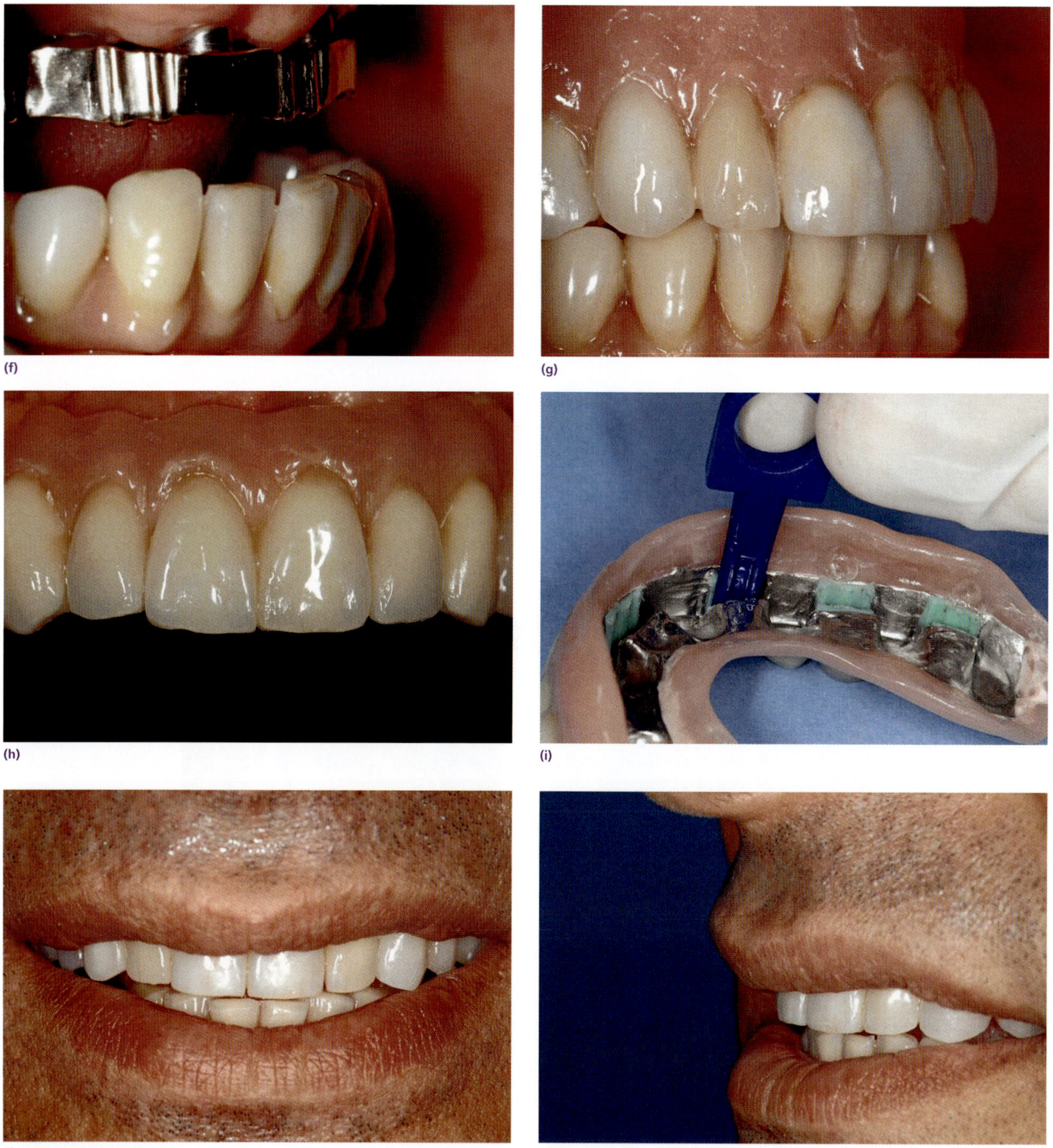

(f) (g) (h) (i) (j) (k)

Figure 17.5 (*Continued*)

contact area has to have a convex contour to allow for oral hygiene, while cleaning access to the abutments can be compromised (Table 17.1d, Figure 17.7a–e).

Porcelain-fused-to-metal implant fixed dental prostheses

With limited or moderate resorption of the alveolar ridge and establishment of average length of the clinical crowns (i.e., 10–11 mm in the anterior[3]), porcelain-fused-to-metal restorations (synonyms "metal ceramic", "implant fixed dental prosthesis", Table 17.1c, Figure 17.6) similar to those made to restore partially edentulous patients have been described in the literature.[15,22–25] To evaluate and optimize esthetics, biology, and function, a fixed provisional restoration should be inserted for a 3–6-month diagnostic period.[25] This temporary FDP is used to mold the tissue in the pontic area and to adjust inter-implant

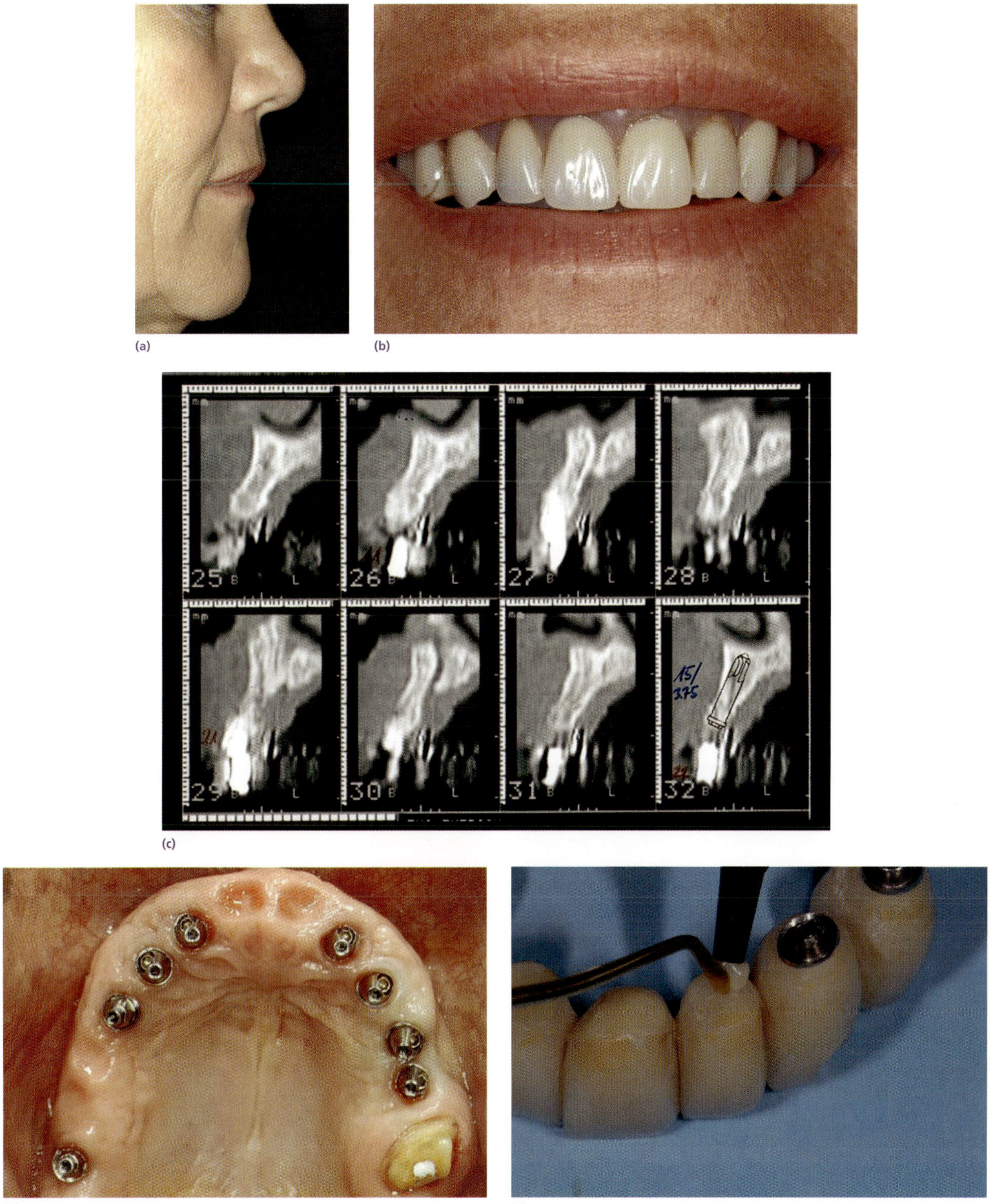

Figure 17.6 (a) Patient's profile with existing removable prosthesis in place showing excessive upper lip support. (b) Anterior view. (c) Reformatted CT scan illustrates close proximity between ideal tooth position (indicated by titanium markers) and underlying maxillary bone with limited bone resorption. (d) Eight implants provided with abutments for screw-retained implant-supported fixed dental prosthesis. (e) Modification of the temporary using composite filling material to mold the soft tissues in the pontic area. (f) Transfer of the ideal temporary situation using a mounted cast. (g) The temporary prosthesis screwed back on the master cast and keyed with silicon. (h) Framework try-in combined with occlusal check using laboratory-prepared stops. (i) Implant fixed dental prosthesis with PFM design (metal–ceramic). (j) Convex pontic contour in the area of the central incisors. (k) Clinical situation with closure of the screw access holes using a little cotton, white gutta percha, and composite filling material. (l, m) Anterior view. (n) Periapical radiographs. (Technician: Anna Sutter, Zürich.)

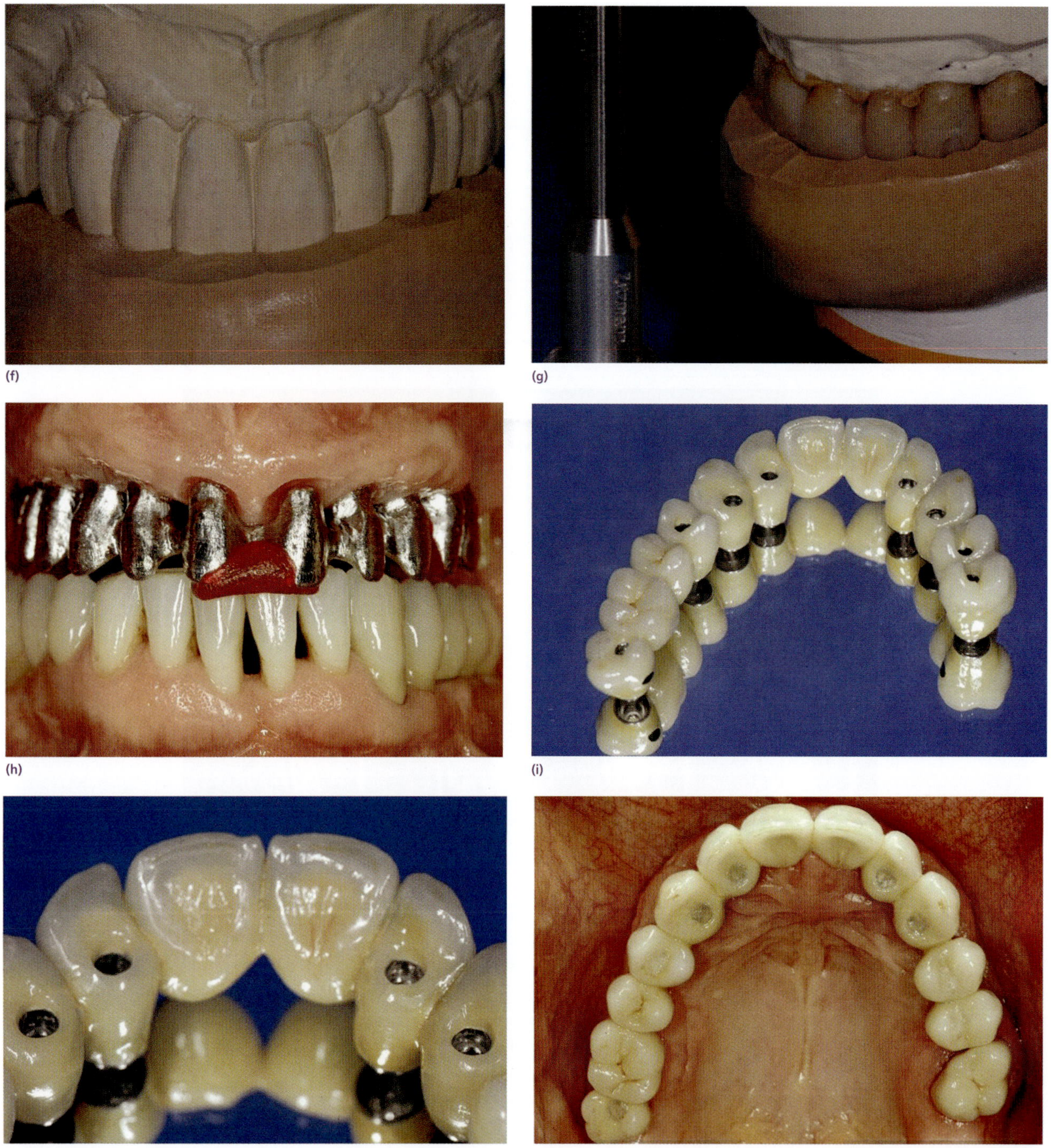

Figure 17.6 (*Continued*)

spaces according to phonetic and cleaning requirements; the ideal morphological contours are then duplicated into the final restoration (Figure 17.6e–g). Fixed implant-supported restorations can be further stratified according to the following parameters (Table 17.1d).[9,25]

- The mode of retention is either screw-retained or cemented. Both options offer a limited compensation of angulation by prefabricated or individualized angulated abutments. Screw retention facilitates retrieval and adaptation of the restoration in case of complications or renewal. Cementation of implant restorations is challenging, due to the risk of cement penetration in a submucosal position, in which the hardened rough cement surface acts as basis for biofilm adherence. Cementation has been found to be frequently associated with

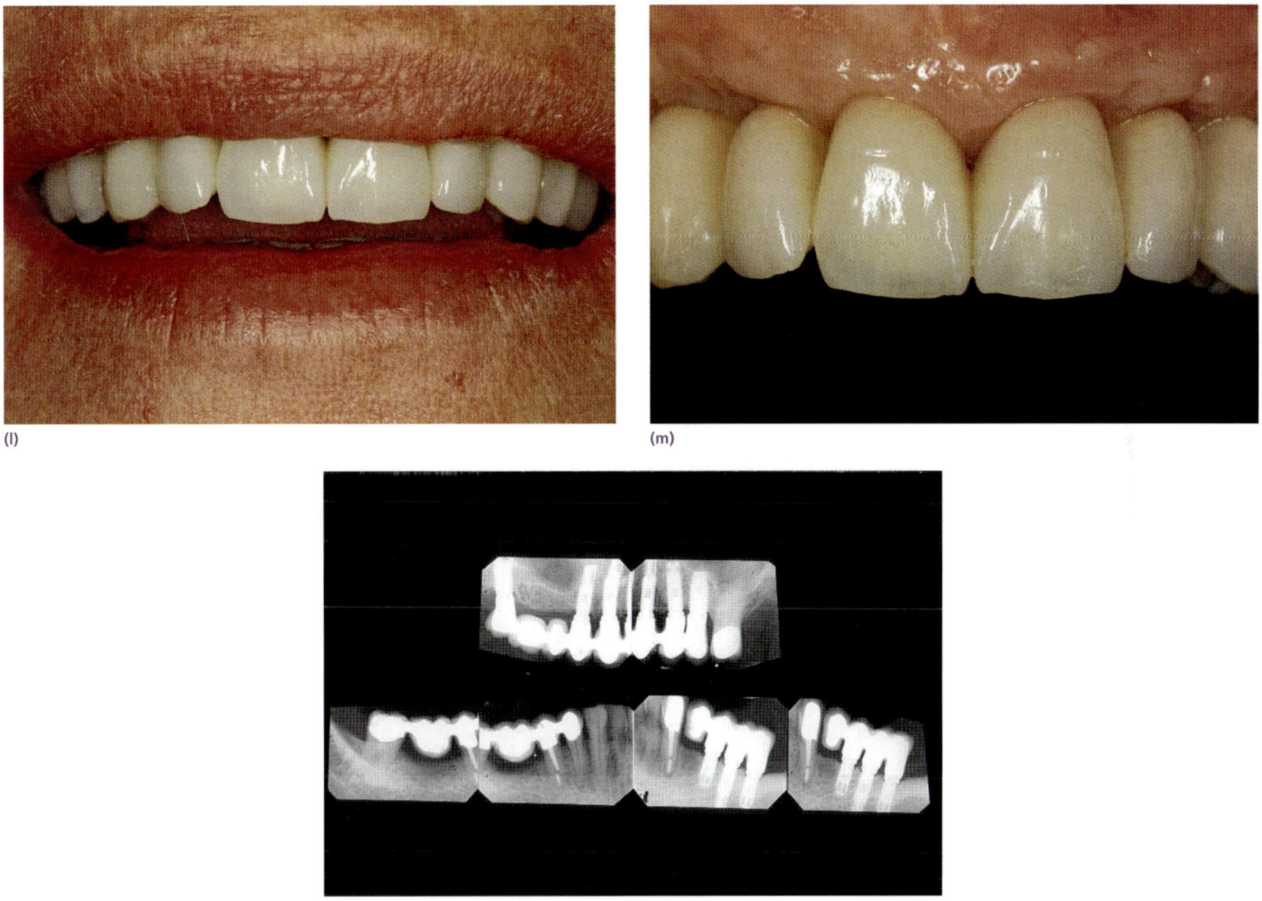

(l) (m) (n)

Figure 17.6 (*Continued*)

cement remnants and subsequent peri-implant disease.[26–28] To allow adequate removal of excess cement in the posterior region, individualized abutments are frequently required so crown margins are located at the mucosal margin.[29]

- The framework is designed in one piece or segmented, and both designs have demonstrated successful long-term results.[30] While casting a full-arch restoration in one piece is technically sensitive in achieving perfect fit, milling techniques in combination with copings luted into the framework facilitate a passive fit. Segmented restorations offer ease of casting and repair, but require strategic implant positioning according to the intended segmentation (e.g., anterior segment with implants in the lateral incisor position, and two posterior segments with implants in the canine and second premolar and/or molar region).
- Prosthetic material blend (metal, zirconium, porcelain, acrylic resin, composite resin) with monolithic design or veneering of the framework.
- Gingiva-colored prosthetic material (gingiva-colored porcelain, composite resin).

According to recent consensus statements, six or more implants were mainly used to retain a one-piece or a segmented maxillary implant-retained fixed prosthesis and the need for prosthetically-driven surgical planning was highlighted. For IFCDs with gingiva-colored prosthetic material, rehabilitation can also be provided with as few as four splinted implants, which are either equally spread in the anterior and posterior regions, or necessitate long posterior cantilevers.[31,32] Greater numbers of implants are frequently recommended to account for generalized cancellous bone in the maxilla, greater function or unbalanced loading (e.g., bruxers, dentate antagonist), and/or segmentation of the fixed dental prosthesis, and to reduce the risk of catastrophic prosthesis failure.[33] While good long-term data are available for survival of implants with moderately rough surfaces and 10 mm implant length placed in autogenous bone,[34,35] reduced success rates were reported when sinus elevation (lateral antrostomy) or vertical bone augmentation with autogenous bone grafts had been performed (3-year implant survival of 90%).[36] Further, adverse events in sinus grafting have been reported with perforation of the sinus membrane, graft infection and sinusitis, and graft loss, resulting in inability to place implants.[36,37] Depending on patient preferences and accounting for the additional burden of autogenous bone grafts used for augmentation procedures, particularly in medically

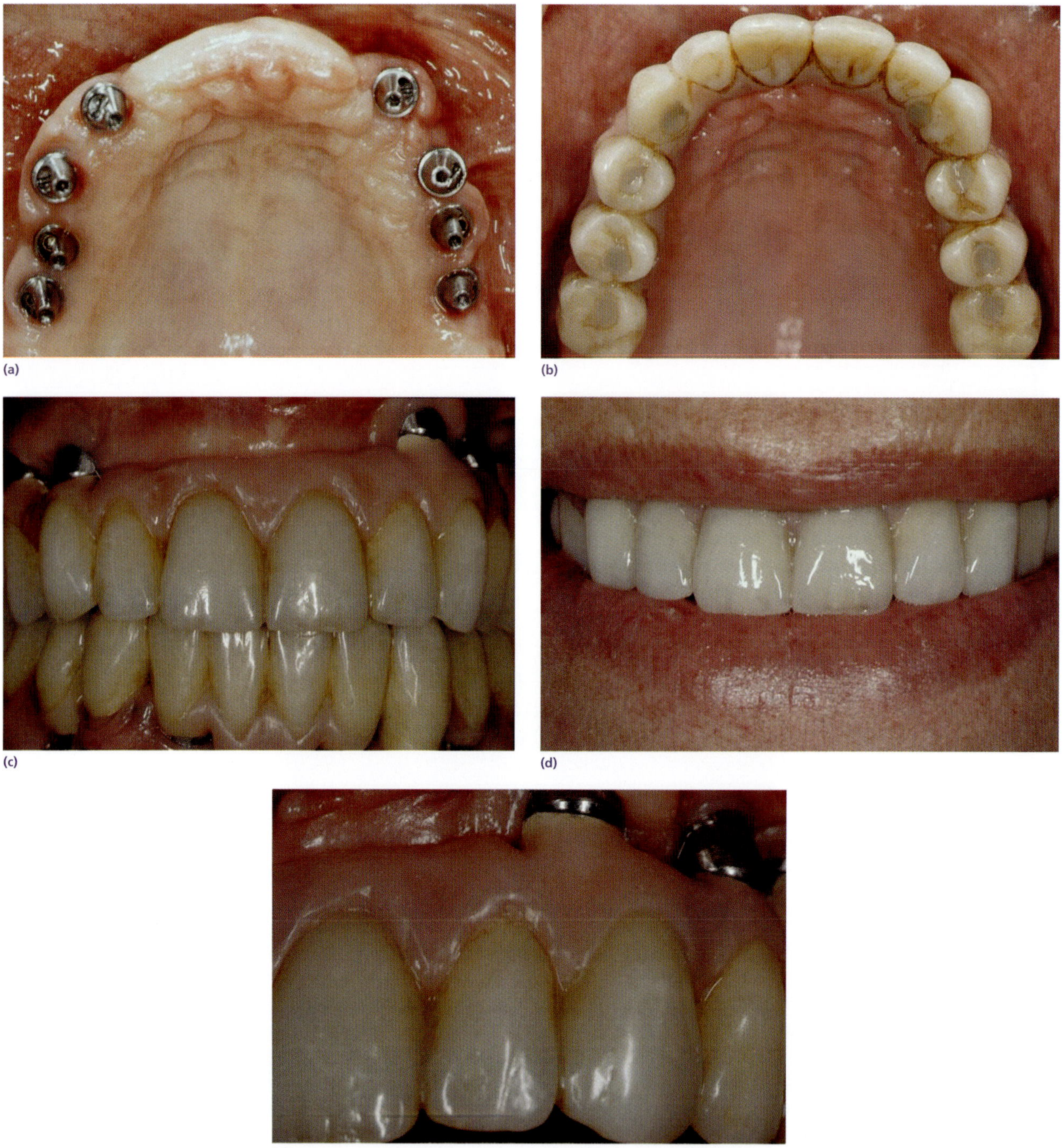

(a) (b) (c) (d) (e)

Figure 17.7 (a) Clinical situation with eight implants provided with angulated abutments. (b) Screw-retained implant fixed complete denture. (c) Denture designed with acrylic resin and gingiva compartment. (d) Anterior view. (e) Detailed view at 2-year follow-up.

compromised patients, efforts can be made to avoid alveolar ridge augmentation and/or lateral antrostomy by using short implants. According to a review, implants with moderately rough surfaces and 6 mm length, had a cumulative survival rate of 94.7% in the maxilla (versus 98.6% in the mandible, 1–8 years of observation), and failures occurred mainly during healing before prosthesis insertion.[38] Further attempts have been made to bypass the area of the maxillary sinus and to avoid long distal cantilevers by placing implants either in the zygomatic region, or along the anterior sinus wall in a tilted position with angulations varying between 30° and 75° in relation to the anterior implants. Such implant positioning with 2 distally inclined and 2 anterior axial implants (also described as "all-on four concept") has been used for immediately loaded maxillary restorations. Short-term (4–33 months) implant survival of 97% has been reported, with the majority of failing implants (78%) in a tilted position.[33] A meta-analysis including fixed maxillary and mandibular prostheses failed to support the hypothesis that tilted implants had more marginal bone loss or a higher incidence of biomechanical complications than straight implants.[39] However, complications have been reported to be more frequent when tilted implants are used for fixed implant prostheses; 37% of patients had esthetic problems, 42% had phonetic disturbances, while mucositis was found in 47% of the patients and related to the difficulties of maintaining good oral hygiene.[40] Further, the clinician must be aware that handling of prosthetic components is challenging and personal oral hygiene may be restricted with bulky contours and distally inclined implants and/or implants placed in the zygomatic or pterygoid region.[41]

Implant overdenture prosthesis

The use of implants in combination with removable prostheses was initially intended to improve denture stability, or applied as a rescue operation when the implant number was limited after early implant failures and fabricating a fixed restoration was no longer feasible.[15,22,42] Hence, the maxillary IOD was frequently selected in cases of severe bone resorption, allowing only short machined implant lengths in dominantly cancellous bone, offering minimal primary stability for implants with machined surfaces used in early studies.[7,15] Due to the fact that the maxillary IOD was often not planned at the outset of treatment but selected after implant failure, risk factors were potentiated, leading to higher implant failure rates and prosthetic complications. For instance, interarch space allowance, and inter-implant distances and angulations were frequently not considered, leading to material fatigue and inadequate bar clip length (Table 17.1c).[43] To keep costs low, ball attachments were connected to the implants and plastic matrices were fixed to the existing complete denture.[7] Today, the implant-supported overdenture prosthesis is well established as the treatment of choice for the atrophic maxilla.[41,44] Removable implant overdentures can be further stratified according to the following parameters:

- attachment system: single attachments or bar splint (bars can be provided with distal extension when implant position is restricted to the anterior region and especially in class II jaw relations, Table 17.1d);
- type of prosthesis support: depending on the implant number and distribution, the tuberosities and the hard palate (full or reduced palatal coverage) can be used for additional mucosal support;
- extension of the denture base: the buccal flange extension is determined during set-up try-in in relation to the smile line and the need for facial support; the contour and reduction of palatal coverage is adjusted according to phonetic requirements;
- prosthesis design and material: while a minimum of 10 mm intermaxillary space is required for most retentive systems, a metal reinforcement is recommended to avoid prosthesis fractures; limited spaces can be managed by designing the chromium–cobalt reinforcement with a metal backing to obviate an irregular bulge in the phonetic zone.[45]

According to a recent review, four to six implants were frequently applied in successful cohort studies, and placing a minimum of four implants with a wide anterior–posterior distribution (AP spread) was recommended for IODs.[43] A meta-analysis including studies with at least 1 year of observation, revealed a 98.2% survival rate per year for IODs with six implants and bar splinting, 96.3% for four implants with bar anchorage, and 95.2% for four implants with ball abutments.[46] It must be noted that the risk of implant loss increased when four or fewer implants with a non-splinted anchorage were applied.[47] Placing only two implants with a hinging prosthesis seems to be associated with a higher risk of implant failures.[41,44] For instance, for IODs with complete palatal coverage, Sanna *et al.* reported a 74% cumulative survival rate at 16 years with two implants and ball abutments, while two implants splinted with a bar had 100% survival at 16 years.[48]

Prefabricated or individualized bar designs offer the opportunity to correct divergent implant angulations, to splint the implants, and to provide a distinct path of insertion that facilitates simple and competent prosthesis insertion and retrieval by the patient without assistance. Bar-retained superstructures should be constructed with a metal reinforcement, and are generally more expensive due to the dental technician's work. With prefabricated round Dolder bars (Cendres & Métaux, Biel, Switzerland), maintenance with activation of metal bar clips or exchange of acrylic bar clips (Galak, Cendres & Métaux) is easily conducted when a metal housing is used (Figure 17.1m,n). Care must be taken that the bar design allows oral hygiene performance around the abutments, since increased soft tissue inflammation has been reported under bars.[43] For a bar-retained overdenture prosthesis, using prefabricated systems (e.g. Dolder; Hader, Lifecore Biomedical Inc., Chaska, Minn., or Vario Soft, Bredent, Senden, Germany), distances of 10–14 mm from implant center to center are required and every second tooth position can be selected to allow the clips in between adjacent abutments to be arranged suitably (Table 17.1). However, if implant placement is restricted to particular areas, due to advanced bone resorption, and adjacent tooth positions have to be selected as implant positions, then an individually milled bar (with 2° taper) should be planned (Figure 17.8a–d). In these cases, the inter-implant distance and angulation are less critical because retention is derived from the frictional fit of the implant-borne superstructure. For additional retention security, frictional pins or attachments (e.g., CEKA, Antwerp, Belgium) can be incorporated into the bar, or swivel latches included in the IOD.[25] While single attachments (e.g., balls, locators) offer some degree of compensation for non-aligned implants, there is a risk of shear forces when patients pull more strongly on one side, and maintenance problems from attachment wear may be higher for solitary attachments.[41,43] A similar path of insertion is provided by telescopes, but these individualized abutments result in higher costs and possibly higher prosthodontic maintenance compared to bar and locator attachments.[41,49]

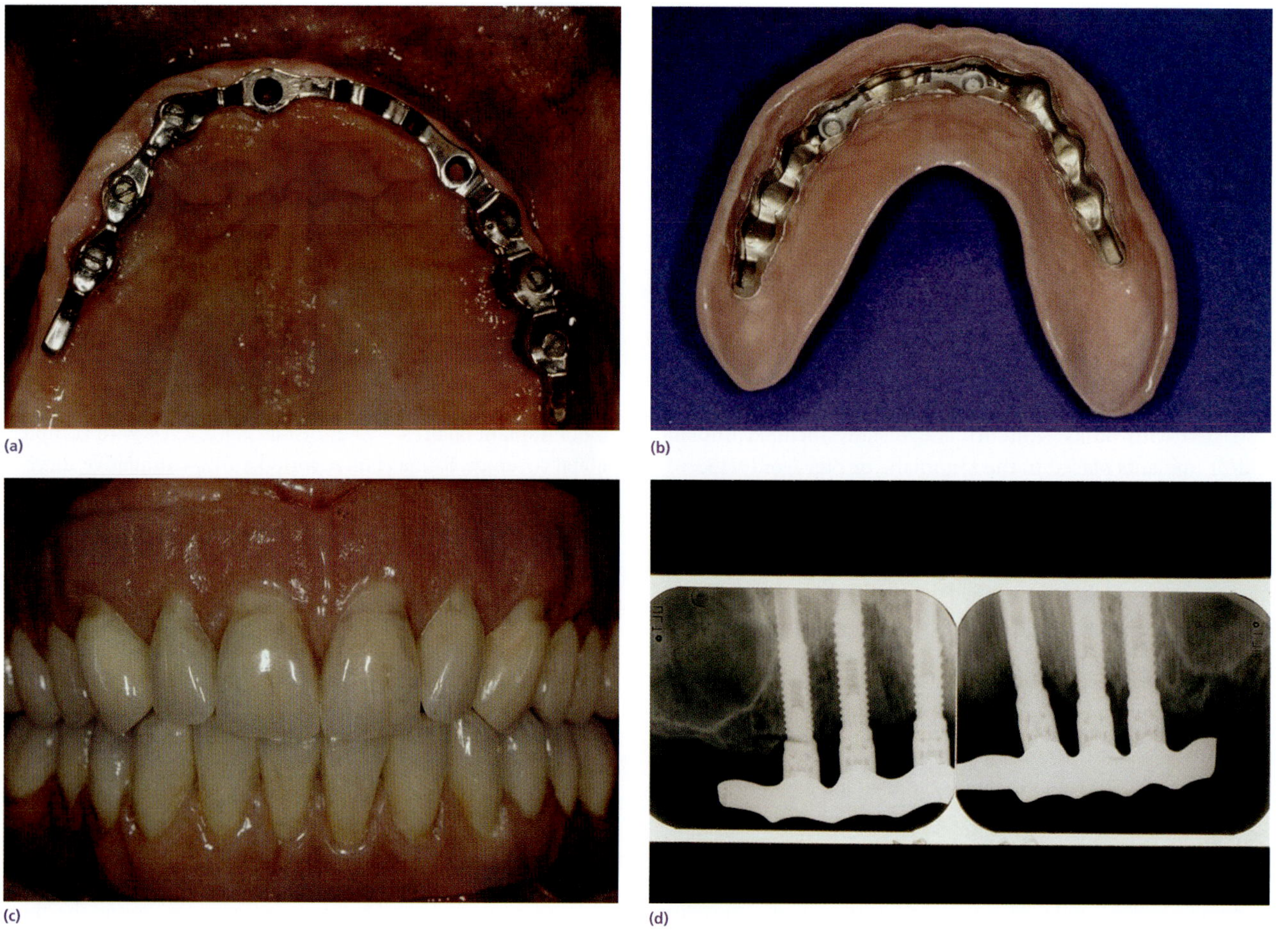

Figure 17.8 (a) Clinical situation of an individually milled bar with 2° taper. (b) IOD with gold overcast. (c) Anterior view. (d) Periapical radiographs. (Technician: Densart Urs Rohner, Wil St. Gallen.)

Maintenance for fixed and removable restorations

To prevent complications and failures of implants and restorations, the clinical examination includes the peri-implant soft tissues, by assessing probing pocket depth and bleeding on probing, and the superstructure, and should be performed once a year, while professional supportive care should be provided according to the individual needs of the patient (e.g. 3-, 6- or 12-month recall intervals).[29] Baseline data should be recorded approximately 2 weeks following prosthesis insertion to enable patient's functional adaptation in phonetics and mastication, and to allow for peri-implant soft tissue healing. Besides the clinical parameters, the baseline examination includes radiographs to provide reference measures. Examination of the fixed or removable superstructure generally includes assessment of the retention and stability, occlusion, and function (and possible adjustments of premature contacts). While retention of fixed restorations is assessed bimanually, IODs are removed and replaced and matrices activated, if required. Further, any wear or fracture of the veneering material, fracture of the framework or any implant component, are recorded and adjusted or repaired. With removable restorations the prosthesis-bearing mucosal tissues are thoroughly examined in order to avoid pressure spots or food impaction.

For fixed implant restorations the most common technical complications are loosening or fracture of the abutment screws or the retaining screws (in screw-retained prostheses), loss of retention (in cemented prostheses), loss of cover of the access hole (in screw-retained prostheses), and chipping or fracture of the veneering material (PFM design), while fracture of the abutment or the framework are less frequent. For the IFCD design applying metal–acrylic, prosthesis tooth wear has been observed as a frequent complication (besides fractured screws and abutments), which occurred after several years of prosthesis function (mean 14 years) and usually required more than two visits to address.[50] Two reviews investigated the long-term complication rates of screw-retained and cemented restorations and found that among maxillary full-arch restorations the vast majority was screw-retained.[27,51] While overall (irrespective of the indication in partially or edentulous jaws) screw-retained FDPs revealed a higher risk for porcelain chipping, this could not be confirmed specifically for full-arch FDPs, and there was a trend towards less total technical complications with screw-retained reconstructions compared to the cemented ones.[27,51] Among the biological complications, the presence of fistula/suppuration

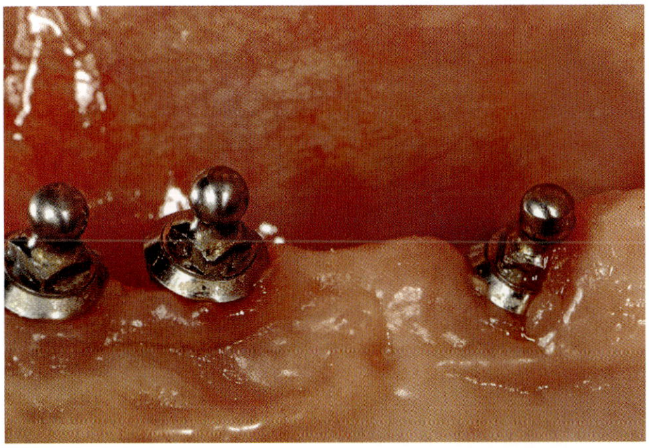

(a)

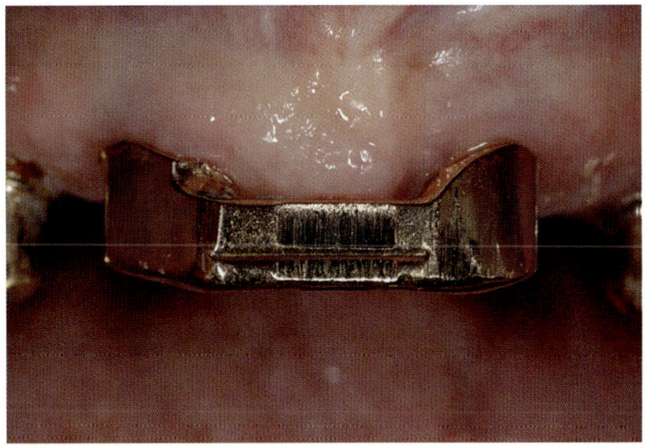

(b)

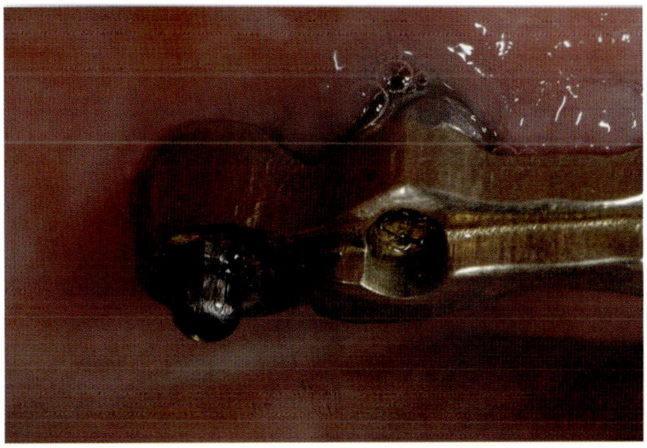

(c)

Figure 17.9 (a) Signs of wear of ball abutments on implants with non-parallel angulation, hyperplasia around posterior tissue-level implant. (b) Wear of individually milled bar with a Bredent element. (c) Wear of individually milled bar and an additional Ceka attachment.

and bone loss (as a sign of peri-implantitis) occurred significantly more often at cemented than at screw-retained restorations, and were possibly related to excess cement.[27,51] Due to the advantages of retrievability to handle biological and technical complications, screw-retained restorations were recommended, in particular, for full-arch FDPs.[31]

For removable overdenture prostheses the most common technical complication is loss of prosthesis retention, which is either related to wear of the matrices within the IOD or results from wear of the retention elements (e.g., balls, bar profile; Figure 17.9). Particularly during the first examination just after prosthesis insertion, the extension of the prosthesis flange is assessed and adjusted if required, and any pressure spots resulting from an incongruence of the prosthesis base fit or from occlusal interference are dealt with. During maintenance, abutment screw or retention screw loosening or fracture, and chipping or fracture of the denture teeth or the denture material are less frequent complications. While the milled bar design demonstrated low maintenance,[52] maintenance efforts and marginal bone loss seem to be generally higher for solitary attachments, particularly when implant angulation is not parallel.[43,53,54] It has been emphasized that an intimate extension base contact with the edentulous residual ridge is essential to minimize stress to the terminal retention unit.[41] Comparing patient groups restored with maxillary fixed and removable implant prostheses, similar maintenance efforts were documented with mean time-until-retreatment of 23 (PFM) and 20 months (IOD). The majority of mechanical complications could be managed chairside during recall visits and did not require additional appointments.[55]

Patient factors and patient-reported outcome measurements

In the mandible, insufficient prosthesis retention and function is the dominant stimulus for patients requesting implant treatment,[56] but in the maxilla, impaired self-esteem is the major motivation for many patients trying to avoid removable appliances, and a perception that missing teeth are recognizable from the outside (Table 17.1a).[57] Further indications for implant restorations are anatomic morphological limitations precluding adequate stability and retention of a CD, including hyposalivation, patient intolerance for palatal coverage, and treatment of refractory gagging.[11,58] It must be noted, however, that the great majority of edentulous patients are adequately restored with maxillary complete dentures and that, in cases of insufficient denture retention, efforts for conventional improvement should be made first to meet patients' expectations.[59,60]

In a recent review, 20 publications were identified reporting patient- and clinician-based data following implant treatment in the maxilla.[43] Among the studies documenting patient-reported outcome measurements (PROMs) before and after implant treatment, there was a clear indication of improvements, particularly in self-esteem, with both fixed and removable implant restorations in comparison to the previous conventional removable prosthesis.[43,57,61–63] Studies comparing fixed and removable implant restorations, in within-subject crossover trials,[64] in self-selected,[57] or in clinician-selected trials,[48,62] indicated that, particularly in patients with more severe alveolar ridge resorption, the ability to speak and ease of cleaning may be restricted with fixed restorations, and subsequently determine personal preferences for IODs. There was a trend to better ratings for retention and fit with fixed than with removable restorations, while food impaction affected both groups.[48] Comparisons on different retentive systems (bar-splint or unsplinted ball attachments) of maxillary IOD did generally not reveal differences in patients' satisfaction, but more difficulty in hygiene with a bar.[54,61] Comparing full and reduced palatal coverage of maxillary IOD, there was a trend to preference of a reduced design over a complete palatal coverage, mainly due to a better perception of taste.[61,65–67]

In implant treatment, financial estimates are related to the number of implants and the materials selected for the implant restoration, giving highest costs when the laboratory work involves porcelain-fused-to-metal implant FDPs, while a simple complete denture converted into an implant overdenture offers minimal costs.[55] Further patient-mediated factors possibly limiting implant placement are the need for adjunctive procedures (e.g., bone augmentation), which increase the risks, aftercare burden, treatment time, and morbidity (Table 17.1a). According to a recent questionnaire among patients seeking implant treatment, only 61% would accept autologous bone grafts (mainly favoring the retromolar area), while only 23% were willing to undergo grafting from the iliac crest. The majority (88%) was not willing to accept an increased risk of implant failure to shorten the total treatment duration.[68] In general, esthetic and phonetic requirements as well as hygiene access considering patient's individual dexterity for personal oral hygiene, may influence the implant treatment considerations. While most patients initially demand a fixed implant restoration[57], it is the practitioner's obligation to conduct thorough diagnostics to provide the patient with an adequate recommendation for the indicated prosthesis design. For some patients, the maxillary IOD is most appropriate because it provides facial scaffolding, covers the prosthesis-tissue junction particularly in patients with a wide smile and/or high smile line, assists in reconciling adverse ridge relations or discrepancies, and allows more latitude in adjusting palatal contour for adequate phonation.[69,70]

Summary

In order to address the exacting functional and esthetic demands of rehabilitating the edentulous maxilla with implant-borne prostheses, the practitioner should follow clinical decision-making and systematically analyze extra- and intraoral factors. A thorough initial diagnosis with an adequate complete denture or a new set-up is required and used for 3-D radiographic visualization of the relationship between the anterior incisor position and the underlying soft and hard tissues. The crucial factors in deciding, whether a fixed or removable prosthesis is indicated, are related to osseous and/or soft tissue deficiencies, the need for facial and lip support, speech disruption, esthetic problems, and/or the patient's willingness to undergo additional surgical procedures. If bone and soft tissue deficiencies cannot be compensated for, a removable implant overdenture (IOD) is the most desirable solution, which allows extending the buccal flange according to the need for facial support as well as covering the prosthesis–tissue junction, and adjusting the palatal coverage according to the phonetic requirements. In addition to the objective clinical indicators, practitioners should provide the option of a maxillary IOD, particularly to those patients who are unable to adapt to maxillary complete denture use (psychological or physiological), who have a desire for, or will benefit from, greater denture stability, and/or who cannot afford the expense of implant fixed prosthesis. According to the literature, four to six implants are successfully applied for IOD, and placing a minimum of four implants with a wide anterior–posterior distribution (AP spread) is recommended. Placing only two implants with a hinging prosthesis seems to be associated with a higher risk of implant failures.

While single attachments are less costly and easier to clean, prefabricated or individualized bar designs offer the opportunity to correct divergent implant angulations, to splint the implants, and to provide a distinct path of insertion that facilitates simple prosthesis insertion and retrieval by the patient.

If a fixed implant prosthesis with a PFM design is feasible in patients with minimal resorption and limited intermaxillary space, six to eight implants should be placed meticulously in the intended tooth position. The prosthesis may be constructed using cement retention or screw retention. The latter offers retrievability and easier adaptation of the restoration in case of complications. Cementation of implant restorations is challenging due to the risk of cement remnants, and crown margins positioned at the mucosal margin are recommended to ensure accessability for cement removal. With more advanced resorption and increased intermaxillary space, fixed restorations can be designed as IFCD prostheses with gingiva-colored prosthetic material and as few as four splinted implants. Provided that the clinical indicators for fixed implant restorations are met, the practitioner may provide a PFM or an IFCD design to patients who are unable to adapt to a removable prosthesis (psychological or physiological), have a desire for or will benefit from a fixed solution, and who can afford the expense of acquiring an implant-supported fixed prosthesis, along with maintaining it for their lifetime.

Any decision to proceed with maxillary implant-retained fixed or removable prosthesis should be a joint decision made by the surgeon, the restorative dentist and the informed patient, who understands the possible difficulties and limitations related to implant treatment in the edentulous maxilla.

References

1. Dye BA, Tan S, Smith V, *et al.* Trends in oral health status: United States, 1988–1994 and 1999–2004. *Vital Health Stat 11* 2007; **248**: 1–92.
2. Wu B, Liang J, Plassman BL, *et al.* Oral health among white, black, and Mexican-American elders: an examination of edentulism and dental caries. *J Public Health Dent* 2011; **71**(4): 308–317.
3. Nelson SJ. Introduction to dental anatomy. In: *Wheeler's Dental Anatomy, Physiology and Occlusion*, 10th edn. Philadelphia: Elsevier 2014; Chapter 1.
4. Atwood DA. Bone loss of edentulous alveolar ridges. *J Periodontol* 1979; **50**(4 Spec No): 11–21.
5. Desjardins RP. Prosthesis design for osseointegrated implants in the edentulous maxilla. *Int J Oral Maxillofac Implants* 1992; **7**(3): 311–320.
6. Parel SM. Implants and overdentures: the osseointegrated approach with conventional and compromised applications. *Int J Oral Maxillofac Implants* 1986; **1**(2): 93–99.
7. Smedberg JI, Lothigius E, Nilner K, *et al.* A new design for a hybrid prosthesis supported by osseointegrated implants: 2. Preliminary clinical aspects. *Int J Oral Maxillofac Implants* 1991; **6**(2): 154–159.
8. AbuJamra NF, Stavridakis MM, Miller RB. Evaluation of interarch space for implant restorations in edentulous patients: a laboratory technique. *J Prosthodont* 2000; **9**(2): 102–105.
9. Bidra AS. Three-dimensional esthetic analysis in treatment planning for implant-supported fixed prosthesis in the edentulous maxilla: review of the esthetics literature. *J Esthetic Restorative Dent* 2011; **23**(4): 219–236.
10. Zitzmann NU, Marinello CP. Treatment plan for restoring the edentulous maxilla with implant-supported restorations: removable overdenture versus fixed partial denture design. *J Prosthet Dent* 1999; **82**(2): 188–196.
11. Sadowsky SJ, Fitzpatrick B, Curtis DA. Evidence-based criteria for differential treatment planning of implant restorations for the maxillary edentulous patient. *J Prosthodont* 2015; **24**(6): 433–446.
12. Vig RG, Brundo GC. The kinetics of anterior tooth display. *J Prosthet Dent* 1978; **39**(5): 502–504.
13. Mecall RA, Rosenfeld AL. Influence of residual ridge resorption patterns on fixture placement and tooth position. Part III: Presurgical assessment of ridge augmentation requirements. *Int J Periodontics Restorative Dent* 1996; **16**(4): 322–337.
14. Tjan AH, Miller GD, The JG. Some esthetic factors in a smile. *J Prosthet Dent* 1984; **51**(1): 24–28.
15. Taylor TD. Fixed implant rehabilitation for the edentulous maxilla. *Int J Oral Maxillofac Implants* 1991; **6**(3): 329–337.
16. Bidra AS, Agar JR. A classification system of patients for esthetic fixed implant-supported prostheses in the edentulous maxilla. *Comp Cont Educ Dent* 2010; **31**(5): 366–374.
17. Schwarz MS, Rothmann SL, Rhodes ML, *et al.* Computed tomography. Part II. Preoperative assessment of the maxilla for endosseous implant surgery. *Int J Oral Maxillofac Implants* 1987; **2**: 143–148.
18. Kühl S, Payer M, Zitzmann NU, *et al.* Technical accuracy of printed surgical templates for guided implant surgery with the coDiagnostiX software. *Clin Implant Dent Relat Res* 2015; **17**(Suppl1): e177–182.
19. Zitzmann NU, Schärer P. *Oral Rehabilitation with Dental Implants. A Clinical Compendium*, 1st edn. Zürich: KBM 1997; 128.
20. Lewis S, Sharma A, Nishimura R. Treatment of edentulous maxillae with osseointegrated implants. *J Prosthet Dent* 1992; **68**(3): 503–508.
21. Zitzmann NU, Marinello CP. Fixed or removable implant-supported restorations in the edentulous maxilla: literature review. *Pract Periodontics Aesthet Dent* 2000; **12**(6): 599–608.
22. DeBoer J. Edentulous implants: overdenture versus fixed. *J Prosthet Dent* 1993; **69**(4): 386–390.
23. Sadowsky SJ. The implant-supported prosthesis for the edentulous arch: design considerations. *J Prosthet Dent* 1997; **78**(1): 28–33.
24. Wicks RA. A systematic approach to definitive planning for osseointegrated implant prostheses. *J Prosthodont* 1994; **3**(4): 237–242.
25. Zitzmann NU, Marinello CP. Clinical and technical aspects of implant-supported restorations in the edentulous maxilla: the fixed partial denture design. *Int J Prosthodont* 1999; **12**(4): 307–312.
26. De la Rosa M, Rodriguez A, Sierra K, *et al.* Predictors of peri-implant bone loss during long-term maintenance of patients treated with 10-mm implants and single crown restorations. *Int J Oral Maxillofac Implants* 2013; **28**(3): 798–802.
27. Sailer I, Mühlemann S, Zwahlen M, *et al.* Cemented and screw-retained implant reconstructions: a systematic review of the survival and complication rates. *Clin Oral Implants Res* 2012; **23**(Suppl6): 163–201.
28. Wilson TG, Jr. The positive relationship between excess cement and peri-implant disease: a prospective clinical endoscopic study. *J Periodontol* 2009; **80**(9): 1388–1392.
29. Jepsen S, Berglundh T, Genco R, *et al.* Primary prevention of peri-implantitis: managing peri-implant mucositis. *J Clin Periodontol* 2015; **42**(Suppl16): S152–157.
30. Lambert FE, Weber HP, Susarla SM, *et al.* Descriptive analysis of implant and prosthodontic survival rates with fixed implant-supported rehabilitations in the edentulous maxilla. *J Periodontol* 2009; **80**(8): 1220–1230.
31. Gotfredsen K, Wiskott A, Working Group. Consensus report – reconstructions on implants. The Third EAO Consensus Conference 2012. *Clin Oral Implants Res* 2012; **23**(Suppl 6): 238–241.
32. Heydecke G, Zwahlen M, Nicol A, *et al.* What is the optimal number of implants for fixed reconstructions: a systematic review. *Clin Oral Implants Res* 2012; **23**(Suppl6): 217–228.
33. Parel SM, Phillips WR. A risk assessment treatment planning protocol for the four implant immediately loaded maxilla: preliminary findings. *J Prosthet Dent* 2011; **106**(6): 359–366.
34. Att W, Bernhart J, Strub JR. Fixed rehabilitation of the edentulous maxilla: possibilities and clinical outcome. *J Oral Maxillofac Surg* 2009; **67**(11Suppl): 60–73.
35. Kotsovilis S, Fourmousis I, Karoussis IK, *et al.* A systematic review and meta-analysis on the effect of implant length on the survival of rough-surface dental implants. *J Periodontol* 2009; **80**(11): 1700–1718.
36. Tonetti MS, Hammerle CH, European Workshop on Periodontology Group C. Advances in bone augmentation to enable dental implant placement: Consensus Report of the Sixth European Workshop on Periodontology. *J Clin Periodontol* 2008; **35**(8Suppl): 168–172.
37. Chiapasco M, Casentini P, Zaniboni M. Bone augmentation procedures in implant dentistry. *Int J Oral Maxillofac Implants* 2009; **24**(Suppl): 237–259.

38. Srinivasan M, Vazquez L, Rieder P, *et al.* Survival rates of short (6 mm) micro-rough surface implants: a review of literature and meta-analysis. *Clin Oral Implants Res* 2014; **25**(5): 539–545.
39. Monje A, Chan HL, Suarez F, *et al.* Marginal bone loss around tilted implants in comparison to straight implants: a meta-analysis. *Int J Oral Maxillofac Implants* 2012; **27**(6): 1576–1583.
40. Rosen A, Gynther G. Implant treatment without bone grafting in edentulous severely resorbed maxillas: a long-term follow-up study. *J Oral Maxillofac Surg* 2007; **65**(5): 1010–1016.
41. Sadowsky SJ. Treatment considerations for maxillary implant overdentures: a systematic review. *J Prosthet Dent* 2007; **97**(6): 340–348.
42. Ricketts RM. Esthetics, environment, and the law of lip relation. *Am J Orthod* 1968; **54**(4): 272–289.
43. Sadowsky SJ, Zitzmann NU. Protocols for the maxillary implant overdenture. *Int J Maxillofacial Implants* 2015; submitted.
44. Chan MF, Narhi TO, de Baat C, *et al.* Treatment of the atrophic edentulous maxilla with implant-supported overdentures: a review of the literature. *Int J Prosthodont* 1998; **11**(1): 7–15.
45. Zitzmann NU, Marinello CP. Implant-supported removable overdentures in the edentulous maxilla: clinical and technical aspects. *Int J Prosthodont* 1999; **12**(5): 385–390.
46. Slot W, Raghoebar GM, Vissink A, *et al.* A systematic review of implant-supported maxillary overdentures after a mean observation period of at least 1 year. *J Clin Periodontol* 2010; **37**(1): 98–110.
47. Raghoebar GM, Meijer HJ, Slot W, *et al.* A systematic review of implant-supported overdentures in the edentulous maxilla, compared to the mandible: how many implants? *Eur J Oral Implantol* 2014; **7**(2): 191–201.
48. Sanna A, Nuytens P, Naert I, *et al.* Successful outcome of splinted implants supporting a 'planned' maxillary overdenture: a retrospective evaluation and comparison with fixed full dental prostheses. *Clin Oral Implants Res* 2009; **20**(4): 406–413.
49. Zou D, Wu Y, Huang W, *et al.* A 3-year prospective clinical study of telescopic crown, bar, and locator attachments for removable four implant-supported maxillary overdentures. *Int J Prosthodont* 2013; **26**(6): 566–573.
50. Dhima M, Paulusova V, Lohse C, *et al.* Practice-based evidence from 29-year outcome analysis of management of the edentulous jaw using osseointegrated dental implants. *J Prosthodont* 2014; **23**(3): 173–181.
51. Wittneben JG, Millen C, Bragger U. Clinical performance of screw- versus cement-retained fixed implant-supported reconstructions – a systematic review. *Int J Oral Maxillofac Implants* 2014; **29**(Suppl): 84–98.
52. Krennmair G, Krainhofner M, Piehslinger E. Implant-supported maxillary overdentures retained with milled bars: maxillary anterior versus maxillary posterior concept – a retrospective study. *Int J Oral Maxillofac Implants* 2008; **23**(2): 343–352.
53. Ekfeldt A, Johansson LA, Isaksson S. Implant-supported overdenture therapy: a retrospective study. *Int J Prosthodont* 1997; **10**(4): 366–374.
54. Narhi TO, Hevinga M, Voorsmit RA, *et al.* Maxillary overdentures retained by splinted and unsplinted implants: a retrospective study. *Int J Oral Maxillofac Implants* 2001; **16**(2): 259–266.
55. Zitzmann NU, Marinello CP. Treatment outcomes of fixed or removable implant-supported prostheses in the edentulous maxilla. Part II: clinical findings. *J Prosthet Dent* 2000; **83**(4): 434–442.
56. Zitzmann NU, Marinello CP. [Survey of treatment-seeking complete denture wearers concerning tooth loss, retention behavior and treatment expectations]. *Schweiz Monatsschr Zahnmed* 2006; **116**(3): 229–236.
57. Zitzmann NU, Marinello CP. Treatment outcomes of fixed or removable implant-supported prostheses in the edentulous maxilla. Part I: patients' assessments. *J Prosthet Dent* 2000; **83**(4): 424–33.
58. Visser A, Raghoebar GM, Meijer HJ, *et al.* Implant-retained maxillary overdentures on milled bar suprastructures: a 10-year follow-up of surgical and prosthetic care and aftercare. *Int J Prosthodont* 2009; **22**(2): 181–192.
59. Allen PF, McMillan AS, Walshaw D. Patient expectations of oral implant-retained prostheses in a UK dental hospital. *Br Dent J* 1999; **186**(2): 80–84.
60. Thalji G, McGraw K, Cooper LF, *et al.* Maxillary Complete Denture Outcomes. A systematic review of patient-based outcomes. *Int J Maxillofacial Implants* 2015; submitted.
61. Al-Zubeidi MI, Alsabeeha NH, Thomson WM, Payne AG. Patient satisfaction with maxillary 3-implant overdentures using different attachment systems opposing mandibular 2-implant overdentures. *Clin Implant Dent Relat Res* 2012; **14**(Suppl1):e11–19.
62. Kronstrom M, Widbom C, Soderfeldt B. Patient evaluation after treatment with maxillary implant-supported overdentures. *Clin Implant Dent Relat Res* 2006; **8**(1): 39–43.
63. Naert I, Gizani S, van Steenberghe D. Rigidly splinted implants in the resorbed maxilla to retain a hinging overdenture: a series of clinical reports for up to 4 years. *J Prosthet Dent* 1998; **79**(2): 156–164.
64. Heydecke G, Boudrias P, Awad MA, *et al.* Within-subject comparisons of maxillary fixed and removable implant prostheses: Patient satisfaction and choice of prosthesis. *Clin Oral Implants Res* 2003; **14**(1): 125–130.
65. de Albuquerque RF Jr, Lund JP, Tang L, *et al.* Within-subject comparison of maxillary long-bar implant-retained prostheses with and without palatal coverage: patient-based outcomes. *Clin Oral Implants Res* 2000; **11**(6): 555–565.
66. Zembic A, Tahmaseb A, Wismeijer D. Within-subject comparison of maxillary implant-supported overdentures with and without palatal coverage. *Clin Implant Dent Relat Res* 2015; **17**(3): 570–579.
67. Zembic A, Wismeijer D. Patient-reported outcomes of maxillary implant-supported overdentures compared with conventional dentures. *Clin Oral Implants Res* 2014; **25**(4): 441–450.
68. Hof M, Tepper G, Semo B, *et al.* Patients' perspectives on dental implant and bone graft surgery: questionnaire-based interview survey. *Clin Oral Implants Res* 2014; **25**(1): 42–45.
69. de Bruyn H, Collaert B, Linden U, *et al.* Patient's opinion and treatment outcome of fixed rehabilitation on Brånemark implants. A 3-year follow-up study in private dental practices. *Clin Oral Implants Res* 1997; **8**(4): 265–271.
70. Lundqvist S, Carlsson GE. Maxillary fixed prostheses on osseointegrated dental implants. *J Prosthet Dent* 1983; **50**(2): 262–270.

CHAPTER 18

Implant Restoration of the Mandibular Edentulous Patient

Steven J. Sadowsky
University of the Pacific Arthur A. Dugoni School of Dentistry, San Francisco, California, USA

In 2009, the British Society for the Study of Prosthetic Dentistry met in York, UK to follow up the McGill Consensus of 2002 on the most appropriate restoration of the edentulous mandible.[1,2] The York statement concluded that there is a substantial body of evidence of high rigor with patient-centered outcomes to demonstrate that the two-implant overdenture, while not the gold standard of implant therapy, is the minimum prosthetic modality that should be rendered to this class of patients. This statement, in conjunction with Fitzpatrick's treatise[3] on the standard of care for the edentulous mandible, underscores the fact that there is no single universally superior treatment for the edentulous mandible. In fact, patient acceptance of specific implant treatment designs is predicated on a multiplicity of factors, such as educational background, cultural/regional influences, age, and socioeconomic influences. Therefore, the decision to restore the edentulous mandible with either an implant overdenture (IOD), an implant fixed complete denture (IFCD), or fixed dental prosthesis (FDP) requires an in-depth analysis of patient-mediated factors and also systemic and local considerations for a cohort that is not quite becoming an endangered species.

Incidence of edentulism and demographic trends on implant treatment acceptance

Across a 5-decade observation period, edentulous prevalence has declined from 18.9% in the mid-1950s to 4.9% in 2010 (12.2 million patients), and is projected to be 2.6% by 2050 (6.8 million patients) in the US.[4] With its highest incidence in states with disproportionately high poverty, edentulism is a rare condition in high-income households. Thus, those most affected by this debilitation may be the least able to afford implant treatment modalities. This is in spite of the fact that higher initial fees for an implant-borne versus a conventional prosthesis are compensated by cost effectiveness, especially given longer life expectancies.[5] The prospect for more affordable implant treatment has been fueled by the number of implant companies offering competitive pricing and the expansion of delivery of implant rehabilitative care across the spectrum of practitioners.[6] However, compounding the present economic barrier is the lack of knowledge about implants in the geriatric cohort. Promotion of oral health with an emphasis on implant therapy education would address concerns about suitability, morbidity, and quality-of-life improvement.[7] When patients are in good health and live independently, regardless of the age, dental implant therapy offers a sustained benefit.[8]

Systemic factors

There is an established association between edentulism and advancing age.[9] A number of studies have addressed the impact of implant placement in the geriatric cohort.[10–12] Engfors *et al.*[13] compared patients older and younger than 79 years treated with mandibular implant fixed complete dentures (IFCD) and, after 5 years, implant survival was above 99% for each group. Notwithstanding these results, 10% of older patients have difficulties with adaptation and muscle control with implant prostheses.[14] While old age is not a contraindication, patients over 65 years of age should receive an in-depth evaluation because of potential medical complications and psychosocial considerations. Absolute contraindications to implant placement include recent myocardial infarction, recent cerebrovascular accident, uncontrolled diabetes, intravenous use of bisphosphonates, severe immunocompromise, irreversible bleeding dyscrasias, alcohol/drug addiction, and significant psychiatric disorders or unrealistic expectations.[15,16] While individual relative contraindications do not preclude implant placement, combinations of chronic disease states have been implicated in cluster failures of implants.[17,18] A recent systematic review reported a positive association between multimorbidity and age and lower socioeconomic status.[19] There is a number of specific disorders that have their onset later in life.

Evidence-based Implant Treatment Planning and Clinical Protocols, First Edition. Edited by Steven J. Sadowsky.

Companion website: www.wiley.com/go/sadowsky/implant

Osteoporosis affects 16% of women and 4% of men in the femur neck or lumbar spine after the age of 50.[20] There is no evidence of high rigor that dental implants in osteoporotic patients have a higher failure rate.[21] Moreover, the anterior mandible has not been reported to suffer an age-related osteopenia.[22] The influence of oral bisphosphonate (alendronate) use for osteoporosis on dental implant survival was recently evaluated in a multicentered prospective study, including completely edentulous patients.[23] After a 6-month cessation of drug treatment, the use of preoperative antibiotic prophylaxis, and 4-month healing time, no implant failures resulted.

Menopause has been associated with increased bone resorption. While nonestrogen replacement postmenopausal women have been reported to have lower implant survival in the maxilla (13.6%), no significant differences were noted on the mandible.[24]

Other relative contraindications not necessarily related to the aging population, such as smoking, use of antidepressants, steroid medications, controlled diabetes, or therapeutic ionizing radiation, need to be assessed in concert with a complete medical/dental work-up.[16,18,25,26]

Local factors

As only a small percentage of patients are precluded from implant therapy because of systemic factors, clinician- and patient-mediated considerations become an important gate for predicting implant success, not just survival. It is essential that the practitioner make an assessment of hard and soft tissue status, arch form, jaw classification, applied forces, antagonist dentition, and interarch space allowance, which may predicate the decision regarding implant number, position, anchorage system, and restorative superstructure design and material on the edentulous mandible.

The advent of low-radiation, low-cost cone-beam computed tomography (CBCT) and illustrative software has enabled the implant team to assess three-dimensionally the bony foundation for implant placement. This affords a cross-sectional view which may unveil otherwise undetected hourglass bone (Figure 18.1a) (3.89% incidence)[27] and/or posterior lingual concavities (Figure 18.1b) (estimation of lingual plate perforation 1.1–1.2%),[28] which increase the risk of surgical complications.

When an overdenture is planned for a V-shaped arch, a two-implant design potentiates rotational movement in the sagittal plane (Figure 18.2a), while a three-implant tripod resists it (Figure 18.2b). The cantilever of the IFCD design was historically limited by the anterior–posterior (AP) span of the implants and, if square arch forms were restored with this modality, the occlusal table was shortened, before the advent of tilted implants (Figure 18.3).

Class II overdenture patients may be best treated with an anchorage system that includes distal extension retentive units to stabilize the preferential posterior loading (Figure 18.4). However, caution should be used when fabricating cantilever extensions without robust connectors to the primary bar, as a high fracture incidence has been reported.[29]

Parafunction and/or antagonist natural dentition may dictate additional implant support to resist increased stresses (Figure 18.5a).[30–32] Four to seven times the maximum bite force has been quantified in bruxers.[33] An opposing natural dentition may be difficult to equilibrate for a harmonious occlusal scheme, which may potentiate preferential loading (Figure 18.5b, c).[34]

Space allowance varies with prosthetic design.[35,36] An overdenture retained by Locator® abutments (Zest Anchors LLC, Escondido, CA) (Figure 18.6a), resilient Dolder bar (Figure 18.6b),

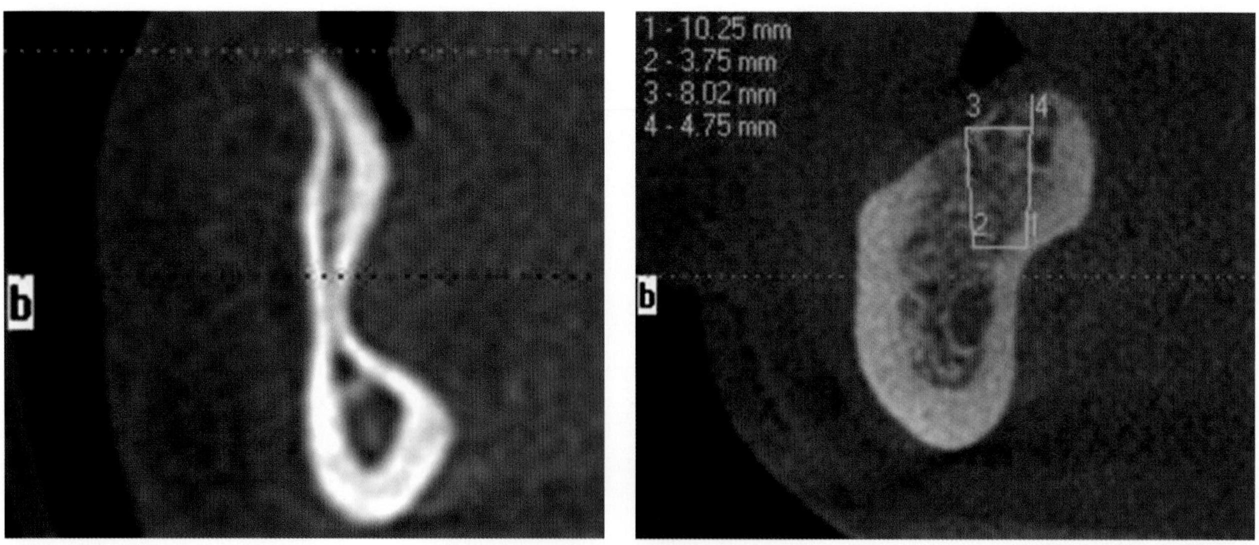

(a) (b)

Figure 18.1 **(a)** Hourglass morphology of anterior mandibular bone as seen on CBCT. **(b)** Mandibular lingual concavity as seen on CBCT.

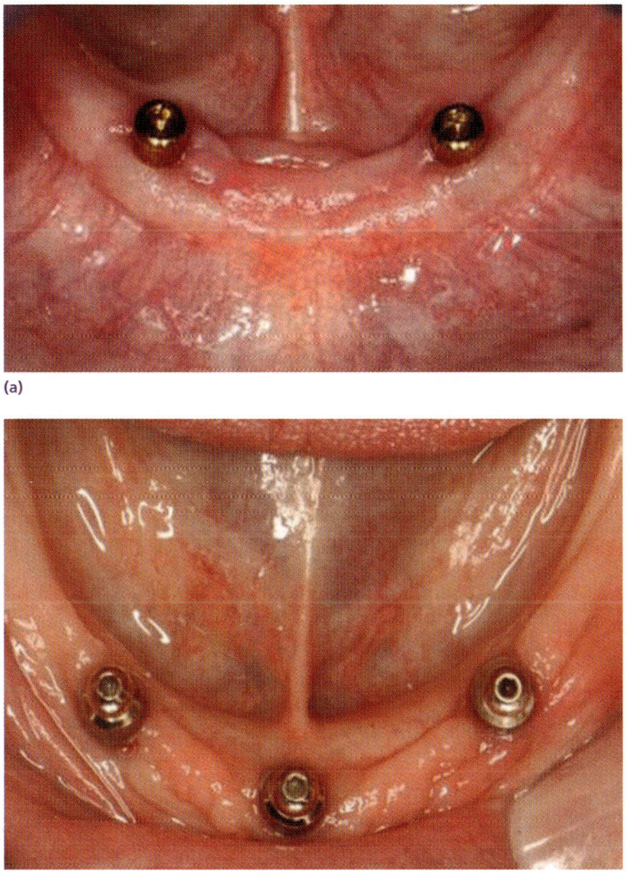

(a)

(b)

Figure 18.2 (a) U-shaped arch restored with two solitary anchors which may demonstrate anterior–posterior rotation on incisal biting. (b) V-shaped arch managed with three implants to resist anterior lever arm.

or spark-eroded milled bar (Figure 18.6c, d) requires 8–9 mm, 12 mm, and 12–15 mm, respectively, from the crest of the tissue to the incisal/occlusal table. An IFCD (Figure 18.6e) will require 12–15 mm and an IFDP (Figure 18.6f, g) may need 7 mm interarch space on the mandible.[37] A mounted resilient cast technique is helpful to visually assess the interarch space available, if the patient has been restored with an equilibrated mandibular complete denture. In preparation, the vertical dimension of occlusion must be verified by subtracting 3 mm from the vertical dimension of rest (class I scenario) along with adequate speaking space and esthetic evaluation. In an edentulous patient, the maxillary denture is mounted on an articulator with a facebow or facial analyzer (Kois Dento-Facial Analyzer, Panadent Corporation, Colton, CA) (Figure 18.7a) after laboratory putty (Splash Putty, DenMat, Lompoc CA) is placed in the intaglio surface of the denture and reinforced for mounting with paperclips (Figure 18.7b). The mandibular denture is prepared similarly with laboratory putty in the intaglio aspect and hand articulated to the maxillary denture, affixed with glue sticks. After mounting is complete, a vertical space analysis can be accomplished when the denture is removed from the resilient cast (Figure 18.7c–e). If the existing mandibular denture is satisfactory, for the vertical dimension of occlusion, occlusal and esthetic harmony, and fit, it may be used as a blueprint for a radiographic template. Otherwise a new wax try-in is required. In either case, the use of the Denture Duplicator Kit (Lang Dental Mfg Co Inc., Wheeling, IL) facilitates fabrication of a radiographic/surgical template. The former will require a ratio of 4:1 clear orthodontic resin (Caulk Orthodontic Resin, Dentsply, York, PA) to barium sulfate (Barium Sulfate, Henry Schein, San Francisco) for the tooth forms (Figure 18.7f–h).

Duplication of the dentures without the anterior flange may also be needed to assess the importance of mimicking the same facial scaffolding (Figure 18.7i). The patient is seen with her dentures in place (Figure 18.7j). The nasolabial and the labiomental angles are too acute, revealing excessive lip support. With the flangeless dentures in place, the facial anatomy is restored (Figure 18.7k). Therefore, an IFCD would be esthetically acceptable. Once the analysis is complete, determination of available bone, requirement for alveoplasty, and planning for implant position can commence to satisfy the clinician- and patient-mediated factors (Figure 18.7l–n).

When a patient presents with a terminal dentition (Figure 18.8a), the use of digital workflow software allows implant placement planning, along with the fabrication of sequenced stereolithographic templates (Figure 18.8b–e). The teeth assist in orienting the cross-pins that will standardize the position of all the templates in three dimensions (Figure 18.8f). The second template is placed after extractions to guide the alveoplasty (Figure 18.8g). The third template will guide the implant placement (Figure 18.8h). This allows for either an immediate- or delayed-loading protocol (Figure 18.8i, j).

Patient-mediated factors

Patient preferences in the final analysis may dictate treatment, given that the implant rehabilitation meets sound prosthodontic principles. These include cost, treatment time, maintenance considerations, and fixed versus removable designs.[38] Implant overdentures (IOD) are either implant supported (ISOD) or implant-retained and tissue-assisted (IROD). Mean incremental costs of a two-implant retained overdenture (IROD) and a four-implant supported overdenture (ISOD) were compared to a complete denture.[39] The ISOD was found to be three times the initial cost of the IROD, but with modest improvement in chewing ability. When ISODs were compared to IFCDs in long-term studies, the initial cost, maintenance, and clinical time were significantly higher with the IFCDs.[40,41] Comparative long-term cost analysis of metal–ceramic implant restorations for the edentulous mandible is lacking in the literature. Contrary to conventional wisdom, cross-over studies and psychometric analyses have failed to demonstrate significant differences in patient satisfaction between removable (implant retained or

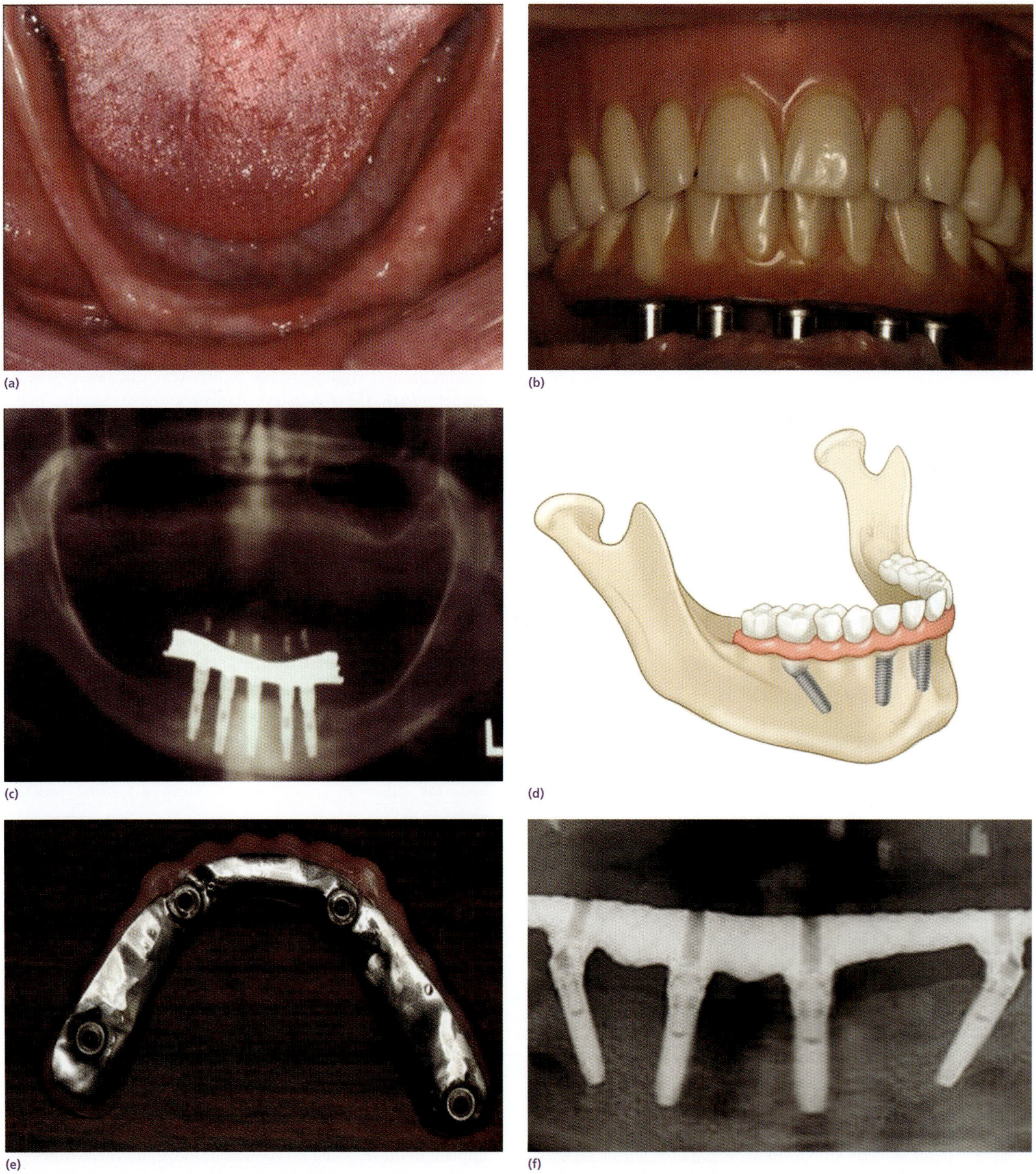

Figure 18.3 (a) Square-shaped arch with limited projected anterior–posterior (AP) span for vertically placed implants. (b) Limited cantilever extension for implant fixed complete denture due to minimal AP span generated by vertically placed implants and adhering to formula (cantilever = 1.5AP span). (c) Radiographic depiction of shortened cantilever IFCD. (d) Graphic illustrating the extended occlusal table and reduced cantilever afforded by tilted terminal implants. (e) Square arch reconciled by tilted implants. (f) Radiographic depiction of All-on-4 prosthesis in (e). *Source*: © 2016, Chris Gralapp.

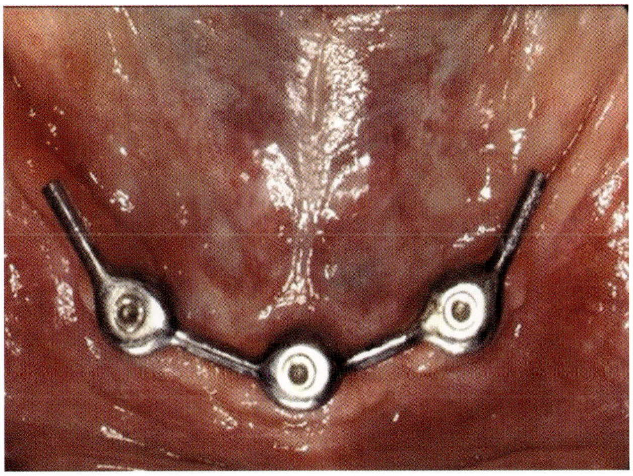

Figure 18.4 Cantilever extension implant overdenture anchorage system designed to improve stability with class II patients, improve retention with intransigent gaggers, or/and protect sensitive mucosa over mental foramina region.

supported) overdentures and IFCDs.[42,43] Patients over 50 years old, experienced denture users, and those with hygiene accessibility priorities favored a removable implant prosthesis.

The implant overdenture versus a conventional denture

When comparing patient satisfaction and oral health-related quality-of-life (QOL) outcomes before and after implants are placed and restored in the edentulous mandible, a number of studies with up to a 10-year follow-up demonstrates advantages of the IROD versus the CD in chewing ability, stability, and comfort, irrespective of mandibular bone height.[44–48] Furthermore, when compared to a CD, the IROD was responsible for a greater self-confidence and satisfaction in social interactions.[49] While 51% of denture patients reported discomfort on chewing significantly impacting their diet,[50] surprisingly,

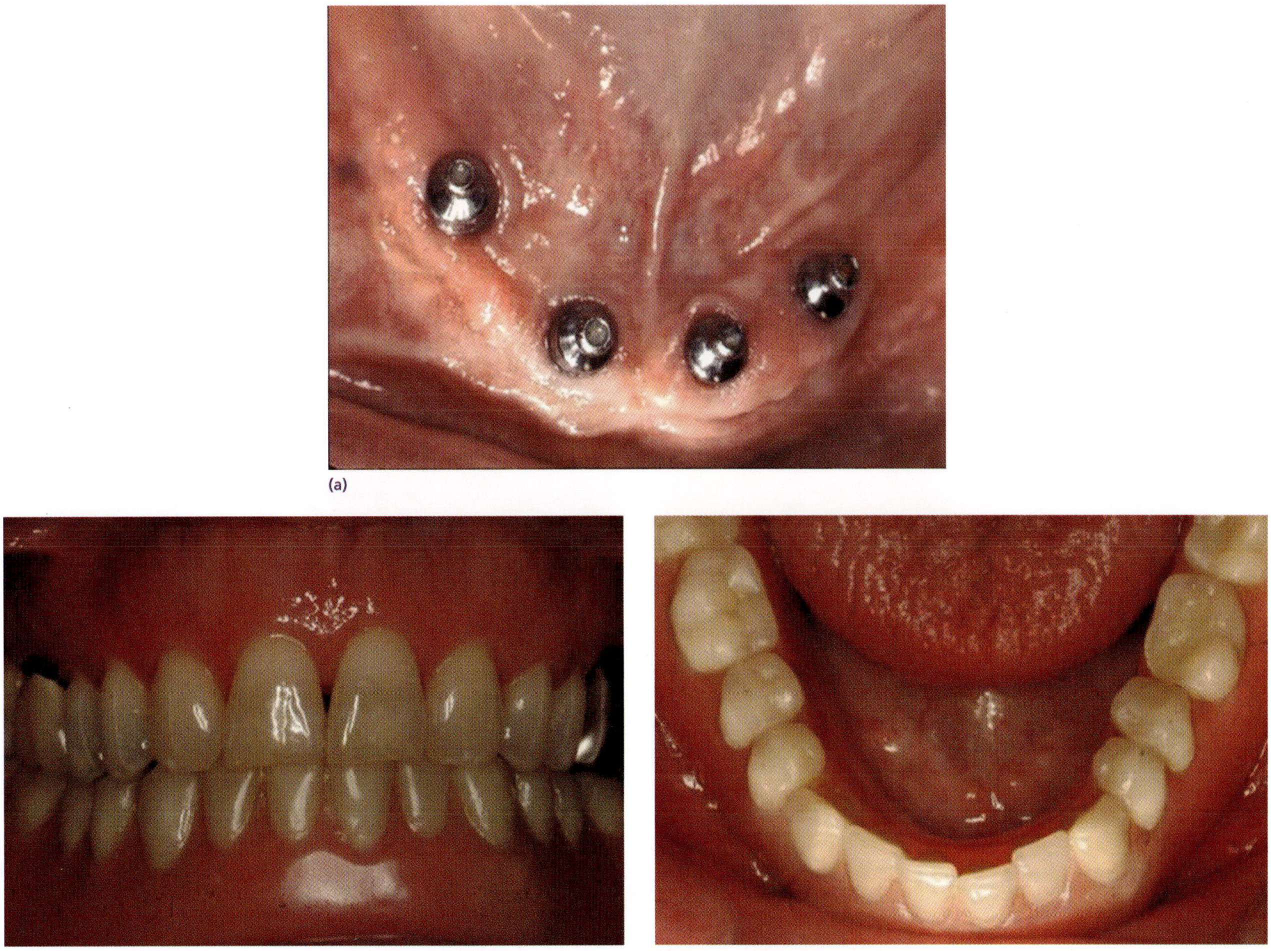

(a)

(b)

(c)

Figure 18.5 (a) Multiple implants placed in edentulous mandible opposing a natural dentition. (b) Frontal view of mandibular implant overdenture opposing natural dentition. (c) Occlusal view of mandibular implant overdenture opposing natural dentition.

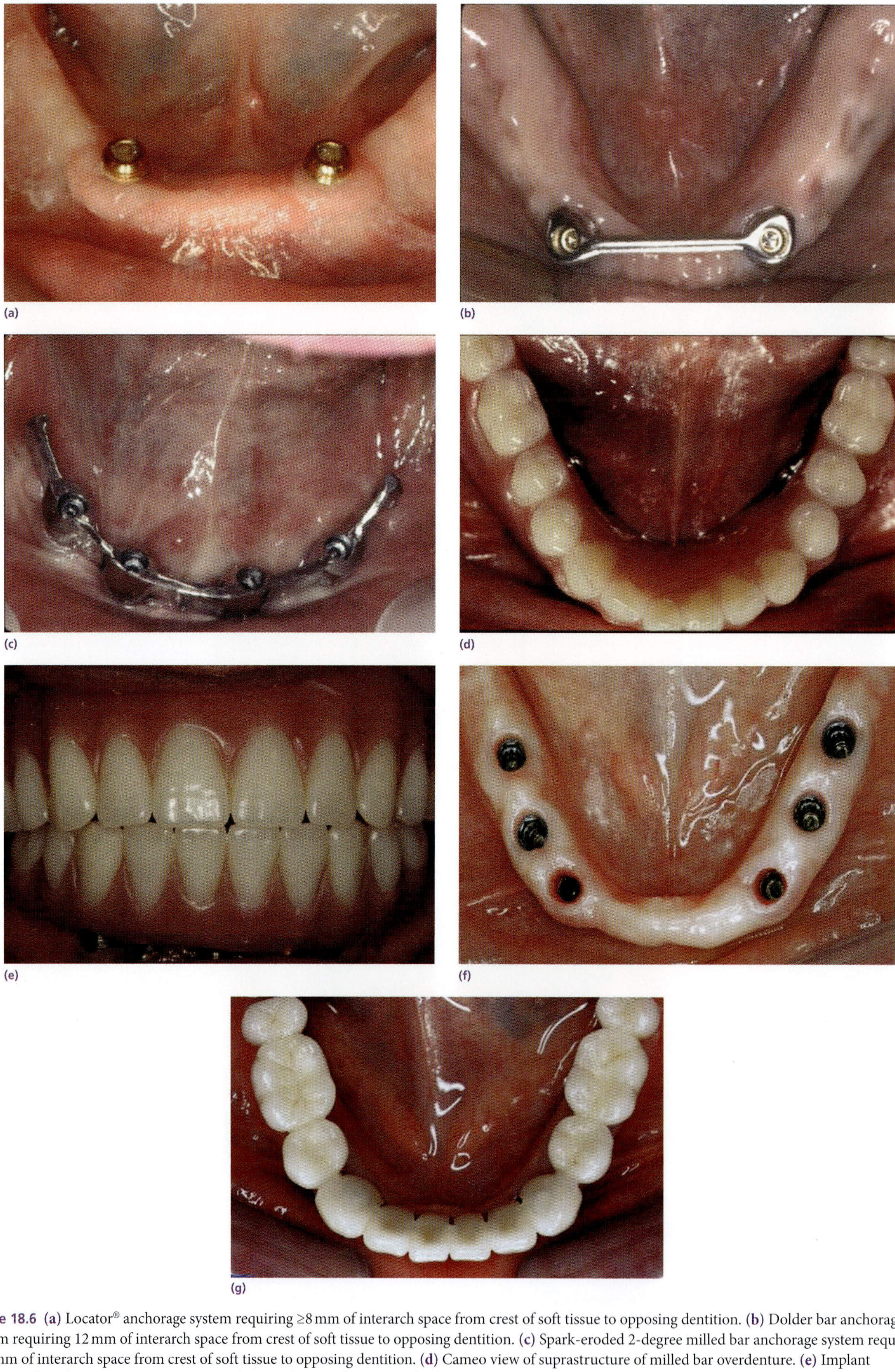

Figure 18.6 (a) Locator® anchorage system requiring ≥8 mm of interarch space from crest of soft tissue to opposing dentition. (b) Dolder bar anchorage system requiring 12 mm of interarch space from crest of soft tissue to opposing dentition. (c) Spark-eroded 2-degree milled bar anchorage system requiring ≥12 mm of interarch space from crest of soft tissue to opposing dentition. (d) Cameo view of suprastructure of milled bar overdenture. (e) Implant fixed complete denture requiring ≥12 mm of interarch space from crest of soft tissue to opposing dentition. (f) Limited resorption of ridge allowing for a porcelain-fused-to-metal design (implant fixed dental prosthesis). Placement of implants is critical to be congruent with restorative design. (g) Porcelain-fused-to-metal implant reconstruction requiring 8–10 mm of interarch space. *Source for* (f, g): Reproduced with permission from Charles Goodacre.

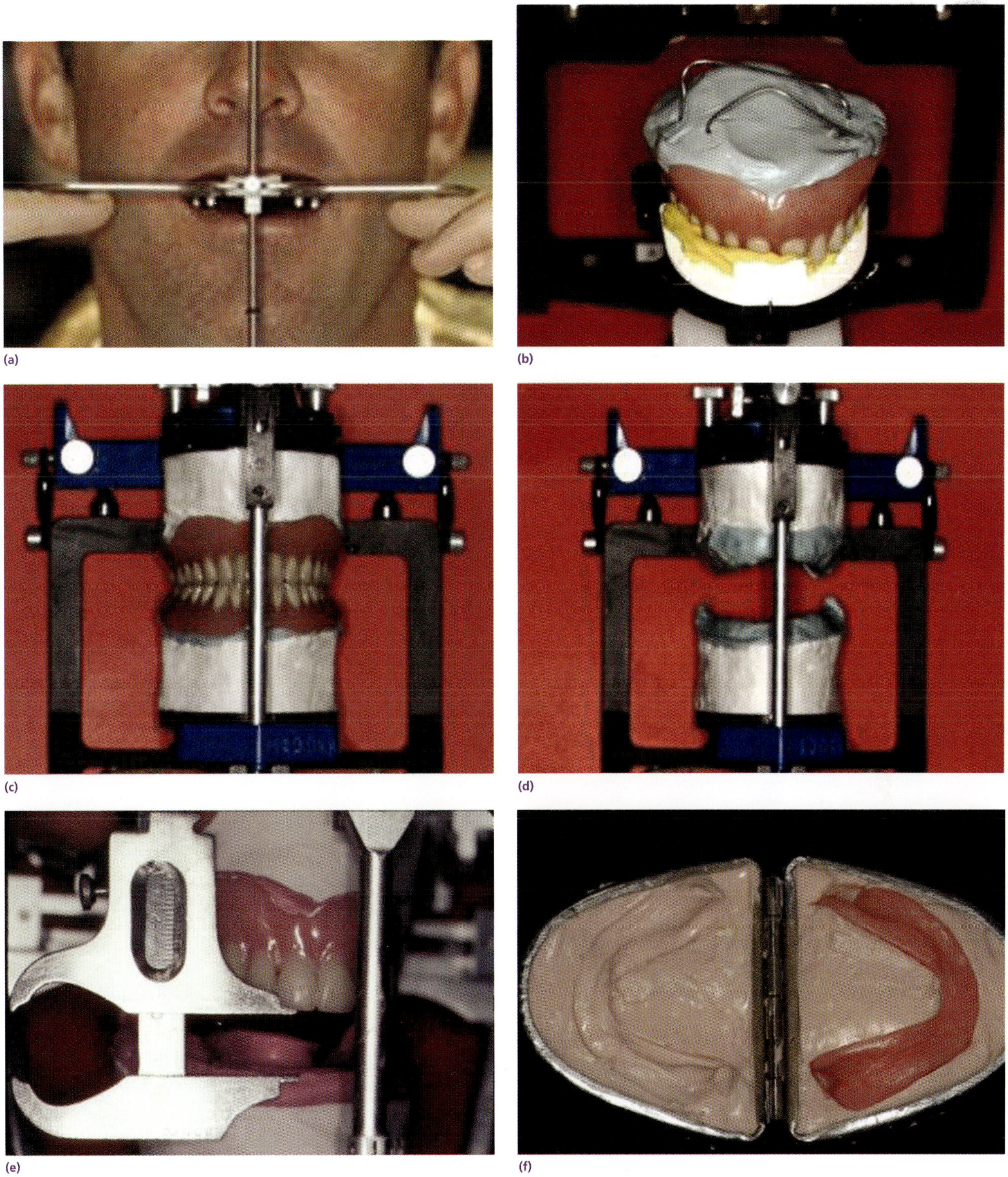

Figure 18.7 (a) Kois Facial Analyzer in place to transfer, three-dimensionally, the position of the maxillary denture to the articulator. (b) Maxillary denture positioned on mounting stand via registration material. The intaglio surface of the denture is filled with laboratory putty and paper clips are engaged in the putty to provide retention for mounting stone. (c) The maxillary denture is mounted on the articulator and the mandibular denture is hand articulated to it (given vertical and horizontal records are appropriate). The intaglio surface of the mandibular denture is filled with laboratory putty and reinforced with paper clips in preparation for mounting on the articulator. (d) Dentures are removed to reveal mounted resilient casts. (e) Vertical measurement determined between occlusal aspect of maxillary denture and mandibular ridge crest. (f) Lang Denture Duplicator with alginate, used to create a replica of existing denture or ideal wax-up for radiographic/surgical template. (g) Radiographic/surgical template. (h) CBCT scan with software program orienting the implants in three dimensions with radiographic template in place for a two-implant overdenture design. (i) Duplicate dentures with anterior flanges removed. (j) Profile of patient with complete dentures in place, demonstrating excessive lip support from anterior flanges. (k) Profile of patient with flangeless duplicates of dentures in place demonstrating natural lip contours. (l) Preoperative evaluation of orthopantomogram for available bone for implant placement. Need for alveoplasty was dictated by the resilient cast measurement. (m) Implant placement after alveoplasty. (n) Definitive implant fixed complete dentures in place.

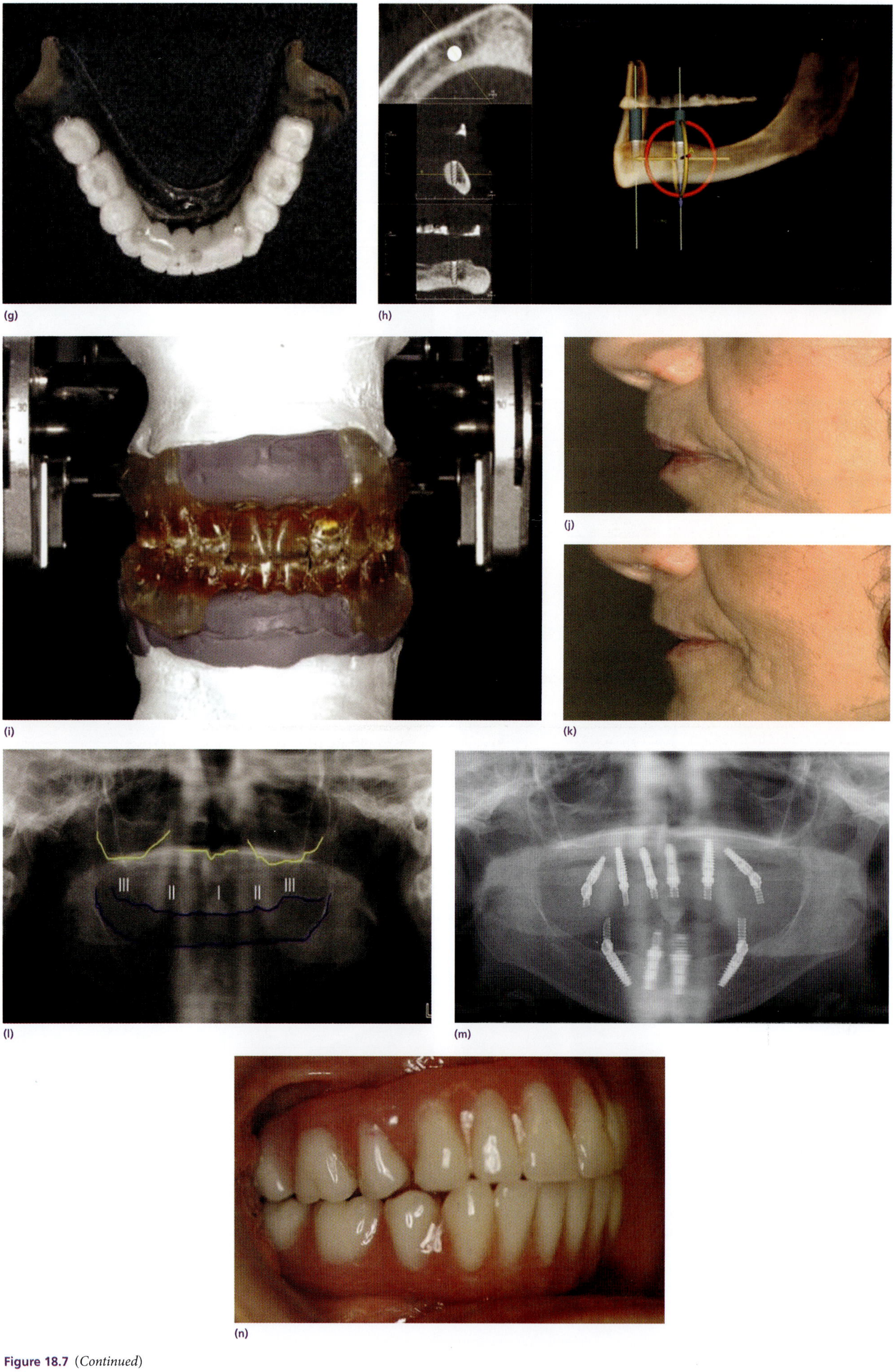

Figure 18.7 (*Continued*)

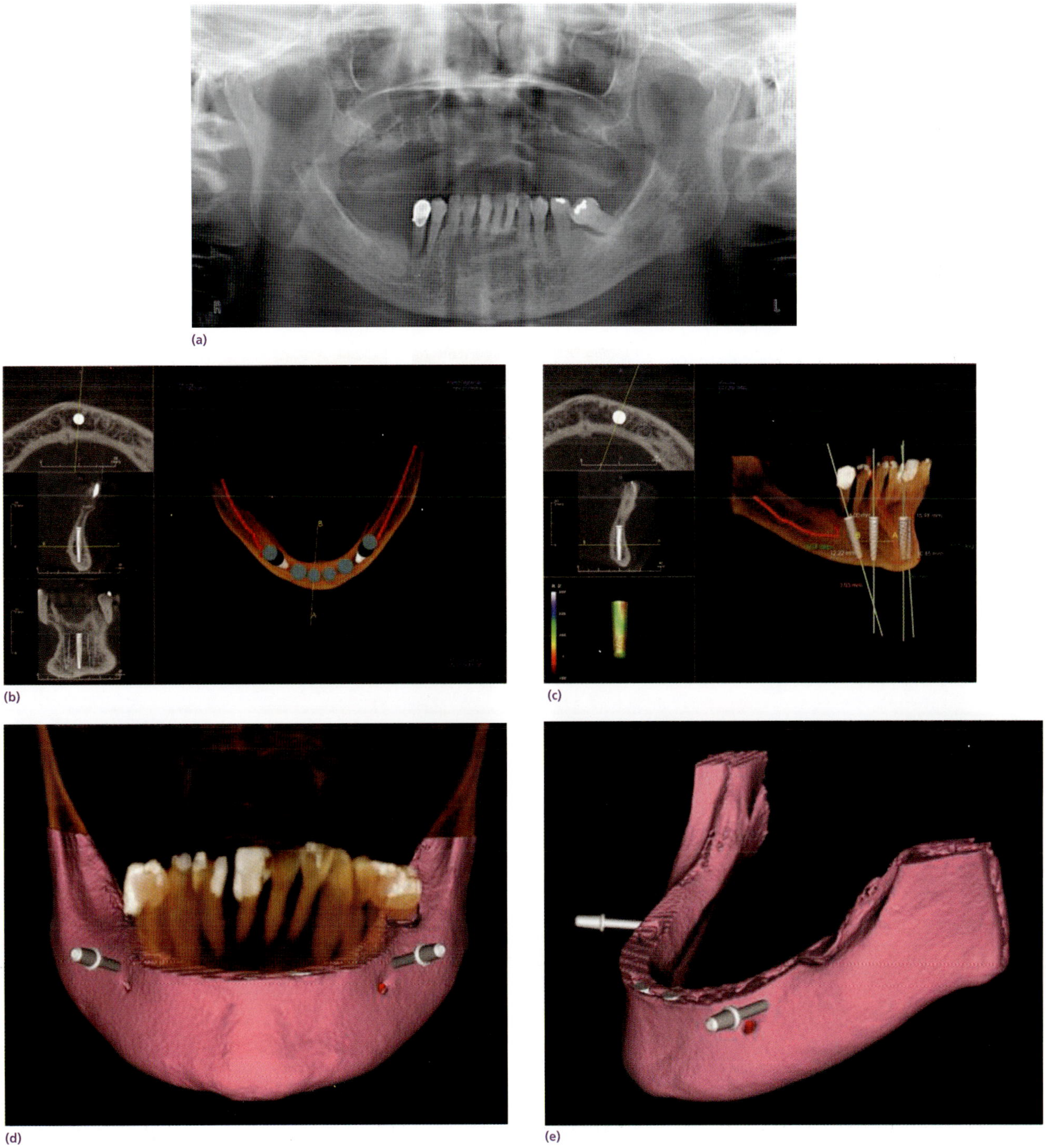

Figure 18.8 (a) Preoperative orthopantomogram of edentulous maxilla and terminal mandibular dentition. (b) CBCT scan displaying potential sites for implants using software program. (c) CBCT scan of implant positions using three anterior vertical implants and two tilted terminal implants. (d) 3-D rendering of preoperative mandible with two cross pins established for referencing templates. (e) Virtual alveoplasty. (f) First template keyed to the existing dentition to orient osteotomy for cross pins. (g) Second template oriented by cross pins for alveoplasty. (h) Third template oriented by cross pins for implant placement. (i) Orthopantomogram of implant placement and immediate provisional prosthesis. (j) Definitive prostheses. *Source*: Courtesy of Fawas Alzoubi; reproduced with permission.

no improvement in nutritional status, body mass index, or serum albumin values has been reported with the IROD.[51]

Given that the annual mandibular bone loss in the edentulous patient averages 0.4 mm,[52] it is of note that, after 12 years, only an average 1.7 mm of bone loss has been observed around implants retaining a hinging overdenture.[53] Similar long-term peri-implant outcomes in two-implant overdenture patients have been documented, with splinted or nonsplinted

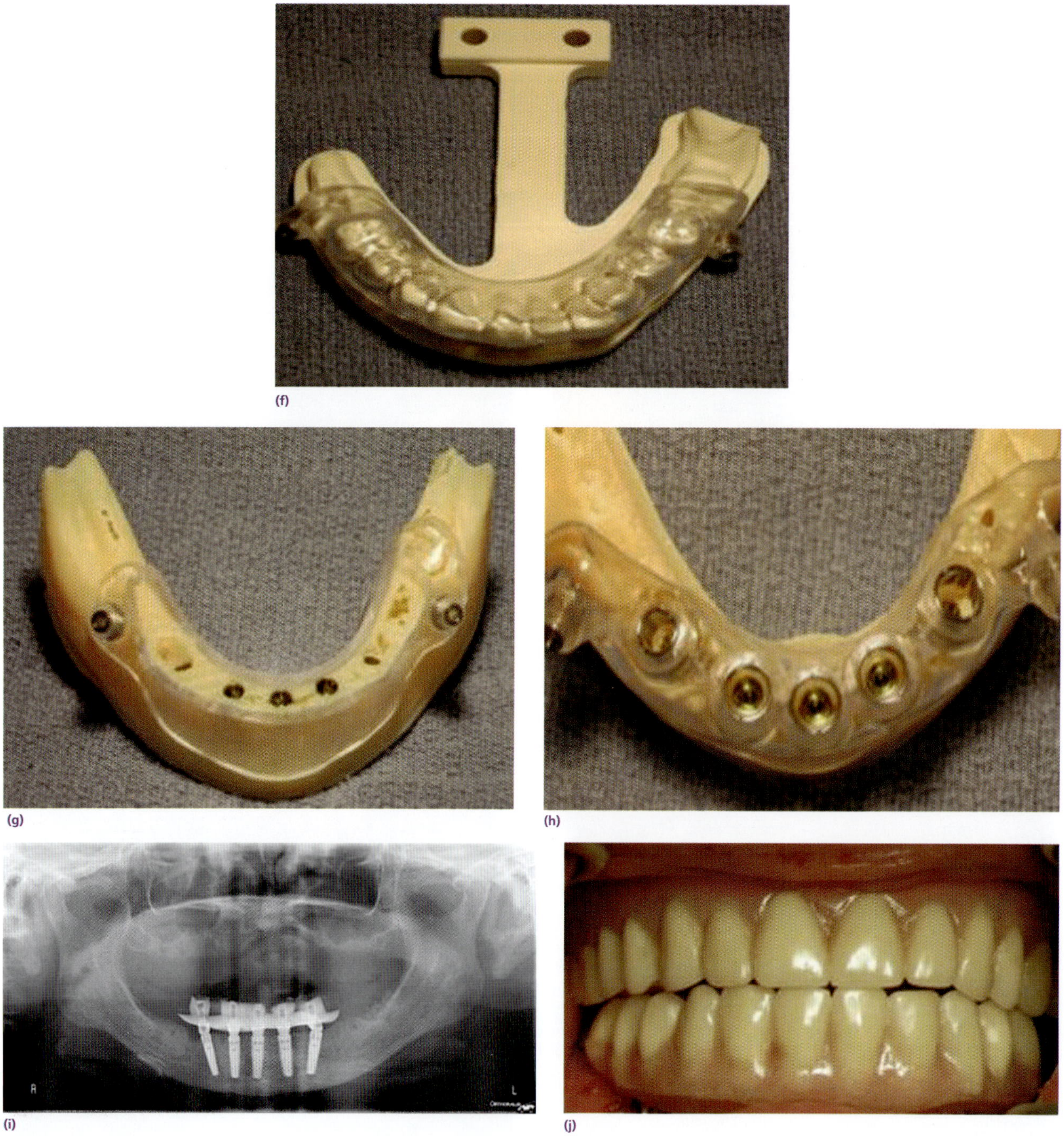

Figure 18.8 (*Continued*)

anchorage systems or different loading protocols.[54–56] However, the two-implant IROD has not been found to be protective of posterior bone levels.[57] In fact two to three times the bone resorption was reported after 2 years of IROD use as compared to CD use.[58] Considering patient preferences, when patients have highly atrophied mandibular posterior alveolar bone and/or they are young, an IFCD would be preferable to an IROD.[59]

Number of implants, anchorage system, and maintenance of the implant overdenture

Number of implants

When comparing two- and four-implant designs with at least a 5-year follow-up, patient satisfaction or peri-implant health were not influenced by the number or type of anchorage system (Figure 18.9a, b).[31,60–62] However, the indication for more than

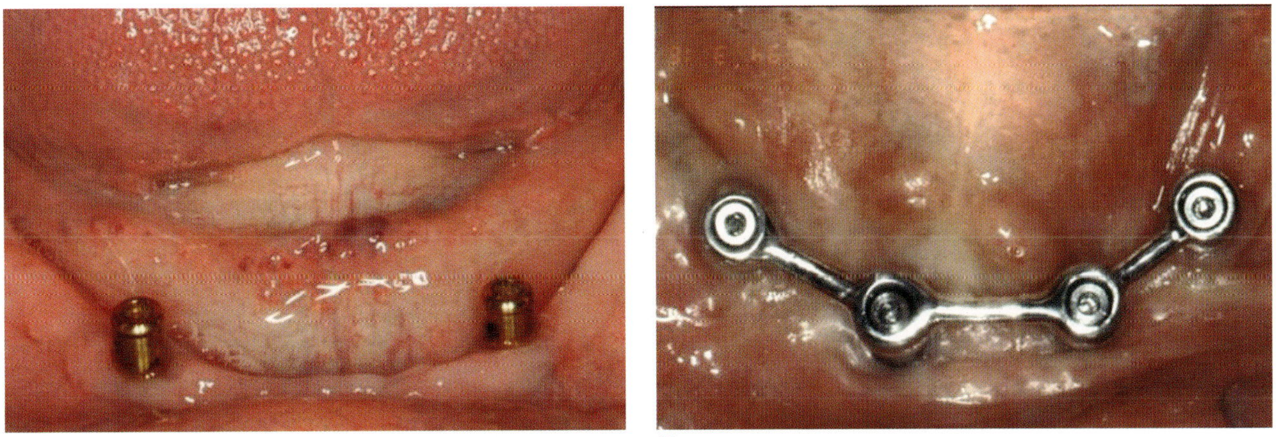

(a) (b)

Figure 18.9 **(a)** Two-implant solitary anchor design (Locator®) for overdenture. **(b)** Four-implant splinted bar design for overdenture.

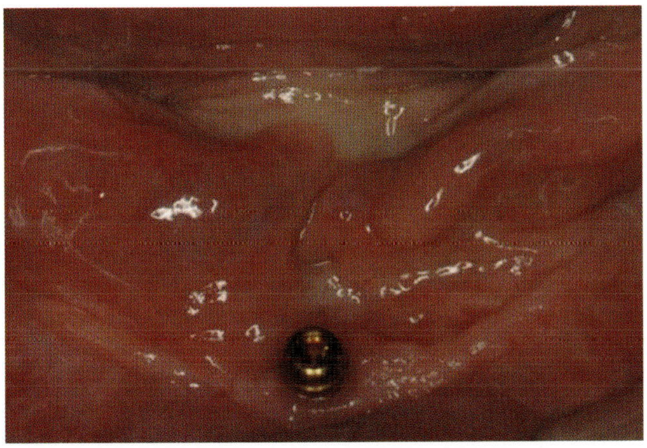

Figure 18.10 Single symphyseal design (Locator®) for overdenture.

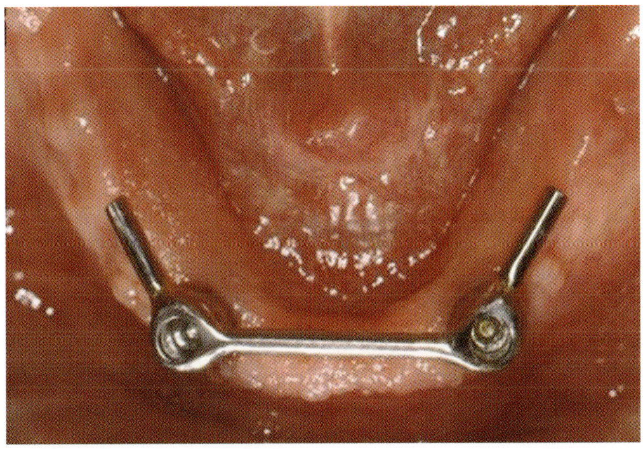

Figure 18.11 Two-implant splinted bar design with distal cantilever extensions.

two implants and type of anchorage system should be predicated on clinician- and patient-related factors. For example, in patients with a dentate maxilla, narrow tapered arches, high muscle attachments, and sharp mylohyoid ridges, more than two implants are recommended for prosthetic stability.[38,63] A recent 5-year randomized clinical trial also discerned no statistically significant differences in patient satisfaction, implant survival, or maintenance with a one- or two-implant mandibular overdenture modality (Figure 18.10).[64] This alternative appears to be appropriate for septuagenarians and octogenarians with surgical morbidity and financial concerns. However, a metal-reinforced prosthesis for the solitary anchor design was recommended to thwart a higher incidence of fracture in this design.

Anchorage system

When considering splinted versus solitary anchors, local and patient-mediated factors often prevail. A splinted bar with a distal extension is recommended for patients with sensitive mucosa over the superficial mental foramina area.[38] Distal bars also provide additional retention for enhanced prosthetic stability when this feature is at a premium for the patient, such as in the intransigent gagger. When two implants are used to retain a bar with cantilever extensions, the distal bars should not extend beyond the first premolar position and together should be no longer than the central bar (Figure 18.11).[63] On the other hand, solitary anchors are preferred in patients with lack of keratinized tissue, interarch space limitations, and hygiene or economic concerns.

Maintenance

Ball attachments have been documented with less incidence of hyperplasia but more mechanical maintenance than bars, increasing ultimate patient costs for ball IRODs.[65–68] On the other hand, when comparative maintenance outcomes were investigated with bars, telescopes, and Locator® attachments (Zest Anchors LLC), the latter performed superiorly over a 3-year observation period.[69] This coupled with the ease of changing the attachments and the low-profile abutment/housing (3.2 mm) explains the popularity of the Locator® system, although in a cross-over study, no patient preference was given to the Locator® attachment.[70] The clinician can expect the two-Locator® IROD over 3 years to require a reline in less than 20% of patients, and two sets of changes in the retentive attachments.

There also has been a troubling finding of food impaction in the occlusal well of the abutment in 47% of patients after 7 years (Figure 18.12).[71] A simple solution is to change the nylon attachments to the extended-range set which has no internal doughnut (Figure 18.13). In a review of literature, there was a wide range of incidence of required relines from 8% to 40% for both IROD and ISOP designs.[72,73] A functional wax refit technique[74] using Adaptol wax sticks (Kaye Research Laboratories, Ashaway, RI) with 10 drops of vegetable oil, which can be heated up to 123 °F (50.5 °C) can facilitate an accurate pick-up of attachments and the extension base tissue zone, which may reduce the frequency for this procedure (Figure 18.14a, b). This technique is also effective for other types of overdenture attachments (Figure 18.14c). A prospective maintenance evaluation of two-, three-, and four-implant bar anchorage systems revealed 1.5 times more retention clip activation in the two-implant (single round bar) design, as compared to the three-implant (double round bar) or four-implant (triple round bar) design.[73] However, retention clip fracture occurred twice as much with three or four implants than with two implants. In response to the frequent maintenance issues seen in the four-implant design, a rigid milled bar mesostructure intimately supporting a reinforced metal suprastructure retained with swivel latches[75] (Figure 18.15) required three times less prosthodontic aftercare over 5 years when compared to resilient bar designs such as the Dolder or Hader bar systems (Figure 18.16).[76,77] The reduction of micromotion in the rigid milled bar design compared to the resilient bar anchorage systems appears to be responsible for the reduced maintenance. When selecting a multiple-implant design, although the rigid milled bar system with latches requires a higher initial investment, it is more cost effective than the resilient bar, while offering retention security.

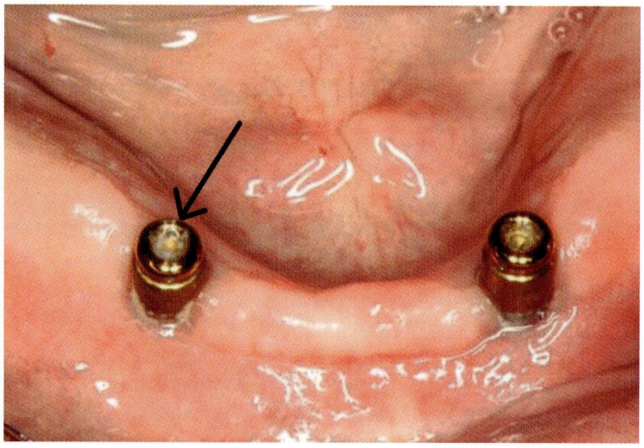

Figure 18.12 Food impaction disclosed in internal well of the Locator® abutment.

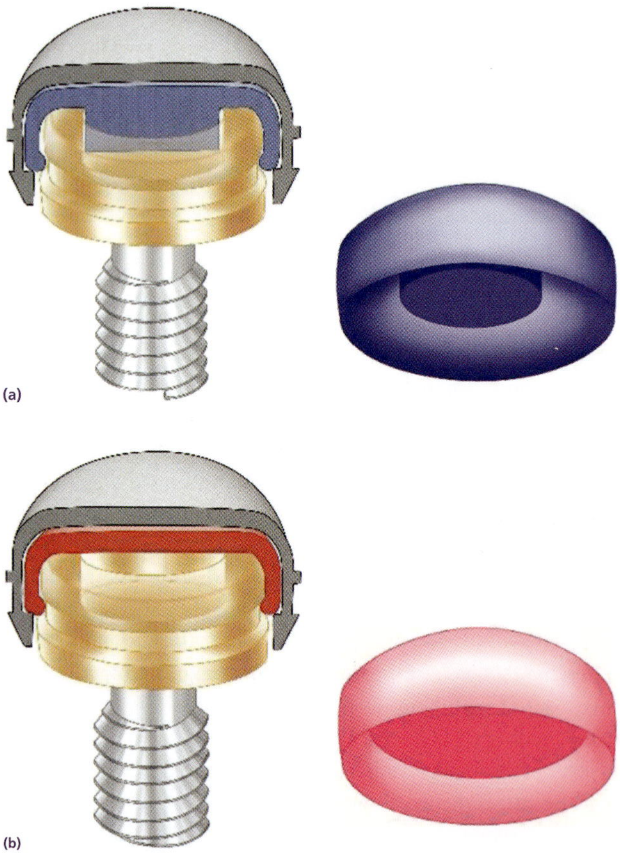

Figure 18.13 **(a)** Nylon attachment inside metal housing engaging the internal well of Locator® abutment. **(b)** Extended-range nylon attachment inside metal housing not engaging the internal well of Locator® abutment. *Source*: Courtesy of Jeff Miles.

Immediate-load protocols

Patients with a terminal dentition that will be transitioning to an implant overdenture are often beleaguered, functionally and psychologically, with a tissue-supported provisional prosthesis during the integration period. An immediate-load implant prosthesis offers patients a stable and retentive alternative, despite such conditions as compromised ridge height, poor soft tissue anatomy, retruded tongue, high muscle attachments, xerostomia, somatogenic gagging, and a highly active floor of the mouth.[78]

Legitimacy for the immediate-load modality for mandibular overdentures has been established with a number of studies considering implant survival and patient-centered outcomes.[79–82] A systematic review revealed that immediate loading (1–2 days) of the edentulous mandible is scientifically and clinically validated with two to four implants, splinted or solitary, all showing implant survival rates above 96% with up to 13 years' follow-up (Figure 18.17).[83] However, the immediately loaded group has been shown to require higher prosthetic maintenance than the delayed group, such as overdenture remakes, and 74% required relines to improve the denture seal around the bar housing, in the first year.[84] Most frequent aftercare problems in the non-splinted design were replacement of the attachment inserts, abutment loosening, dislodgement of the attachment housing,

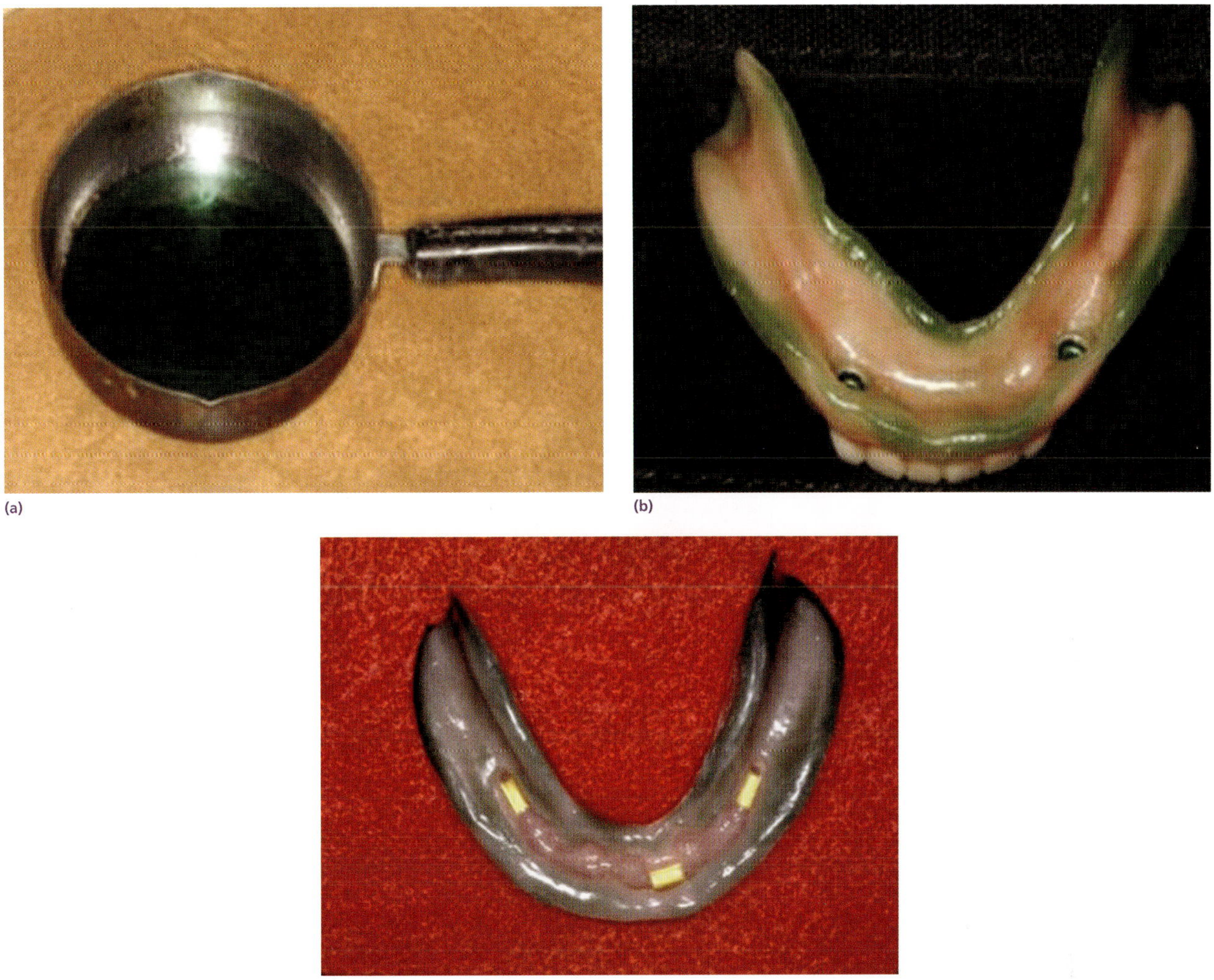

(a) (b) (c)

Figure 18.14 (a) Melted Adaptol® wax sticks (10 drops vegetable oil per stick) fusing at 123 °F (50.5 °C) in small pan. (b) Place heated wax in intaglio of implant overdenture with a #7 spatula, temper in 120 °F (48.8 °C) water bath, and place in mouth. Remove and add or subtract wax as needed to allow uniform seating on extension base and attachments. Have the patient reproduce functional movements and chew on a small cube of foam. Fins are evidence of underextensions. Show-throughs in the flange area may be overextensions. Once the intaglio of the prosthesis is optimized, have the patient rinse with ice water, and remove and seal in a baggie of ice water for transport to lab for reline. (c) Functional wax technique for Hader bar overdenture design.

reline, denture tooth fracture, and overdenture base fracture.[85] A reinforced metal base may thwart fracture and add rigidity to the prosthesis. Marzola *et al.*[86] underscored the importance of precise adaptation and equilibration of the denture before the surgical procedure, no removal of the prosthesis for 1 week, and minimal flap reflection. In an effort to reduce mechanical maintenance, other researchers of immediately loaded solitary abutments have tailored the prosthetic connection at the time of placement to include using a flexible polyether lining in the metal housings for 3 months or adapting tissue conditioner over high-profile healing abutments.[87,88] Immediate load of a free-standing symphyseal IROD has been investigated by Liddelow *et al.*,[89] who followed patients with a mean age of 68 years for 3 years. They noted a 100% implant survival on 25 implants that were oxidized and achieved primary stability, but more studies are needed with high methodological rigor.

Patient selection

Patients with systemic conditions that would challenge wound healing or implant stability should be excluded from immediate-load protocols. Poor candidates are those with a history of diabetes, hyperparathyroidism, alcohol/drug abuse, heavy smoking (over 20 cigarettes/day), therapeutic ionizing radiation, or are currently being treated with antiblastic chemotherapy or steroids.[78,90] Other patient habits such as heavy parafunction,[91,92] poor oral hygiene control,[60] and lack of compliance with a soft diet and a strict recall schedule have also been implicated in implant failure with this regimen. Aside from these factors, the quantity and quality of native bone will predicate primary stability, which has been considered a *sine qua non* for immediate loading. While some have suggested a range of 35–60 Ncm insertion torque[93] (resonance frequency analysis >54[94]) with a medium roughened implant of at least 10 mm in length, others

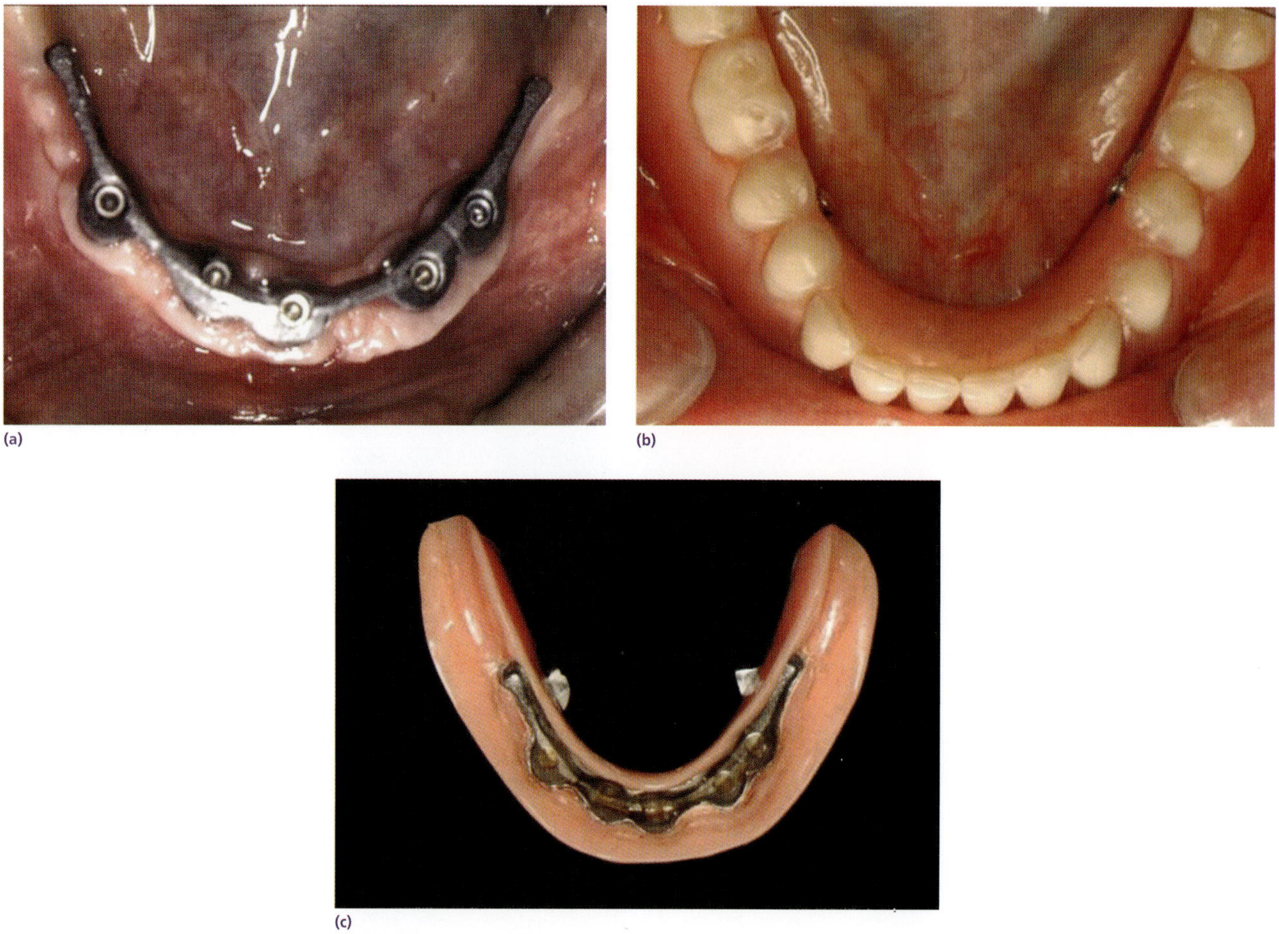

Figure 18.15 (a) Spark-eroded milled bar anchorage system. (b) Milled bar overdenture suprastructure. (c) Intaglio of milled bar overdenture suprastructure revealing secondary bar and reinforcement.

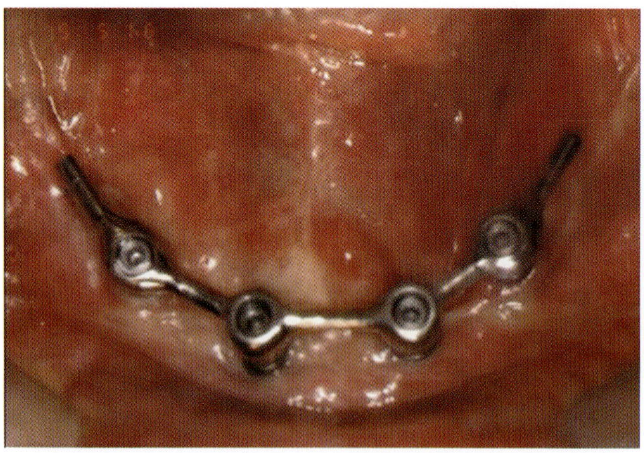

Figure 18.16 Resilient cantilevered Dolder bar anchorage system.

have deemed 20–25 Ncm to be sufficient.[86,95] Modifications in surgical protocol to enhance primary stability, such as underpreparation of the osteotomy site, using the osteotome technique, engaging bicortical stabilization, and avoidance of countersinking and/or tapping, have not been shown to be critical because of the healing capacity of the anterior mandible.[96] However, surgical expertise has been linked to successful immediate protocols.[97]

Implant fixed complete dentures

A metal–resin implant fixed complete denture (MRIFCD), rather than an IROD or ISOD, is indicated in patients with combination syndrome,[98] temporomandibular dysfunction,[99] and marked posterior residual resorption,[100] assuming the patient will be satisfied with the dental and facial esthetics, hygiene access, and cost considerations (Figure 18.18). The *ad modum* Branemark prototype or MRIFCD was first installed over 50 years ago and has the benefit of the most longitudinal retrospective follow-up of any implant modality. Thirty-year outcomes have demonstrated 100% implant survival with 2.6 ± 0.5 mm of average marginal bone loss at the final recall.[101] These data are in keeping with other long-term studies with larger populations.[102,103] To address the success (length of time before requiring an intervention), Dhima *et al.*[104] reported a 29-year outcome analysis tracking over 200

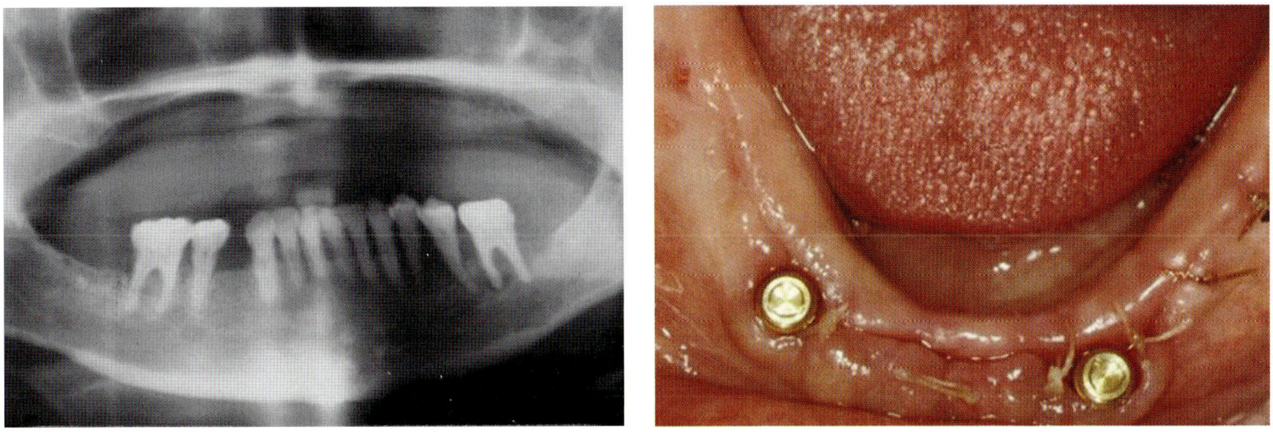

(a) (b)

Figure 18.17 (a) Preoperative panoramic film of patient with terminal dentition on mandible. (b) Immediate placement/loading of two implants.

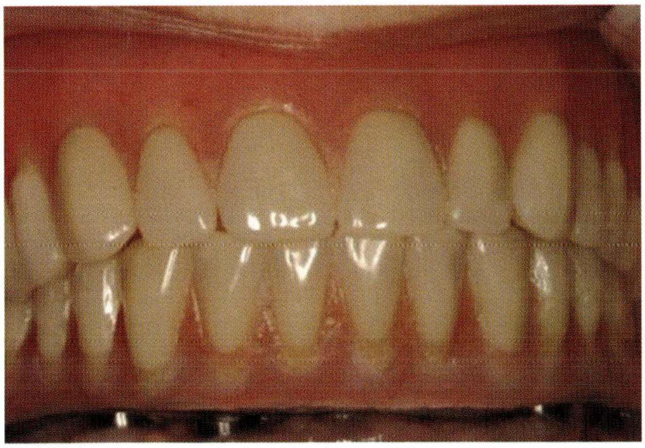

Figure 18.18 Metal–resin implant fixed complete denture.

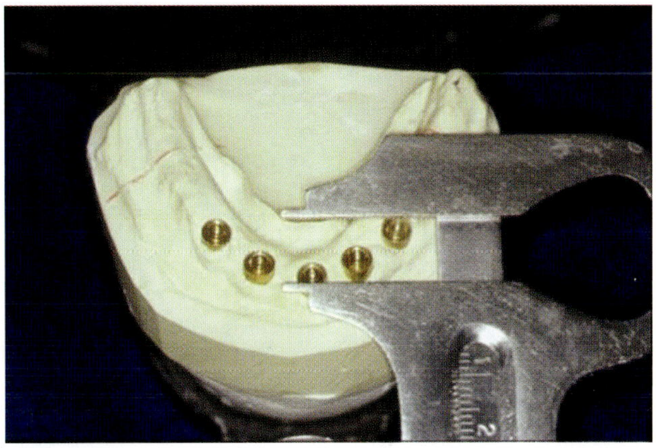

Figure 18.19 Measurement of anterior–posterior span (AP) to establish cantilever length (CL) using formula: CL = 1.5AP.

mandibular MRIFCDs. With a mean follow-up of 13 years, they found that prosthetic (mechanical) complications occurred later and exceeded biologic events (notably hyperplasia) by a factor of almost four. Only 15% of the prostheses survived without a maintenance event and 8.6% required a remake. Other authors have acknowledged that the most predominant mechanical complications were fracturing of the veneering and/or tooth material, tooth wear, maxillary denture relines, and screw loosening/fractures.[105–107] Edentulous patients treated with a MRIFCD should be informed of the high aftercare burden accompanying this modality.[107]

In an effort to reduce the aftercare burden, guidelines for treatment planning and fabricating an IFCD have evolved. A minimum of 15 mm from the crest of the soft tissue to the incisal edge anteriorly and 12 mm from the crest of the soft tissue to the posterior occlusal table.[108] This span allows for a 15 mm cantilever (CL) based on a recommended empirical formula, CL = 1.5AP (Figure 18.19).[109] Historically, square arches would dictate a short cantilever for the IFCD and, when untenable functionally or esthetically, an overdenture design would be selected. With the advent of tilted terminal implants, an extended occlusal table was facilitated with an enhanced distribution of implants.[110–112] Systematic reviews have compared the marginal bone loss around straight and tilted implants and reported no significant differences with up to a 5-year recall.[113,114]

Design considerations for fabricating the MRIFCD have evolved from 30 years ago.[115] Originally, frameworks were waxed and cast with noble alloys to engage standard intermediate abutments with prosthetic screws via gold cylinders. The "high water" prosthesis (Figure 18.20a, b) has been replaced with a "profile" prosthesis that either engages directly to the implant or to a multi-unit abutment that allows a slightly supragingival emergence (Figure 18.20c). Biomechanical principles have driven advances in framework design and materials. An I- or L-beam configuration (Figure 18.21) of at least 4 mm dimensional height (fracture resistance to withstand 900 N force, T. Salinas unpublished data) with adequate retentive components and adhesive treatment is recommended.[116] A wax set-up will dictate the 3-D position of the frame to provide support for the prosthetic teeth (Figure 18.22). The use of palladium–silver

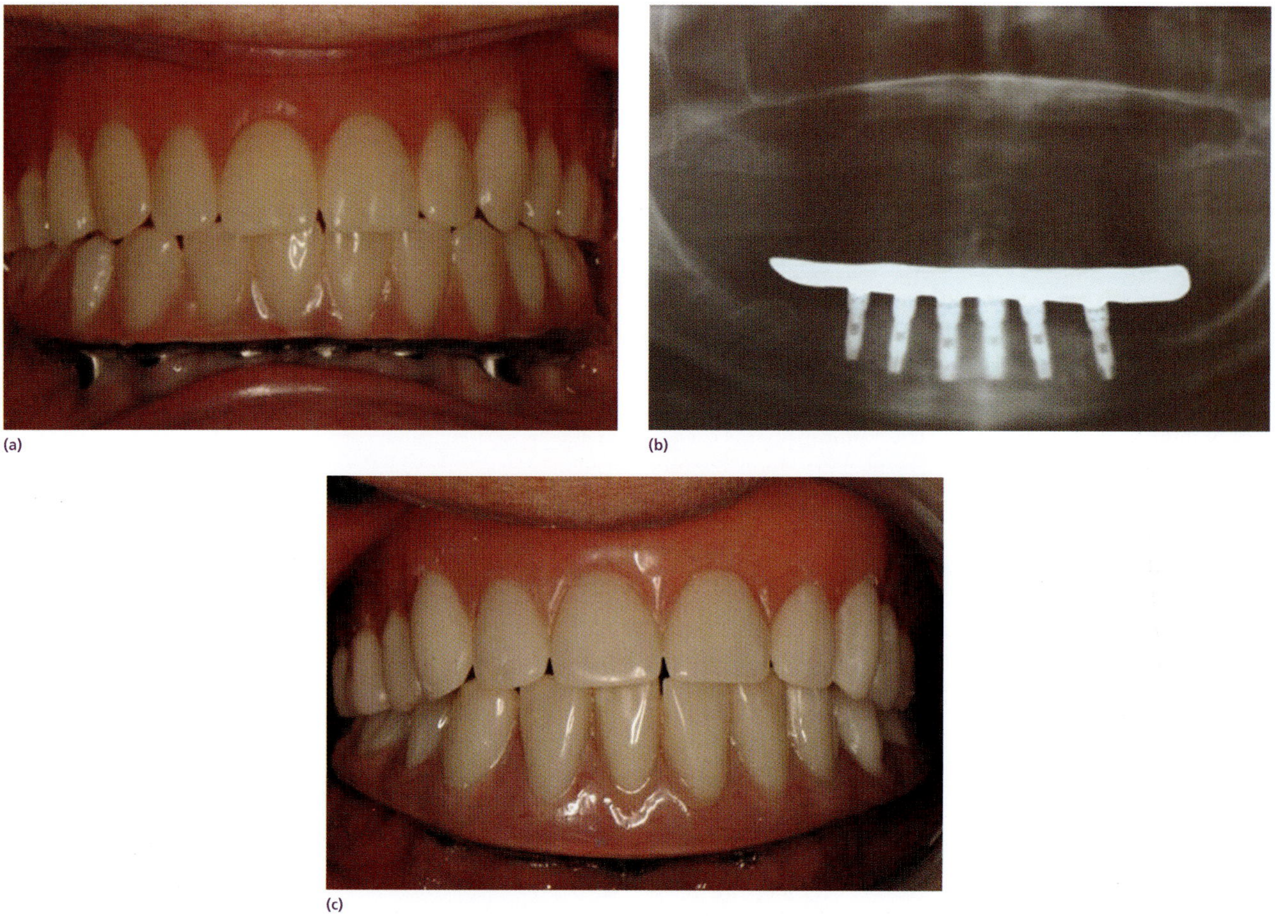

Figure 18.20 (a) Implant fixed complete denture with a high water design using standard abutments. (b) Radiograph of (a). (c) Profile prosthesis design with minimal space under the flange.

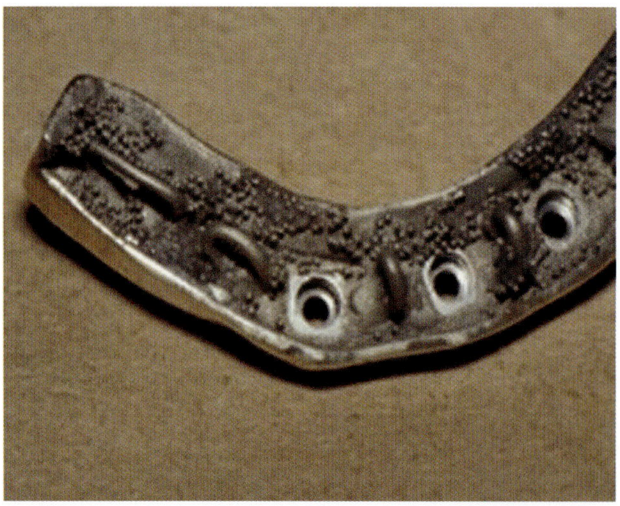

Figure 18.21 L-beam configuration of metal framework for implant fixed complete denture.

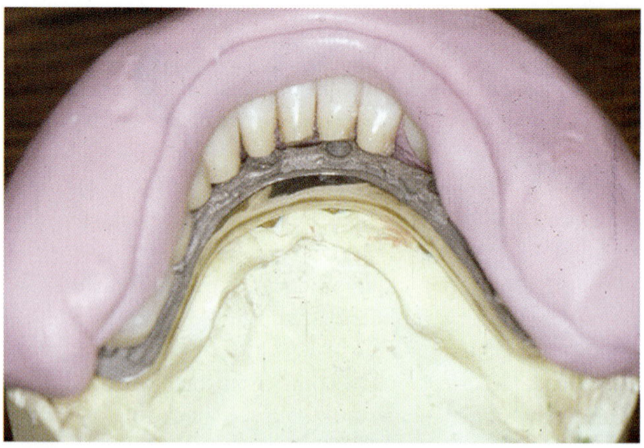

Figure 18.22 Putty cameo of denture tooth position and arrangement to confirm framework support.

alloys (50–60% palladium) has been shown to offer good rigidity, corrosion resistance, reduced cost, and favorable clinical comparisons to gold alloy after 5 years.[117] Milled CAD/CAM or CNC titanium frameworks have gained popularity as they facilitate a virtual review of design, which can incorporate nailhead retention units for each tooth (increasing fracture resistance of the denture teeth) and have been found to fit more precisely than frameworks fabricated by the lost wax technique (Figure 18.23a–g).[118–120] However, misfit of 100 μm has not been conclusively linked to marginal bone loss although it may encourage screw complications.[121,122] Notwithstanding the clinical insignificance of the precision of fit of the milled versus cast frameworks, efforts continue to improve the accuracy of impression techniques, such as minimizing the distortion of luting materials when splinting impression copings (Figure 18.23h–l),[123] digital scanning of the implants with polymer scan bodies,[124] and stereophotogrammetry.[125,126] The latter two techniques avoid the inconvenience of conventional impressions and ultimately promise more efficiency.

Another iteration using a milled component titanium framework to retain all-ceramic crowns (Figure 18.24a, b) has been clinically evaluated with favorable outcomes for up to 10 years of follow-up.[127] While crown fractures were not uncommon, they were more easily replaced because of the design and CAD/CAM fabrication. Despite these developments, patients with antagonist implant-supported restorations and/or high masticatory forces (parafunction) preferentially have had mechanical complications or heavy attrition (Figure 18.25a–c).[128] Anterior tooth fracture can be potentiated by a lack of horizontal overlap in the original occlusal scheme. Late mechanical failures of anterior tooth fracture are often due to attrition of the posterior teeth causing a collapse of the anterior coupling. Replacement of the teeth with nanofilled composite tooth materials has been recommended (Figure 18.25d) or, in the case of preferential posterior tooth wear, monolithic lithium disilicate onlays have been milled after a digital scan and bonded to the prepared denture teeth (Figure 18.25e–g).

Zirconia-based materials have recently gained traction as a replacement material for MRIFCDs in response to veneer/tooth fracture and attrition (Figure 18.26a–c). Aside from superior physical properties and biocompatibility, zirconia prostheses can be fabricated through a CAD/CAM process.[129] This feature allows an assessment by the clinician in the virtual design space and the facility of generating prototypes with polymethyl methacrylate to confirm and adjust intraoral fit, phonetics, occlusion, and esthetics (Figure 18.26c).[130] Evaluation of a replica of the definitive prosthesis is critical to refine the functional, phonetic, and esthetic parameters. Stress-generated surface treatment, such as grinding, will trigger the tetragonal and monoclinic phase transformation which may lead to higher incidence of mechanical complications.[131] Short-term biologic, prosthetic, and patient-centered outcomes have been reported. Limmer *et al.*[132] reported on 1-year results on 17 mandibular monolithic zirconia prostheses, finding a 99% implant and 88% prosthesis survival rate, but a concerning 59% complication rate. Technical problems prevailed over biologic events, most notably chipped antagonist denture teeth, fractured abutment, and fracture of one zirconia framework (1.7:1 CL:AP distance, 9 mm vertical height compared to a mean of 13.2 mm). A catastrophic failure could be the result of porosity in the zirconia blank, post-sintering damage (adjustments), or possibly a cantilever exceeding a 1.5 cantilever to AP distance or less than 10 mm in vertical height. Despite these findings, overall patient satisfaction scores reflected a significant improvement in therapy when compared to a properly fitted denture, which was corroborated in study with up to a 4-year follow-up.[130] In summary, the zirconia-based IFCD holds promise for a more maintenance-free restoration. Furthermore, the prospect of milling out a replica of the prosthesis to replace the problem prosthesis is also attractive. However, until longer-term studies divulge design and fabrication specifications, some caution should be exercised.

Immediate-load protocols

The All-on-4 concept for the edentulous mandible has capitalized on optimal foundation (>30 Ncm initial insertion torque) and the increased AP span offered by tilted terminal implants (Figure 18.27). Longitudinal reports of up to 10 years have been encouraging.[133–135] Prosthesis survival has been reported at 10 years to be 99.2% and the mean marginal bone loss (MBL) at 5 years was 1.81 mm. Smoking was associated with MBL 2.8 mm or greater. Mechanical complications were more common during the initial provisional phase with the all-acrylic conversion prosthesis.[136] This appears to be less frequent on the mandible because of the reduced integration time, but if it occurs, it may be damaging to the implants due to local loading. An analog index cast fabricated at the time of implant placement will facilitate repairs extraorally. In addition, quartz fiber (RTD Dental, Louisville, KY) or open-lattice metal mesh incorporated in the initial prosthesis may retard fracture. More recently, a digitally planned and fabricated (titanium bar reinforced) mandibular prosthesis has been reported to aid in a more efficient workflow and reduced fracture incidence.[137] When comparing single and double complete-arch All-on-4 prostheses over 5 years, Malo *et al.*[128] reported a majority of the complications occurred in the interim prostheses when opposing a similar prosthesis. Overall, mechanical complications, including fracture and abutment screw loosening were 16% and 13% for the double and single configurations, with 37.5% suspected of being heavy bruxers. Adjustment of occlusion at multiple appointments and manufacture of an orthotic was recommended. Biologic complications were not significantly different for the single and double implant reconstructions, at 5–6%.

Immediately restored complete-arch restorations in fresh extraction sites have been retrospectively evaluated over 3 years.[138] No significant differences were reported in implant survival or crestal bone levels compared to healed sites, unless cervical augmentation was introduced. Strub *et al.*[97] have underscored the

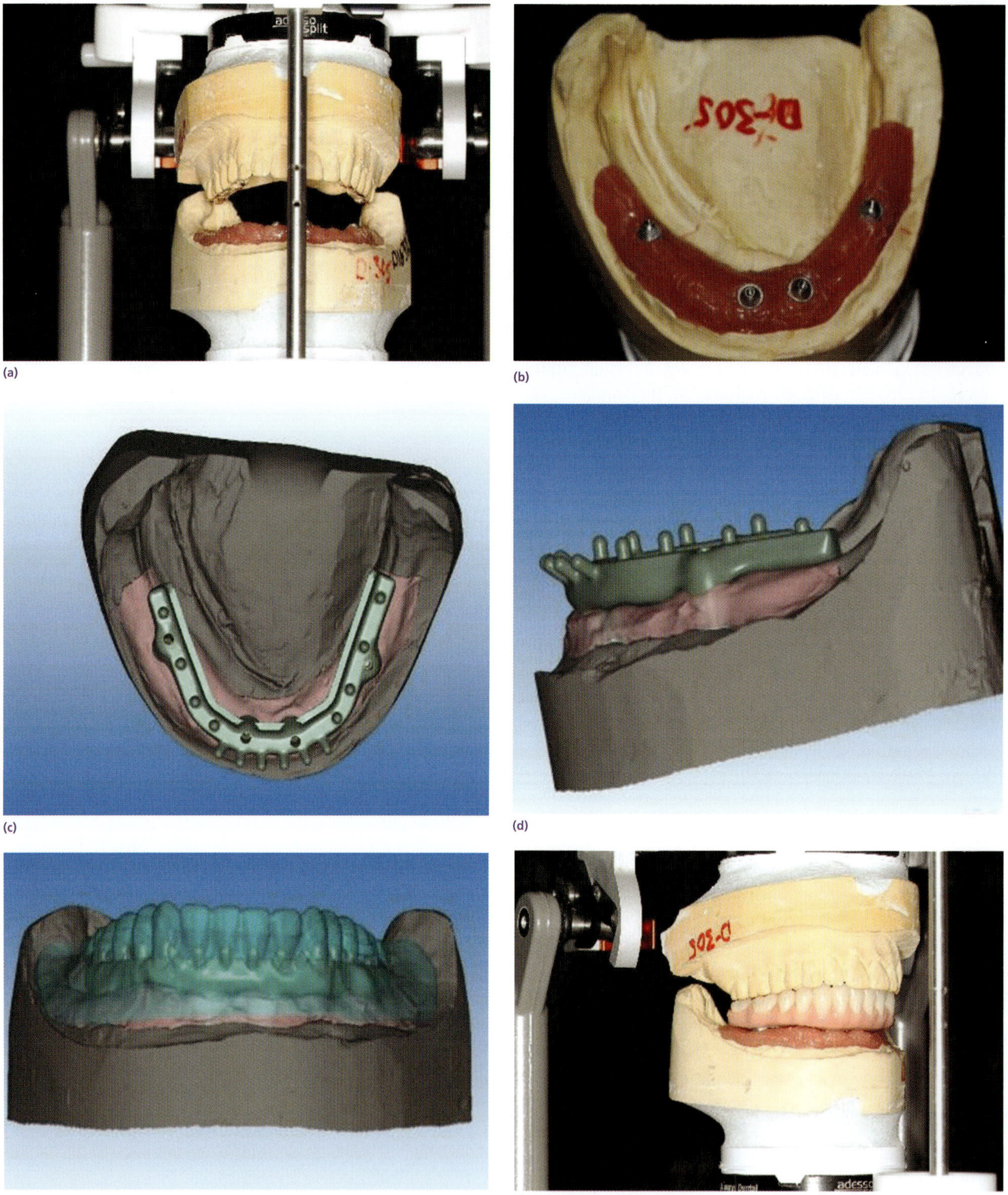

Figure 18.23 **(a)** Articulator mounting of soft tissue master cast for All-on-4 implant fixed complete denture design. **(b)** Soft tissue master cast of multi-unit abutment analogs (angled abutments in terminal positions). **(c)** Occlusal view of virtual milled bar design using nailhead retention for denture teeth. **(d)** Sagittal view of virtual milled bar design. **(e)** Frontal view of prosthesis superimposed over framework. **(f)** Processed implant fixed complete denture on articulator. **(g)** Intraoral view of implant fixed complete denture. **(h)** Alginate impression of open tray impression copings. **(i)** GC Pattern Resin (GC America, Alsip, IL) injected in alginate impression with reinforcing pins to incorporate in stone cast. **(j)** Fabrication of a Triad visible light-cured sheet material (Dentsply Int, York, PA) for impression tray and a second sheet to create a bridge around the impression copings without contacting them, to allow a minimal amount of luting material for splinting impression copings intraorally. **(k)** Triad bridge in place in preparation for GC Pattern Resin luting to each impression coping. **(l)** Definitive polyether. *Source for* **(h–l):** Bergin *et al.*, 2013.[126] Reproduced with permission from *The Journal of Prosthetic Dentistry*.

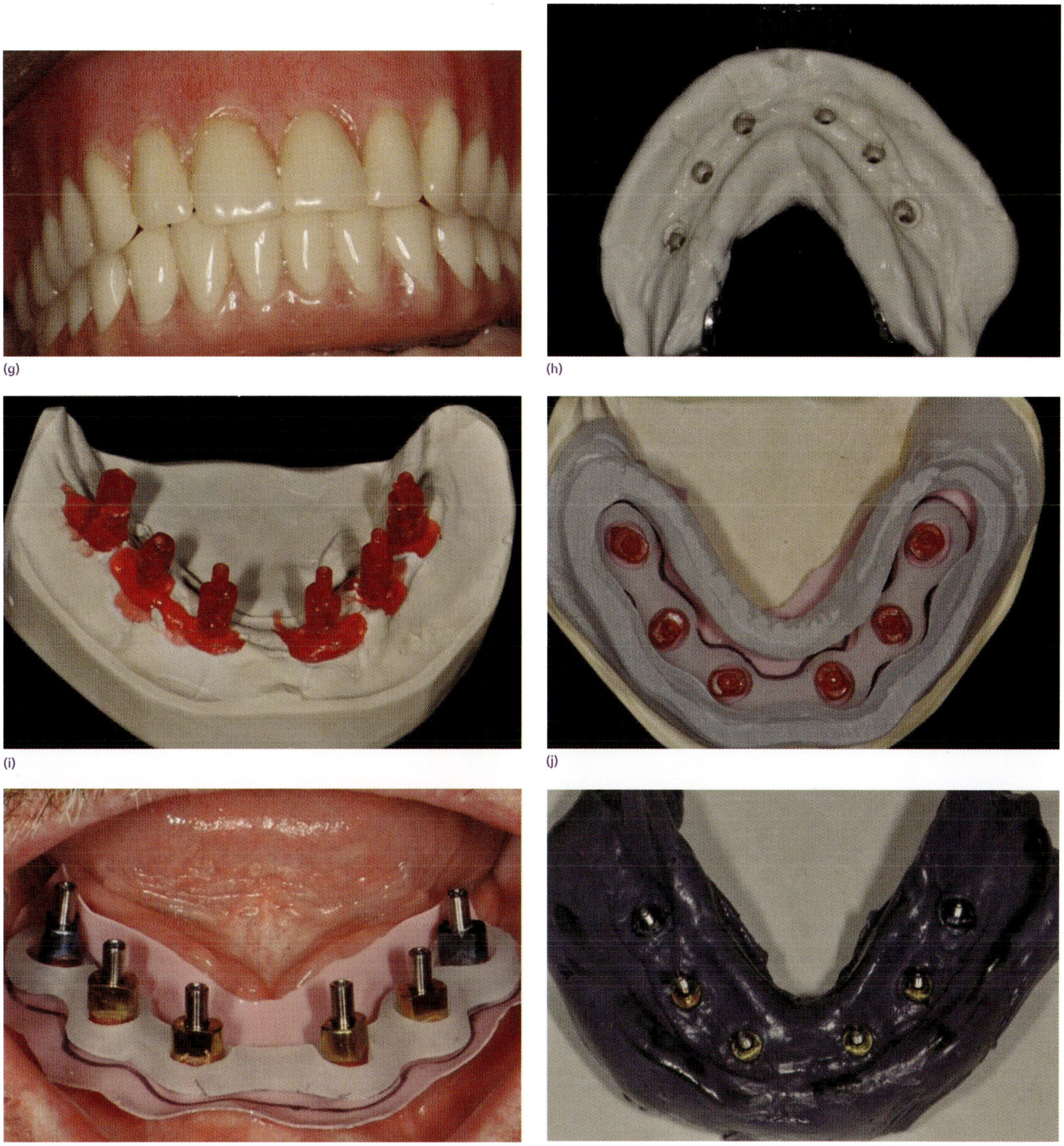

(g) (h) (i) (j) (k) (l)

Figure 18.23 (*Continued*)

importance of patient/operator selection (as elaborated earlier in chapter), primary implant stability, cross-arch stabilization, and at least 10 mm long implants for predictable long-term success. When eliciting patient-centered outcomes for this protocol, such as subjective feelings about comfort, function, speech, social image, social inhibitions, psychological discomfort, and overall satisfaction, 95% responded by being extremely satisfied (74%) or satisfied (21%).[139] In summary, the use of four mandibular splinted textured implants (10% failure with three implants), widely distributed in the appropriate patient, and executed with a careful protocol, has been shown to result in 0–3.3% implant failure rate and excellent patient-centered outcomes.[140]

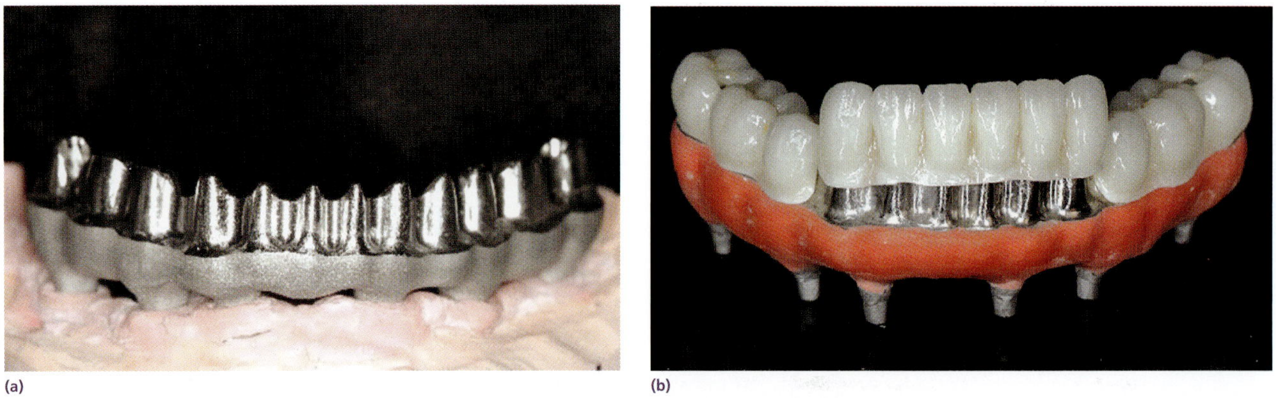

Figure 18.24 (a) Component framework design of implant fixed complete denture with individual copings fabricated for crowns. (b) Monolithic crown segments to be cemented to titanium milled framework. *Source:* Reproduced with permission from IDOC Dental Lab, Orange, CA.

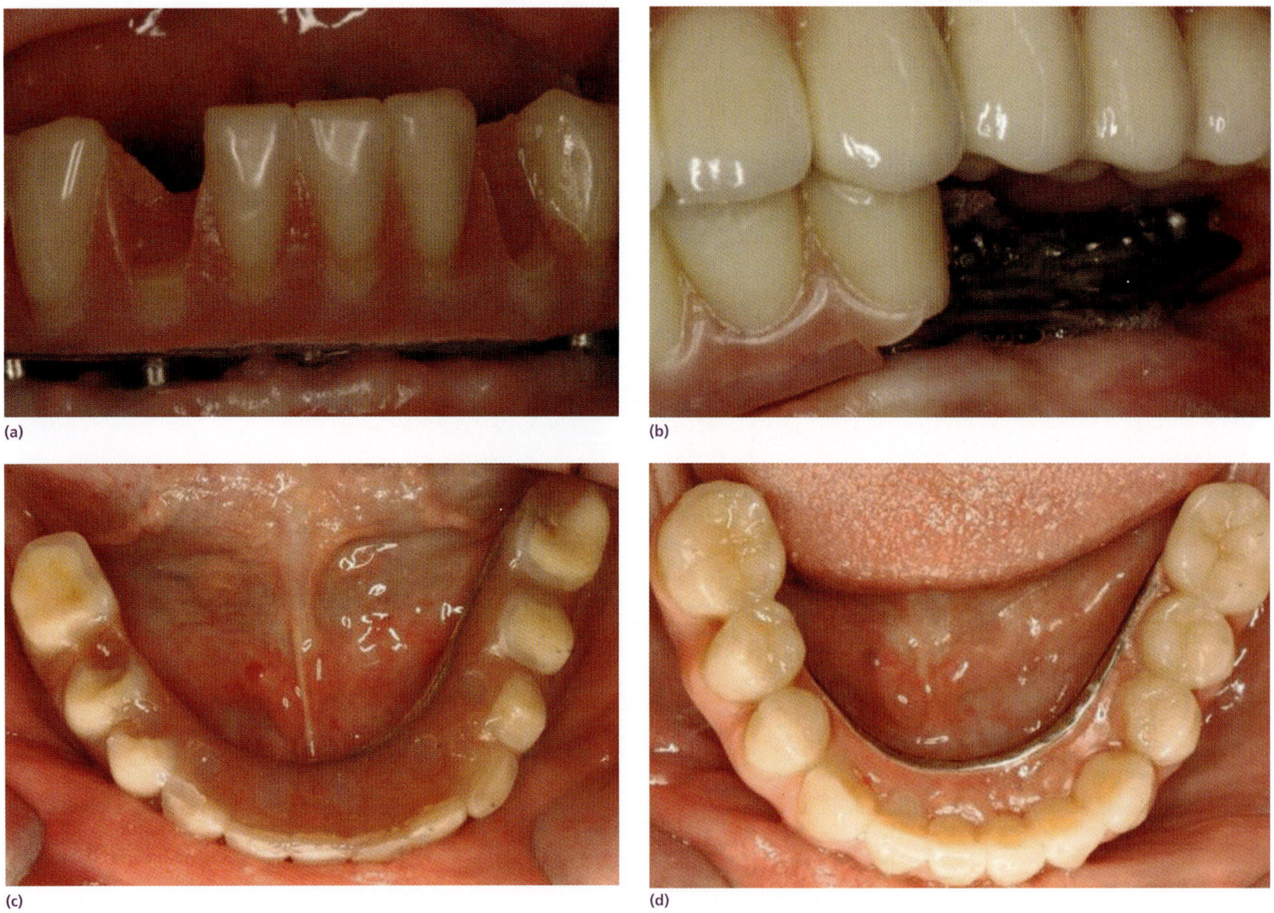

Figure 18.25 (a) Fractured denture teeth, most likely due to preferential anterior contact, protrusive interceptive contacts, and/or "food as a weapon". Processing error would show entire denture tooth lost from resin base. (b) Resin veneer fracture, most likely due to lack of framework support under teeth. (c) Heavy attrition of implant fixed complete denture after 6 years of service. (d) Replacement of all denture teeth with nano-filled composite denture tooth material. (e) Preferential wear noted on posterior denture teeth after 5 years of service. Posterior denture teeth were prepared and scanned for digital milling of onlay restorations. (f) Lithium disilicate splinted onlay crowns. (g) Restored posterior teeth on implant fixed complete denture.

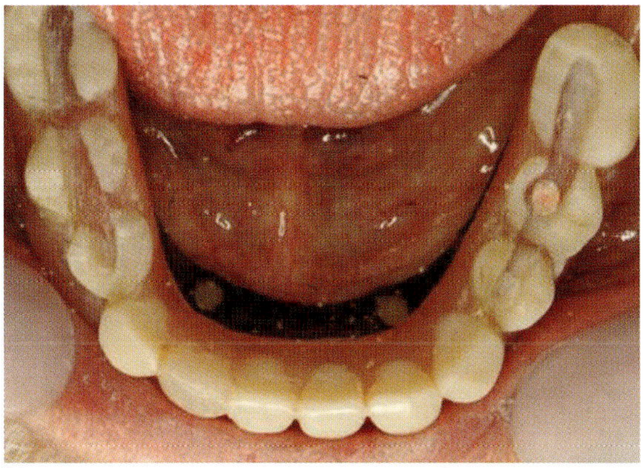

(e)

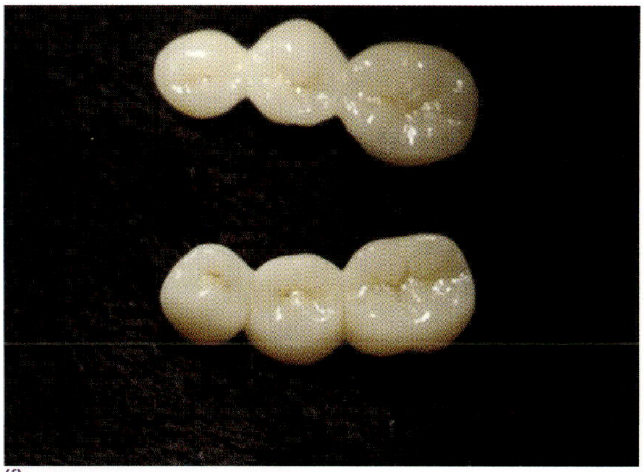

(f)

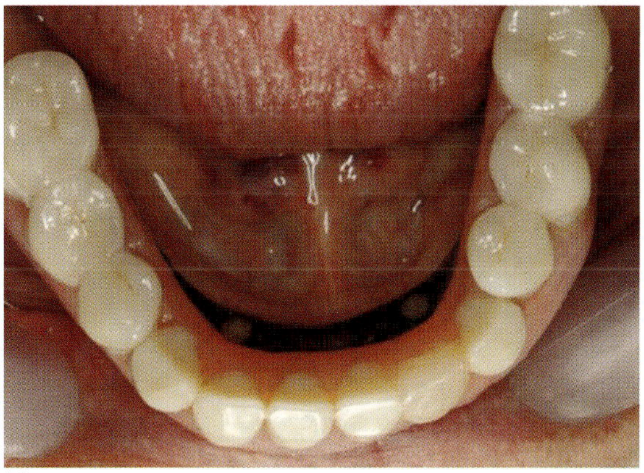

(g)

Figure 18.25 (*Continued*)

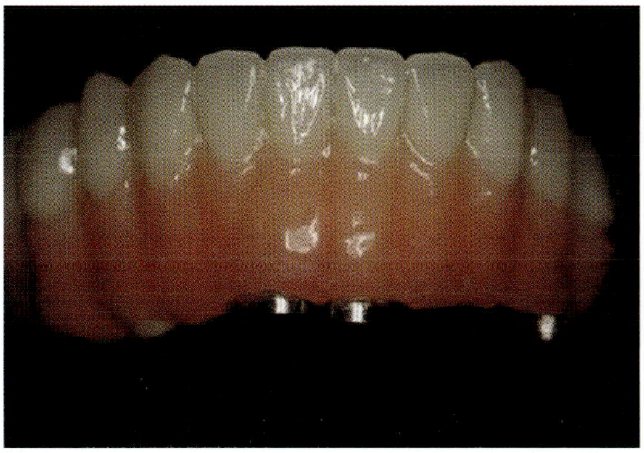

(a)

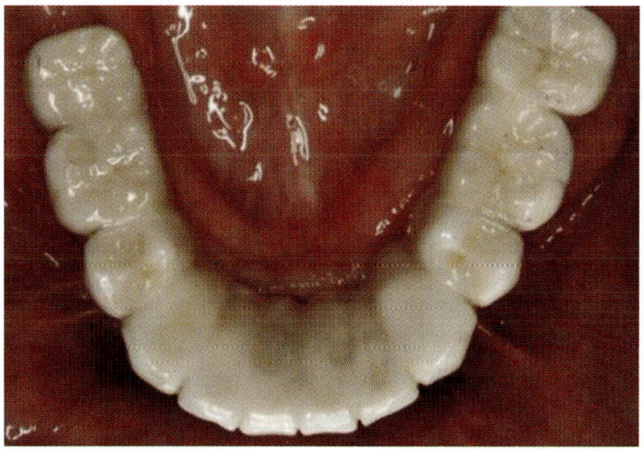

(b)

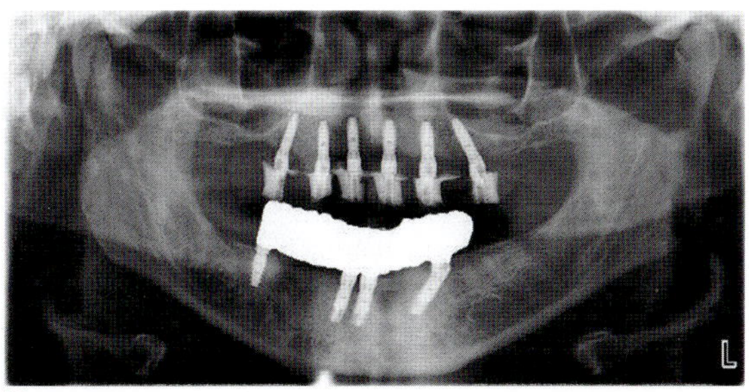

(c)

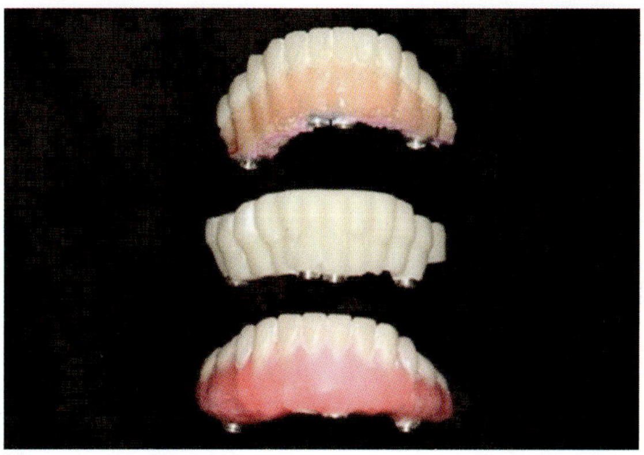

(d)

Figure 18.26 (**a**) Frontal view of zirconia implant fixed complete denture. (**b**) Intraoral occlusal view of zirconia implant fixed complete denture. (**c**) Orthopantomogram of mandibular zirconia implant fixed complete denture opposing an immediate provisional implant fixed complete denture. (**d**) Prototypes of zirconia implant fixed complete denture. The bottom view is in wax, the middle view is polymethyl methacrylate, and the top view is polymethyl methacrylate with gingival stain, and a low viscosity polyvinyl silicone impression pick-up of the soft tissue for the laboratory to scan.

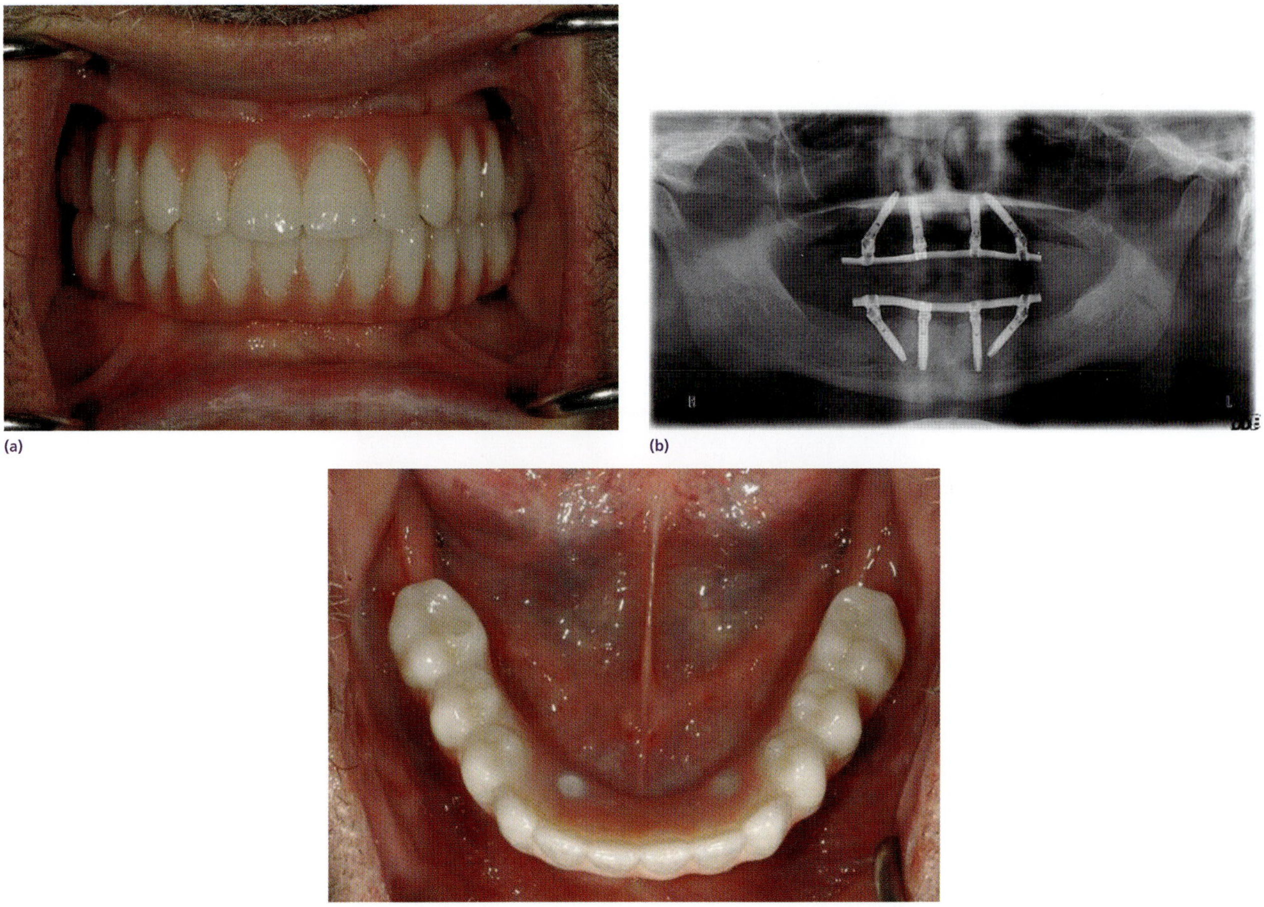

(a) (b) (c)

Figure 18.27 (a) All-on-4 mandibular and maxillary immediate prostheses. (b) Orthopantomogram of All-on-4 prostheses. (c) Definitive implant fixed complete denture. *Source:* Reproduced with permission from Daniel Galindo.

Fixed dental prostheses

For patients with limited alveolar resorption, a fixed dental prosthesis (FDP) accommodates a tooth-only defect with only 7 mm of interocclusal space. This design, while offering optimal esthetics, is more challenging because of the priority on placement of the implants congruent with the abutment crowns. Here the implant placement requires cantilevers and limits the number of segments for the prosthetic design (Figure 18.28). There is a paucity of longitudinal studies reporting on complete-arch metal–ceramic (MC) reconstructions, but Rasmusson *et al.*[141] reported a cumulative implant survival rate of 97.2% and an annual 0.15 mm bone loss after 10 years of tracking 10 mandibular MC prostheses. A 5-year investigation of MC reconstructions also revealed a similar high implant survival rate when the mean number of implants was greater than seven, and mean diameter 3.8 mm.[142] However, in square arches, it is appropriate to plan six micro-textured implants of 8–10 mm length in the cuspid, first bicuspid, and first molar region.[143] In tapered arches, an additional implant in the central incisor position will counter an anterior lever arm, especially important with cement-retained restorations.[144] In both scenarios, short-span FDPs (one six-unit and two three-unit segments) will facilitate casting and repair. Given that the number of segments is not related to implant survival (87%/15 years) in the completely edentulous scenario,[145] this design is especially helpful given the high incidence (38.7%/5 years) of technical failures reported.[146] Ceramic fracture, abutment loosening, and loss of retention were identified as most prevalent in that order. The lack of proprioception, minimal shock absorbing effect, presence of bruxism, and technical failure in the manufacturing process have all been implicated in high incidence of ceramic fracture of implant restorations. Kinsel *et al.*[147] reported that FDPs have seven times the ceramic fracture rate when opposed by another implant-supported restoration, or in bruxers, and two times higher odds when compared to patients without bruxism and not wearing an occlusal guard.

Zirconia has been suggested as a substitute for metal–ceramic materials when restoring a complete-arch implant restoration.[148] A recent systematic review suggests that while the 3–5-year implant survival rate is excellent, there was a 30.5% incidence of complications, mostly mechanical fractures, when monolithic

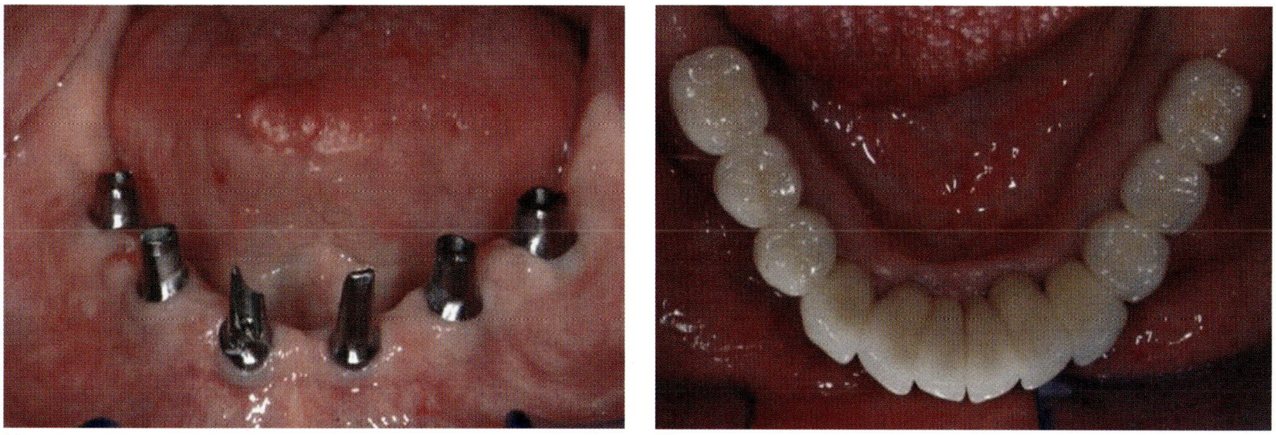

(a) (b)

Figure 18.28 (a) Implant placement limiting the design of the prosthetic sections. (b) Two prosthetic sections with cantilevers in the central incisor position. Implants placed in the cuspid rather than lateral incisor position would have facilitated three sections without cantilevers.

zirconium was veneered with feldspathic porcelain, a 10% increase from tooth-borne zirconia-based restorations.[149] Analysis of crack propagation showed that the chipping failure was due to roughness of the ceramic at the level of the cusps.[148] Occlusal adjustments should follow a strict sequence, beginning with fine-grain diamonds, followed by a series of polishing wheels (Dialite line [including ZR and LD], Brasseler USA, Savannah, GA). Moreover, Venezia *et al.*[150] noted that when veneering porcelain was limited to nonfunctional areas rather than covering the incisal margin, this led to more robust connectors and increased resistance to occlusal loading. With that being said, high wear rates have been reported on the antagonist natural dentition from monolithic zirconia. The hardness and thickness of enamel, chewing behavior, bruxism patterns, maximum bite force, and abrasive nature of food all may potentiate clinical attrition. However, some reports have shown that polished zirconia has the lowest wear rate on enamel as compared to veneered zirconia, glazed zirconia, monolithic base alloy, or glazed zirconia using glazed ceramic.[151,152] In summary, the vast majority of the studies on zirconia-based implant restorations are not controlled clinical trials and have limited follow-up. Thus, interpretation of the results should be made with caution.

Immediate-load protocols

The immediate loading concept for the edentulous mandible has been reported for fixed restorations, at an implant survival rate of 90–100% with up to 10 years of follow-up.[153] No differences have been documented when immediate, early, and delayed loading are compared. Primary stability of at least 30 Ncm has been reported as a prerequisite for immediate loading. Resonance frequency analysis (Osstell/Integration Diagnostics, Goteborg, Sweden) has also been employed (65 ± 6.5 ISQ units) to assess adequate initial stability before loading.[154] The use of a cast reinforced provisional restoration to thwart fracture has been recommended, but is controversial.[154–156] The design most prevalently used is a one-piece provisional prosthesis for cross-arch stabilization during the integration phase. However, six to eight implants allow for more easily cast and repaired segmented prostheses when the definitive restoration is placed.[145] Periodic removal of provisional restorations during the 3-month healing period for suture removal, implant stability assessment, soft tissue evaluation, adjustment of contours, and professional cleaning has been recommended but not unanimously embraced.[154,157,158] Newer studies document prosthetic complications of the definitive MC restoration as between 3.2% and 25.5% fracture of the veneer material over a 5-year observation period.[159] Screw-retained designs have been documented to have overall fewer complications than cement-retained restorations.[160] Conversion from a polymethyl methacrylate resin provisional restoration to zirconia FDPs with limited veneering porcelain on the facial surfaces, to both retard fracture incidence and improve esthetics, has shown promise.[131] Longitudinal comparative studies are needed to evaluate various material and design differences for the definitive FDP restoration.

Summary

The mandibular denture cripple was the first and foremost beneficiary of Branemark's serendipitous discovery of osseointegration. What has been equally impressive has been the cascade of permutations of design, materials, and loading protocols that have continued the innovative chain to meet patient needs. Treatment planning decisions are more nuanced than ever before as we exceed the promise of implant survival to arrive at cost-effective and high quality-of-life outcomes for patients. The best available externally valid literature will continue to refine our ability to treat predictably our patients, taking account of an array of systemic, local, and socioeconomic factors.

References

1. Thomason JM, Kelly SA, Bendkowski A, *et al.* Two implant retained overdentures – a review of the literature supporting the McGill and York consensus statements. *J Dent* 2012; **40**(1): 22–34.
2. Feine JS, Carlsson GE, Awad MA, *et al.* The McGill consensus statement on overdentures. Mandibular two-implant overdentures as first choice standard of care for edentulous patients. Montreal, Quebec, May 24–25, 2002. *Int J Oral Maxillofac Implants* 2002; **17**(4): 601–602.
3. Fitzpatrick B. Standard of care for the edentulous mandible: a systematic review. *J Prosthet Dent* 2006; **95**(1): 71–78.
4. Slade GD, Akinkugbe AA, Sanders AE. Projections of US edentulism prevalence following 5 decades of decline. *J Dent Res* 2014; **93**(10): 959–965.
5. Dudley J. Implants for the ageing population. *Aust Dent J* 2015; **60**(Suppl 1): 28–43.
6. Calvert G, Thomason JM, Ellis JS. Are implant supported overdentures too complex to be included in the undergraduate curriculum? *Eur J Prosthodont Restor Dent* 2012; **20**(4): 176–180.
7. Muller F, Salem K, Barbezat C, *et al.* Knowledge and attitude of elderly persons towards dental implants. *Gerodontology* 2012; **29**(2): e914–923.
8. Thomason JM. The use of mandibular implant-retained overdentures improve patient satisfaction and quality of life. *J Evid Based Dent Pract* 2012; **12**(3 Suppl): 182–184.
9. Muller F, Naharro M, Carlsson GE. What are the prevalence and incidence of tooth loss in the adult and elderly population in Europe? *Clin Oral Implants Res* 2007; **18**(Suppl 3): 2–14.
10. Bryant SR, Zarb GA. Osseointegration of oral implants in older and younger adults. *Int J Oral Maxillofac Implants* 1998; **13**(4): 492–499.
11. Al Jabbari Y, Nagy WW, Iacopino AM. Implant dentistry for geriatric patients: a review of the literature. *Quintessence Int* 2003; **34**(4): 281–285.
12. de Baat C. Success of dental implants in elderly people – a literature review. *Gerodontology* 2000; **17**(1): 45–48.
13. Engfors I, Ortorp A, Jemt T. Fixed implant-supported prostheses in elderly patients: a 5-year retrospective study of 133 edentulous patients older than 79 years. *Clin Implant Dent Relat Res* 2004; **6**(4): 190–198.
14. Jemt T. Implant treatment in elderly patients. *Int J Prosthodont* 1993; **6**(5): 456–461.
15. Hwang D, Wang HL. Medical contraindications to implant therapy. Part I: absolute contraindications. *Implant Dent* 2006; **15**(4): 353–360.
16. Bornstein MM, Cionca N, Mombelli A. Systemic conditions and treatments as risks for implant therapy. *Int J Oral Maxillofac Implants* 2009; **24**(Suppl): 12–27.
17. Ekfeldt A, Christiansson U, Eriksson T, *et al.* A retrospective analysis of factors associated with multiple implant failures in maxillae. *Clin Oral Implants Res* 2001; **12**(5): 462–467.
18. Hwang D, Wang HL. Medical contraindications to implant therapy. Part II: relative contraindications. *Implant Dent* 2007; **16**(1): 13–23.
19. Violan C, Foguet-Boreu Q, Flores-Mateo G, *et al.* Prevalence, determinants and patterns of multimorbidity in primary care: a systematic review of observational studies. *PLoS One* 2014; **9**(7): e102149.
20. Looker AC, Borrud LG, Hughes JP, *et al.* Total body bone area, bone mineral content, and bone mineral density for individuals aged 8 years and over: United States, 1999–2006. *Vital Health Stat 11* 2013; **253**: 1–78.
21. Giro G, Chambrone L, Goldstein A, *et al.* Impact of osteoporosis in dental implants: a systematic review. *World J Orthop* 2015; **6**(2): 311–315.
22. Bryant SR, Zarb GA. Crestal bone loss proximal to oral implants in older and younger adults. *J Prosthet Dent* 2003; **89**(6): 589–597.
23. Tallarico M, Canullo L, Xhanari E, *et al.* Dental implants treatment outcomes in patient under active therapy with alendronate: 3-year follow-up results of a multicenter prospective observational study. *Clin Oral Implants Res* 2015.
24. August M, Chung K, Chang Y, *et al.* Influence of estrogen status on endosseous implant osseointegration. *J Oral Maxillofac Surg* 2001; **59**(11): 1285–1289.
25. Wu X, Al-Abedalla K, Rastikerdar E, *et al.* Selective serotonin reuptake inhibitors and the risk of osseointegrated implant failure: a cohort study. *J Dent Res* 2014; **93**(11): 1054–1061.
26. Moy PK, Medina D, Shetty V, *et al.* Dental implant failure rates and associated risk factors. *Int J Oral Maxillofac Implants* 2005; **20**(4): 569–577.
27. Butura CC, Galindo DF, Cottam J, *et al.* Hourglass mandibular anatomic variant incidence and treatment considerations for all-on-four implant therapy: report of 10 cases. *J Oral Maxillofac Surg* 2011; **69**(8): 2135–2143.
28. Chan HL, Benavides E, Yeh CY, *et al.* Risk assessment of lingual plate perforation in posterior mandibular region: a virtual implant placement study using cone-beam computed tomography. *J Periodontol* 2011; **82**(1): 129–135.
29. den Dunnen AC, Slagter AP, de Baat C, *et al.* Adjustments and complications of mandibular overdentures retained by four implants. A comparison between superstructures with and without cantilever extensions. *Int J Prosthodont* 1998; **11**(4): 307–311.
30. Topkaya T, Solmaz MY. The effect of implant number and position on the stress behavior of mandibular implant retained overdentures: a three-dimensional finite element analysis. *J Biomech* 2015; **48**(10): 2102–2109.
31. Sadowsky SJ. Mandibular implant-retained overdentures: a literature review. *J Prosthet Dent* 2001; **86**(5): 468–473.
32. Sarmento HR, Dantas RV, Pereira-Cenci T, *et al.* Elements of implant-supported rehabilitation planning in patients with bruxism. *J Craniofac Surg* 2012; **23**(6): 1905–1909.
33. Glaros AG, Rao SM. Effects of bruxism: a review of the literature. *J Prosthet Dent* 1977; **38**(2): 149–157.
34. Parel SM, Phillips WR. A risk assessment treatment planning protocol for the four implant immediately loaded maxilla: preliminary findings. *J Prosthet Dent* 2011; **106**(6): 359–366.
35. Phillips K, Wong KM. Vertical space requirement for the fixed-detachable, implant-supported prosthesis. *Compend Contin Educ Dent* 2002; **23**(8): 750–756.
36. Phillips K, Wong KM. Space requirements for implant-retained bar-and-clip overdentures. *Compend Contin Educ Dent* 2001; **22**(6): 516–522.
37. Hunt K, Turk M. Bioesthetic dentistry, part 4. *Dent Today* 2012; **31**(6): 102–107.
38. Sadowsky SJ, Hansen PW. Evidence-based criteria for differential treatment planning of implant restorations for the mandibular edentulous patient. *J Prosthodont* 2014; **23**(2): 104–111.
39. Zitzmann NU, Sendi P, Marinello CP. An economic evaluation of implant treatment in edentulous patients-preliminary results. *Int J Prosthodont* 2005; **18**(1): 20–27.

40. Attard N, Wei X, Laporte A, *et al.* A cost minimization analysis of implant treatment in mandibular edentulous patients. *Int J Prosthodont* 2003; **16**(3): 271–276.
41. Attard NJ, Zarb GA, Laporte A. Long-term treatment costs associated with implant-supported mandibular prostheses in edentulous patients. *Int J Prosthodont* 2005; **18**(2): 117–123.
42. de Grandmont P, Feine JS, Tache R, *et al.* Within-subject comparisons of implant-supported mandibular prostheses: psychometric evaluation. *J Dent Res* 1994; **73**(5): 1096–1104.
43. Feine JS, de Grandmont P, Boudrias P, *et al.* Within-subject comparisons of implant-supported mandibular prostheses: choice of prosthesis. *J Dent Res* 1994; **73**(5): 1105–1111.
44. Cochran DL, Schou S, Heitz-Mayfield LJ, *et al.* Consensus statements and recommended clinical procedures regarding risk factors in implant therapy. *Int J Oral Maxillofac Implants* 2009; **24**(Suppl): 86–89.
45. Emami E, Heydecke G, Rompre PH, *et al.* Impact of implant support for mandibular dentures on satisfaction, oral and general health-related quality of life: a meta-analysis of randomized-controlled trials. *Clin Oral Implants Res* 2009; **20**(6): 533–544.
46. Awad MA, Lund JP, Shapiro SH, *et al.* Oral health status and treatment satisfaction with mandibular implant overdentures and conventional dentures: a randomized clinical trial in a senior population. *Int J Prosthodont* 2003; **16**(4): 390–396.
47. Raghoebar GM, Meijer HJ, van 't Hof M, *et al.* A randomized prospective clinical trial on the effectiveness of three treatment modalities for patients with lower denture problems. A 10 year follow-up study on patient satisfaction. *Int J Oral Maxillofac Surg* 2003; **32**(5): 498–503.
48. Pan S, Dagenais M, Thomason JM, *et al.* Does mandibular edentulous bone height affect prosthetic treatment success? *J Dent* 2010; **38**(11): 899–907.
49. Pan YH, Lin TM, Liang CH. Comparison of patient's satisfaction with implant-supported mandibular overdentures and complete dentures. *Biomed J* 2014; **37**(3): 156–162.
50. Lin YC, Chen JH, Lee HE, *et al.* The association of chewing ability and diet in elderly complete denture patients. *Int J Prosthodont* 2010; **23**(2): 127–128.
51. Khoo HD, Chai J, Chow TW. Prosthetic outcome, patient com plaints, and nutritional effects on elderly patients with magnet-retained, implant-supported overdentures – a 1-year report. *Int J Oral Maxillofac Implants* 2013; **28**(5): 1278–1285.
52. Tallgren A. The continuing reduction of the residual alveolar ridges in complete denture wearers: a mixed-longitudinal study covering 25 years. 1972. *J Prosthet Dent* 2003; **89**(5): 427–435.
53. van Steenberghe D, Quirynen M, Naert I, *et al.* Marginal bone loss around implants retaining hinging mandibular overdentures, at 4-, 8- and 12-years follow-up. *J Clin Periodontol* 2001; **28**(7): 628–633.
54. Naert I, Alsaadi G, van Steenberghe D, *et al.* A 10-year randomized clinical trial on the influence of splinted and unsplinted oral implants retaining mandibular overdentures: peri-implant outcome. *Int J Oral Maxillofac Implants* 2004; **19**(5): 695–702.
55. Cehreli MC, Karasoy D, Kokat AM, *et al.* A systematic review of marginal bone loss around implants retaining or supporting overdentures. *Int J Oral Maxillofac Implants* 2010; **25**(2): 266–277.
56. Ma S, Tawse-Smith A, Thomson WM, *et al.* Marginal bone loss with mandibular two-implant overdentures using different loading protocols and attachment systems: 10-year outcomes. *Int J Prosthodont* 2010; **23**(4): 321–332.
57. Chen J, Ahmad R, Suenaga H, *et al.* A comparative study on complete and implant retained denture treatments: a biomechanics perspective. *J Biomech* 2015; **48**(3): 512–519.
58. Jacobs R, Schotte A, van Steenberghe D, Quirynen M, *et al.* Posterior jaw bone resorption in osseointegrated implant-supported overdentures. *Clin Oral Implants Res* 1992; **3**(2): 63–70.
59. Davis WH, Lam PS, Marshall MW, *et al.* Using restorations borne totally by anterior implants to preserve the edentulous mandible. *J Am Dent Assoc* 1999; **130**(8): 1183–1189.
60. Mumcu E, Bilhan H, Geckili O. The effect of attachment type and implant number on satisfaction and quality of life of mandibular implant-retained overdenture wearers. *Gerodontology* 2012; **29**(2): e618–623.
61. Batenburg RH, Raghoebar GM, Van Oort RP, *et al.* Mandibular overdentures supported by two or four endosteal implants. A prospective, comparative study. *Int J Oral Maxillofac Surg* 1998; **27**(6): 435–439.
62. Visser A, Raghoebar GM, Meijer HJ, *et al.* Mandibular overdentures supported by two or four endosseous implants. A 5-year prospective study. *Clin Oral Implants Res* 2005; **16**(1): 19–25.
63. Mericske-Stern RD, Taylor TD, Belser U. Management of the edentulous patient. *Clin Oral Implants Res* 2000; **11**(Suppl 1): 108–125.
64. Bryant SR, Walton JN, MacEntee MI. A 5-year randomized trial to compare 1 or 2 implants for implant overdentures. *J Dent Res* 2015; **94**(1): 36–43.
65. Stoker GT, Wismeijer D, van Waas MA. An eight-year follow-up to a randomized clinical trial of aftercare and cost-analysis with three types of mandibular implant-retained overdentures. *J Dent Res* 2007; **86**(3): 276–280.
66. Klemetti E. Is there a certain number of implants needed to retain an overdenture? *J Oral Rehabil* 2008; **35**(Suppl 1): 80–84.
67. Dudic A, Mericske-Stern R. Retention mechanisms and prosthetic complications of implant-supported mandibular overdentures: long-term results. *Clin Implant Dent Relat Res* 2002; **4**(4): 212–219.
68. Bressan E, Tomasi C, Stellini E, *et al.* Implant-supported mandibular overdentures: a cross-sectional study. *Clin Oral Implants Res* 2012; **23**(7): 814–819.
69. Zou D, Wu Y, Huang W, *et al.* A 3-year prospective clinical study of telescopic crown, bar, and locator attachments for removable four implant-supported maxillary overdentures. *Int J Prosthodont* 2013; **26**(6): 566–573.
70. Krennmair G, Seemann R, Fazekas A, *et al.* Patient preference and satisfaction with implant-supported mandibular overdentures retained with ball or locator attachments: a crossover clinical trial. *Int J Oral Maxillofac Implants* 2012; **27**(6): 1560–1568.
71. Mackie A, Lyons K, Thomson WM, *et al.* Mandibular two-implant overdentures: three-year prosthodontic maintenance using the locator attachment system. *Int J Prosthodont* 2011; **24**(4): 328–331.
72. Payne AG, Solomons YF. The prosthodontic maintenance requirements of mandibular mucosa- and implant-supported overdentures: a review of the literature. *Int J Prosthodont* 2000; **13**(3): 238–243.
73. Payne AG, Solomons YF. Mandibular implant-supported overdentures: a prospective evaluation of the burden of prosthodontic maintenance with 3 different attachment systems. *Int J Prosthodont* 2000; **13**(3): 246–253.
74. Sadowsky SJ. The bilateral distal extension base removable partial denture. *J Calif Dent Assoc* 1992; **20**(1): 59–62.

75. Toljanic JA, Antoniou D, Clark RS, *et al.* A longitudinal clinical assessment of spark erosion technology in implant-retained overdenture prostheses: a preliminary report. *J Prosthet Dent* 1997; **78**(5): 490–495.
76. Weinlander M, Piehslinger E, Krennmair G. Removable implant-prosthodontic rehabilitation of the edentulous mandible: five-year results of different prosthetic anchorage concepts. *Int J Oral Maxillofac Implants* 2010; **25**(3): 589–597.
77. Krennmair G, Krainhofner M, Piehslinger E. The influence of bar design (round versus milled bar) on prosthodontic maintenance of mandibular overdentures supported by 4 implants: a 5-year prospective study. *Int J Prosthodont* 2008; **21**(6): 514–520.
78. Sadowsky SJ. Immediate load on the edentulous mandible: treatment planning considerations. *J Prosthodont* 2010; **19**(8): 647–653.
79. Alfadda SA, Attard NJ, David LA. Five-year clinical results of immediately loaded dental implants using mandibular overdentures. *Int J Prosthodont* 2009; **22**(4): 368–373.
80. Attard NJ, Laporte A, Locker D, *et al.* A prospective study on immediate loading of implants with mandibular overdentures: patient-mediated and economic outcomes. *Int J Prosthodont* 2006; **19**(1): 67–73.
81. Assad AS, Hassan SA, Shawky YM, *et al.* Clinical and radiographic evaluation of implant-retained mandibular overdentures with immediate loading. *Implant Dent* 2007; **16**(2): 212–223.
82. Chiapasco M, Gatti C. Implant-retained mandibular overdentures with immediate loading: a 3- to 8-year prospective study on 328 implants. *Clin Implant Dent Relat Res* 2003; **5**(1): 29–38.
83. Gallucci GO, Morton D, Weber HP. Loading protocols for dental implants in edentulous patients. *Int J Oral Maxillofac Implants* 2009; **24**(Suppl): 132–146.
84. Attard NJ, David LA, Zarb GA. Immediate loading of implants with mandibular overdentures: one-year clinical results of a prospective study. *Int J Prosthodont* 2005; **18**(6): 463–470.
85. Roe P, Kan JY, Rungcharassaeng K, *et al.* Immediate loading of unsplinted implants in the anterior mandible for overdentures: 3-year results. *Int J Oral Maxillofac Implants* 2011; **26**(6): 1296–1302.
86. Marzola R, Scotti R, Fazi G, *et al.* Immediate loading of two implants supporting a ball attachment-retained mandibular overdenture: a prospective clinical study. *Clin Implant Dent Relat Res* 2007; **9**(3): 136–143.
87. Ormianer Z, Garg AK, Palti A. Immediate loading of implant overdentures using modified loading protocol. *Implant Dent* 2006; **15**(1): 35–40.
88. Cooper LF, Scurria MS, Lang LA, *et al.* Treatment of edentulism using Astra Tech implants and ball abutments to retain mandibular overdentures. *Int J Oral Maxillofac Implants* 1999; **14**(5): 646–653.
89. Liddelow G, Henry P. The immediately loaded single implant-retained mandibular overdenture: a 36-month prospective study. *Int J Prosthodont* 2010; **23**(1): 13–21.
90. Esposito M, Grusovin MG, Willings M, *et al.* The effectiveness of immediate, early, and conventional loading of dental implants: a Cochrane systematic review of randomized controlled clinical trials. *Int J Oral Maxillofac Implants* 2007; **22**(6): 893–904.
91. Zarb GA, Albrektsson T. Consensus report: towards optimized treatment outcomes for dental implants. *J Prosthet Dent* 1998; **80**(6): 641.
92. Wismeijer D, Van Waas MA, Vermeeren JI, *et al.* Patient satisfaction with implant-supported mandibular overdentures. A comparison of three treatment strategies with ITI-dental implants. *Int J Oral Maxillofac Surg* 1997; **26**(4): 263–267.
93. Misch CE, Wang HL, Misch CM, *et al.* Rationale for the application of immediate load in implant dentistry: part II. *Implant Dent* 2004; **13**(4): 310–321.
94. Nedir R, Bischof M, Szmukler-Moncler S, *et al.* Predicting osseointegration by means of implant primary stability. *Clin Oral Implants Res* 2004; **15**(5): 520–528.
95. Norton MR. Multiple single-tooth implant restorations in the posterior jaws: maintenance of marginal bone levels with reference to the implant-abutment microgap. *Int J Oral Maxillofac Implants* 2006; **21**(5): 777–784.
96. Nikellis I, Levi A, Nicolopoulos C. Immediate loading of 190 endosseous dental implants: a prospective observational study of 40 patient treatments with up to 2-year data. *Int J Oral Maxillofac Implants* 2004; **19**(1): 116–123.
97. Strub JR, Jurdzik BA, Tuna T. Prognosis of immediately loaded implants and their restorations: a systematic literature review. *J Oral Rehabil* 2012; **39**(9): 704–717.
98. Henry PJ, Bower RC, Wall CD. Rehabilitation of the edentulous mandible with osseointegrated dental implants: 10 year follow-up. *Aust Dent J* 1995; **40**(1): 1–9.
99. Bergendal T, Magnusson T. Changes in signs and symptoms of temporomandibular disorders following treatment with implant-supported fixed prostheses: a prospective 3-year follow up. *Int J Prosthodont* 2000; **13**(5): 392–398.
100. Wright PS, Glantz PO, Randow K, *et al.* The effects of fixed and removable implant-stabilised prostheses on posterior mandibular residual ridge resorption. *Clin Oral Implants Res* 2002; **13**(2): 169–174.
101. Turkyilmaz I, Tozum TF. 30-Year outcomes of dental implants supporting mandibular fixed dental prostheses: a retrospective review of 4 cases. *Implant Dent* 2015; **24**(5): 620–624.
102. Astrand P, Ahlqvist J, Gunne J, *et al.* Implant treatment of patients with edentulous jaws: a 20-year follow-up. *Clin Implant Dent Relat Res* 2008; **10**(4): 207–217.
103. Priest G, Smith J, Wilson MG. Implant survival and prosthetic complications of mandibular metal-acrylic resin implant complete fixed dental prostheses. *J Prosthet Dent* 2014; **111**(6): 466–475.
104. Dhima M, Paulusova V, Lohse C, *et al.* Practice-based evidence from 29-year outcome analysis of management of the edentulous jaw using osseointegrated dental implants. *J Prosthodont* 2014; **23**(3): 173–181.
105. Purcell BA, McGlumphy EA, Holloway JA, *et al.* Prosthetic complications in mandibular metal-resin implant-fixed complete dental prostheses: a 5- to 9-year analysis. *Int J Oral Maxillofac Implants* 2008; **23**(5): 847–857.
106. Bozini T, Petridis H, Garefis K, *et al.* A meta-analysis of prosthodontic complication rates of implant-supported fixed dental prostheses in edentulous patients after an observation period of at least 5 years. *Int J Oral Maxillofac Implants* 2011; **26**(2): 304–318.
107. Papaspyridakos P, Chen CJ, Chuang SK, *et al.* A systematic review of biologic and technical complications with fixed implant rehabilitations for edentulous patients. *Int J Oral Maxillofac Implants* 2012; **27**(1): 102–110.
108. Cooper LF, Limmer BM, Gates WD. "Rules of 10" – guidelines for successful planning and treatment of mandibular edentulism using dental implants. *Compend Contin Educ Dent* 2012; **33**(5): 328–334.
109. English CE. Critical A-P spread. *Implant Soc* 1990; **1**(1): 2–3.

110. Kim KS, Kim YL, Bae JM, *et al.* Biomechanical comparison of axial and tilted implants for mandibular full-arch fixed prostheses. *Int J Oral Maxillofac Implants* 2011; **26**(5): 976–984.
111. Bellini CM, Romeo D, Galbusera F, *et al.* Comparison of tilted versus nontilted implant-supported prosthetic designs for the restoration of the edentuous mandible: a biomechanical study. *Int J Oral Maxillofac Implants* 2009; **24**(3): 511–517.
112. Krekmanov L, Kahn M, Rangert B, *et al.* Tilting of posterior mandibular and maxillary implants for improved prosthesis support. *Int J Oral Maxillofac Implants* 2000; **15**(3): 405–414.
113. Monje A, Chan HL, Suarez F, *et al.* Marginal bone loss around tilted implants in comparison to straight implants: a meta-analysis. *Int J Oral Maxillofac Implants* 2012; **27**(6): 1576–1583.
114. Del Fabbro M, Ceresoli V. The fate of marginal bone around axial vs. tilted implants: a systematic review. *Eur J Oral Implantol* 2014; **7**(Suppl 2): S171–189.
115. Zarb GA, Zarb FL. Tissue integrated dental prostheses. *Quintessence Int* 1985; **16**(1): 39–42.
116. Drago C, Howell K. Concepts for designing and fabricating metal implant frameworks for hybrid implant prostheses. *J Prosthodont* 2012; **21**(5): 413–424.
117. Murphy WM, Absi EG, Gregory MC, *et al.* A prospective 5-year study of two cast framework alloys for fixed implant-supported mandibular prostheses. *Int J Prosthodont* 2002; **15**(2): 133–138.
118. Takahashi T, Gunne J. Fit of implant frameworks: an in vitro comparison between two fabrication techniques. *J Prosthet Dent* 2003; **89**(3): 256–260.
119. Al-Fadda SA, Zarb GA, Finer Y. A comparison of the accuracy of fit of 2 methods for fabricating implant-prosthodontic frameworks. *Int J Prosthodont* 2007; **20**(2): 125–131.
120. Ortorp A, Jemt T. CNC-milled titanium frameworks supported by implants in the edentulous jaw: a 10-year comparative clinical study. *Clin Implant Dent Relat Res* 2012; **14**(1): 88–99.
121. Jemt T, Book K. Prosthesis misfit and marginal bone loss in edentulous implant patients. *Int J Oral Maxillofac Implants* 1996; **11**(5): 620–625.
122. McGlumphy EA, Mendel DA, Holloway JA. Implant screw mechanics. *Dent Clin North Am* 1998; **42**(1): 71–89.
123. Ma J, Rubenstein JE. Complete arch implant impression technique. *J Prosthet Dent* 2012; **107**(6): 405–10.
124. Papaspyridakos P, Gallucci GO, Chen CJ, *et al.* Digital versus conventional implant impressions for edentulous patients: accuracy outcomes. *Clin Oral Implants Res* 2016; **27**(4): 465–472.
125. Agustin-Panadero R, Penarrocha-Oltra D, Gomar-Vercher S, *et al.* Stereophotogrammetry for recording the position of multiple implants: technical description. *Int J Prosthodont* 2015; **28**(6): 631–636.
126. Bergin JM, Rubenstein JE, Mancl L, *et al.* An in vitro comparison of photogrammetric and conventional complete-arch implant impression techniques. *J Prosthet Dent* 2013; **110**(4): 243–251.
127. Malo P, de Araujo Nobre M, Borges J, *et al.* Retrievable metal ceramic implant-supported fixed prostheses with milled titanium frameworks and all-ceramic crowns: retrospective clinical study with up to 10 years of follow-up. *J Prosthodont* 2012; **21**(4): 256–264.
128. Malo P, Araujo Nobre MD, Lopes A, *et al.* Double full-arch versus single full-arch, four implant-supported rehabilitations: a retrospective, 5-year cohort study. *J Prosthodont* 2015; **24**(4): 263–270.
129. Ozkurt Z, Kazazoglu E. Clinical success of zirconia in dental applications. *J Prosthodont* 2010; **19**(1): 64–68.
130. Papaspyridakos P, Lal K. Computer-assisted design/computer-assisted manufacturing zirconia implant fixed complete prostheses: clinical results and technical complications up to 4 years of function. *Clin Oral Implants Res* 2013; **24**(6): 659–665.
131. Cheng CW, Chien CH, Chen CJ, *et al.* Complete-mouth implant rehabilitation with modified monolithic zirconia implant-supported fixed dental prostheses and an immediate-loading protocol: a clinical report. *J Prosthet Dent* 2013; **109**(6): 347–352.
132. Limmer B, Sanders AE, Reside G, *et al.* Complications and patient-centered outcomes with an implant-supported monolithic zirconia fixed dental prosthesis: 1 year results. *J Prosthodont* 2014; **23**(4): 267–275.
133. Malo P, de Araujo Nobre M, Lopes A, *et al.* A longitudinal study of the survival of All-on-4 implants in the mandible with up to 10 years of follow-up. *J Am Dent Assoc* 2011; **142**(3): 310–320.
134. Malo P, de Araujo Nobre M, Lopes A, *et al.* All-on-4® treatment concept for the rehabilitation of the completely edentulous mandible: a 7-year clinical and 5-year radiographic retrospective case series with risk assessment for implant failure and marginal bone level. *Clin Implant Dent Relat Res* 2015; **17**(Suppl 2): e531–541.
135. Balshi TJ, Wolfinger GJ, Slauch RW, *et al.* A retrospective analysis of 800 Branemark System implants following the All-on-Four protocol. *J Prosthodont* 2014; **23**(2): 83–88.
136. Hinze M, Thalmair T, Bolz W, *et al.* Immediate loading of fixed provisional prostheses using four implants for the rehabilitation of the edentulous arch: a prospective clinical study. *Int J Oral Maxillofac Implants* 2010; **25**(5): 1011–1018.
137. Kattadiyil MT, Goodacre CJ, Lozada JL, *et al.* Digitally planned and fabricated mandibular fixed complete dentures. Part 2. Prosthodontic phase. *Int J Prosthodont* 2015; **28**(2): 119–123.
138. Artzi Z, Kohen J, Carmeli G, *et al.* The efficacy of full-arch immediately restored implant-supported reconstructions in extraction and healed sites: a 36-month retrospective evaluation. *Int J Oral Maxillofac Implants* 2010; **25**(2): 329–335.
139. Babbush CA. Posttreatment quantification of patient experiences with full-arch implant treatment using a modification of the OHIP-14 questionnaire. *J Oral Implantol* 2012; **38**(3): 251–260.
140. De Bruyn H, Raes S, Ostman PO, *et al.* Immediate loading in partially and completely edentulous jaws: a review of the literature with clinical guidelines. *Periodontol 2000* 2014; **66**(1): 153–187.
141. Rasmusson L, Roos J, Bystedt H. A 10-year follow-up study of titanium dioxide-blasted implants. *Clin Implant Dent Relat Res* 2005; **7**(1): 36–42.
142. Schwartz-Arad D, Chaushu G. Full-arch restoration of the jaw with fixed ceramometal prosthesis. *Int J Oral Maxillofac Implants* 1998; **13**(6): 819–825.
143. Gallucci GO, Bernard JP, Belser UC. Treatment of completely edentulous patients with fixed implant-supported restorations: three consecutive cases of simultaneous immediate loading in both maxilla and mandible. *Int J Periodontics Restorative Dent* 2005; **25**(1): 27–37.
144. Ogawa T, Dhaliwal S, Naert I, *et al.* Impact of implant number, distribution and prosthesis material on loading on implants supporting fixed prostheses. *J Oral Rehabil* 2010; **37**(7): 525–531.
145. Lambert FE, Weber HP, Susarla SM, *et al.* Descriptive analysis of implant and prosthodontic survival rates with fixed implant-supported rehabilitations in the edentulous maxilla. *J Periodontol* 2009; **80**(8): 1220–1230.

146. Pjetursson BE, Tan K, Lang NP, *et al.* A systematic review of the survival and complication rates of fixed partial dentures (FPDs) after an observation period of at least 5 years. *Clin Oral Implants Res* 2004; **15**(6): 625–642.
147. Kinsel RP, Lin D. Retrospective analysis of porcelain failures of metal ceramic crowns and fixed partial dentures supported by 729 implants in 152 patients: patient-specific and implant-specific predictors of ceramic failure. *J Prosthet Dent* 2009; **101**(6): 388–394.
148. Guess PC, Att W, Strub JR. Zirconia in fixed implant prosthodontics. *Clin Implant Dent Relat Res* 2012; **14**(5): 633–645.
149. Le M, Papia E, Larsson C. The clinical success of tooth- and implant-supported zirconia-based fixed dental prostheses. A systematic review. *J Oral Rehabil* 2015; **42**(6): 467–480.
150. Venezia P, Torsello F, Cavalcanti R, *et al.* Retrospective analysis of 26 complete-arch implant-supported monolithic zirconia prostheses with feldspathic porcelain veneering limited to the facial surface. *J Prosthet Dent* 2015; **114**(4): 506–512.
151. Sherif S, Susarla HK, Kapos T, *et al.* A systematic review of screw-versus cement-retained implant-supported fixed restorations. *J Prosthodont* 2014; **23**(1): 1–9.
152. Nissan J, Narobai D, Gross O, *et al.* Long-term outcome of cemented versus screw-retained implant-supported partial restorations. *Int J Oral Maxillofac Implants* 2011; **26**(5): 1102–1107.
153. Papaspyridakos P, Chen CJ, Chuang SK, *et al.* Implant loading protocols for edentulous patients with fixed prostheses: a systematic review and meta-analysis. *Int J Oral Maxillofac Implants* 2014; **29**(Suppl): 256–270.
154. Gallucci GO, Bernard JP, Bertosa M, *et al.* Immediate loading with fixed screw-retained provisional restorations in edentulous jaws: the pickup technique. *Int J Oral Maxillofac Implants* 2004; **19**(4): 524–533.
155. Horiuchi K, Uchida H, Yamamoto K, *et al.* Immediate loading of Branemark system implants following placement in edentulous patients: a clinical report. *Int J Oral Maxillofac Implants* 2000; **15**(6): 824–830.
156. Tarnow DP, Emtiaz S, Classi A. Immediate loading of threaded implants at stage 1 surgery in edentulous arches: ten consecutive case reports with 1- to 5-year data. *Int J Oral Maxillofac Implants* 1997; **12**(3): 319–324.
157. Grunder U. Immediate functional loading of immediate implants in edentulous arches: two-year results. *Int J Periodontics Restorative Dent* 2001; **21**(6): 545–551.
158. Jaffin RA, Kumar A, Berman CL. Immediate loading of implants in partially and fully edentulous jaws: a series of 27 case reports. *J Periodontol* 2000; **71**(5): 833–838.
159. Pjetursson BE, Asgeirsson AG, Zwahlen M, *et al.* Improvements in implant dentistry over the last decade: comparison of survival and complication rates in older and newer publications. *Int J Oral Maxillofac Implants* 2014; **29**(Suppl): 308–324.
160. Wittneben JG, Millen C, Bragger U. Clinical performance of screw- versus cement-retained fixed implant-supported reconstructions – a systematic review. *Int J Oral Maxillofac Implants* 2014; **29**(Suppl): 84–98.

CHAPTER 19

Material Considerations in the Fabrication of Prostheses for Completely Edentulous Patients

James A. Kelly and Thomas J. Salinas
Mayo Clinic College of Medicine, Rochester, Minnesota, USA

The scope of this chapter is to provide the reader with information related to material science in construction of implant prosthetics for patients with complete edentulism. The last decades have experienced a plethora of biomaterial and surgical sequencing developments, which have led to a modified approach in treating edentulous patients with dental implants. While evidence-based information on this approach is not robust, some protocols with varying degrees of success will be reviewed for case application according to patient-specific factors.

Origin of material selection for implant prostheses

The early decades preceding osseointegration had identified a challenge in meeting the need for treating patients with prostheses that were mucosally supported and retained.[1] The edentulous patient demographic represented the greatest need to improve prosthesis support and retention. Using cast alloys and combining these with polymethylmethacrylate seemed to be the logical choice, as most removable dental prostheses were linked to fixed anchorage by precision or semi-precision means. There seemed to be concerns about using base metals for this purpose as some galvanic potential[2] was considered detrimental to health of the implant, so the use of noble alloys with a high elastic modulus likewise seemed logical. Knowing the cascade of events leading to osseointegration, it was also of concern that the implant–bone interface be protected from the impact of occlusal forces.[3] The choice of using acrylic resin was intended to shield the bone interface from impact load.

The use of this design was published as being successful surgically and prosthodontically without the need for major prosthesis redesign.[4] Even with additional experience of medium-term success, results did not indicate that prosthesis redesign was a major factor in time to retreatment.[5] Many other treatment centers that were conducting duplicate population studies seemed to find quite a high "survival" with what was being interpreted as synonymous implant and prosthesis survival.[6,7] Survival of osseointegrated implants, even with first-generation implant design, was quite predictable and it remains a reliable surgical technique. The reality is that surgical survival and prosthesis survival are quite different. As with other restorative interfaces, the servicing needs for materials that are chosen will be evident in some fashion. Goodacre *et al.*[8] conducted a review of complications cited for these prostheses and identified the overdenture as requiring significant servicing needs. As literature accumulated, Purcell *et al.*,[9] Gallucci *et al.*,[10] and Dhima *et al.*[11] all cited concerns with this type of design's long-term cost effectiveness. The problems encountered were fractured teeth, loosened screws, fractured screws, and failure of the veneering material in some form. Although some of the problems with implant components were addressed after a redesign, the balance of these complications seemed to happen on average 7–14 years after initial placement. The follow-up requirement begged for an improvement of material performance, design testing, and improved space-allocation techniques.

The advent of osseointegration has revolutionized the treatment of those who have acquired and congenital absence of teeth and associated maxillofacial structures. The treatment paradigm used for this demographic had historically been based upon unique factors of presentation. While many piloted centers had approached treatment of edentulous patients on a large scale, the demographics of these patients have changed considerably, with many patients keeping their teeth for a longer time.[12,13]

The oral conditions of patients who present with the affliction of decades-old edentulism may differ considerably from those who present with a failing dentition (Figure 19.1). In these circumstances, it is imperative to understand spatial consideration with regard to diagnosis and treatment planning with specific prosthesis design. Treatment planning from both a surgical[14,15] and prosthetic[16] basis should be given due consideration as each will have specific requisites for successful outcomes.

Evidence-based Implant Treatment Planning and Clinical Protocols, First Edition. Edited by Steven J. Sadowsky.

Companion website: www.wiley.com/go/sadowsky/implant

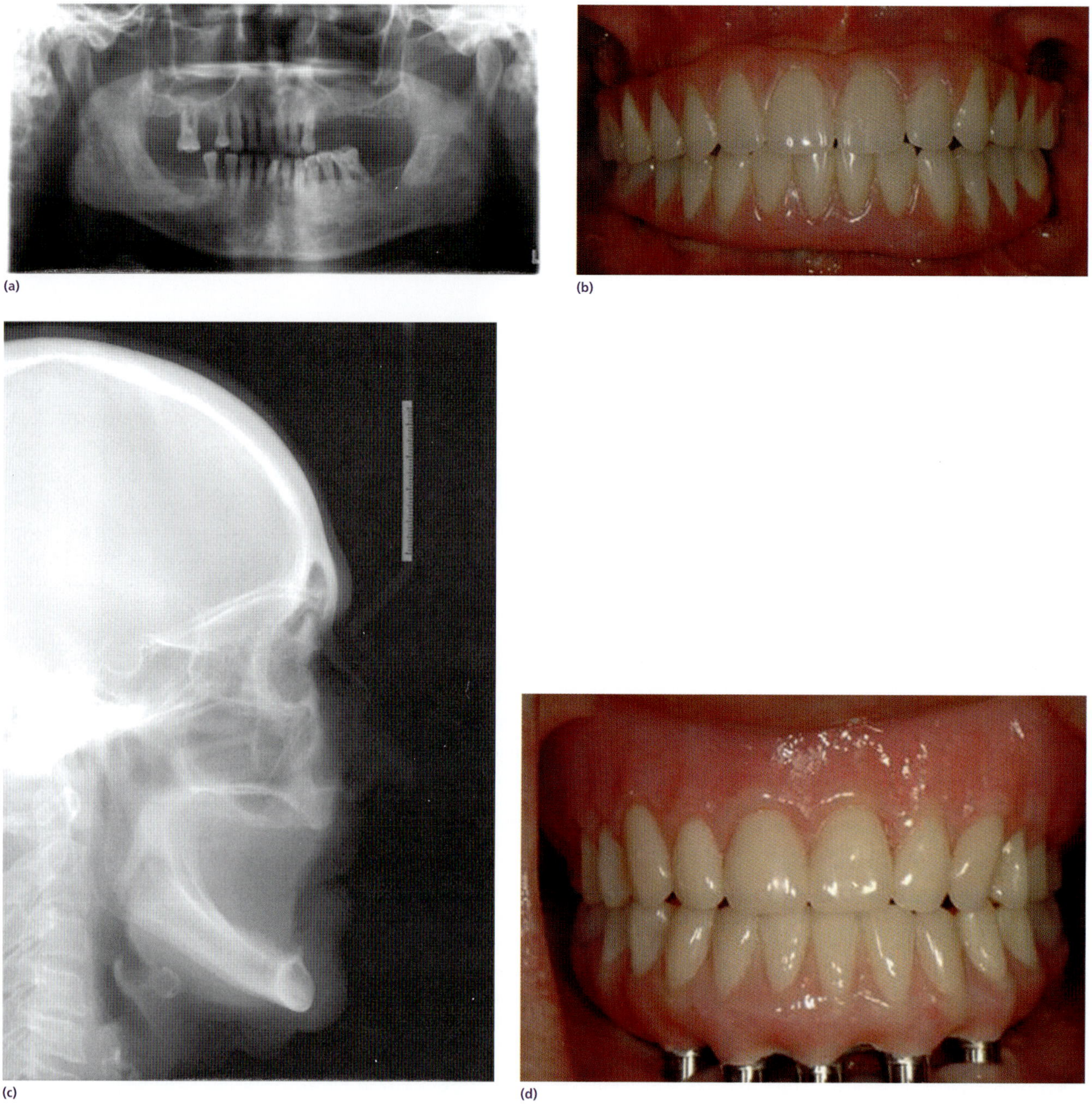

Figure 19.1 (a) Patient presenting for implant prosthetic reconstruction months prior to (b) definitive implant fixed reconstruction. (c) Patient presenting decades after tooth loss for (d) mandibular implant fixed reconstruction.

Initial evaluation and treatment planning

Patients presenting edentulous or in need of strategic edentulation should be evaluated for treatment goals and expectations.[4,17] In some cases, patient expectations of treatment should be revisited to ascertain objectives, which may be nonachievable given their circumstances. Many instruments that evaluate expectations have been proposed for patient-perceived outcomes with complete dentures.[18–21] Although these instruments can give insight into behavioral ideals, they do not make provision for those who do not have appropriate perception of their edentulous state. In some cases, the use of the Diagnostic and Statistical Manual of Mental Disorders can assist with identification of body dysmorphic disorder or other similar perceptive deficits.[22] If expectations are realistic and achievable, the initial treatment phase may be with conventional prosthetics or with provisional implant-assisted prosthetics.

Facial form, orthognathic profile, and interocclusal distances will also give important information for gaining an understanding of the available restorative volume. Analog or digital

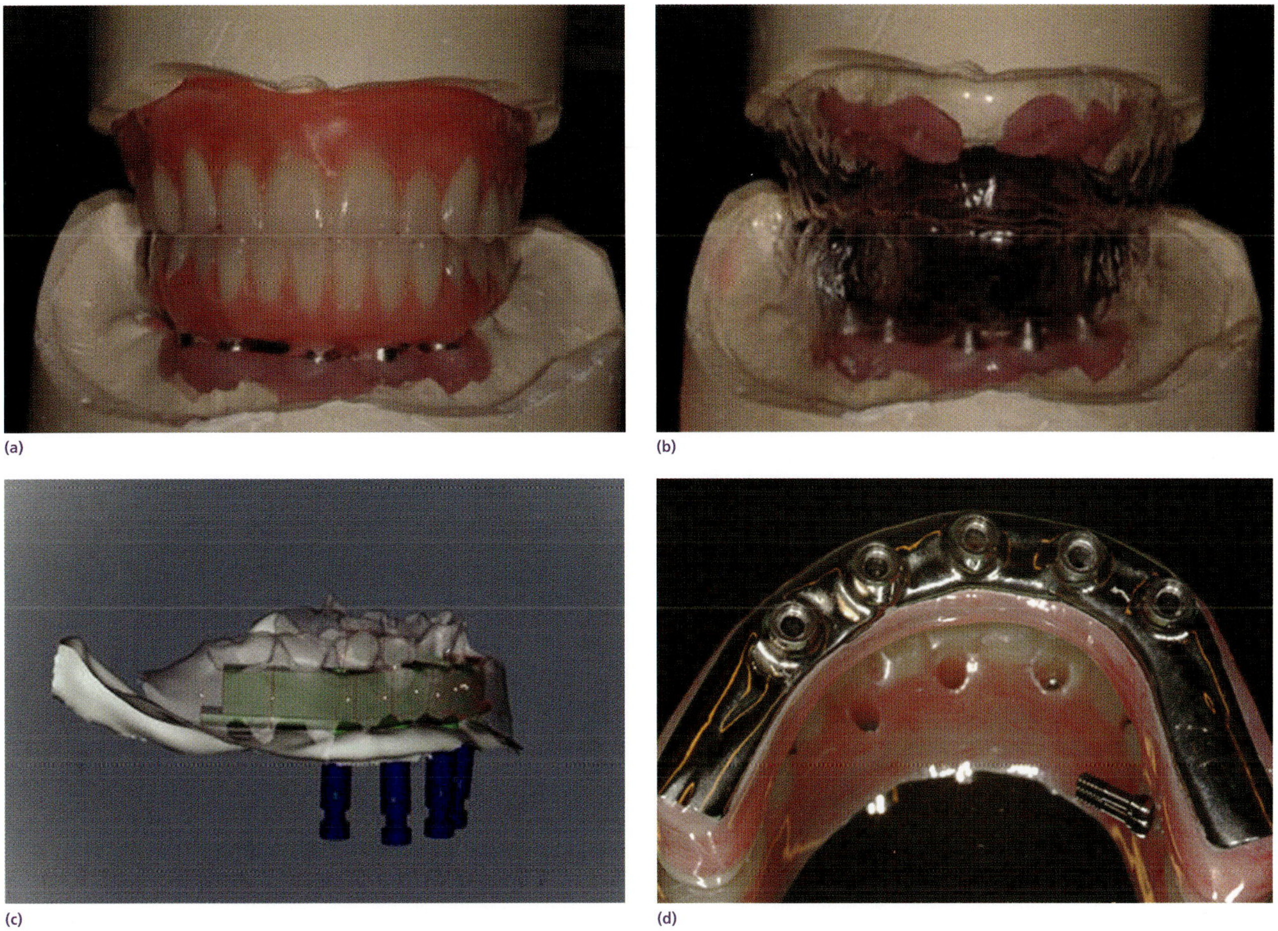

Figure 19.2 (a) Analog wax-up. (b) Wax-up permits spatial considerations for planning and fabricating maxillary and mandibular prostheses. (c) Virtual bar design after scan of wax-up to produce bar structure. (d) Both techniques produce information to determine spatial constraints and proper design of prostheses.

analysis prior to extractions or implant placement is essential and will give the basis for sound treatment objectives (Figure 19.2). A further understanding of the patient's concerns will direct proper planning to satisfy these requirements, be it fixed or removable prosthodontics.

Once patient-mediated factors are considered, space availability and expected applied forces may be pivotal in the design selection. After a decision has been made, an understanding of material properties will aid further in making these decisions.

Mandibular edentulism has been approached from a number of different vantage points, and has been treated from a variety of approaches. Although there are limited studies which indicate specific protocols for treating patients with mandibular edentulism,[16] some evidence of improvement in function does exist when using bone-anchored prostheses. Patients who are dissatisfied with their mandibular dentures can be treated with new prostheses, or have treatment with dental implant anchorage with overdentures or fixed prostheses; these may have different outcomes.[23] Treatment with implant-assisted prostheses is preferable for patients with regard to efficient function. In fact, dietary choices are very different in those treated with a maxillary complete denture and implant-supported mandibular prostheses in comparison to those treated with conventional complete dentures.[24]

Maxillary edentulism appears to be well treated with conventional complete dentures, as supported by many randomized studies, which have used the maxillary complete denture as a standard treatment. If patients express a level of satisfaction with a conventional maxillary complete denture, there is little evidence of any advantages of offering further treatment with implant stabilization. However, if stability or retention is not met, the patient may be offered a variety of treatment alternatives. The use of four well distributed dental implants for retention of a maxillary overdenture has met with success and substantial improvement in support and retention. With reduced palatal coverage and alloy-reinforced bases, this seems to be a popular treatment alternative for patient satisfaction (Figure 19.3).[25] Acceptance by patients, of a fixed dental prosthesis for maxillary edentulism versus a removable prosthesis, is variable, and requirements in facial, orthognathic, and phonetic forms are likewise variable. The approach to using four strategically placed and angled implants for a fixed prosthesis was introduced some years ago and

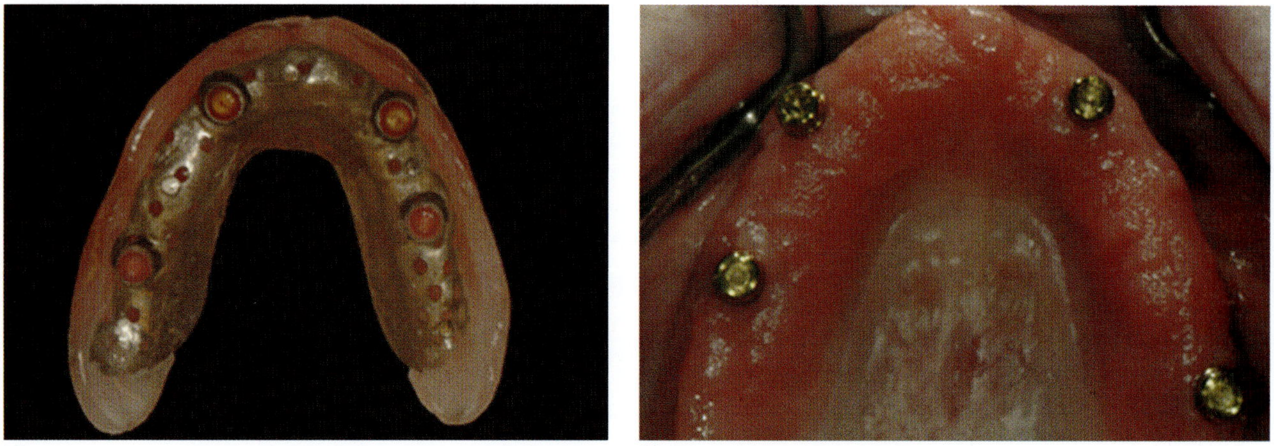

(a) (b)

Figure 19.3 (a) Design of overdenture with reduced palatal coverage and metal-reinforced base. (b) Stud abutments well spaced with potential for servicing.

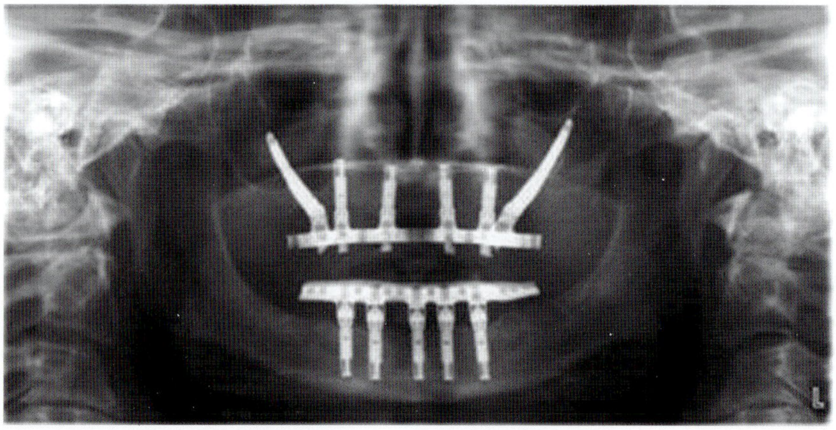

(a)

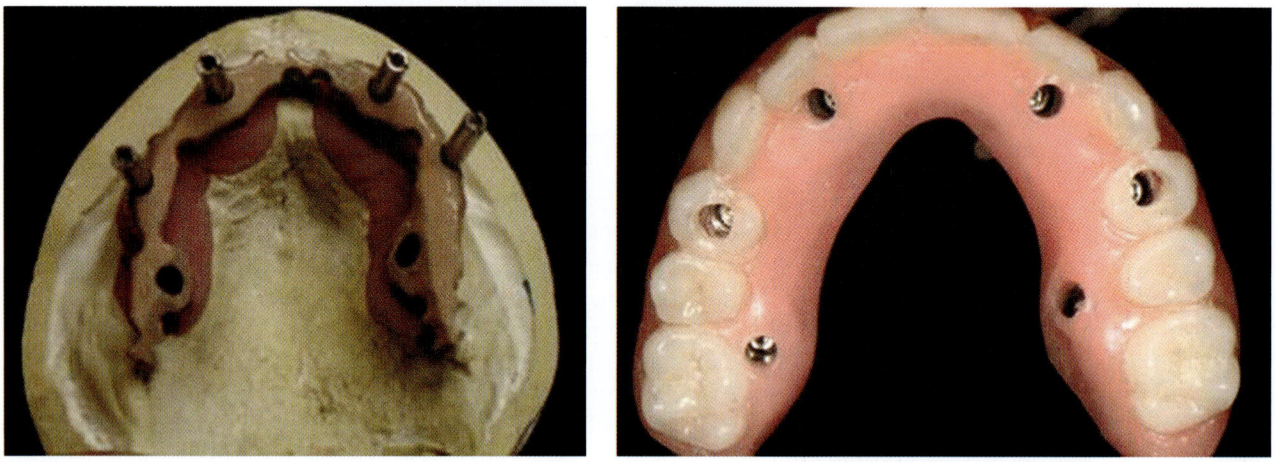

(b) (c)

Figure 19.4 (a) Patient treated for anhidrotic ectodermal dysplasia and 10-year follow-up indicates some servicing need with multiple acrylic tooth replacements. Good surgical success with zygoma and conventional implants. (b) Silicoated TiAl6V4 frameworks. (c) Laminated with compression-molded acrylic resin and denture teeth.

has been replicated with a high degree of success.[26,27] Other authors have reported good success rates with extended implants into the zygoma with auxiliary anchorage in the anterior maxilla for treatment of maxillary posterior atrophy (Figure 19.4),[14,28] and, more recently, with extramaxillary orientation.[29] Where there is additional deficiency of the premaxillary bone, the use of four zygomatic-anchored implants has also been advocated as a potential treatment scenario (Figure 19.5).[30] Strategies developed for these specialized protocols have targeted reduction of cantilever design, along with angulation of anterior and posterior implants,

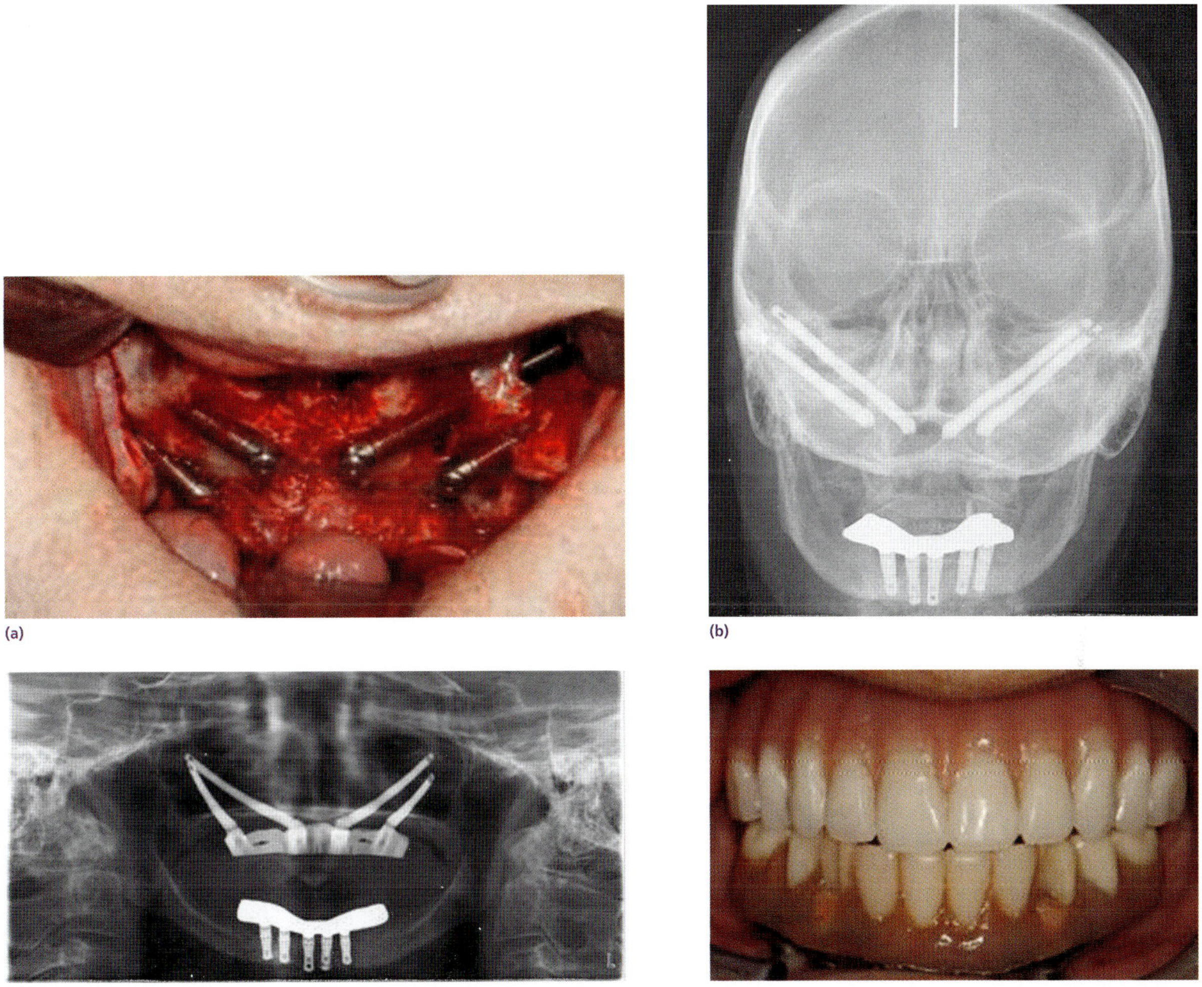

(a) (b) (c) (d)

Figure 19.5 **(a)** Extended-length zygoma implants placed adjacent to atrophic maxilla. **(b)** Follow-up cephalogram indicates stable placement. **(c)** Radiograph showing subsequent bar attachment. **(d)** Clinical view with precision-fit electrical-discharged machined metal-based overdenture.

and a shortened arch form. In any case, systematic reviews indicate a high degree of success using four to six dental implants to restore an arch using a fixed dental prosthesis.[31]

Basic material properties

The range of dental materials has grown considerably over the last decade, with development in polymethylmethacrylate, composite resin, and dental ceramics. A comparison of the materials commonly used for veneering and base construction of implant prosthodontics will give a basic understanding of the gamut of physical properties (Table 19.1). Although methacrylate resin may seem inferior, the ease of repair is attractive, allowing the esthetics, vertical dimension, and occlusal schemes to be redesigned relatively easily.

While these materials can be used for a variety of prosthetic constructions, it should be realized that there are fundamental differences in behavior between alloys and ceramics. As stress is applied to metals, it becomes evident that an elastic and plastic deformation occurs. With regard to ceramics, however, this behavior is quite different and, despite high yield strengths of these materials, they may fail abruptly under an increased load (Figure 19.6).[32]

Although material consideration is important for understanding construction requirements, thorough diagnosis and design principles will also need consideration. Patients requiring full-arch prosthesis replacement of a dentition can be treated in a variety of pathways. The primary diagnostic sequences should give a general vision of patient expectations, available anatomy, interarch distances, and biomechanical design. Available anatomy is evaluated in a three-dimensional (3-D) form to give some correlation between diagnosis and treatment planning (Figure 19.7). In correlating this phase with patient expectations, the treatment team can properly plan the treatment sequencing to arrive at a predictable result. The first part of this anatomical consideration is to assure sufficient bone volume exists to meet the foundational need in planning implant location.

Table 19.1 Comparison of different restorative material physical properties (PMMA, polymethyl methacrylate).

Restorative material	Compressive strength[1] (MPa)	Elastic modulus[2] (GPa)	Flexural strength[3] (MPa)	Ultimate tensile strength[4] (MPa)
Cobalt–chromium alloy		220		520–820
Feldspathic porcelain	149	70	65	25
Composite resin	225	21	139	–
PMMA	124	1.8–3.1	137	75
Zirconia	–	210	1087	–
Ti-6Al-4 V	970	114	903	930

[1] Compressive strength: tested in standard cylinder that has a length of twice its diameter.
[2] Elastic modulus: stiffness of a material in elastic range of stress/strain curve.
[3] Flexural strength: three-point bending test of a standard supported beam of material.
[4] Ultimate tensile strength: maximum stress material can withstand before failure in tension.

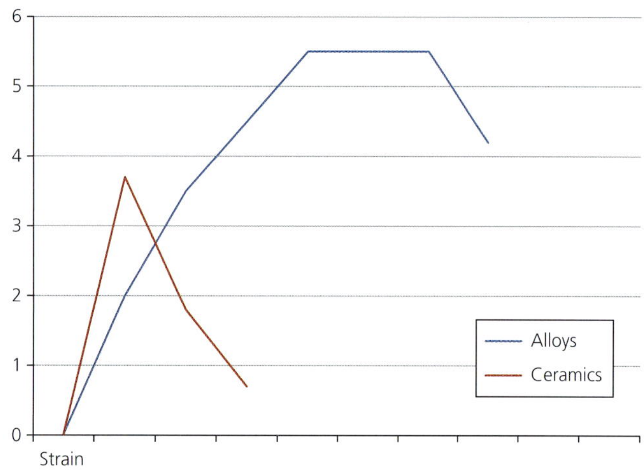

Figure 19.6 Stress/strain diagram indicating the brittle nature of ceramics in comparison to alloys.

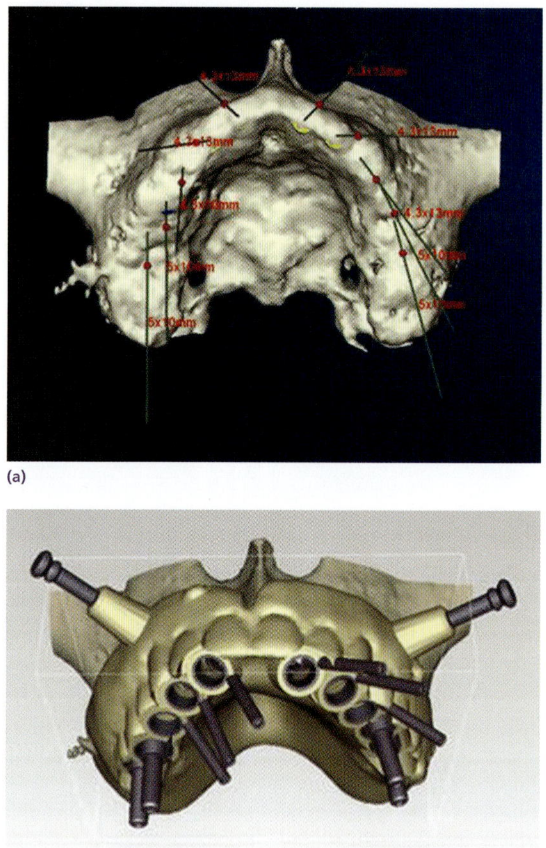
(a)
(b)

Figure 19.7 A patient presented with significant alveolar bone, desiring a fixed prosthesis. **(a)** Digital surgical planning with CT scan for site selection and implant angulation for screw-retained prosthesis. **(b)** Surgical template fabrication from plan to carry out surgery supportive of prosthesis design.

On this basis, biomechanical design and interarch distance can prompt material selection, so that the surgical and prosthodontic disciplines are synergistically linked (Figure 19.8).

Once patient-mediated factors are considered, space availability and expected applied forces may be pivotal in the material selection. After foundational planning, a working knowledge of biomechanics should help the treatment team to understand the advantages that a screw joint imparts to the stability of multiple implant interfaces.

Basic screw joint mechanics

In the interests of efficient workflow and understanding the potential need for retreatment, consideration of screw joint mechanics is essential when constructing dental prostheses. Force transmission from the prosthesis to the implant platform is of primary concern. The surfaces that will participate in this will be those that are intended for force transfer and those that are orientation features.[33] The most common configurations have been force transfer to a flat or conical implant connection, and, despite a trend to the conal variety, these do not demonstrate superior mechanical resistance in the long term.[33,34] *Preload*, the compressive force between the platform and abutment, is important to allow sufficient generation of clamping force.[36] This is generated by internal tensile stress in the screw, called *pretension*. When two surfaces are clamped together, the total zone of contact will transmit the applied load, making this successful

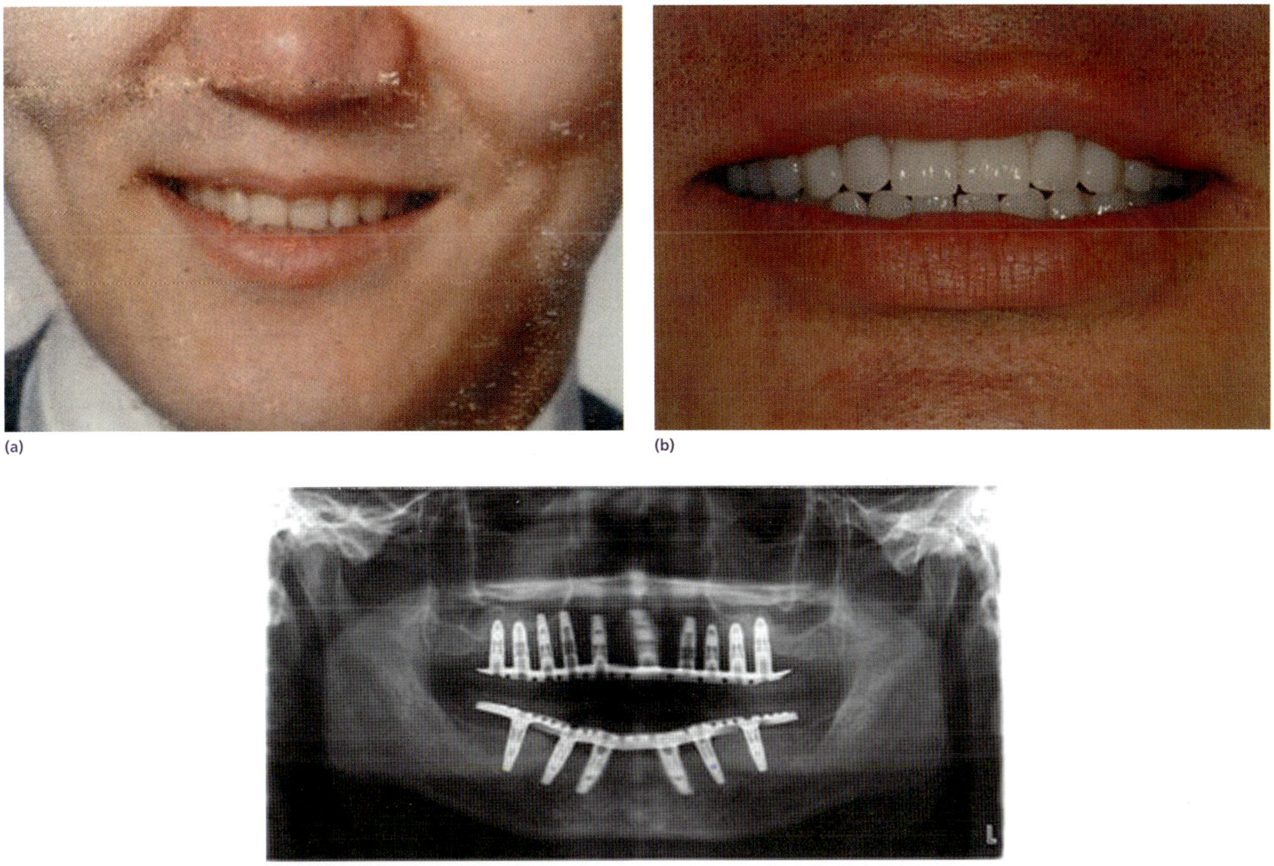
(a) (b) (c)

Figure 19.8 Prosthodontic treatment of patient planned in Figure 18.7. (a) High school graduation photo of patient with desired esthetics. (b) Definitive prostheses with satisfactory lip support and achieved esthetics. (c) Radiographic survey of definitive prostheses.

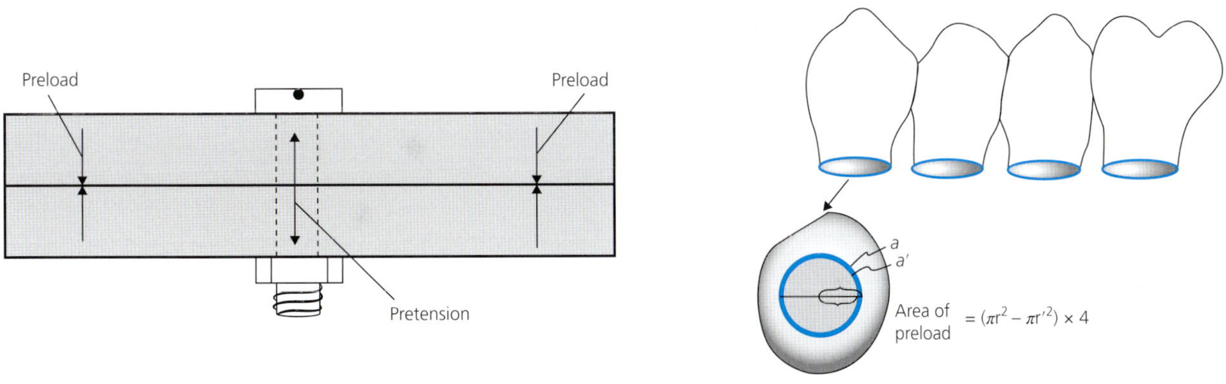

(a) (b)

Figure 19.9 Clamping forces exerted between two surfaces when torque is applied to a screw securing two surfaces. (a) Pre-tension in the screw is created that is shielded from the compression forces (preload) stabilizing the two plates. (b) The measure of load-bearing surface area between implant platform and prosthesis is optimal when maximized for force transfer.

long term (Figure 19.9). By this principle, the contact surfaces bear the primary load (up to 90%) and shield transfer of the load to the screw, making the components act as one. To accomplish the goal of a sufficiently strong screw joint, a standard application of torque is essential, and this should be applied with a calibrated torque delivery device. As mentioned, preload generated by a screw joint creates a clamping force, which stabilizes over the surface area of prosthetic abutment-to-implant connection. Between 2% and 10% of this clamping force will attenuate after flattening and loading of these surfaces under function.[37]

Force transfer and biomechanics

Force transfer from the prosthesis to the abutment or implant interface places emphasis on consideration of the available bone support. For instance, using a specific implant number, ideally and widely distributed throughout an edentulous arch with available restorative distance, results in little need for cantilevering where direct prosthesis-to-implant connections might be used (Figure 19.10). In these circumstances, the use of screw- or cement-retained abutments, or a combination thereof, is feasible.

The use of screw retention versus cementation appears controversial, but it certainly is advantageous to make the restoration retrievable, as it can be better serviced for technical complications if needed.[38] Because of technique, material, and component developments, modern survival statistics for screw-retained reconstructions are very different compared to those from studies prior to 2001.[39] This paper reported updated prosthetic survival results for screw- and cement-retained restorations, documenting similar 5-year rates. The use of cemented prostheses seems to be problematic and associated with more biologic complications.[40] Larger implant diameters seem to be associated with a greater chance of extravasated cement.[41]

In other circumstances, where there is limited bone or inability to distribute implants widely throughout the arch, the use of cantilevering or angle correction design may become necessary (Figure 19.11). The choice of using a direct implant connection to maximize preload is preferable, as this will reduce the likelihood of overloading the prosthetic screw assembly, a problem considered more likely with reduced screw diameter. Cantilever design has been controversial with implant prosthodontics. Two independent systematic reviews[42,43] indicate that distal cantilevers on fixed implant prostheses do not carry a high risk of mechanical complications; other observational reports indicate an apposition of bone in arches restored with cantilevered prosthetics.[44] Other reports indicate that, although biologic complications appear to be absent, technical complications, including veneer fracture, were common[10,45] and may be related to deflection of the connector under load. In these cases, the deflection of a beam is inversely related to the third power of the occlusal gingival thickness. Use of stiffer materials imparts

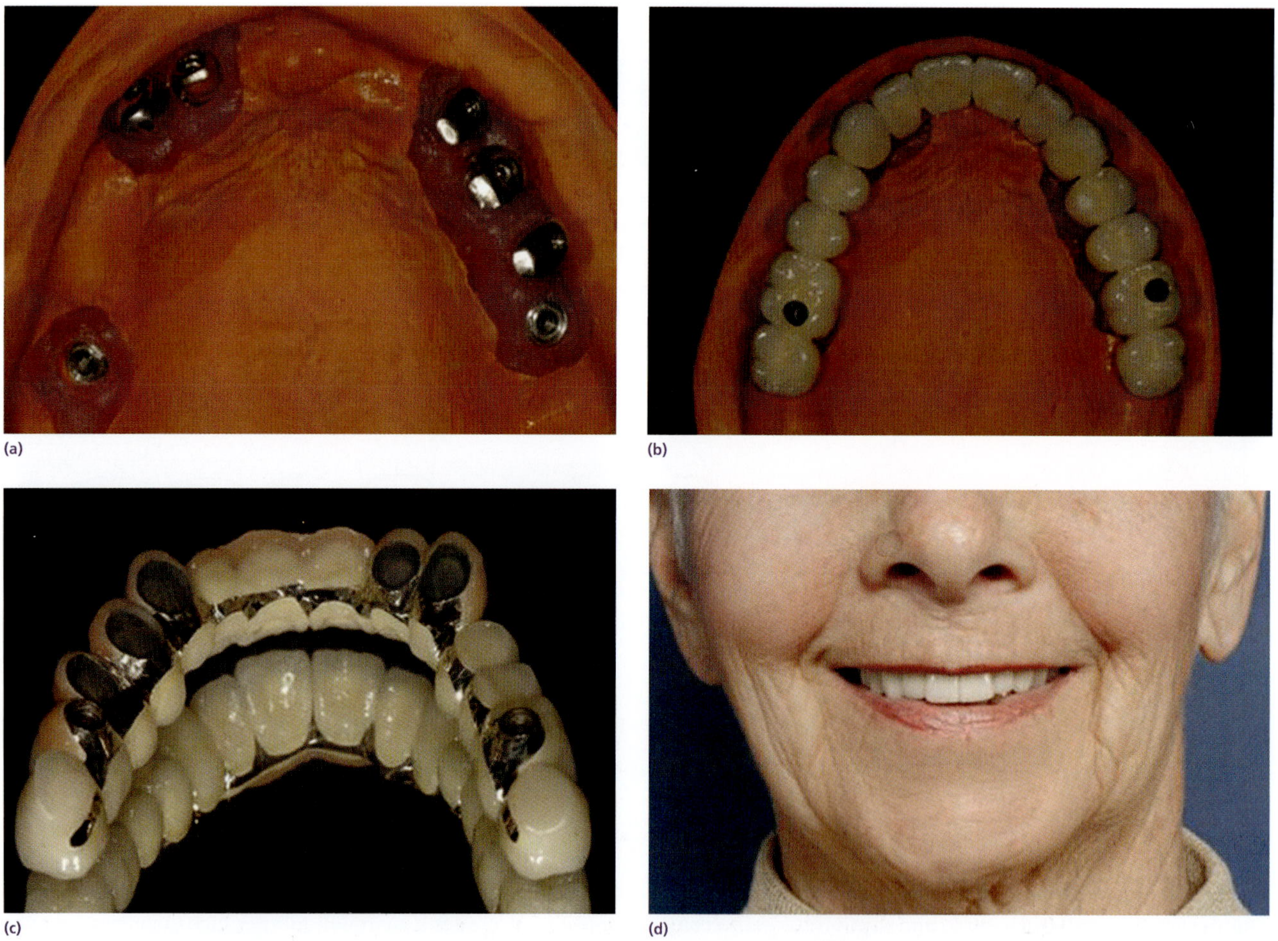

Figure 19.10 Patient with failing maxillary dentition presented with limited bone and sites selected with available bone. (a) Telescopic abutment design for angle correction and auxiliary screw retention on posterior implants. (b) Metal–ceramic design with cross arch splinting. (c) Intaglio of prosthesis showing telescopic retainers and direct-to-fixture screw connections. (d) Final esthetic result with fixed dental prosthesis.

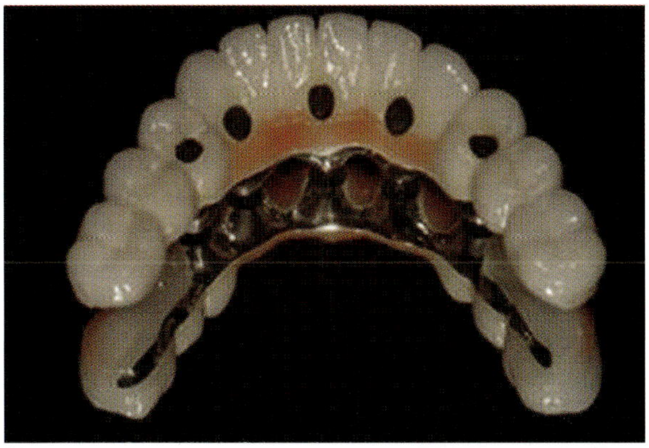

(a)

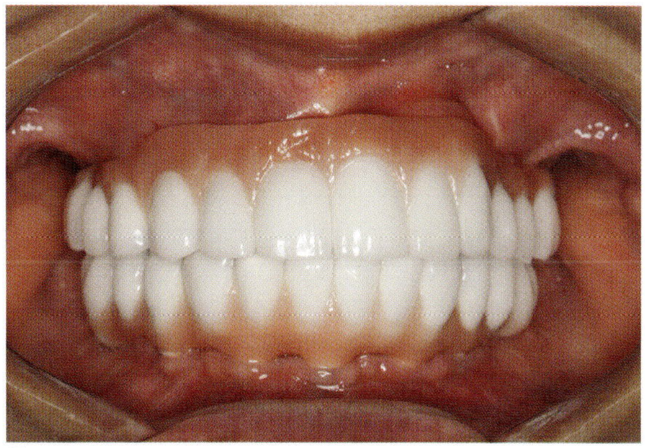

(b)

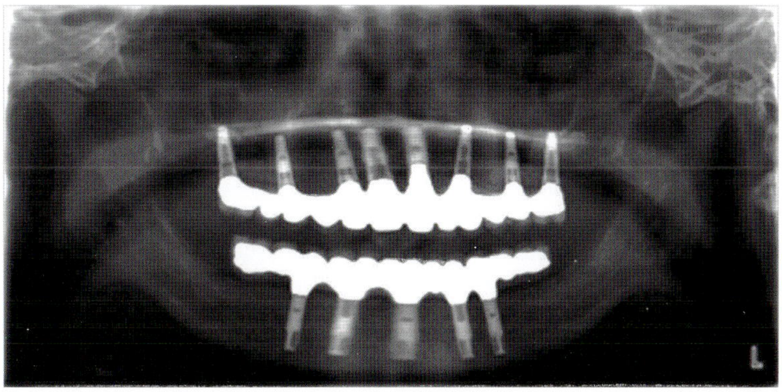

(c)

Figure 19.11 (a, b, c) Prosthesis construction included direct-to-fixture connection to secure cantilever design as sole osseous anchorage in interforaminal mandible opposing a maxillary fixed dental prosthesis. Palladium–copper framework used to obtain maximal resistance to stress on cantilevered area.

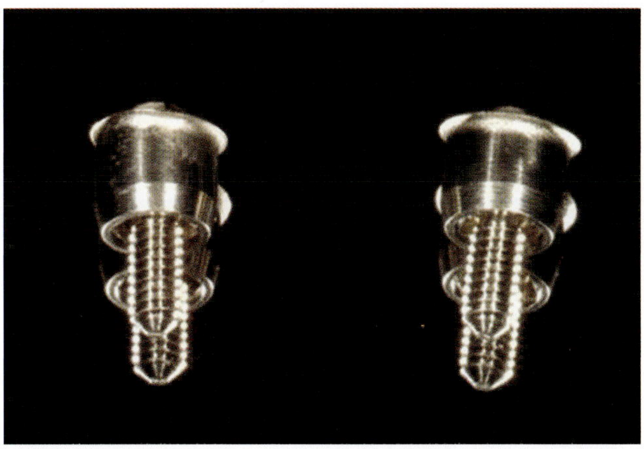

Figure 19.12 Standard abutments removed after 10 years of functioning beneath a fixed dental prosthesis with cantilevered design. Note the lip formed at the supporting portion of the abutments.

more tension to the most anterior screw joint, in which case a direct connection to the implant platform may be desirable for maximum resistance. The deformation of implant components beneath cantilever segments has also been controversial, as this clearly does occur, as demonstrated in laboratory studies (Figure 19.12).[46] Some of this can be attributed to the differential hardness between the prosthetic alloy and components, where stiff alloys, such as palladium–copper, cobalt–chromium, or ceramic, may deform titanium after years of functioning. Supplying new components in these cases can be difficult as manufacturers redesign restorative systems, making original implant components obsolete and unavailable. It is a challenge to use stiffer materials to overcome this flexure of cantilever design, but it may be met with the alternative of alloyed titanium. Although alloyed titanium may be less likely to deform the underlying abutment or implant platform, continued high cycle flexure may have tendency to delaminate the veneering material.

Prosthesis design

Overdentures

Traditionally, overdenture design was a classic approach for treatment of complete edentulism. Although minimal changes have been evident in methacrylate resin composition, aside of plasticizers and coloring agents, processing methods by continuous injection and low heat curing have resulted in a significant reduction in the amount of total dimensional changes upon polymerization.[47] Spatial considerations for overdenture design have been suggested from an empirical approach.[48] More specifically, the overdenture minimum thickness should be at least 2 mm[49] (with a stock denture tooth requiring at least 3 mm of thickness).[50] Spatial requirements of the resin base, prosthetic denture teeth, and attachment mechanisms should provide sufficient resistance under load where at least 2 mm of resin base is a foundation for the other components.[51] Vertical restorative space is the primary consideration, and has a bearing on base reinforcement, alveoloplasty, intentional vertical dimension increase, occlusal plane repositioning, and overdenture attachment selection.

Some reviews have given rise to understanding resistant design in the long-term management of these prostheses, and have led to the use of a cast reinforced framework (Figure 19.13).[52] The reinforced base is more resistant to crack propagation and ultimate failure. The use of this reinforced design in patients with parafunctional activity and opposing natural or implant-borne dentition may also be useful in reducing crack development and propagation. Resin-to-metal bonding is also beneficial, by making this union more chemically based, further enhancing the long-term stability and resistance to microleakage, which occurs where an inherent gap exists between the two phases of materials.[53,54]

Attachment mechanisms between the infrastructure and superstructure can be either stud-based abutments or bar attachments with incorporated stud attachments or precision electrical-discharged machined components. Implant parallelism has the potential to reduce attachment maintenance in solitary anchors/abutments. Implant proximity and length may also dictate the use of a bar attachment. Although patient satisfaction does not typically favor one over the other, the choice of using bar attachments is typically indicated where implant positioning trajectories are either convergent or divergent, rendering stud attachments problematic. Long-term attachment intimacy seems to be the primary servicing need in overdentures supported in part or completely by dental implants.[8] The vertical height requirement may be highly variable and partly dependent upon the system used. The minimum suggested height for simple Hader bar efficiency is at least 2 mm, to the more precise electrical-discharged machined primary bar at 4 mm, with a standard 2° taper.[55,56] There should be some degree of relief (1 mm) below the bar attachment to allow for hygiene and soft tissue management. The support by a bar infrastructure creates a large point fulcrum in the overdenture base which can give rise to crack origin. In cases where bar attachments are used, it is important to consider a corresponding metal reinforcement in the overdenture base.

Fixed implant complete denture

Fixed dental prosthetic reconstruction should be first approached with consideration of the biomechanical design. As mentioned, the first decade of osseointegration implementation considered the usual presenting conditions of patients who had been edentulous for some time and utilized the available bone for innovative design. This was engineered by Skalak[57] and others, who estimated a favorable biomechanical response with a thoughtfully planned cantilevered fixed prosthesis design (Figure 19.14). The paradigm shift came with understanding that the biomechanical demands placed upon bone led to a physiologic response,[58] and in some cases an exaggerated response to bone apposed in the posterior edentulous mandible.[44] The most common treatment scenario for patients who presented with edentulism was a maxillary complete denture opposing a fixed mandibular prosthesis supported by four to six dental implants in the anterior mandible. This had been described extensively and duplicated in many studies worldwide.[1,59]

The traditional design of the acrylic resin-to-metal fixed prosthesis has been documented extensively with systematic reviews[60] and long-term databases, rendering the treatment very predictable. Prosthodontic intervention-free survival is quite low as many of these prostheses require care for loosened/fractured

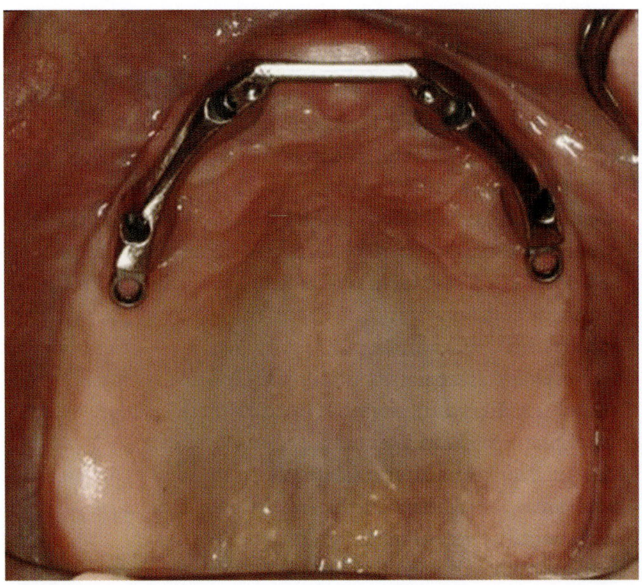

(a)

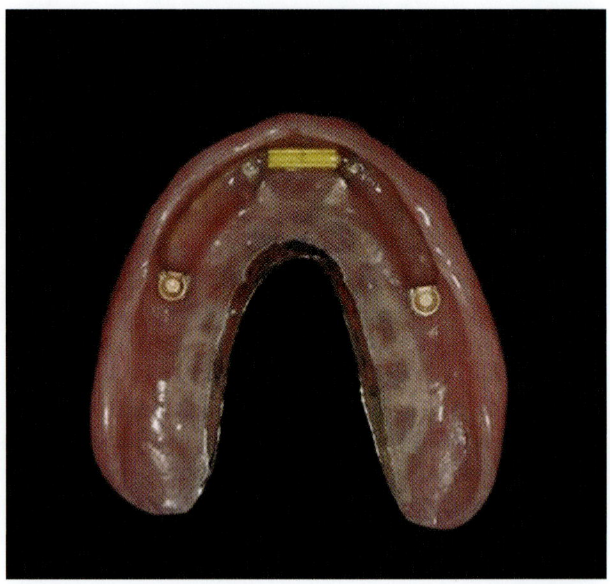

(b)

Figure 19.13 (a) Hader bar attachment in support and retention for (b) metal-based overdenture design. This feature has advantages of intaglio integrity, patient comfort, and ability for servicing attachments.

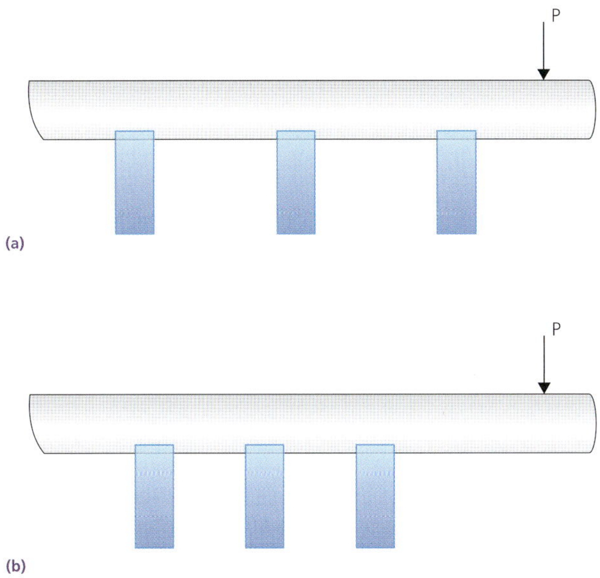

Figure 19.14 (a) Standard beam cantilever with well-spaced implants and minimal cantilever as force "P" is applied. (b) Closely spaced implants with extended cantilever creates almost double resultant force on implant adjacent to cantilever. *Source:* Adapted from Skalak, 1986.[57]

implant components or patient-specific biologic complications, such as soft tissue hypertrophy.[11,61] It is understood that many of these studies included patients with first-generation implant components that had undergone redesign some 15 years after their introduction. Second-generation and later implant component design dramatically changed the outcomes of cases treated with fixed dental prostheses. Acrylic resin tooth wear is commonly encountered and addressed by retrieval and resurfacing with new acrylic resin teeth. This typically occurs after 5–7 years, and they can either be resurfaced or augmented by onlays of gold or lithium disilicate, which may be more cost effective in the long term. Failure of the veneering material seems to be the most common complication, and this is difficult to predict, despite optimal thicknesses of material. Some of this can be attributed to proprioceptive deficiency, because of implant restorations being static, and dynamic fatigue of the material itself. Others theorize that the interocclusal relationships change rapidly due to wear, and create unfavorable positioning leading to fracture or delamination (Figure 19.15).

Aside from expert opinion,[50,62] there are very limited outcome data on specific recommendations for the spatial dimensions to which fixed implant resin-to-metal prostheses should be constructed. However, the best available evidence should dictate

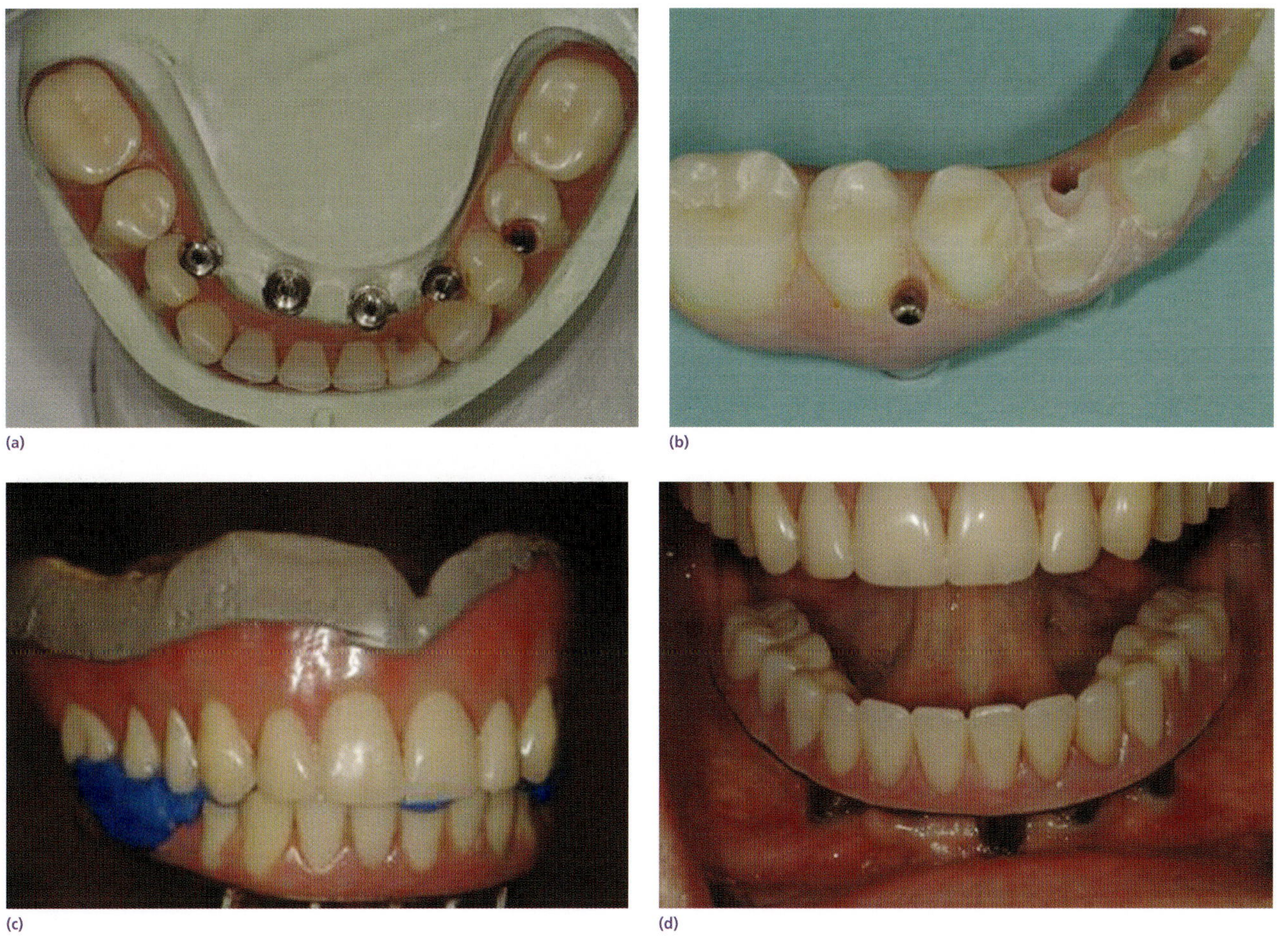

Figure 19.15 Patients treated with acrylic resin-to-metal prostheses illustrating servicing needs over time. (a) Worn acrylic resin teeth which have functioned for over 8 years. (b) Fractured composite resin layered denture teeth opposing a fixed dental prosthesis. (c, d) Rebasing of opposing complete denture and replacement of worn mandibular denture teeth are commonly required in this treatment group.

optimal function correlated to material thickness. For example, Choi *et al.*[51] indicated a minimum of 2 mm of resin base for standard resistance. This study also stated that the presence of resinous denture teeth substantially reduced the resistance of the resin to resist failure. Therefore, resin thickness would need to be at least 3 mm or more to best support resistance to failure. The choice of using cast alloy or CAD/CAM titanium frameworks is philosophical, as many advantages exist for each. The ease in making the framework by computer numeric controlled (CNC) means may be an advantage, since it can be designed virtually, with gross contouring accomplished by the software. Subsequent production into titanium alloys or cobalt–chromium can be very predictable, with incorporation of retentive features for acrylic resin. The use of commercially pure titanium (grades 1–5) was part of the initial production scope of many manufacturers (Table 19.2). Although the modulus of elasticity of grade 5 titanium is similar to commercially pure titanium, it can withstand high cyclic elastic deformation while maintaining its integrity. More contemporary approaches in using Ti-6Al-4 V (grade 5 titanium alloy) and cobalt–chromium have resulted in frameworks with higher flexural strengths, making them further resistant to deformation. These stiffer alloys may be especially useful where cantilever designs are planned. Although the resistance to deformation is much improved with stiffer alloys, few parameters exist within current software indicating critical material heights and thicknesses. The treatment team is encouraged to consider the unfavorable loading concepts that accompany cantilever designs when used in the edentulous model (Figure 19.16). Extrapolation of this treatment paradigm to a restored opposing arch of natural teeth or dental implants can be fraught with risk and mechanical complications. Cross-sectional area and configuration,[63] especially height, are critical to performance of cantilever resistance. Standardized testing of Ti-6Al-4V bars of various cross-sectional areas indicates that a minimum height of 4 mm and width of 4 mm is recommended for maximum resistance to deformation (Figures 19.17 and 19.18).

In taking these spatial recommendations of 3 mm or greater resin thickness, 4 mm bar height, and artificial tooth stock of 3 mm minimum, 10–15 mm of available restorative dimension should be planned for a resin-to-metal fixed implant complete denture.

Metal–ceramic fixed dental prosthesis

Metal castings have some order of 10-fold less accuracy than do computer numeric controlled (CNC) machined frameworks.[64] Although long-term follow-up of cast frameworks shows similar survival rates to those for CNC frameworks,[65] the importance of

Table 19.2 Comparison of physical properties of various grades of titanium. Data from American Society for Testing and Materials (ASTM international Standards).

Alloy	Yield strength[1] (MPa)	Tensile strength[2] (MPa)	Modulus of elasticity[3] (GPa)
Commercially pure titanium grade 1	172	241	103
Commercially pure titanium grade 2	276	345	103
Commercially pure titanium grade 3	379	448	103
Commercially pure titanium grade 4	483	552	104
Ti-6Al-V4	828	897	114

[1] The stress at which the material plastically deforms.
[2] The maximum stress the material withstands prior to failure in tension.
[3] The slope of the material's resistance to elastic deformation along the stress/strain curve.

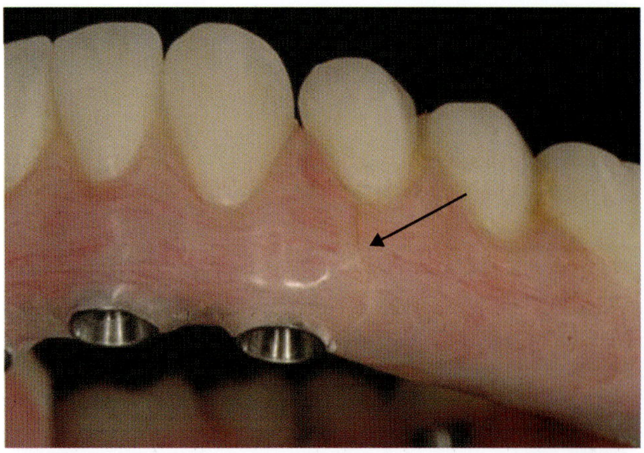
(a)

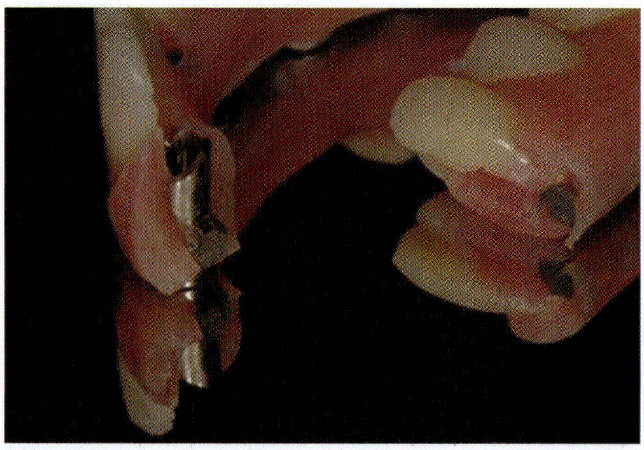
(b)

Figure 19.16 **(a)** Resin veneer failure indicative of framework flexure distal to posterior implant. **(b)** Subsequent failure of CNC machined titanium framework.

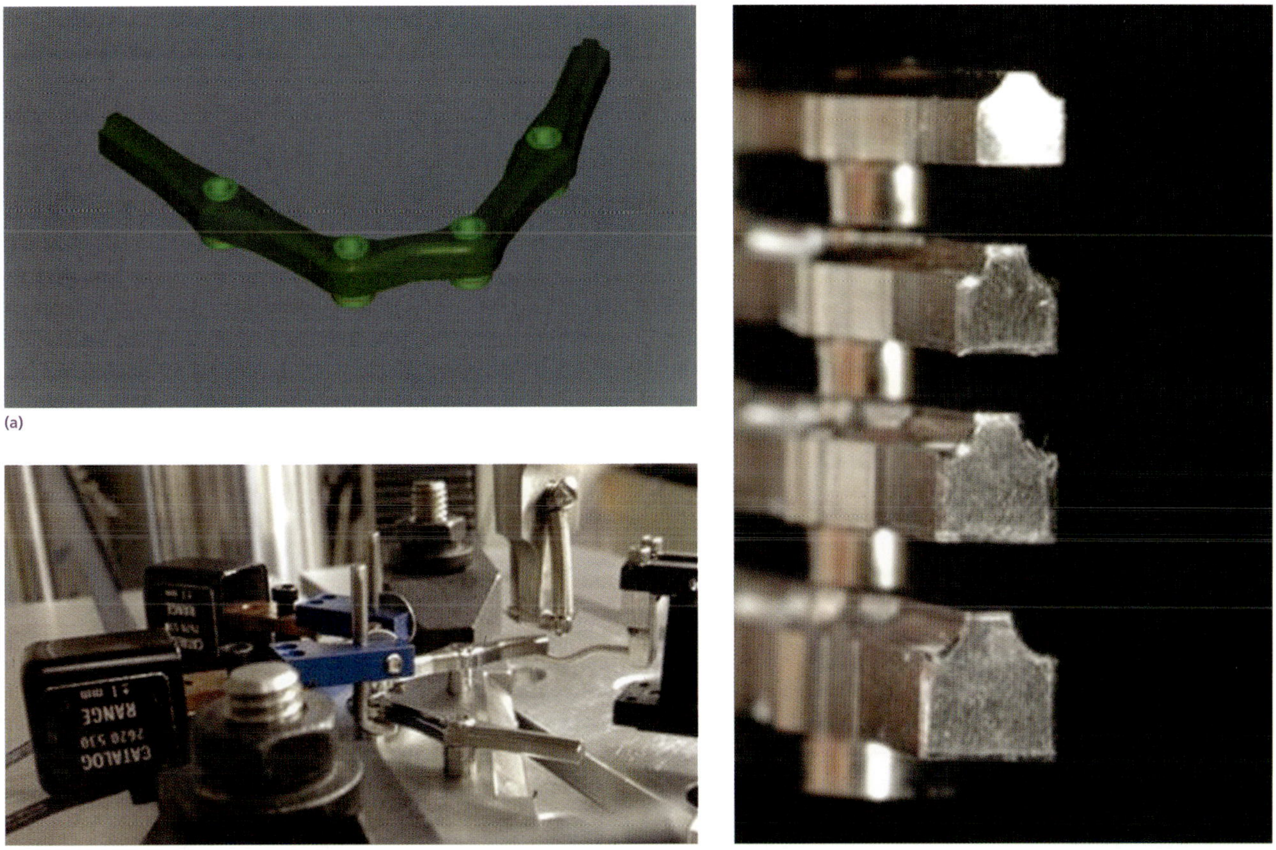
(a)
(c)
(b)

Figure 19.17 (**a**) Testing of Ti-6Al-4V titanium bar construct. (**b**) Testing carried out with standardized loading of cantilevered beams with varying cross-sectional areas of 2.5 × 2.5, 3.0 × 3.0, 3.5 × 3.5, and 4.0 × 4.0 mm. (**c**) Apparatus for static and dynamic testing.

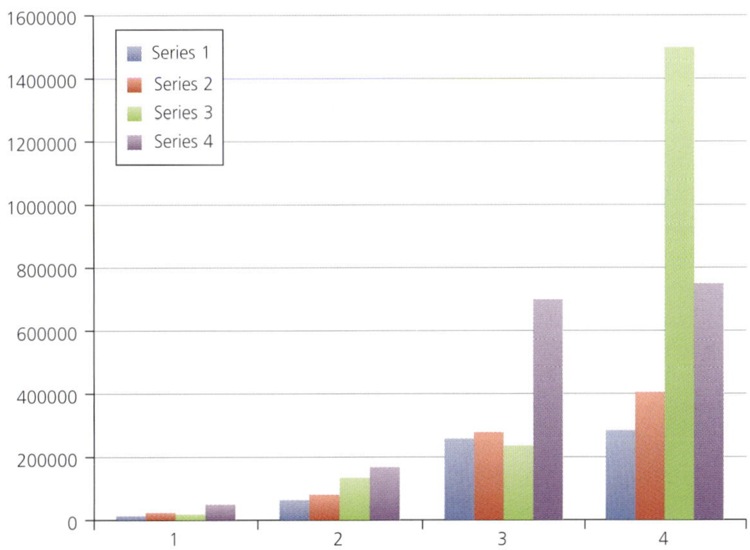

Figure 19.18 Standardized laboratory test results illustrate the number of cycles to failure of cantilevered bars, indicating that the 4 × 4 mm exhibited the greatest resistance to deformation.

passive fit appears to be elusive,[66] and, despite these technologies being more accurate, they do not appear to make a difference in animal models[67] and in medium-term follow-up.[68] If a cantilevered design is anticipated, it may be prudent to consider using an alloy with a high tensile strength. Palladium–copper is a good choice since its flexural strength is nearly 900 MPa.

Where the interarch distance is limited, construction of a prosthesis with a metal–ceramic design may be a prudent choice. In cases where this choice is not clear, construction of a diagnostic prosthesis may be beneficial to ascertain where acrylic resin-to-metal design is appropriate (Figure 19.19). The use of a conventional metal–ceramic design has particular advantages,

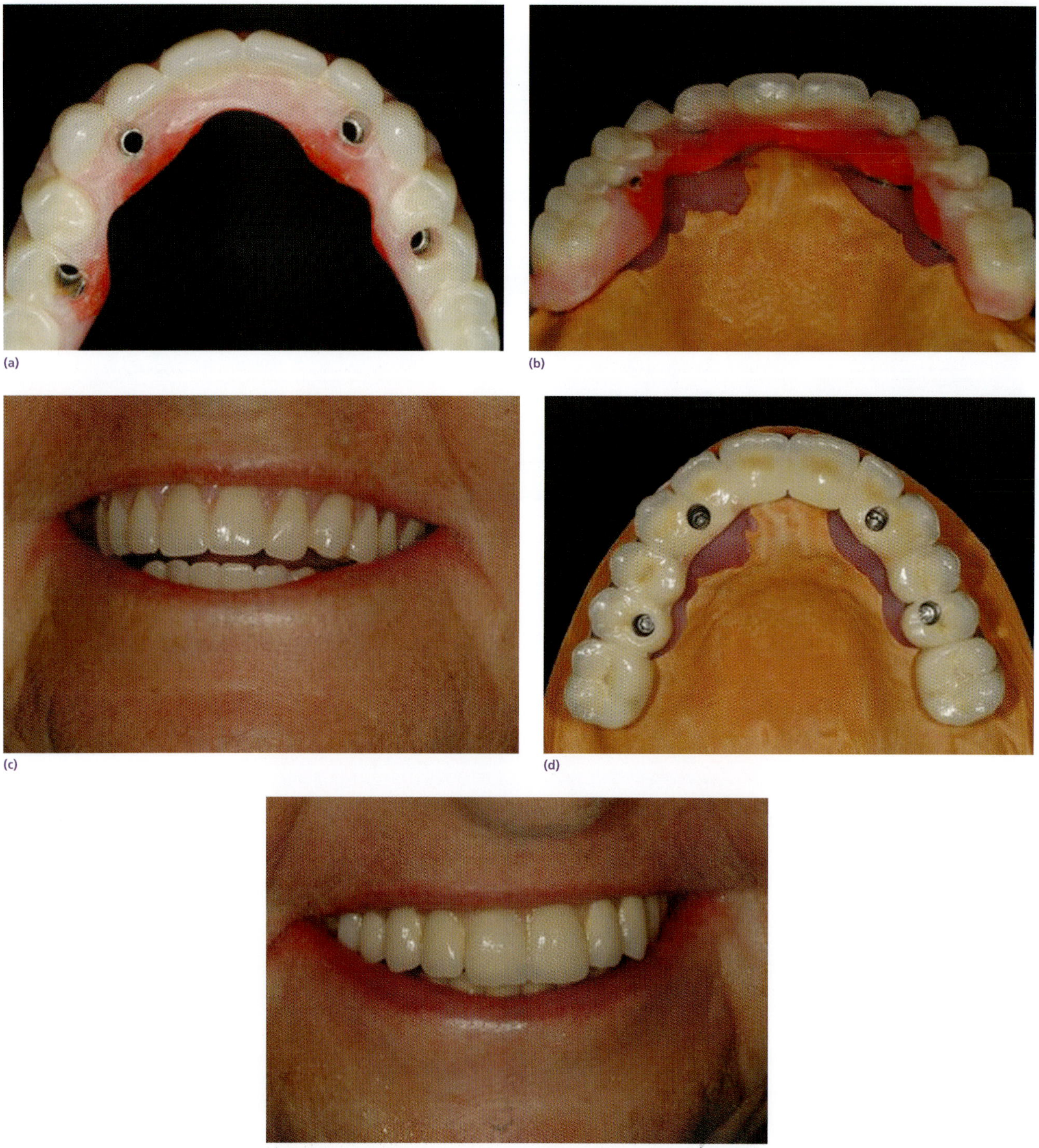

Figure 19.19 Constrained interarch distance may preclude acrylic resin to metal design. **(a)** Construction of diagnostic prosthesis using impression verification index. **(b)** Illustrated restriction of interarch distance. **(c)** Satisfactory esthetic and functional trial of diagnostic prostheses. **(d)** Resultant construction of metal–ceramic fixed dental prosthesis. **(e)** Clinical view of definitive prostheses.

in that the slight differences in thermal expansion coefficients and contraction between metal and porcelain creates compression of the ceramic upon cooling, giving it significant strength. The choice of a particular alloy for the framework has significance in multiple-unit restorations of this type. Prerequisites for choosing an appropriate alloy will depend partly upon prosthesis design and partly on the veneering porcelain chosen. Gold–palladium has been a popular choice for years due to the high resistance to corrosion. The tensile strength of the alloy is desirable for multiple-unit fixed partial dentures as it approaches 50% gold and 40% palladium. In recent years with the increasing cost of gold, the use of this alloy has become cost prohibitive. Silver–palladium alloy (Ag 37.7%, Pd 53.3%, In >1.0%, Sn 8.5%, Ru >1.0%, Li >1.0%) is another alternative, which gives significant flexural strength (450 MPa) and is highly compatible with most feldspathic porcelains. Some critique of the alloy has been a greenish hue, that can leach into the porcelain, associated with silver content. Alternatively palladium–copper (80% Pd, 10% Cu, 9% Ga) has been used, since resistance to corrosion is still high and it has more significant resistance to deformation than most other noble alloys (Table 19.3). A disadvantage of this alloy is an intense oxide accumulation that is difficult to mask with opaque porcelain application,[69] so it is better used with acrylic resin-to-metal prostheses. Without sandblasting some of the dark, heavy oxide away, the potential for delamination appears higher than with other alloys. An additional disadvantage of palladium-based alloys is the high cross-reactivity with those who manifest an allergy to nickel.[70,71] Although decreasing, the general incidence of nickel hypersensitivity has been quoted to be as much as 10–15% and it is usually associated with hand eczema. A screening questionnaire to include nickel hypersensitivity is appropriate in the planning stage to avoid any difficulty with metal allergy.

Table 19.3 Alloy selection for metal–ceramic prostheses.

Alloy	Flexural strength (MPa)	Elastic modulus (MPa)
Palladium–copper	795	97
Palladium–silver	415	98
Gold–palladium	505	118
Cobalt–chromium	500	198

Designing the metal substructure is also of importance, where anatomic cut back and classic trestle frame designs prevail, to minimize distortion during firing and cooling (Figure 19.20). This has been described extensively and is foundational for porcelain-fused-to-metal restorations.[72] This, in itself, is also a tremendous advantage, as each case can be designed for specific contours where current digital technology software fails to meet this customized need. The use of casting techniques, where metal–ceramic technology will be employed, is of significant consideration, as the fit of castings in multi-unit applications can be very challenging to achieve. Some of the work by White[73] has given strategies in sprueing and obtaining a metal casting that fits the mating surfaces well with little need for brazing techniques to compensate for cooling contraction.

Digital technology is developing to allow controlled design to better achieve the desired contours and configurations. It may be appealing to mill ceramics and titanium since control of spatial orientation and opposing occlusion allows development of a unique customized occlusal design. However, machined ceramics for multi-unit restorations require significant interproximal cross-sectional area for maximum resistance. Comparatively, the interproximal connectors with a cast metallic framework are much stronger than most machined high-strength ceramics. Due to the costs involved, it is not currently viable to machine noble alloys. Where resorption has taken place, creating esthetic tooth proportions will necessitate creating some form of gingival architecture.[74] With cases of advanced resorption, this may require a significant amount of gingival porcelain lamination

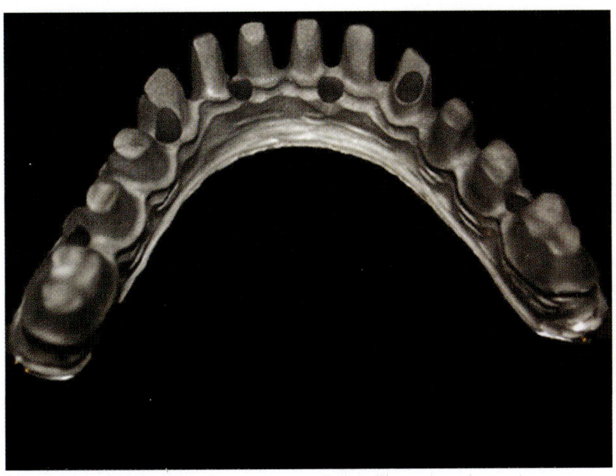

(a)

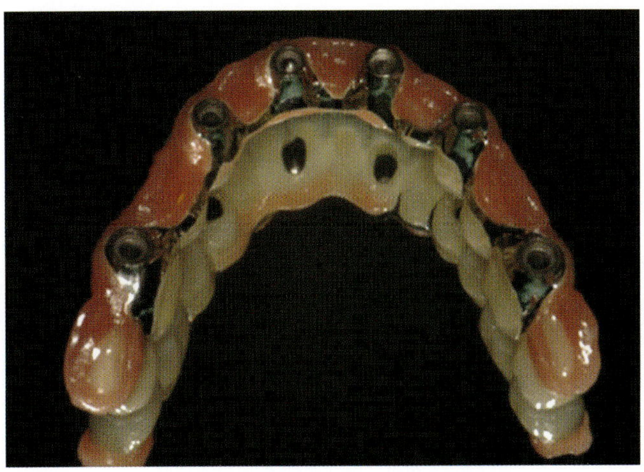

(b)

Figure 19.20 **(a)** Trestle framework design. **(b)** This design used to uniformly support porcelain and minimize framework strain contraction upon cooling.

to give correct tooth-to-tooth proportion and create an esthetic appearance (Figure 19.21). A multitude of materials can be used for this purpose and combinations of a bulk gingiva-colored ceramic with a thin composite resin veneer has been advocated in the partially dentate patient where a visible interface may be evident.[75] However, the use of laminated resin gives rise to servicing needs as it wears and becomes less color stable. In edentulous arches, this "hybrid approach" of using both types of materials is not needed unless the residual ridge changes within the esthetic zone (Figure 19.22). As with the variety of colors evident in teeth, gingival ceramics should emulate the subtleties of the various elements of different gingival tissues. This requires a strategic approach to color development and texture.[76,77]

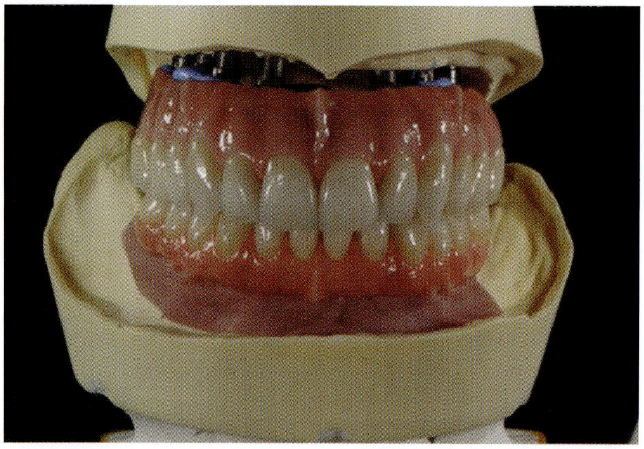

Figure 19.21 Gingival porcelain on component prosthesis where significant gingival architecture is required. This allows creation of correct tooth-to-tooth proportion. *Source:* Riera *et al.*, 2010.[82] Reproduced with permission from Quintessence Publishing Company Inc.

Attachment strategies for these restorations can be quite varied: either connection direct to the implant or in combination with custom telescopic abutment support. As with any laminated restoration, the possibility of veneer fracture still exists and should be minimized. Additional strategies for limiting the risk of ceramic fracture include minimizing surface roughness, thermal tempering, ion exchange, reducing number of firing cycles, and progressive layering of ceramic with gradual differences in coefficients of thermal expansion.[78]

Component fixed dental prosthesis

The use of component prostheses is a more contemporary approach to managing long-term servicing of fixed dental prostheses.[79–81]

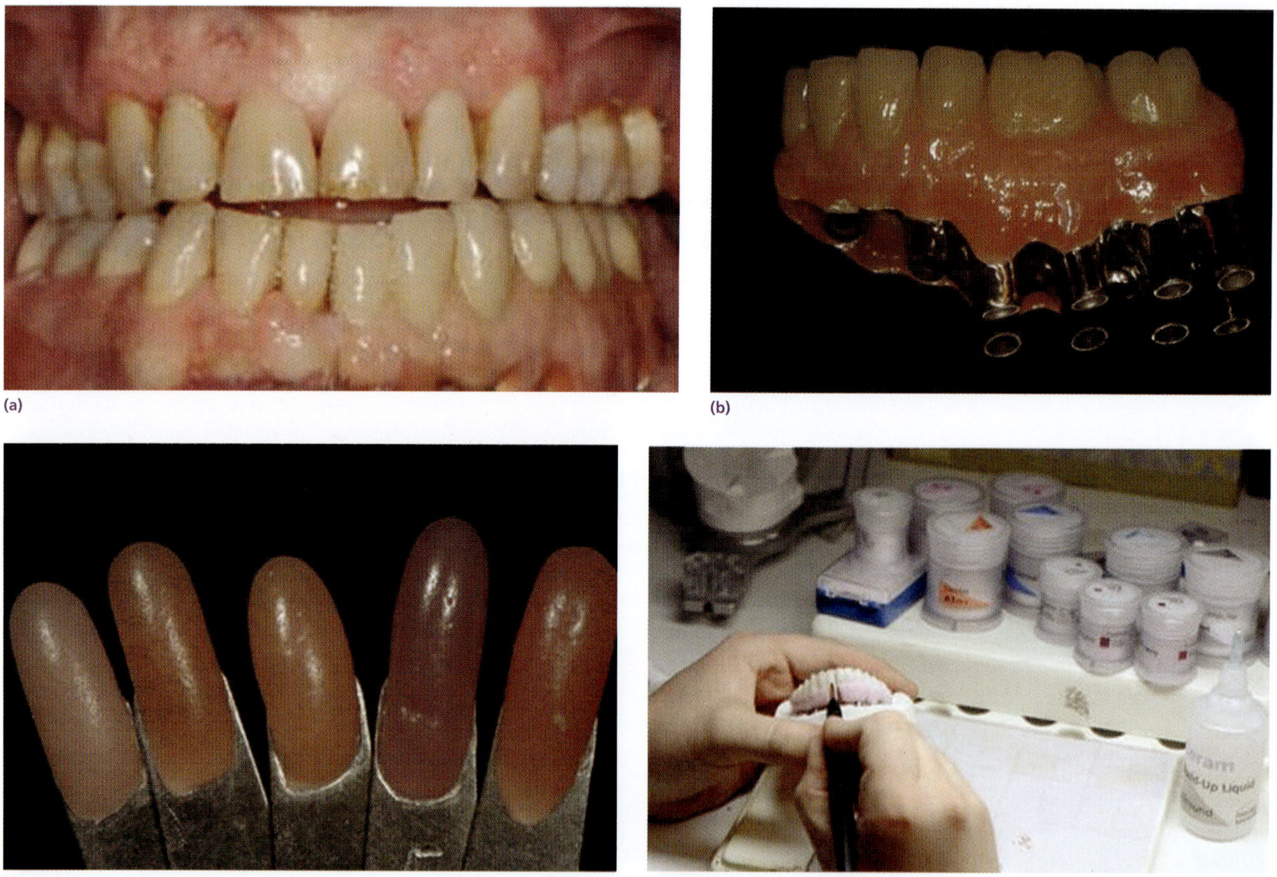

(a) (b) (c) (d)

Figure 19.22 (a, b) Patient treated for mandibular resection with metal–ceramic prosthesis where topography of arch is abruptly different. (c) Customized gingival shade tabs. (d) Technique of gingival porcelain lamination. *Source:* Reproduced with permission from Peter Angelus, M.D.T.

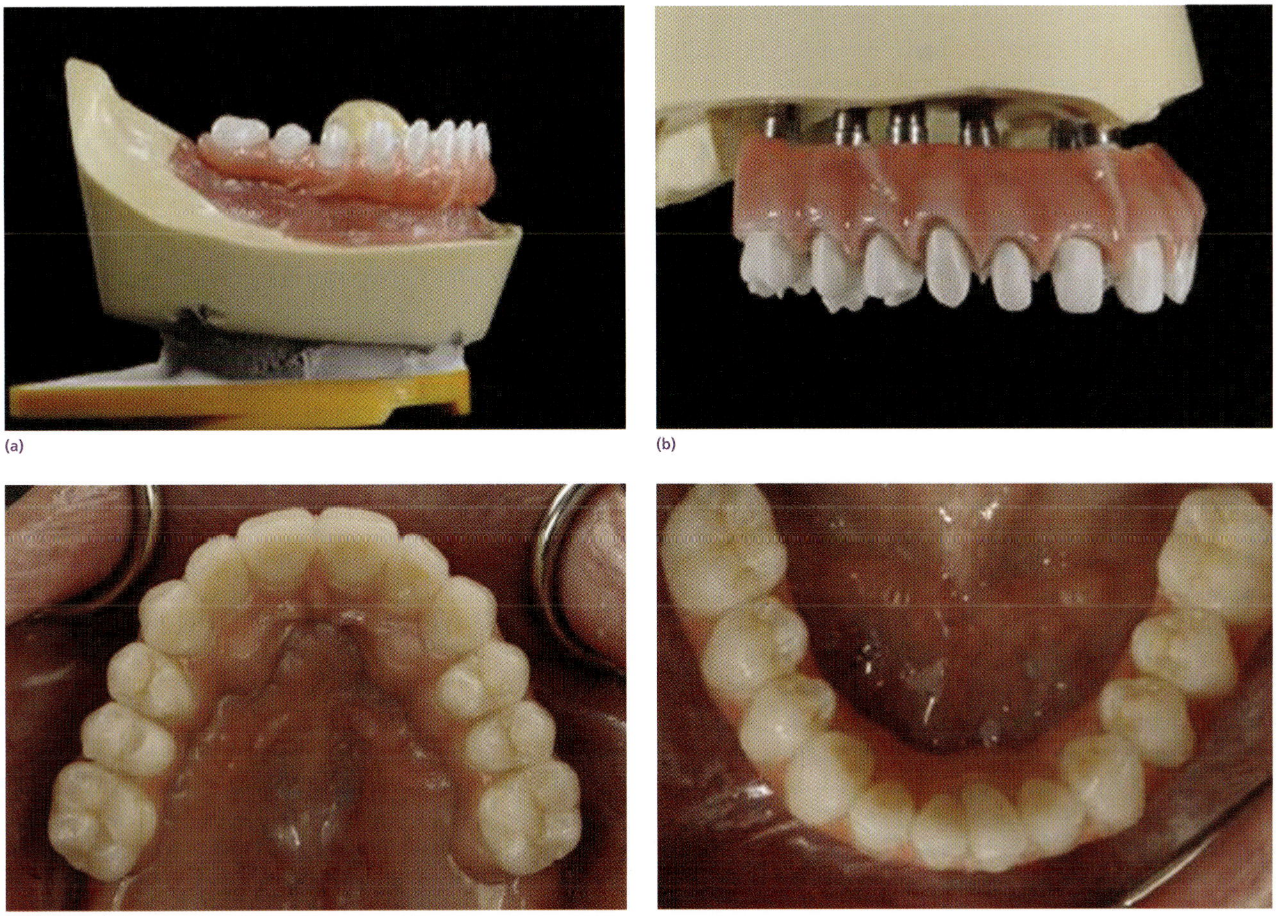

(a) (b) (c) (d)

Figure 19.23 (a, b) Component prosthesis constructed of laminated zirconia primary frameworks with zirconia copings that are CAD and can be retrieved for retreatment. (c, d) Occlusal views of finished prostheses after securing occlusal units by bonding. *Source:* Riera *et al.*, 2010.[82] Reproduced with permission from Quintessence Publishing Company Inc.

It has been proposed to address the recent difficulty of finding trained dental technicians to provide a restoration that can be fabricated by mostly digital means and easily serviced long term. The construction of the primary framework can be either titanium or zirconia,[82] which is subsequently veneered with simulated gingival material (Figure 19.23). The final contour allows a supportive preparation area for construction of individual "crowns" which can be subsequently cemented to the primary framework. Failure of any of the units can allow retrieval and "retreatment" of the single unit without subjecting the entire prosthesis to repeated firings.

Monolithic fixed dental prosthesis

Additional strategies to minimize prosthesis servicing have incorporated the use of monolithic zirconia with specialized staining techniques.[83,84] The machining size available for copy-milled zirconia discs is quite accommodating, and can be up to 30 mm thick to comply with the interarch spacing needed for monolithic design. As development of translucent zirconia continues, lamination of the anterior portion of these prostheses is still essential to maintain maximum esthetic potential (Figure 19.24). Monolithic zirconia restorations have an excellent prognosis at least in short-term follow-up, as the main concerns are outcomes of the opposing prosthesis.[84] Some concerns over the servicing of layered zirconia restorations have identified factors associated with its use.[85] Chipping and delamination are the primary mode of complication,[86] it is theorized that this is due to large differences in coefficients of thermal expansion of the veneering material upon cooling.[87] Luting yttria-stabilized zirconia has been somewhat problematic, as it is easily phase-transformed to a monoclinic (weaker) form upon the use of high pressure/speed abrasives in an attempt to etch or roughen its surface. However, low air pressure particle abrasion can be helpful, without undue risk of phase-transformation, and may result in better long-term cementation survival.[88]

The use of zirconia direct to the implant platform has raised concern over its abrasive potential under loading. The connection has been shown in laboratory studies[89,90] to potentially damage the implant platform and also create titanium debris within the tissue, potentially creating tattooing phenomena.[91] For this and

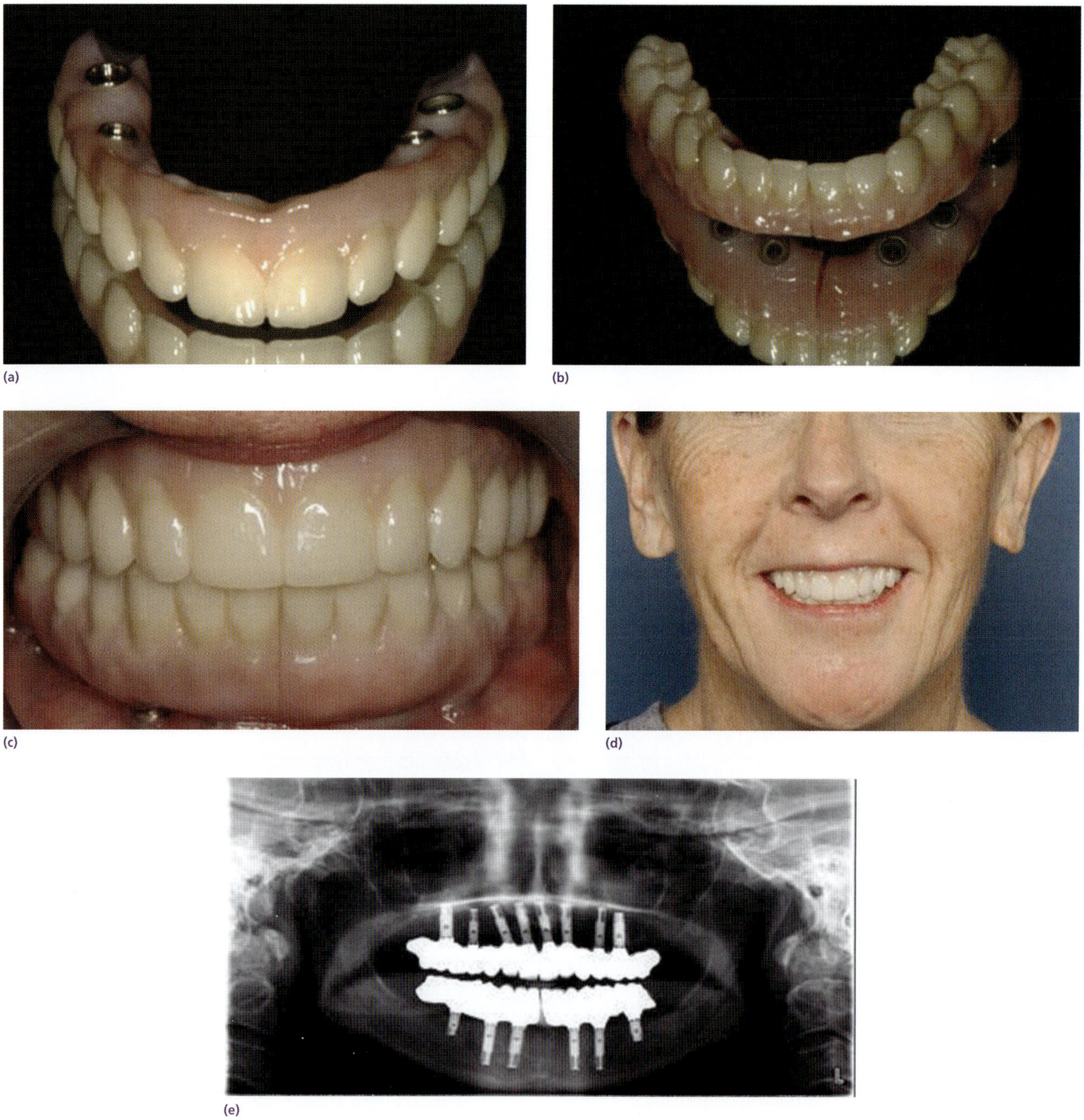

Figure 19.24 Predominantly zirconia full-arch restorations. (a) Maxillary prosthesis with screw-retained posterior abutment support and telescopic anterior support. (b) Mandibular segmental restoration with screw-retained design. (c) Intraoral view. (d) Extraoral view. (e) Post-treatment panoramic radiographic survey.

other reasons related to fit, it is advocated to use a titanium base prior to construction of these types of restorations. Luting the main zirconia construct to titanium bases is advantageous for a variety of reasons, including the inherent disparity between milled implant surfaces after sintering and the 3-D varied positions of abutments. This specialized technique was introduced for casting inaccuracies years ago and accounted for a more accurate fit as it was accomplished on the patient.[92,93] Risks in this procedure are debonding of the titanium base under function, cement extravasation or residual excess cement that occurs easily without soft tissue attachment to the abutments. Recognizing the signs and symptoms of residual excess cement is important to reverse any associated pathology.[94] Some recent strategies propose the use of vented restorations and internally vented abutments.[95]

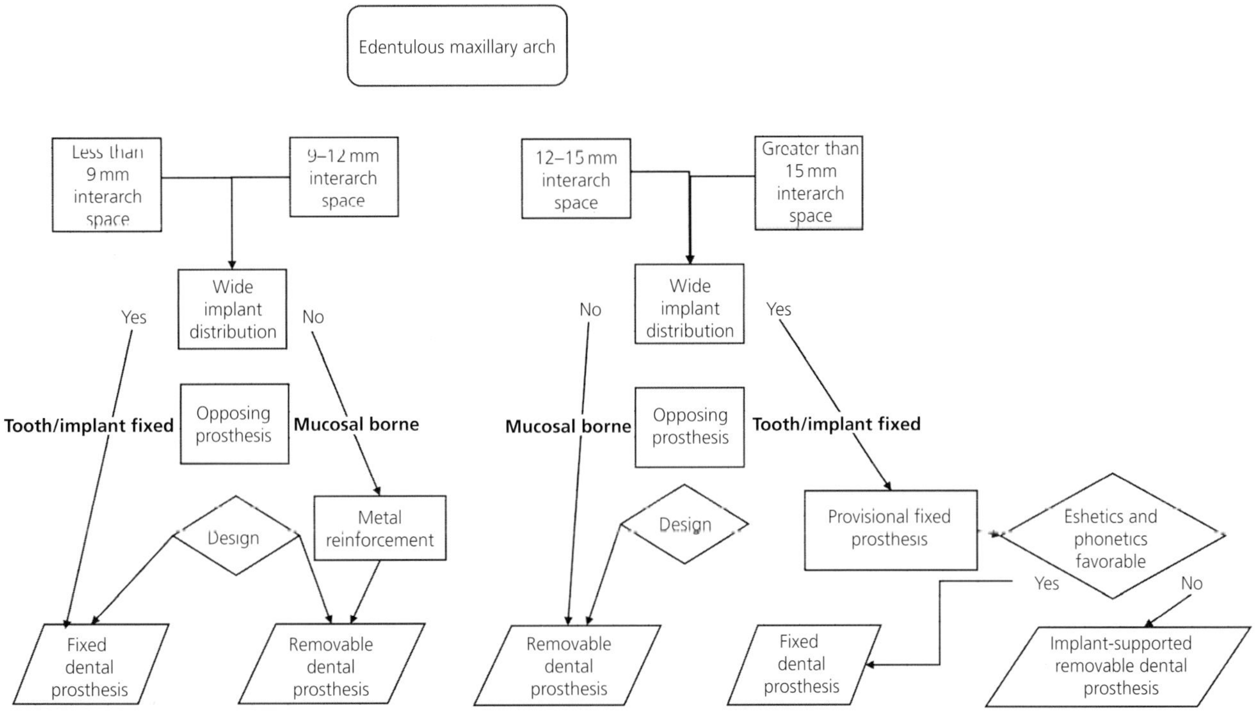

Figure 19.25 Algorithm for designing a maxillary implant prosthesis for an edentulous arch.

Proposed design algorithm

Basic tenets of oral physiology should be considered prior to designing prostheses for edentulous patients. Some additional patient-specific factors are speech, ease of hygiene, interarch distance, implant location, orthognathic relationship, and patient preference.

The prosthetic requirements for the edentulous maxilla are multifactorial and consideration must be given to esthetics, phonetics, interarch distance, opposing design, and implant distribution. Some guidelines for a systematic approach are given in Figure 19.25. The process is guided by first considering the available space and then secondary consideration is given to the other factors concerning implant distribution and opposing design. Additional consideration for advanced resorption of the maxilla incorporates the use of a provisional prosthesis to trial phonetics and esthetics. In some cases a precision detachable prosthesis is indicated to best serve a phonetic seal while facilitating esthetics and hygiene.

Designing the mandibular prosthesis is likewise multifactorial, with function and physiologic considerations based on interarch distance, opposing design, and implant distribution, as the esthetic and phonetic variables are less influential (Figure 19.26). The tenet of designing the mandibular prosthesis to be equivalent or slightly greater in support to the maxillary prosthesis is important, in that a maxillary fixed dental prosthesis should not oppose a mucosal-based mandibular prosthesis. This design works poorly with respect to maintenance and overall prosthesis stability.

Material choices for prosthetics

After local and patient-mediated factors are established for a selected design, choice of material for the construction can be recommended and should address long-term maintenance.

Overdentures that oppose either other implant-supported restorations or restored dentitions, or are constructed in constrained interarch distances, should contain some metal reinforcement in the base, and consideration should be given to maintaining posterior vertical dimension with metal or ceramic onlays.

In general, a retrievable metal–ceramic design can be used where a fixed dental prosthesis is planned in a constricted interarch distance. This is a reliable design that allows a level of repair, and which is esthetically versatile and strong. Cantilevering should be limited as metal–ceramic designs function poorly in tension. Where parafunctional activity exists, the use of component design or monolithic zirconia may be a more appropriate selection. Larger interarch distances may allow the use of metal–acrylic designs in applications where equivalent to lower powering is needed in the opposing occlusal design. Of course, the clinician may choose a departure from these suggestions, as case variability does not dictate that one material choice is superior over the other.

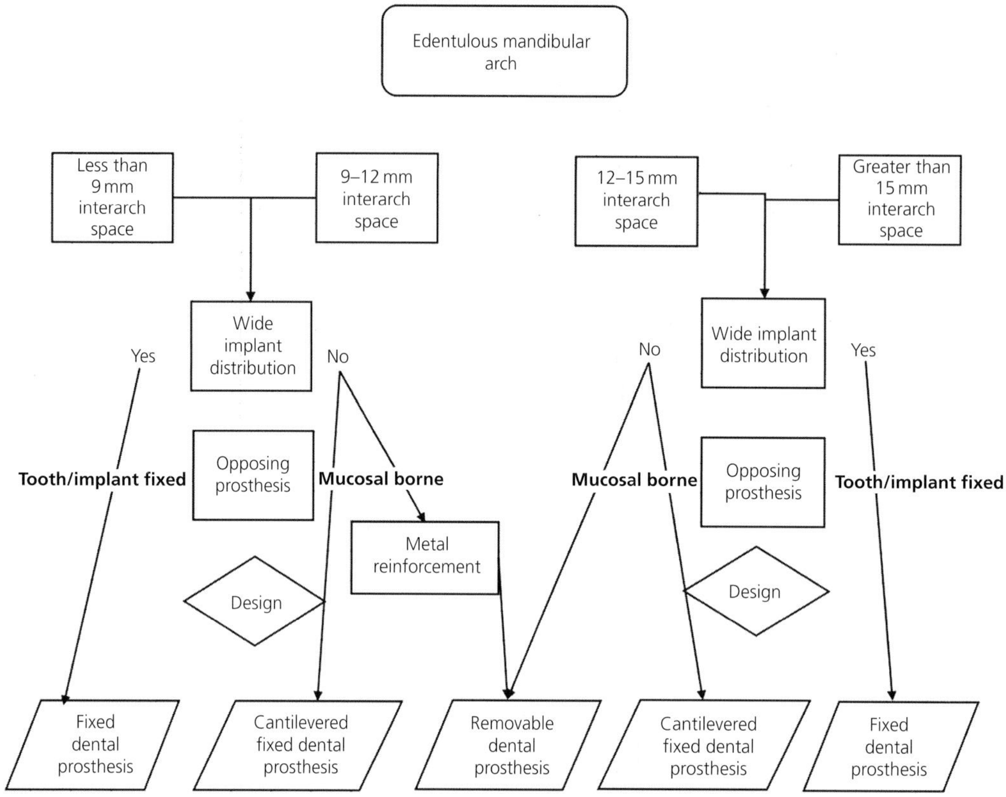

Figure 19.26 Algorithm for designing a mandibular implant prosthesis for an edentulous arch.

Repair techniques

The use of a variety of materials for full-arch implant prosthodontics can be, in part, based on the available laboratory support of the dental practice for repairs. For instance, support needed to effectively repair a dislodged acrylic resin tooth might be a consideration when designing the prosthesis. Prostheses of this sort can be effectively repaired easily with on-site lab support, while other expertise/support may allow one to consider adding porcelain, which is more complex and involves more risk.

The overdenture design, either a stud- or bar-retained attachment, has required the most maintenance in comparison to all other prostheses.[8] Frequently, the attachments must be changed, the intaglio surfaces relined, the prosthetic teeth changed, or the base repaired due to fracture. Although some studies consider the stud attachment superior to bar attachment design,[96] other studies find that certain attachments are easier to care for than alternatives.[97] Some systematic reviews cite that the high variability associated with implant distribution does not substantiate a specific recommendation, but some information on resistance of the base design has been advocated.[98]

Resurfacing of acrylic veneered prostheses, an expected medium-term maintenance procedure, is rather simplistic with an idea of opposing occlusal surfaces and adaptation of denture bases as well if applicable. If a single tooth will need replacing, it has been suggested to add minimal autopolymerizing acrylic resin and keep the ridge lap portion intact to support the repair vertically and make the repair as robust as possible.[99] Other strategies to maintain vertical dimension are to laminate the posterior acrylic resin teeth with metal or ceramic onlays, thereby maintaining overbite/overjet relationships in anterior teeth. If mucosally supported, the base adaptation should also be maintained so as to preserve occlusal relationships. Along with reaffirmation of the vertical dimension of occlusion and occlusal plane, re-establishing bilateral balance to favor the weaker of the two arches is recommended. Finally, confirmation of the esthetic parameters will complete the servicing. If bruxism is of concern, the use of a mouthguard is recommended, which can be made of a thermoplastic material and designed as a flat plane (Figure 19.27).

For porcelain veneer failures, a conservative approach can involve either recontouring or polishing for minor chips; preparing a porcelain laminate veneer may be needed for more extensive failures (Figure 19.28). A ceramic–metal veneering failure (i.e., exposing metal) may prompt segmental refiring or reveneering of the entire construct. It is of utmost importance to desiccate the ceramic prior to refiring, as any residual moisture content will cause a catastrophic breakdown of the ceramic. Each firing cycle will convert more of available ceramic to leucite, increasing the coefficient of thermal expansion of the ceramic, resulting in changes to the residual compressive stress imparted to the metal substructure.[78] Repeated firings or

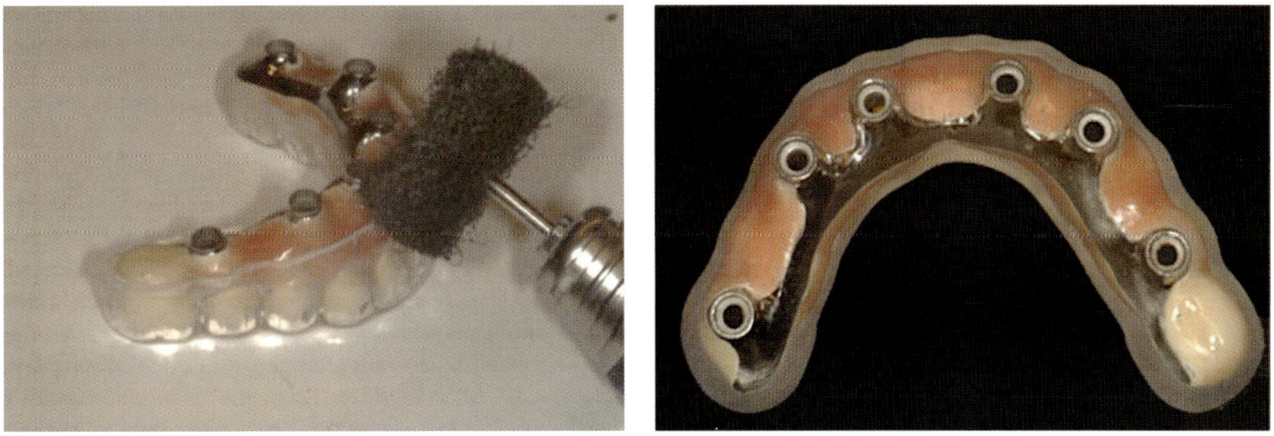
(a) (b)

Figure 19.27 Occlusal guard fabricated of polyethylene material. (a) Finishing on prosthesis with foam abrasive wheels. (b) Final finish of occlusal guard illustrating maximal adaptation.

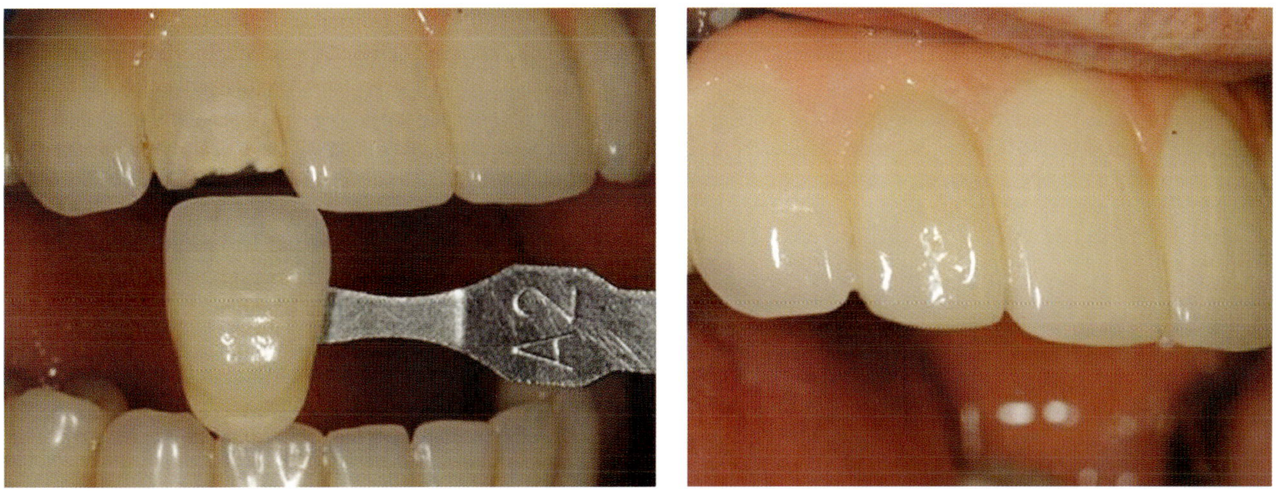

(a) (b)

Figure 19.28 Patient presenting with fractured metal–ceramic prosthesis. (a) Light veneer preparation with shade selection. (b) Lithium disilicate pressed veneer adhesively luted to etched porcelain surface.

segmental repair will considerably change the resistance properties of the ceramic and it may be worth considering re veneering the entire structure.

Repair of a component prosthesis can be anticipated by storing the occlusal/crown unit components in a digital database that can rapidly reproduce the unit, so that it is readily available to be attached by adhesive means inside or outside of the mouth.

Segmentation versus single-piece prosthetic design is also somewhat controversial and depends upon operator preferences. The trend toward placement of fewer implants for a complete arch of prosthetics may dictate single-piece prosthetic design. However, segmentation has merit based on retrievability and retreatment of potential veneer failure. Long-span metal–ceramic units may be more difficult to fabricate in the laboratory without multiple firings which will convert more available ceramic to leucite, increasing the coefficient of thermal expansion of the ceramic, resulting in changing the residual compressive stress imparted to the metal substructure. Lambert *et al.*[100] have reported the number of prostheses per arch had no influence on the prosthodontic survival rate. Segmented prosthetic units would also avail the end-provider with greater ease in repair and replacement if an implant is lost.

Summary

The development of many materials in dentistry has undergone a renaissance in the last decade. The choice of materials for treatment of edentulous patients is dependent upon patient-specific factors of interarch distances, bone volume, and indicated biomechanical design. A thorough approach to this decision-making process should start with diagnosis and treatment planning by all team members, to insure that the desired outcome can be achieved. Volume of restorative material is often one factor which can give indication as to design. Occasionally making a diagnostic prosthesis can be a pilot reference for design before constructing a definitive prosthesis. Although an algorithm can be helpful, the decision on using specific material combinations is not empiric and should be met with consideration for esthetic and functional requirements. The restorative dentist should be prudent with these choices but should also discuss servicing responsibilities with the patient and their commitment to maintenance of the prostheses.

References

1. Adell R. Clinical results of osseointegrated implants supporting fixed prostheses in edentulous jaws. *J Prosthet Dent* 1983; **50**(2): 251–254.
2. Tagger Green N, Machtei EE, Horwitz J, *et al.* Fracture of dental implants: literature review and report of a case. *Implant Dent* 2002; **11**(2): 137–143.
3. Misch CE. Progressive loading of bone with implant prostheses. *J Dent Symp* 1993; **1**: 50–53.
4. Laney WR, Tolman DE, Keller EE, *et al.* Dental implants: tissue-integrated prosthesis utilizing the osseointegration concept. *Mayo Clin Proc* 1986; **61**(2): 91–97.
5. Tolman DE, Laney WR. Tissue-integrated dental prostheses: the first 78 months of experience at the Mayo Clinic. *Mayo Clin Proc* 1993; **68**(4): 323–331.
6. Sekine H, Yoshida K, Komiyama Y, *et al.* Functioning survival rate of the fixture and superstructure of osseointegrated implants (first report). *Bull Tokyo Dent Coll* 1993; **34**(4): 177–181.
7. Henry PJ, Bower RC, Wall CD. Rehabilitation of the edentulous mandible with osseointegrated dental implants: 10 year follow-up. *Aust Dent J* 1995; **40**(1): 1–9.
8. Goodacre CJ, Bernal G, Rungcharassaeng K, *et al.* Clinical complications with implants and implant prostheses. *J Prosthet Dent* 2003; **90**(2): 121–132.
9. Purcell BA, McGlumphy EA, Holloway JA, *et al.* Prosthetic complications in mandibular metal-resin implant-fixed complete dental prostheses: a 5- to 9-year analysis. *Int J Oral Maxillofac Implants* 2008; **23**(5): 847–857.
10. Gallucci GO, Doughtie CB, Hwang JW, *et al.* Five-year results of fixed implant-supported rehabilitations with distal cantilevers for the edentulous mandible. *Clin Oral Implants Res* 2009; **20**(6): 601–607.
11. Dhima M, Paulusova V, Lohse C, *et al.* Practice-based evidence from 29-year outcome analysis of management of the edentulous jaw using osseointegrated dental implants. *J Prosthodont* 2014; **23**(3): 173–181.
12. Zarb GA, Symington JM. Osseointegrated dental implants: preliminary report on a replication study. *J Prosthet Dent* 1983; **50**(2): 271–276.
13. Zarb G. *Nature and Significance of the Edentulous State. Tissue Integrated Dental Prosthesis.* **1**, 1st edn. Chicago: Quintessence 1986; 77–88.
14. Bedrossian E, Sullivan RM, Fortin Y, *et al.* Fixed-prosthetic implant restoration of the edentulous maxilla: a systematic pretreatment evaluation method. *J Oral Maxillofac Surg* 2008; **66**(1): 112–122.
15. Steigmann M. Treatment sequencing for the multiunit restoration: hard and soft tissue considerations. *J Oral Maxillofac Surg* 2007; **65**(7 Suppl 1): 53–63.
16. Sadowsky SJ, Hansen PW. Evidence-based criteria for differential treatment planning of implant restorations for the mandibular edentulous patient. *J Prosthodont* 2014; **23**(2): 104–111.
17. Newton JT, Cunningham SJ. Great expectations: what do patients expect and how can expectations be managed? *J Orthod* 2013; **40**(2): 112–117.
18. Hobkirk JA, Abdel-Latif HH, Howlett J, *et al.* Prosthetic treatment time and satisfaction of edentulous patients treated with conventional or implant-supported complete mandibular dentures: a case-control study (part 1). *Int J Prosthodont* 2008; **21**(6): 489–495.
19. Hobkirk JA, Abdel-Latif HH, Howlett J, *et al.* Prosthetic treatment time and satisfaction of edentulous patients treated with conventional or implant-stabilized complete mandibular dentures: a case-control study (part 2). *Int J Prosthodont* 2009; **22**(1): 13–19.
20. Nuttall NM, Slade GD, Sanders AE, *et al.* An empirically derived population-response model of the short form of the Oral Health Impact Profile. *Community Dent Oral Epidemiol* 2006; **34**(1): 18–24.
21. Slade GD, Spencer AJ. Development and evaluation of the Oral Health Impact Profile. *Community Dent Health* 1994; **11**(1): 3–11.
22. American Psychiatric Association. *Diagnostic and Statistical Manual of Mental Disorders.* Washington DC: American Psychiatric Association, 1994.
23. Fueki K, Kimoto K, Ogawa T, *et al.* Effect of implant-supported or retained dentures on masticatory performance: a systematic review. *J Prosthet Dent* 2007; **98**(6): 470–477.
24. Tajbakhsh S, Rubenstein JE, Faine MP, *et al.* Selection patterns of dietary foods in edentulous participants rehabilitated with maxillary complete dentures opposed by mandibular implant-supported prostheses: a multicenter longitudinal assessment. *J Prosthet Dent* 2013; **110**(4): 252–258.
25. Dudley J. The 2-implant maxillary overdenture: a clinical report. *J Prosthet Dent* 2014; **112**(2): 104–107.
26. Malo P, Rangert B, Nobre M. All-on-4 immediate-function concept with Branemark System implants for completely edentulous maxillae: a 1-year retrospective clinical study. *Clin Implant Dent Relat Res* 2005; **7**(Suppl 1): S88–94.
27. Malo P, de Araujo Nobre M, Lopes A, *et al.* "All-on-4" immediate-function concept for completely edentulous maxillae: a clinical report on the medium (3 years) and long-term (5 years) outcomes. *Clin Implant Dent Relat Res* 2012; **14**(Suppl 1): e139–150.
28. Malo P, de Araujo Nobre M, Lopes A, *et al.* Posterior maxillary implants inserted with bicortical anchorage and placed in immediate function for partial or complete edentulous rehabilitations. A retrospective clinical study with a median follow-up of 7 years. *Oral Maxillofac Surg* 2015; **19**(1): 19–27.
29. Malo P, Nobre Mde A, Lopes A, *et al.* Five-year outcome of a retrospective cohort study on the rehabilitation of completely edentulous atrophic maxillae with immediately loaded zygomatic implants placed extra-maxillary. *Eur J Oral Implantol* 2014; **7**(3): 267–281.
30. Wang F, Monje A, Lin GH, *et al.* Reliability of four zygomatic implant-supported prostheses for the rehabilitation of the atrophic maxilla: a systematic review. *Int J Oral Maxillofac Implants* 2015; **30**(2): 293–298.

31. Heydecke G, Zwahlen M, Nicol A, *et al.* What is the optimal number of implants for fixed reconstructions: a systematic review. *Clin Oral Implants Res* 2012; **23**(Suppl 6): 217–228.
32. Gamborena I, Blatz MB. *Evolution: Contemporary Protocols for Anterior Single-Tooth Implants.* Chicago: Quintessence 2014; 440.
33. Wiskott HWA. *Fixed Prosthodontics: Principles and Clinics*, 1st edn. Great Britain: Quintessence Int 2011; 441–475.
34. Theoharidou A, Petridis HP, Tzannas K, *et al.* Abutment screw loosening in single-implant restorations: a systematic review. *Int J Oral Maxillofac Implants* 2008; **23**(4): 681–690.
35. Seetoh YL, Tan KB, Chua EK, *et al.* Load fatigue performance of conical implant–abutment connections. *Int J Oral Maxillofac Implants* 2011; **26**(4): 797–806.
36. *The Glossary of Oral and Maxillofacial Implants*, 1st edn. Chicago: Quintessence 2007; 199.
37. Bakaeen LG, Winkler S, Neff PA. The effect of implant diameter, restoration design, and occlusal table variations on screw loosening of posterior single-tooth implant restorations. *J Oral Implantol* 2001; **27**(2): 63–72.
38. Wittneben JG, Millen C, Bragger U. Clinical performance of screw-versus cement-retained fixed implant-supported reconstructions – a systematic review. *Int J Oral Maxillofac Implants* 2014; **29**(Suppl): 84–98.
39. Pjetursson BE, Asgeirsson AG, Zwahlen M, *et al.* Improvements in implant dentistry over the last decade: comparison of survival and complication rates in older and newer publications. *Int J Oral Maxillofac Implants* 2014; **29**(Suppl): 308–324.
40. Sailer I, Muhlemann S, Zwahlen M, *et al.* Cemented and screw-retained implant reconstructions: a systematic review of the survival and complication rates. *Clin Oral Implants Res* 2012; **23**(Suppl 6): 163 201.
41. Korsch M, Robra BP, Walther W. Predictors of excess cement and tissue response to fixed implant-supported dentures after cementation. *Clin Implant Dent Relat Res* 2015; **17**(Suppl 1): e45–53.
42. Romanos GE, Gupta B, Eckert SE. Distal cantilevers and implant dentistry. *Int J Oral Maxillofac Implants* 2012; **27**(5): 1131–1136.
43. Romeo E, Storelli S. Systematic review of the survival rate and the biological, technical, and aesthetic complications of fixed dental prostheses with cantilevers on implants reported in longitudinal studies with a mean of 5 years follow-up. *Clin Oral Implants Res* 2012; **23**(Suppl 6): 39–49.
44. Dhima M, Balshi T, Wolfinger G, *et al.* A retrospective analysis of mandibular bone height changes associated with 81 screw-retained implant-supported prostheses with distal cantilevers: a long-term follow-up analysis. *Int J Oral Maxillofac Implants* 2013; **28**(3): 854–859.
45. Malo P, de Araujo Nobre M, Lopes A. The prognosis of partial implant-supported fixed dental prostheses with cantilevers. A 5-year retrospective cohort study. *Eur J Oral Implantol* 2013; **6**(1): 51–59.
46. Hecker DM, Eckert SE. Cyclic loading of implant-supported prostheses: changes in component fit over time. *J Prosthet Dent* 2003; **89**(4): 346–351.
47. Nogueira SS, Ogle RE, Davis EL. Comparison of accuracy between compression- and injection-molded complete dentures. *J Prosthet Dent* 1999; **82**(3): 291–300.
48. Ahuja S, Cagna DR. Classification and management of restorative space in edentulous implant overdenture patients. *J Prosthet Dent* 2011; **105**(5): 332–337.
49. Alsiyabi AS, Felton DA, Cooper LF. The role of abutment-attachment selection in resolving inadequate interarch distance: a clinical report. *J Prosthodont* 2005; **14**(3): 184–190.
50. Phillips K, Wong KM. Space requirements for implant-retained bar-and-clip overdentures. *Compendium* 2001; **22**(6): 516–522.
51. Choi M, Acharya V, Berg RW, *et al.* Resinous denture base fracture resistance: effects of thickness and teeth. *Int J Prosthodont* 2012; **25**(1): 53–59.
52. Salvi GE, Bragger U. Mechanical and technical risks in implant therapy. *Int J Oral Maxillofac Implants* 2009; **24**(Suppl): 69–85.
53. Clelland NL, van Putten MC, Brantley WA, *et al.* Adhesion testing of a denture base resin with 5 casting alloys. *J Prosthodont* 2000; **9**(1): 30–36.
54. Mudford L, Curtis RV, Walter JD. An investigation of debonding between heat-cured PMMA and titanium alloy (Ti-6A1-4V). *J Dent* 1997; **25**(5): 415–421.
55. Trakas T, Michalakis K, Kang K, *et al.* Attachment systems for implant retained overdentures: a literature review. *Implant Dent* 2006; **15**(1): 24–34.
56. Van Roekel NB. Prosthesis fabrication using electrical discharge machining. *Int J Oral Maxillofac Implants* 1992; **7**(1): 56–61.
57. Skalak R. Osseointegration biomechanics. *J Oral Implantol* 1986; **12**(3): 350–356.
58. Frost HM. Perspectives: on a "paradigm shift" developing in skeletal science. *Calcif Tissue Int* 1995; **56**(1): 1–4.
59. Jemt T, Lindquist L, Hedegard B. Changes in chewing patterns of patients with complete dentures after placement of osseointegrated implants in the mandible. *J Prosthet Dent* 1985; **53**(4): 578–583.
60. Papaspyridakos P, Chen CJ, Chuang SK, *et al.* A systematic review of biologic and technical complications with fixed implant rehabilitations for edentulous patients. *Int J Oral Maxillofac Implants* 2012; **27**(1): 102–110.
61. Bozini T, Petridis H, Garefis K, *et al.* A meta-analysis of prosthodontic complication rates of implant-supported fixed dental prostheses in edentulous patients after an observation period of at least 5 years. *Int J Oral Maxillofac Implants* 2011; **26**(2): 304–318.
62. Phillips K, Wong KM. Vertical space requirement for the fixed-detachable, implant-supported prosthesis. *Compendium* 2002; **23**(8): 750–756.
63. Stewart RB, Staab GH. Cross-sectional design and fatigue durability of cantilevered sections of fixed implant-supported prostheses. *J Prosthodont* 1995; **4**(3): 188–194.
64. Ortorp A, Jemt T, Back T, *et al.* Comparisons of precision of fit between cast and CNC-milled titanium implant frameworks for the edentulous mandible. *Int J Prosthodont* 2003; **16**(2): 194–200.
65. Ortorp A, Jemt T. CNC-milled titanium frameworks supported by implants in the edentulous jaw: a 10-year comparative clinical study. *Clin Implant Dent Relat Res* 2012; **14**(1): 88–99.
66. Eliasson A, Wennerberg A, Johansson A, *et al.* The precision of fit of milled titanium implant frameworks (I-Bridge) in the edentulous jaw. *Clin Implant Dent Relat Res* 2010; **12**(2): 81–90.
67. Carr AB, Gerard DA, Larsen PE. The response of bone in primates around unloaded dental implants supporting prostheses with different levels of fit. *J Prosthet Dent* 1996; **76**(5): 500–509.
68. Ortorp A. On titanium frameworks and alternative impression techniques in implant dentistry. *Swed Dent J Suppl* 2005; **169**: 3–88.
69. Bertolotti RL. Rational selection of casting alloy. In: Preston JD (ed). *Perspectives in Dental Ceramics.* Proceedings of the Fourth

International Symposium on Ceramics. 1. 1st edn. Chicago: Quintessence 1985; 75–92.
70. Santucci B, Cannistraci C, Cristaudo A, *et al.* Multiple sensitivities to transition metals: the nickel palladium reactions. *Contact Dermatitis* 1996; **35**(5): 283–286.
71. Faurschou A, Menne T, Johansen JD, *et al.* Metal allergen of the 21st century – a review on exposure, epidemiology and clinical manifestations of palladium allergy. *Contact Dermatitis* 2011; **64**(4): 185–195.
72. Miller LL. Framework design in ceramo-metal restorations. *Dent Clin North Am* 1977; **21**(4): 699–716.
73. White G. *Osseointegrated Dental Technology*. London: Quintessence 1993; 233.
74. Tallgren A, Lang BR, Walker GF, *et al.* Roentgen cephalometric analysis of ridge resorption and changes in jaw and occlusal relationships in immediate complete denture wearers. *J Oral Rehabil* 1980; **7**(1): 77–94.
75. Coachman C, Van Dooren E, Gurel G, *et al.* Minimally invasive reconstruction in implant therapy: the prosthetic gingival restoration. *Quintessence Dent Technol* 2010; **33**: 61–75.
76. Cascione D, Aloum A, Takanashi K, *et al.* Artistry and CAD/CAM technology: predictable outcomes in contemporary implant dentistry. *Quintessence Dent Technol* 2011; **34**: 120–132.
77. Jungo E, Aloum A. Pink ceramic: combining esthetics and longevity. *Quintessence Dent Technol* 2013; **36**: 107–120.
78. Anusavice K, Chiayi S, Rawls HR. *Phillips' Science of Dental Materials*, 12th edn. St. Louis, MO: Elsevier 2013; 571.
79. Reshad M, Cascione D, Aalam AA. Fabrication of the mandibular implant-supported fixed restoration using CAD/CAM technology: a clinical report. *J Prosthet Dent* 2009; **102**(5): 271–278.
80. Mehrhof J, Nelson K. Implant-supported fixed restoration based on electroforming for the esthetic rehabilitation of edentulous patients. *Quintessence Dent Technol* 2008; **31**: 9–18.
81. Wohrle PS, Cornell DF. Contemporary maxillary implant-supported full arch restorations combining esthetics and passive fit. *Quintessence Dent Technol* 2008; **31**: 31–47.
82. Riera JG, Flores AR, Rivera FZ, *et al.* Endosseous implant rehabilitation of edentulism using high strength ceramics and component design. *Quintessence Dent Technol* 2010; **33**: 11–30.
83. Rojas-Vizcaya F. Full zirconia fixed detachable implant-retained restorations manufactured from monolithic zirconia: clinical report after two years in service. *J Prosthodont* 2011; **20**(7): 570–576.
84. Limmer B, Sanders AE, Reside G, *et al.* Complications and patient-centered outcomes with an implant-supported monolithic zirconia fixed dental prosthesis: 1 year results. *J Prosthodont* 2014; **23**(4): 267–275.
85. Kolgeci L, Mericske E, Worni A, *et al.* Technical complications and failures of zirconia-based prostheses supported by implants followed up to 7 years: a case series. *Int J Prosthodont* 2014; **27**(6): 544–552.
86. Raigrodski AJ, Hillstead MB, Meng GK, *et al.* Survival and complications of zirconia-based fixed dental prostheses: a systematic review. *J Prosthet Dent* 2012; **107**(3): 170–177.
87. Tan JP, Sederstrom D, Polansky JR, *et al.* The use of slow heating and slow cooling regimens to strengthen porcelain fused to zirconia. *J Prosthet Dent* 2012; **107**(3): 163–169.
88. Attia A, Kern M. Effect of cleaning methods after reduced-pressure air abrasion on bonding to zirconia ceramic. *J Adhes Dent* 2011; **13**(6): 561–567.
89. Klotz MW, Taylor TD, Goldberg AJ. Wear at the titanium-zirconia implant-abutment interface: a pilot study. *Int J Oral Maxillofac Implants* 2011; **26**(5): 970–975.
90. Stimmelmayr M, Edelhoff D, Guth JF, *et al.* Wear at the titanium-titanium and the titanium-zirconia implant-abutment interface: a comparative in vitro study. *Dent Mater* 2012; **28**(12): 1215–1220.
91. Taylor TD, Klotz MW, Lawton RA. Titanium tattooing associated with zirconia implant abutments: a clinical report of two cases. *Int J Oral Maxillofac Implants* 2014; **29**(4): 958–960.
92. Stumpel LJ, 3rd. The adhesive-corrected implant framework. *J Calif Dent Assoc* 1994; **22**(2): 47–53.
93. Stumpel LJ, 3rd, Quon SJ. Adhesive abutment cylinder luting. *J Prosthet Dent* 1993; **69**(4): 398–400.
94. Wadhwani C, Rapoport D, La Rosa S, *et al.* Radiographic detection and characteristic patterns of residual excess cement associated with cement-retained implant restorations: a clinical report. *J Prosthet Dent* 2012; **107**(3): 151–157.
95. Wadhwani C, Pineyro A, Hess T, *et al.* Effect of implant abutment modification on the extrusion of excess cement at the crown-abutment margin for cement-retained implant restorations. *Int J Oral Maxillofac Implants* 2011; **26**(6): 1241–1246.
96. Zou D, Wu Y, Huang W, *et al.* A 3-year prospective clinical study of telescopic crown, bar, and locator attachments for removable four implant-supported maxillary overdentures. *Int J Prosthodont* 2013; **26**(6): 566–573.
97. Turk PE, Geckili O, Turk Y, *et al.* In vitro comparison of the retentive properties of ball and locator attachments for implant overdentures. *Int J Oral Maxillofac Implants* 2014; **29**(5): 1106–1113.
98. Osman RB, Payne AG, Ma S. Prosthodontic maintenance of maxillary implant overdentures: a systematic literature review. *Int J Prosthodont* 2012; **25**(4): 381–391.
99. Clark WA, Hsu YT. The effect of autopolymerizing acrylic resin thickness on the bond strength of a repaired denture tooth. *J Prosthodont* 2014; **23**(7): 528–533.
100. Lambert FE, Weber HP, Susarla SM, *et al.* Descriptive analysis of implant and prosthodontic survival rates with fixed implant-supported rehabilitations in the edentulous maxilla. *J Periodontol* 2009; **80**(8): 1220–1230.

CHAPTER 20

Digital Alternatives in the Implant Restoration of the Edentulous Patient

Mathew T. Kattadiyil
Loma Linda University School of Dentistry, Loma Linda, California, USA

Introduction

There are multiple digital applications that are available for the implant restoration of an edentulous patient. However, they are relatively new, as most applications continue to improve with time and innovative ideas. Some of these applications include digital impressions, computer-aided designing and computer-aided manufacturing (CAD/CAM) of metallic or zirconia-based bar/substructures, and even fabrication of implant-assisted dentures. There is consensus amongst clinicians that a successful implant restoration is planned keeping the final prosthesis in mind. This allows ideal planning and placement of implants. This could not be truer when planning and fabricating an implant-assisted prosthesis for the completely edentulous arch. An appropriately fabricated complete denture serves as an ideal template for this planning.

The history of complete denture fabrication started in the US approximately 250 years ago with dentures being carved from ivory.[1] The wooden dentures worn by President George Washington and his concerns with them have become part of US history. Since those early days, concepts, techniques, and materials involved in the fabrication of complete dentures have evolved and improved over time. An aging population[2] promotes a demand for complete dentures that sustains continued interest in innovations in complete denture fabrications. This has been evidenced by the re-emergence of interest in innovative techniques using digital and computer-aided engineering of complete dentures. There are multiple options available to the clinician in the rehabilitation of the completely edentulous patient (Figure 20.1). These include prostheses made utilizing digital technology at some stage of fabrication. Figure 20.2 shows the steps involved in the fabrication of a fixed complete denture and steps identifying areas where conventional or digital technology can be applied in the process of fabrication.

While digital applications are fairly well entrenched in fixed prosthodontics, it was only recently that published reports on computer-aided engineering emerged, leading, in a sense, to the awakening of digital applications in removable prosthodontics.

Maeda *et al.*[3] in 1994 initially reported the concept of developing computer-aided technology for designing and fabricating complete dentures. In this article, the authors described a rapid prototyping technique to fabricate a complete denture by photopolymerizing a composite resin material. They also predicted the application of a numerical controlled milling process as a potential technique in the digital fabrication of dentures. A few years later, Kawahata *et al.*[4] reported the potential of computer numeric controlled (CNC) milling in the fabrication and duplication of dentures.

Goodacre *et al.*[5] described the development of CAD/CAM technology producing initially a crude "proof-of-concept" denture base milled from leucite with a three-axis milling machine. Denture bases were subsequently milled from prepolymerized poly (methyl methacrylate), a material more commonly used in the fabrication of complete dentures than leucite.[5]

Kattadiyil *et al.*[6] provided a report on the application of the two currently available digital denture systems; the AvaDent Digital Denture (Global Dental Science, LLC (GDS)) and the Dentca™ CAD/CAM denture (Dentca Inc). They reviewed the fabrication protocol involved with both systems. One of the primary advantages of both digital systems is the reduced clinical appointments to two from the traditional five-appointment process associated with the conventional method of fabrication. Other anticipated advantages of the use of CAD/CAM technology in the fabrication of digital complete dentures over conventionally fabricated dentures are reduction in actual treatment time, reduction in fees, lack of polymerization shrinkage, potential for convenient fabrication of replacement dentures from the repository of digital data acquired for fabrication of the first set of dentures, and less patient adaptation time for the replacement dentures due to consistency in morphology with the previous dentures.

Evidence-based Implant Treatment Planning and Clinical Protocols, First Edition. Edited by Steven J. Sadowsky.

Companion website: www.wiley.com/go/sadowsky/implant

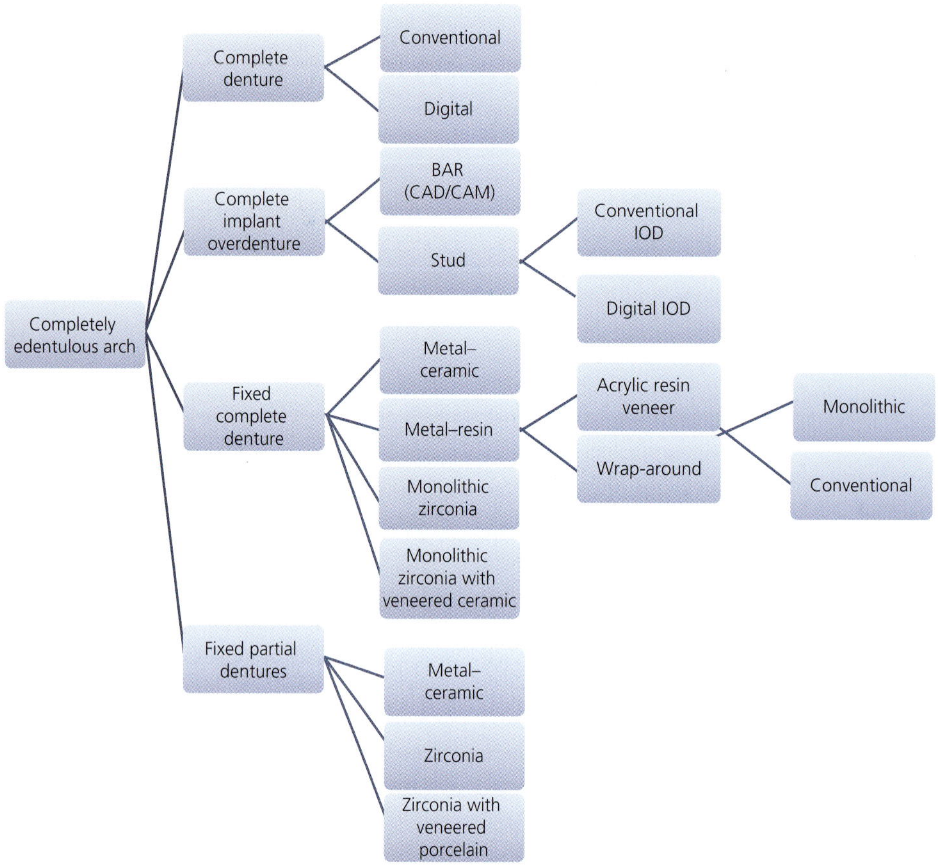

Figure 20.1 Schematic diagram showing the options available in the restoration of the completely edentulous arches. *Source:* Reproduced with permission from Erin Burke, CA.

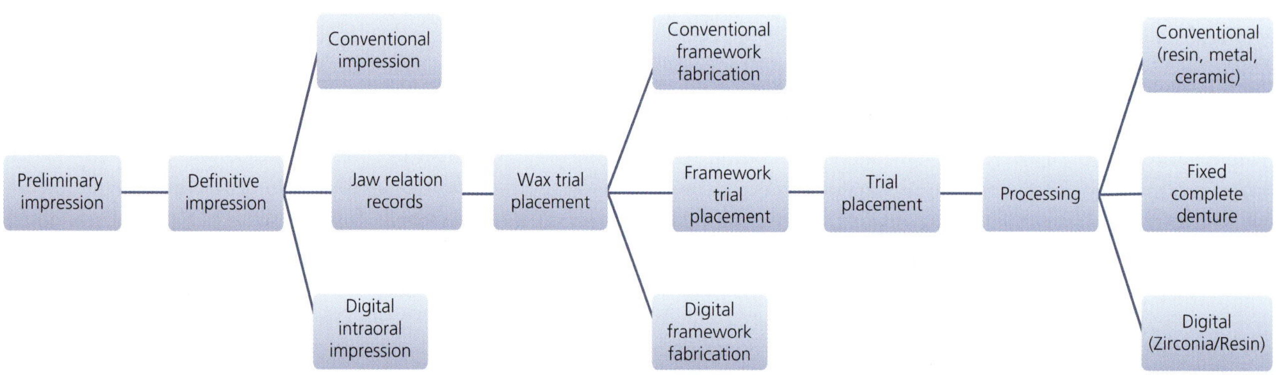

Figure 20.2 Schematic diagram showing the steps involved in the fabrication of a fixed complete denture with areas where digital applications can be an option. *Source:* Reproduced with permission from Erin Burke, CA.

A systematic review on the fabrication of complete dentures with computer-aided technology (CAT) by Bidra *et al.*[7] predicted that the application of CAT in the fabrication of complete removable dental prostheses (CRDP) could significantly impact patient care, dental education, public health, and dental research.

Infante *et al.*[8] reported in detail the technique employed to fabricate milled complete dental prostheses with the utilization of digital scanning technology. They described the method of fabrication involved with one of the more commonly used digital CRDP systems (AvaDent, GDS).

The introduction of implants to improve retention and stability for complete dentures has had a significant impact on the quality of life of the edentulous patient.[9,10] The McGill consensus report,[11] published in 2002, stated that the two-implant mandibular implant overdenture be considered for every completely edentulous patient stating "there is now overwhelming evidence that a two-implant overdenture should become minimally the first choice of treatment for the edentulous mandible." In 2009, the York consensus statement made the same point as the McGill report, saying that "a substantial body of evidence is now available demonstrating that patients' satisfaction and quality of life with implant supported overdentures is significantly greater than for conventional dentures."[12]

This chapter outlines the innovative application of digital technology in the rehabilitation of the edentulous patients with implant-assisted prostheses.

Applications of digital complete dentures with implants

The increasing interest in digital denture fabrication expanded to the exploration of the application of this technology in the rehabilitation of completely edentulous patients with implant-assisted prostheses. Although this should only be considered an early stage in this application, there have been some interesting case reports that show promise in expanding the utilization of the new technology.

Bidra *et al.*[13] described the application of this technology where a two-appointment digital denture process was used to fabricate a complete denture which was subsequently converted to an implant overdenture by picking up the attachments intraorally at the placement appointment. Lozada *et al.*[14] and Kattadiyil *et al.*[15] reported some unique utilization of the digital denture technology to improve efficiency in both the surgical and prosthodontic phases of treatment of the completely edentulous patient. In a two-part series they described in detail the utilization of CAD/CAM technology in the surgical and prosthodontic phases of treatment.

In part 1, for the surgical phase of treatment, Lozada *et al.*[14] described the fabrication of provisional dentures which were fully milled (including both the denture base and teeth) using a proprietary technique. Subsequently, a milled radiographic template was also fabricated by the digital denture manufacturer that was a duplicate of the mandibular provisional denture to which fiduciary markers were attached. A cone-beam computed tomography (CBCT) scan was made of only the radiographic template and then the radiographic template was positioned intraorally using an index and a CBCT scan made of the patient following the NobelGuide™/NobelClinician protocol.[16] The surgical planning for implant placement was performed using NobelClinician software (Figure 20.3), based on the orientation of the denture bases and teeth to the existing bone and vital anatomical structures, so the most appropriate locations could be identified for each implant. Once the plan for implant positions was finalized, a NobelGuide™ surgical template was fabricated.

In a classic model where two companies collaborated together using individual strengths of their different software to achieve successful outcome, the virtual implant positions planned using the Nobel Clinician software were used by Global Dental

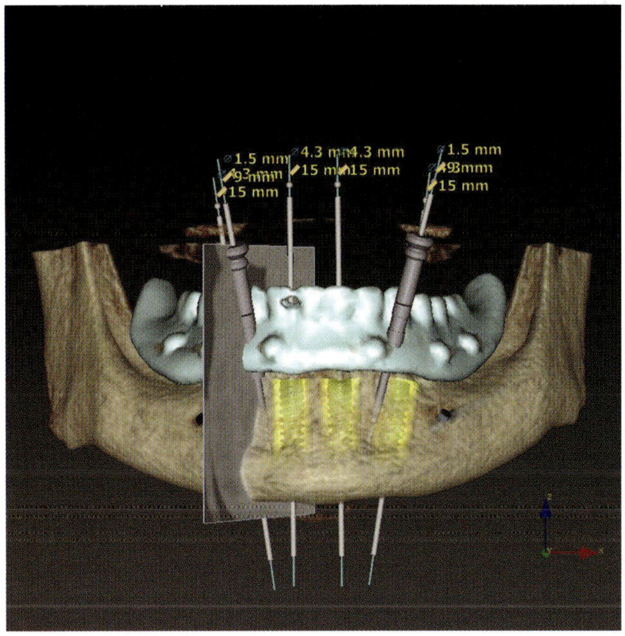

Figure 20.3 Planning for implant surgery accomplished with the Nobel Clinician protocol. The radiographic template is a milled, identical in morphology, replica of the digital provisional denture.

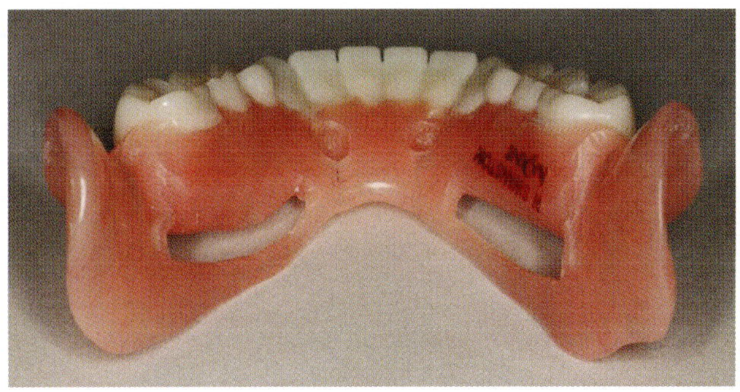

Figure 20.4 Milled conversion denture with slots and recesses to allow easy placement, connection to temporary copings for conversion to a provisional fixed complete denture. *Source:* Reproduced with permission from Ankur Dahiya, Austin, TX.

Science to fabricate an AvaDent™ mandibular conversion complete denture (Figure 20.4). This conversion denture had channels milled through the denture base at the appropriate positions where temporary copings would be located after their attachment to the implant abutments. It also had a pre-milled slot located around the denture base with a small number of struts that connected the peripheral denture base to the central portion of the conversion denture that functioned as the immediate provisional fixed complete denture (CD). The presence of the channels and slot facilitated easy conversion of the denture to a fixed prosthesis, while using the positional stability of the peripheral denture base to accurately orient the prosthesis in the patient's mouth during attachment of the denture to the temporary copings. The AvaDent™ Conversion Denture was connected to temporary copings using autopolymerizing acrylic

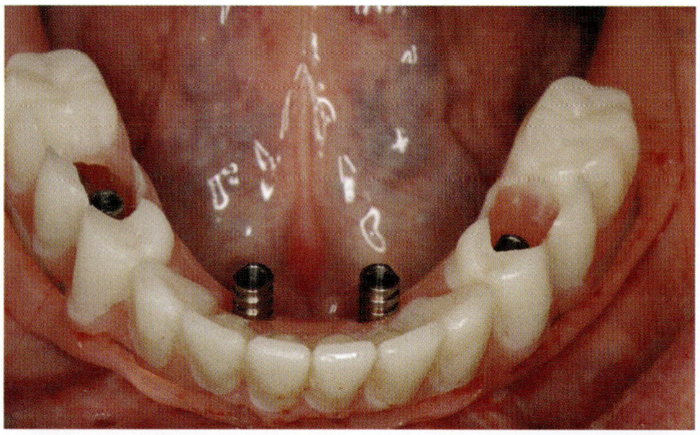

Figure 20.5 Mandibular conversion denture placed easily to seat on to the soft tissues. Access holes had been already fabricated utilizing information from the digital planning for the surgery. Temporary copings had already been placed on the implants and are ready to be attached to the conversion denture. Note the peripheral struts for easy separation.

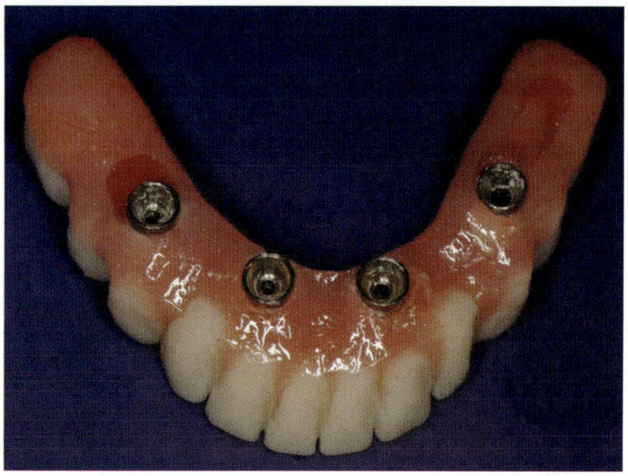

Figure 20.6 Intaglio surface of mandibular conversion denture.

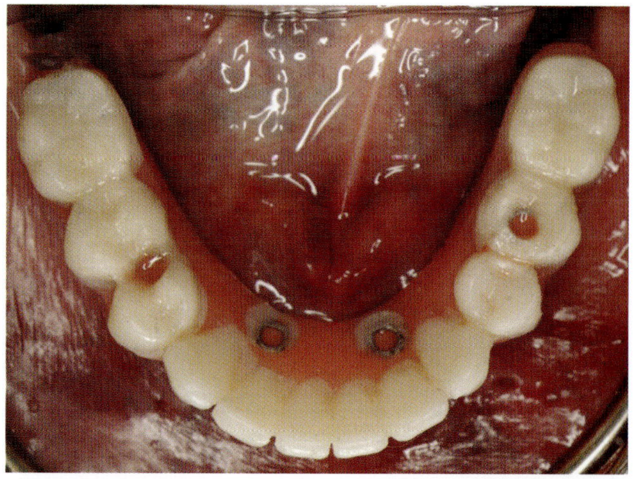

(a)

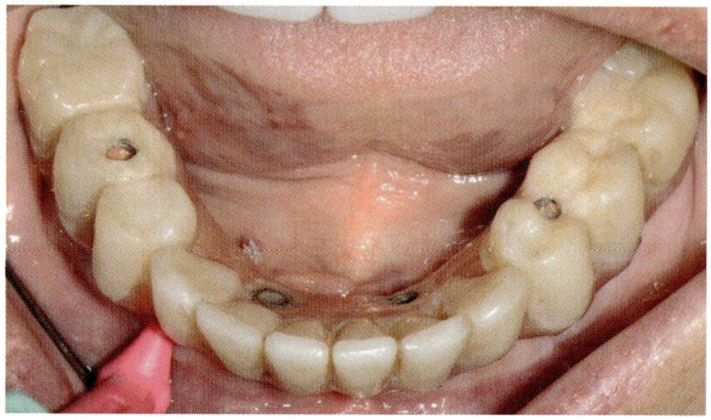

(b)

Figure 20.7 **(a)** Occlusal intraoral view of the mandibular conversion denture. **(b)** Tufted brush (for easy access) used to clean the intaglio surface of the conversion denture.

resin (Figure 20.5). Once the resin had polymerized, the struts were sectioned to efficiently convert the denture to an immediate fixed CD (Figures 20.5, 20.6 and 20.7). This method reduces the time involved in forming the conversion prosthesis during the surgery.

In part two of the two-part series, Kattadiyil *et al.*[15] described the application of digital technology in the prosthodontic phase of treatment by using the digital data previously acquired and stored for the same patient situation reported by Lozada *et al.*[14] in part one. They described how the same previously acquired data could also be utilized in the planning and fabrication of the definitive mandibular fixed complete denture.

In this prosthodontic phase of treatment, a custom impression tray (Figure 20.8a) (duplicate of the provisional denture with recess milled in the center to accommodate the impression coping and the connected verification jig) for the definitive impression for the fixed complete denture was provided by Global Dental Science. They also provide a verification jig template (Figure 20.8b), designed to fit around impression copings fabricated using information from the surgical planning software and allowing efficient connection of the impression copings intraorally.

The verification jig was used to rigidly connect either temporary copings or impression copings, depending on the preference of the clinician. The verification jig was attached to the impression copings with flowable light-polymerizing composite resin. The custom tray was oriented relative to the mucosa via the posterior edentulous ridges and anterior denture borders. The denture teeth present on the tray allowed it to be oriented in relation to the maxillary provisional denture teeth, using occlusal interdigitation prior to making the definitive impression. The positioning of the custom impression tray over the edentulous ridge was confirmed by having the patient close into occlusion with the existing maxillary provisional denture. The long impression coping screws might sometimes need to be sectioned to allow the patient to close into occlusion (Figure 20.9). Definitive impressions were made using the open tray technique. While the impression material polymerized, the patient occluded with

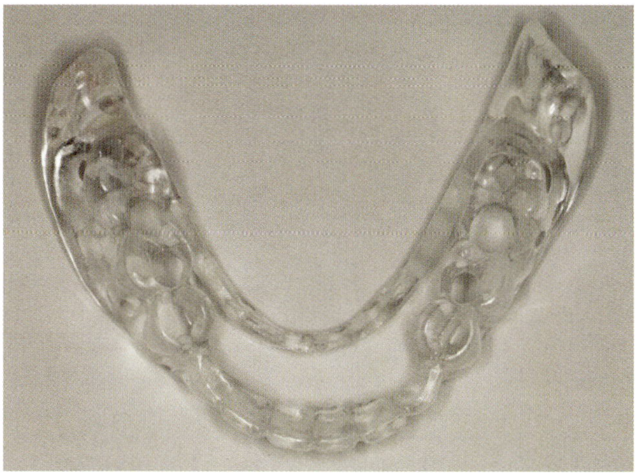

(a)

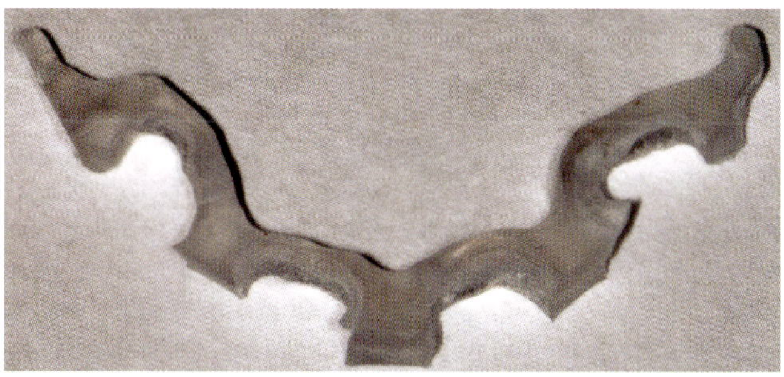

(b)

Figure 20.8 (**a**) Custom impression tray (duplicate of the provisional denture with recess milled in the center to accommodate the impression coping). (**b**) Prefabricated verification jig template.

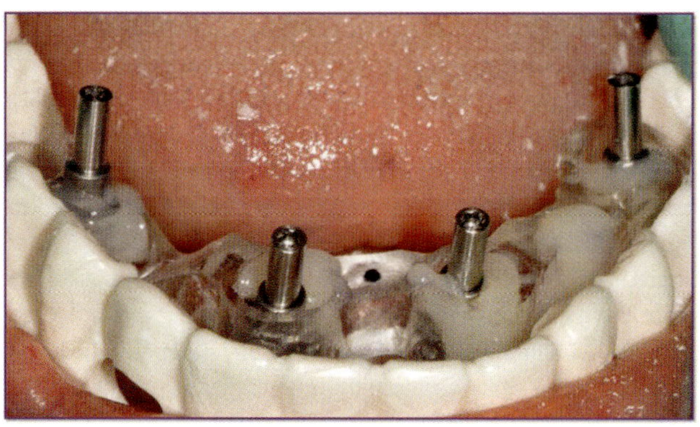

Figure 20.9 An example of a mandibular custom tray seated around the impression copings already connected to the verification jig. The long screws can be sectioned prior to impression making to allow the patient to close into occlusion.

the opposing provisional denture, confirming the proper orientation of the custom tray. This is a critical step in the protocol. The definitive impression (Figure 20.10) recorded the implant positions and part of the edentulous ridge while containing the verification jig with connected copings. Excess impression material that would impede accurate occlusal interdigitation

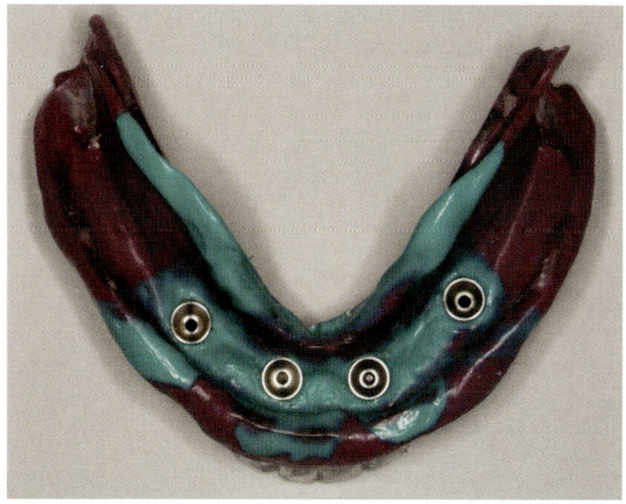

Figure 20.10 Definitive impression.

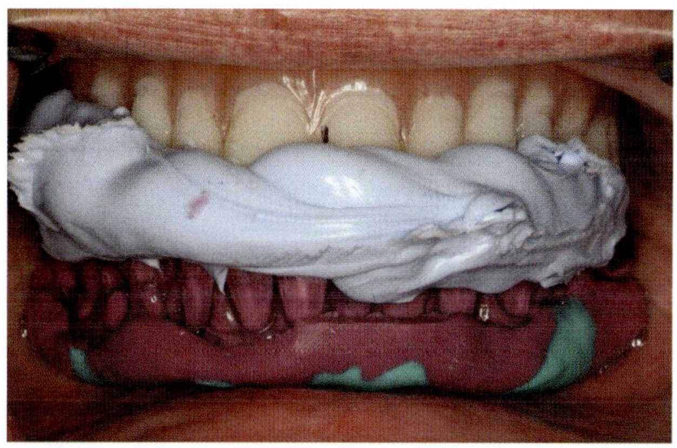

Figure 20.11 Interocclusal record (maxillary provisional denture opposing the impression made with the milled custom tray, which is a duplicate of the mandibular provisional denture).

of the reseated impression against the maxillary denture was removed and an interocclusal record was made between the reseated impression and the provisional maxillary denture (Figure 20.11). The definitive impression was sent to Global Dental Science along with the interocclusal record. The previous digital data that were stored with Global Dental Science allowed for easy fabrication of a new definitive maxillary CD which was identical in base morphology and tooth positions to the provisional maxillary CD. The digital tooth positions and base form data present in the conversion denture were used for the definitive mandibular implant fixed complete denture. The mandibular implant impression made with the custom tray and the interocclusal record were used to identify the proper relationship between the implants and the mandibular prosthetic teeth as well as the relationship between the maxillary and mandibular prosthetic teeth. The implant position data from the impression were used to design and fabricate a NobelProcera™

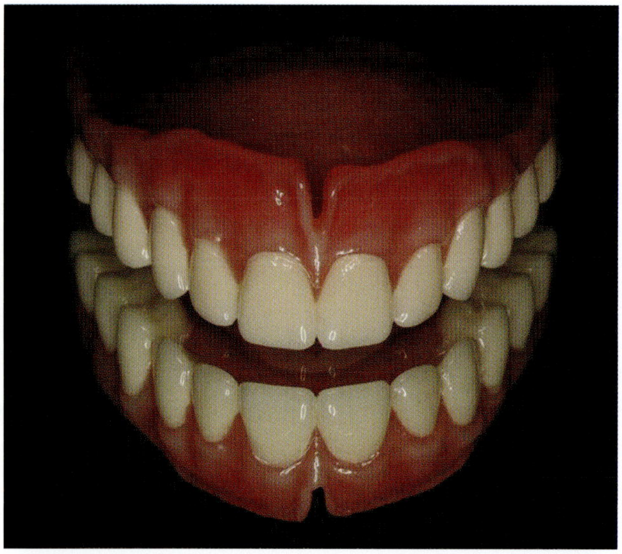

Figure 20.12 Maxillary monolithic complete denture.

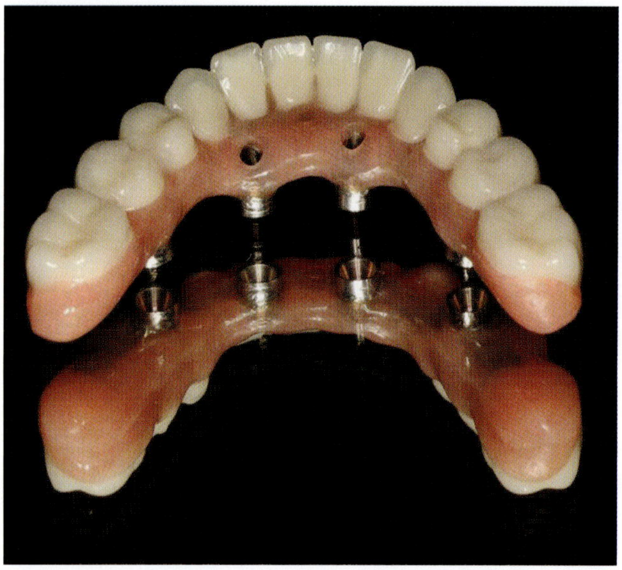

Figure 20.13 Mandibular fixed complete denture with Procera Bar encased in the monolithic acrylic resin.

titanium bar.[16] Global Dental Science fabricated the definitive milled maxillary CD (Figure 20.12) and a milled mandibular fixed CD with the titanium bar (Figures 20.13 and 20.14) incorporated, oriented, and encased precisely into the resin base using a proprietary technique.

This technique has promising applications but is dependent on precise execution of each step to achieve a clinically acceptable result. Further studies also need to be conducted to validate the assumed strength and fracture resistance of the monolithic prosthesis. Though the manufacturer claims the definitive prosthesis to be monolithic, the encasement of the bar with a proprietary technique needs to be studied to confirm that a

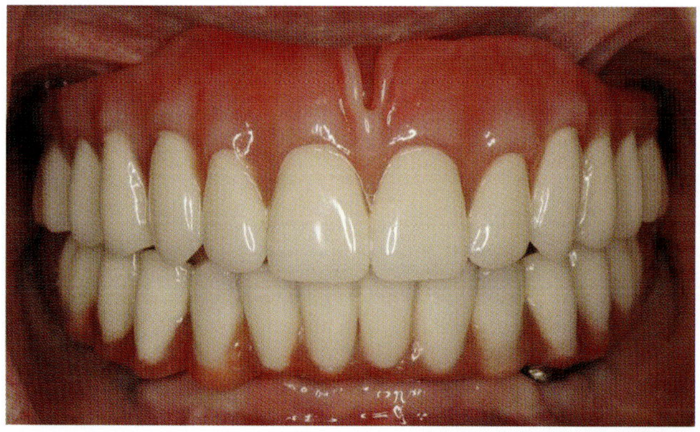

Figure 20.14 Intraoral view of maxillary and mandibular fixed complete dentures.

resin interface does not exist that could negate the perceived strength and advantage of a monolithic prosthesis.

Digital impressions for edentulous arches

The previous section of this chapter described the utilization of digital denture technology and CAD/CAM technology in the efficient fabrication of implant-assisted prostheses. It should be noted that, although the fabrication process for CAD/CAM complete dentures is digitized, the impressions and records are made in a conventional manner. This could be attributed to the fact that, at present, it is not possible to digitally capture an intraoral impression of the edentulous arch with the appropriate peripheral extensions that would be captured with a functional border-molding procedure. Hence, for removable prostheses such as a conventional complete denture or an implant overdenture, conventional impressions will be still required until the available technology is enhanced.

However, there has been increased interest in capturing impressions of already placed implants using digital scanning technology.[17,18,19] Scannable abutments designed for specific implant dimensions are routinely used to fabricate digital or printed models after scanning. Some of the advantages from using this technique have been speculated to be increased accuracy, comfort, efficiency, and even cost effectiveness. Although this application has been usually limited to single-tooth implant situations and partially edentulous arches, Gherlone *et al.*[20] evaluated the accuracy of digital impressions in the fabrication of an All-on-4 prosthesis for the completely edentulous arch. They utilized scannable abutments placed and tightened on to the implant fixtures. Using a calibrated intraoral scanner from Lava COS (3M ESPE) which uses a 3-D video system and active wavefront sampling to obtain the images, they scanned the abutments coated with titanium oxide and created a high-resolution model, the data from which was uploaded to 3M ESPE. A virtual model was then created with the implants in place. The framework or prosthesis could then be designed virtually, and milled using CAD/CAM technology.

They also reported that a physical model was generated which had removable repositionable implant analogs so that restorations and framework could be also fabricated in a conventional manner on a definitive cast. They reported accuracy in fit for the titanium frameworks in all of the 14 patients evaluated in the study. The authors utilized radiographic examination and the Sheffield 1-screw test to check the fit of the titanium framework. A clinical evaluation for up to 1 year did not reveal any significant bone loss around the implants and the authors concluded that intraoral scanning was a viable and acceptable alternative to conventional method of making impressions on implants.

Lin *et al.*[21] published a case report on the rehabilitation of a patient with a completely edentulous maxilla with a fixed complete denture, where they acquired the digital data at the implant body level using scannable abutments/impression copings. After placing the scannable impression copings and torquing them to the recommended value, an intraoral scanner (Cadent iTero) was used to digitally capture the data, which were imported to Straumann software and the information used to fabricate a milled polyurethane definitive cast (Cadent iTero). They reported using a verification jig and fabricated a verification cast, which suggested that there were some inaccuracies from the digital impression.

There are some drawbacks to using scannable abutments. Most abutments currently are placed at the implant fixture level (Figure 20.15). Hence the fixed prosthesis is fabricated to connect to the implant fixture level. This might not be a good option if the height of the soft tissue around each implant is excessive, which is an indication for using abutments that raise the prosthetic platform slightly above the soft tissue. There are ways to overcome this, by placing abutments on the implant replicas (in the cast) and the implant fixtures (intraorally). However, this could reduce accuracy and adds additional features, reducing efficiency.

It is the opinion of the author that there are certain drawbacks with making accurate digital impressions of implants for the complete arch and accuracy needs to be confirmed with a verification jig and corrections made as needed before proceeding with framework fabrication. However, this technology will continue to improve with the introduction of more accurate scanning methods and instrumentation.

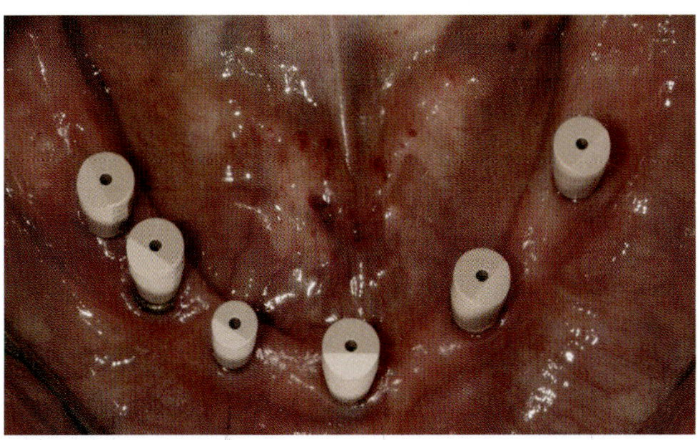

Figure 20.15 Occlusal view of intraoral scannable abutments. *Source:* Reproduced with permission from Ankur Dahiya, Austin, TX.

Digital options for substuctures and monolithic framework prostheses

One area where the digital technology has rapidly progressed in the rehabilitation of the completely edentulous arch and has been embraced by the dental profession is the area of framework fabrication. The shift from the conventional lost wax casting technique for the fabrication of frameworks made from base metal, noble, and high noble alloys has occurred. CAD/CAM frameworks made from titanium alloy or zirconia have gained in popularity.[22–25] The application of CAD/CAM technology in framework fabrication has proven to provide precise fit comparable or even better than the conventional casting and soldering techniques. This has also resulted in more cost-effective frameworks made with titanium compared to the gold alloy frameworks. A review of multiple publications by Abduo[26] reported that fit of CAD/CAM frameworks exceeded the fit of the one-piece cast frameworks and laser-welded frameworks. They also reported a similar fit between CAD/CAM frameworks and those that utilized the bonding of the framework body to prefabricated cylinders and reported acceptable fit for CAD/CAM frameworks.

The application of CAD/CAM technology allows precise utilization of available restorative space designing a framework with appropriate space and access for oral hygiene, while ensuring adequate thickness for the framework so that strength is not compromised. The prosthesis for a metal–acrylic resin can have a metal-veneered acrylic resin design (Figure 20.16) or a wrap-around acrylic resin design (Figure 20.17). The most common complication associated with metal–acrylic resin frameworks is the fracture of the veneering resin.[27] There have been case reports[28,29] that have utilized, to achieve improved strength and esthetics, frameworks with abutments that mimic the form of teeth preparation. Metal–ceramic or ceramic crowns are cemented on these abutments, thereby eliminating the drawback of layering ceramic in bulk, which can compromise strength.

The introduction of the minimally veneered or completely monolithic zirconia fixed complete denture has provided another option for the rehabilitation of the completely edentulous arch. There have been multiple case reports utilizing CAD/CAM technology to fabricate either zirconia frameworks as a substructure, veneered with feldspathic porcelain, or milled monolithic or minimally veneered monolithic zirconia prostheses. Puri *et al.*,[30] in a 4-year follow up of a complete mouth reconstruction with implant-supported fixed partial dental prostheses with zirconia frameworks veneered with feldspathic porcelain, demonstrated the potential risk involved with fracturing the veneering porcelain associated with this approach.

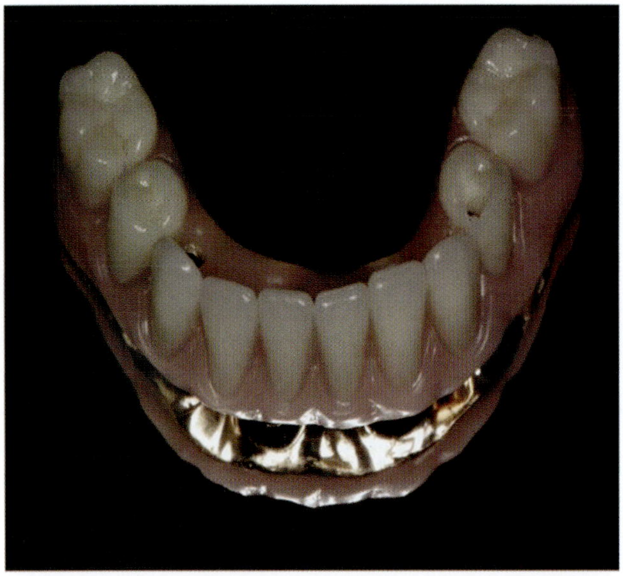

Figure 20.16 Metal–acrylic resin fixed complete denture. Note the intaglio surface is the polished metal alloy framework. *Source:* Reproduced with permission from Montry Suprono, CA.

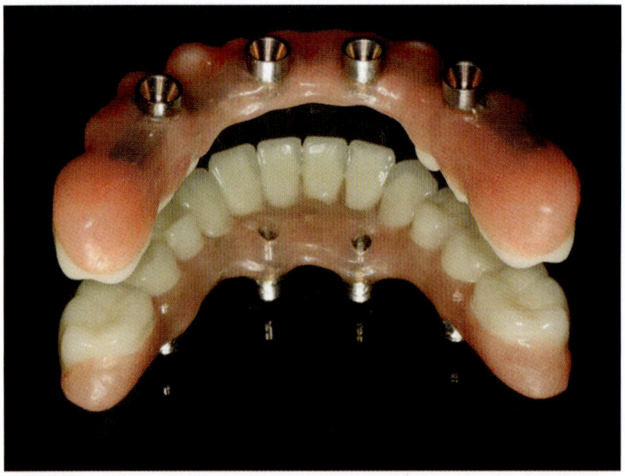

Figure 20.17 Metal–acrylic resin "wrap-around" fixed complete denture. Note the intaglio surface is acrylic resin which wraps around the metal alloy framework.

There are case reports which have utilized monolithic zirconia prostheses and have reported favorable outcomes for a 1–2-year follow-up period.[31,32]

It is the opinion of the author that monolithic prostheses, especially fabricated with ceramic materials such as 3-YTZP zirconia, are gaining popularity and the technology and protocol required to gain predictable long-term results will improve. Long-term outcomes data are lacking and clinicians must be careful with patient selection in utilizing zirconia frameworks with feldspathic porcelain and monolithic zirconia (Figures 20.18 and 20.19) as a predictable option, as complications could be difficult to manage and replacement would be expensive.

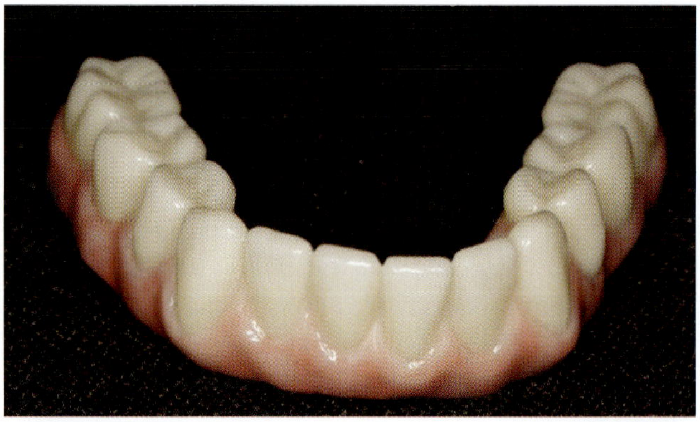

Figure 20.18 Occlusal view of mandibular monolithic zirconia fixed complete denture.

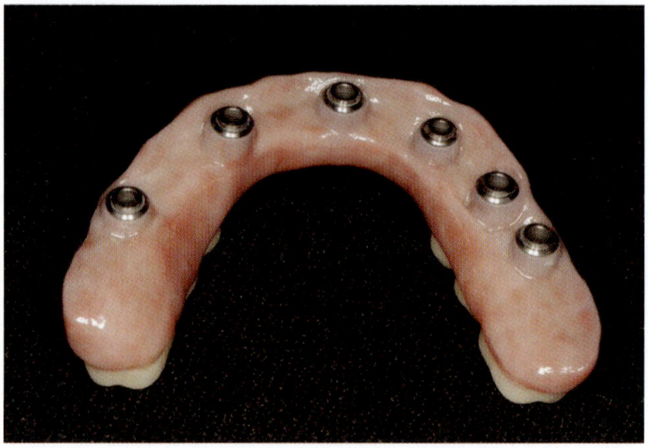

Figure 20.19 Intaglio surface view of the mandibular monolithic zirconia fixed complete denture. *Source:* Reproduced with permission from Ankur Dahiya, Austin, TX.

However, zirconia offers some significant advantages, such as increased esthetics, strength, and biocompatibility, and hence warrants attention as a material with significant potential.

Conclusion

This chapter discusses the digital alternatives currently available in the rehabilitation of the edentulous patient with implants. There is no doubt that, as improvements in digital applications occur, there will be a paradigm shift towards these applications as they achieve more predictability and efficiency.

References

1. Bishop HF. American Academy of Dental Science, a history of dental and oral science in America. *Am J Dent Science* 1867; **1**: 347–352.
2. Douglass CW, Shih A, Ostry L. Will there be a need for complete dentures in the United States in 2020? *J Prosthet Dent* 2002; **87**(1): 5–8.

3. Maeda Y, Minoura M, Tsutsumi S, *et al.* A CAD/CAM system for removable denture: part I: fabrication of complete dentures. *Int J Prosthodont* 1994; **7**(1): 17–21.
4. Kawahata N, Ono H, Nishi Y, *et al.* Trial of duplication procedure for complete dentures by CAD/CAM. *J Oral Rehabil* 1997; **24**(7): 540–548.
5. Goodacre CJ, Garbacea A, Naylor WP, *et al.* CAD/CAM fabricated complete dentures: concepts and clinical methods of obtaining required morphological data. *J Prosthet Dent* 2012; **107**(1): 34–46.
6. Kattadiyil MT, Goodacre CJ, Baba NZ. CAD/CAM complete dentures: a review of two commercial fabrication systems. *J Calif Dent Assoc* 2013; **41**(6): 407–416.
7. Bidra AS, Taylor TD, Agar JR. Computer-aided technology for fabricating complete dentures: systematic review of historical background, current status, and future perspectives. *J Prosthet Dent* 2013; **109**(6): 361–366.
8. Infante L, Yilmaz B, McGlumphy E, *et al.* Fabricating complete dentures with CAD/CAM technology. *J Prosthet Dent* 2014; **111**(5): 351–355.
9. Heydecke G, Locker D, Awad M, *et al.* Oral and general health-related quality of life with conventional and implant dentures. *Com Dent Oral Epidem* 2003; **31**(3): 161–168.
10. Raghoebar G, Meijer H, van't Hof M, *et al.* A randomized prospective clinical trial on the effectiveness of three treatment modalities for patients with lower denture problems. A 10-year follow-up study on patient satisfaction. *Int J Oral Maxillofac Surg* 2003; **32**(5): 498–503.
11. Thomason JM. The McGill consensus statement on overdentures. Mandibular 2-implant overdentures as first choice standard care for edentulous patients. *Eur J Prosthodont Res Dent* 2002; **10**(3): 95–96.
12. Thomason J, Feine J, Exley C, *et al.* Mandibular two implant-supported overdentures as the first choice standard of care for edentulous patients – the York Consensus Statement. *Brit Dent J* 2009; **207**(4): 185–186.
13. Bidra, AS. The 2-visit CAD-CAM implant-retained overdenture: a clinical report. *J Oral Implantol* 2014; **40**(6): 722–728.
14. Lozada JL, Garbacea A, Goodacre CJ, *et al.* Use of a digitally planned and fabricated mandibular complete denture for easy conversion to an immediately loaded provisional fixed complete denture. Part 1. Planning and surgical phase. *Int J Prosthodont* 2014; **27**(5): 417–421.
15. Kattadiyil MT, Goodacre CJ, Lozada JL, *et al.* Digitally planned and fabricated mandibular fixed complete denture. Part 2. Prosthodontic phase. *Int J Prosthodont* 2015; **28**(2): 119–123.
16. Balshi SF, Wolfinger GJ, Balshi TJ. Surgical planning and prosthesis construction using computed tomography, CAD/CAM technology, and the internet for immediate loading of dental implants. *J Esthet Restor Dent* 2006; **18**(6): 312–323.
17. Lee SJ, Galucci GO. Digital vs conventional implant impressions: efficiency outcomes. *Clin Oral Implants Res* 2013; **24**(1): 111–115.
18. Christensen GJ. Impressions are changing: deciding on conventional, digital, or digital plus in-office milling. *J Am Dent Assoc* 2009; **140**(10): 1301–1304.
19. Nayyer N, Yilmaz B, McGlumphy E. Using digitally coded healing abutments and an intraoral scanner to fabricate implant-supported, cement-retained restorations. *J Prosthet Dent* 2013; **109**(4): 210–215.
20. Drago C, Howell K. Concepts for designing and fabricating metal implant frameworks for hybrid implant prostheses. *J Prosthodont* 2012; **21**(5): 413–424.
21. Gherlone EF, Ferrini F, Crespi R, *et al.* Digital impressions for fabrication of definitive "all-on-four" restorations. *Implant Dent* 2015; **24**(1): 125–129.
22. Lin WS, Harris BT, Morton D. The use of a scannable impression coping and digital impression technique to fabricate a customized anatomic abutment and zirconia restoration in the esthetic zone. *J Prosthetic Dent* 2013; **109**(3): 187–191.
23. Sachs C, Groesser J, Stadelmann M, *et al.* Full-arch prostheses from translucent zirconia: accuracy of fit. *Dent Mater* 2014; **30**(8): 817–823.
24. Drago C, Howell K. Concepts for designing and fabricating metal frameworks for hybrid implant prostheses. *J Prosthodont* 2012; **21**(5): 413–424.
25. Katsoulis J, Mericske-Stern R, Enkling N, *et al.* Invitro precision of fit of computer-aided designed and computer-aided manufactured titanium screw-retained fixed dental prostheses before and after ceramic veneering. *Clin Oral Implants Res* 2015; **26**(1): 44–49.
26. Abduo J. Fit of CAD/CAM implant frameworks: a comprehensive review. *J Oral Implantol* 2014; **40**(6): 758–766.
27. Goodacre CJ, Bernal G, Rungcharassaeng K, *et al.* Clinical complications with implants and implant prostheses. *J Prosthet Dent* 2003; **90**(2): 121–132.
28. Kleinman A, Avendano S, Leyva F. Aesthetic treatment option for completely edentulous patients using CAD/CAM technology. *Prac Proced Aesthet Dent* 2008; **20**(3): 185–191.
29. Reshad M, Cascione D, Aalam AA. Fabrication of the mandibular implant-supported fixed restoration using CAD/CAM technology: a clinical report. *J Prosthet Dent* 2009; **102**(5): 271–278.
30. Puri S, Parciak EC, Kattadiyil MT. Complete mouth reconstruction with implant-supported fixed partial dental prostheses fabricated with zirconia frameworks: a 4-year clinical follow-up. *J Prosthet Dent* 2014; **112**(3):397–401.
31. Rojas-Vizcaya F. Full zirconia fixed detachable implant retained restorations manufactured from monolithic zirconia: clinical report after two years in service. *J Prosthodont* 2011; **20**(7): 570–576.
32. Mehra M, Vahidi F. Complete mouth implant rehabilitation with a zirconia ceramic system: a clinical report. *J Prosthet Dent* 2014; **112**(1): 1–4.

CHAPTER 21

Restoration of Acquired Oral Defects with Osseointegrated Implants

John Beumer, III[1], Karl Lyons[2], Jay Jayanetti[1], and Eric C. Sung[1]
[1] University of California, Los Angeles School of Dentistry, Los Angeles, California, USA
[2] University of Otago, Dunedin, New Zealand

Introduction

Treatment of tumors of the oral cavity may result in severe functional disability and cosmetic disfigurement. Not so long ago, it was difficult to rehabilitate these patients on a consistent basis. Today, however, it is possible to restore most patients to near normal form and function, enabling them to lead useful and productive lives. Two advances have made this possible and both were introduced in the 1980s: osseointegrated implants and free vascularized flaps. Implants permitted the prosthodontist to provide additional stability, retention, and support for our intraoral prostheses, and free flaps enabled the surgeon to reconstruct oral tissues, such as the mandible and the tongue, on a consistent basis. Implants have also been a valuable tool for restoring patients presenting with traumatic and congenital defects.

Implant-retained prostheses for acquired hard and soft palate defects

Prosthetic rehabilitation is still the primary and the preferred means of restoring acquired defects of the hard and soft palate following tumor ablation. These prostheses are used to restore the partition between the oral and nasal cavities, restore the palatal contours and the missing dentition, and enable normal velopharyngeal function, permitting the patient to speak and swallow normally. In experienced hands, the clinical outcomes are quite predictable. The principle challenge, especially in edentulous patients, is retention of the prosthesis.

Restoration of hard palate defects

Retention provided by osseointegrated implants can have a dramatic effect on the function of the prosthesis, especially for the edentulous maxillectomy and palatectomy patient (Figure 21.1). Implants are equally impacting for edentulous patients presenting with soft palate defects because the implants retain and precisely position the complete denture–obturator in the velopharyngeal area and permit it to interact effectively with the residual velopharyngeal musculature (Figure 21.2). They have also been used with success in patients with hard and soft palate defects with marginal or failing residual dentition. Implants provide retention, enhance support, and improve the stability of the obturator prosthesis. Mastication performance may be restored to presurgical levels in some patients[2] and, with the retention provided by the implants, the obturator prosthesis restores speech and swallowing to normal limits.

Clinical data

Previous studies[3–5] describe the locations and prognosis for implants used to support and retain maxillary obturator prostheses. In the Roumanas report,[3] 102 implants were placed in 26 patients with acquired maxillary defects secondary to resection of palatal and paranasal sinus tumors. Seventy-eight implants with known status were available for study. The implant survival rate for these 78 implants was 69.2%. The implant survival rates were 63.6% for the irradiated group (67.0% before radiation and 50% after radiation, mean dose of 50 Gy) and 82.6% for the nonirradiated group.

A pattern of failure and bone loss was apparent with implants placed in each of the three most common sites. Failures were grouped into two categories: namely early, when the implants failed to achieve osseointegration within 6 months and following the second-stage surgery, and late, when implants failed after being subjected to clinical function for a year or more. Minimum bone loss was defined as bone loss limited to 1–2 threads, moderate 3–4 threads, and severe more than 4 threads. In the anterior maxilla three failures occurred "late" and were secondary to progressive bone loss around the implants. Almost one half of the implants in the premaxilla currently in function demonstrated severe bone loss. In contrast, in the maxillary tuberosity where the bone quality is generally poorer, virtually all of the implant failures were "early" or prior to functional

Evidence-based Implant Treatment Planning and Clinical Protocols, First Edition. Edited by Steven J. Sadowsky.

Companion website: www.wiley.com/go/sadowsky/implant

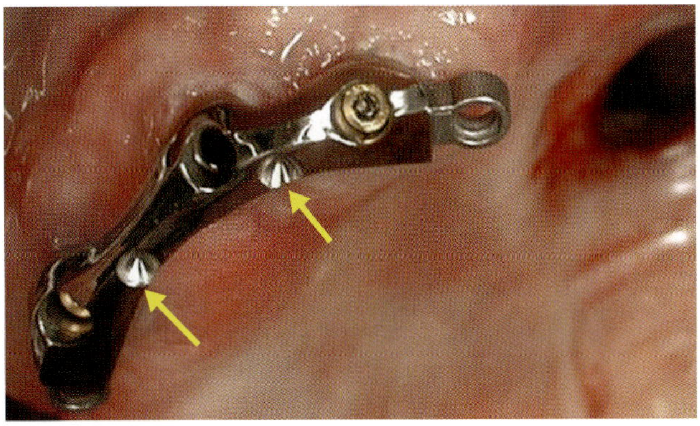

Figure 21.1 Implant connecting bar used to retain a complete denture–obturator in an edentulous maxillectomy patient. Note the rests atop the implant connecting bar. *Source:* Beumer *et al.*, 2011.[1] Reproduced with permission from Quintessence Publishing Company Inc.

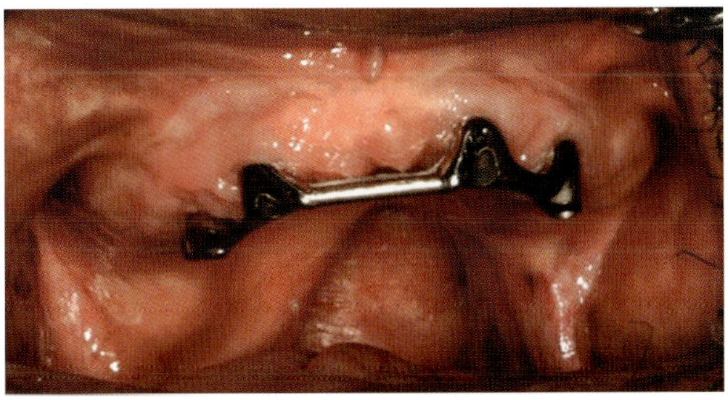

Figure 21.2 Implant connecting bar used to retain a complete denture and soft palate obturator in a patient with a soft palate defect.

loading. However, once osseointegration was achieved and the implants were placed into function, bone levels did not appear to deteriorate over time. The Roumanas report[3] and animal studies[6–13] suggest that implant overload was responsible for the pattern of bone loss and implant failure in these patients. These data prompted a significant change in the design of implant connecting bar.

The implant connecting bar attachment system initially used at UCLA, when implants were clustered in the residual anterior maxillary segment, employed a "Hader" bar extension posteriorly on the unresected side. This implant connecting bar-attachment system did not accommodate for the multiple axes of rotation and forces applied to the implants associated with bolus manipulation, mastication, and eccentric mandibular movements. Chewing forces on the unresected side resulted in significant load magnification of the distal implant because of the cantilevering effect. Thus, this may be the primary reason why so many of the implants placed into the premaxillary segment quickly demonstrated advanced bone loss. In large defects or where only tuberosities remain (Figure 21.3), single implants with "O" ring attachments were used. The solitary implants with an "O" ring attachment permit multiple axes of rotation and so the implants were used

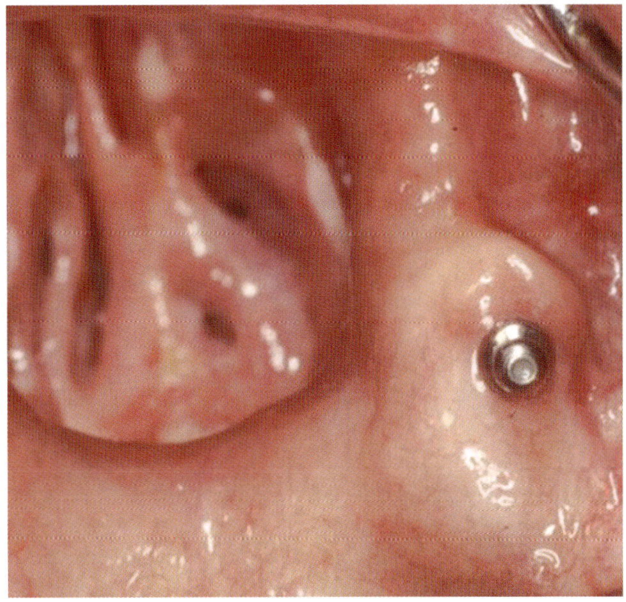

Figure 21.3 Single implant with "O" ring attachment used to retain a large obturator. "O" ring allows prosthesis to rotate around multiple axes.

almost entirely for retention as opposed to providing support and/or stability. As a result the torquing forces delivered to the implant were limited.

Implant sites

The number of implants and their location is determined by the nature of the defect and the available bony sites. The ideal location for implants for most edentulous total maxillectomy patients is the residual premaxillary segment (Figure 21.1). This site is preferred because the anterior maxillary segment is opposite the most retentive portion of the classical skin-lined radical maxillectomy defect, located along its posterior lateral wall. In addition, satisfactory volume and density of bone can be found in the premaxilla in most patients. The maxillary tuberosity site (Figure 21.3) is considered only when there is insufficient bone in the residual premaxilla. Since the bone is not very dense in the maxillary tuberosity, initial implant stabilization is difficult, as evidenced by the high failure rates at stage II surgery. Because of this factor, some clinicians have recommended placing longer, mesially inclined implants in this region. The edentulous posterior alveolar process may serve as an alternative site for implants if there is at least 10 mm of bone available beneath the maxillary sinus. If insufficient bone is present, these sites may be augmented by sinus augmentation.[14,15] This technique has become a popular option when treating conventional patients, but has also been used in patients with large hard palate defects.[1]

Implants of conventional lengths have been used in the residual elements of the zygoma on the defect side of total maxillectomy defects.[1] However, there are important disadvantages to be considered with this approach. First, it is very difficult surgically to create a zone of immobile tissues around the implants.

Second, the implants will exit the tissues high in the defect, making oral hygiene very difficult for the patient. As a result, the risk of peri-implantitis is very high. Third, because the implants are generally positioned parallel to the plane of occlusion they cannot be engaged aggressively. Magnets are often used to minimize lateral torquing forces delivered to the implants. In the authors' limited experience, most implants of conventional lengths used in this site have failed. In defects lined with a skin graft with good posterior lateral undercuts, these implants make only a limited contribution to retention.

Zygomatic implants 20–30 mm long, however, have been used effectively in patients with large maxillectomy or total palatectomy defects. In the UCSF report,[16] 28 zygomatic implants were placed in nine patients with large maxillary defects. Six implants failed (most in irradiated patients), and five of the patients were eventually restored with an implant-retained obturator prosthesis.

Landis *et al.*,[17] reported the use of 36 zygomatic implants in 15 patients. Twenty-four conventional implants were also placed in oral sites in these patients. Twelve of the 15 patients presented status post resection of large tumors of the maxilla and three presented with congenital defects. Nine of the patients were edentulous. Six of the twelve oncology patients received chemotherapy and seven received radiation therapy during the course of their treatments. Radiation doses ranged from 45–61 Gy. Nine of the patients were edentulous. The prostheses were retained with telescopic crowns associated with, when necessary, angled abutments. Follow-up ranged from 13–102 months. Three zygomatic implants were lost secondary to overloading and/or chronic infection and five others were removed secondary to resection of recurrent neoplastic disease.

When restoring total palatectomy defects the authors recommend that, when possible, two implants be placed into each residual zygoma (Figure 21.4) and that all implants be splinted together with an implant connecting bar (Figure 21.5).

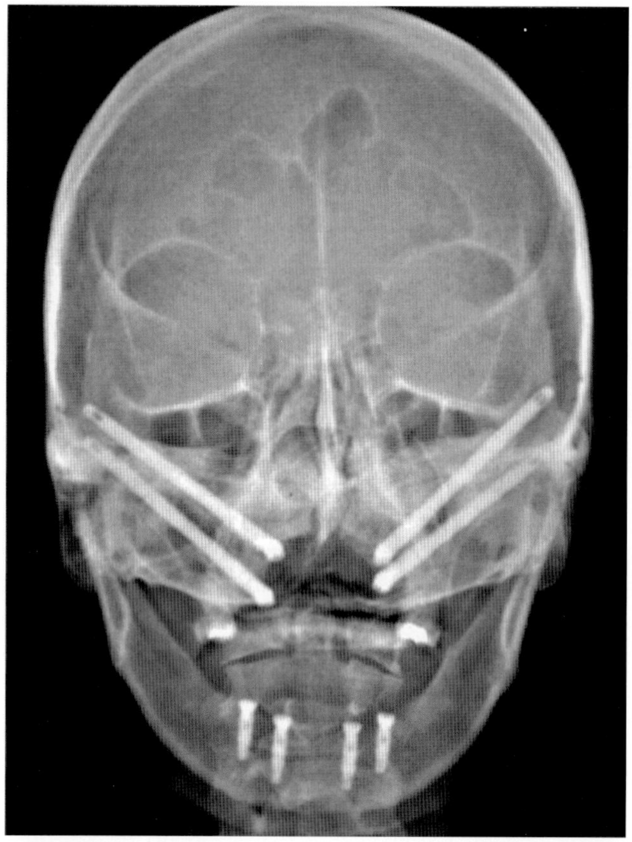

Figure 21.4 When possible two implants should be placed into each zygoma.

Clinical procedures

Following implant placement, the implants are left to heal for several months before they are exposed to functional forces. During this period the patient continues to function with the existing obturator prosthesis. When the implants are exposed at second-stage surgery, the surgeon should carefully thin the mucoperiosteum and create a zone of keratinized, attached mucosa around the implants. If the implants exit in mobile, unattached tissues, an attempt should be made to replace these tissues with keratinized attached tissues. Free grafts from the palatal mucosa are preferred to skin grafts.

Fabrication of the definitive obturator prosthesis begins when the peri-implant soft tissues are well healed. It is desirable to fabricate a trial denture before designing the retention apparatus. The authors prefer to splint multiple implants together with implant-assisted implant connecting bars as opposed to the use of individual attachments. Preliminary impressions are made with transfer (closed tray) impression copings. An edentulous stock tray is chosen and the defect portion of the tray augmented with periphery wax. The impression is made with irreversible hydrocolloid material. Care should be taken to record the lateral wall of the defect and any desirable undercuts which may be engaged by the definitive prosthesis. Following removal of the impression, the impression copings are removed, attached to fixture analogs as required, and inserted into the impression. A preliminary cast is poured with dental stone.

The custom tray for the master impression is designed to record the position and angulation of the implants, as well as the residual normal tissues and those associated with the palatal defect. When the border molding is completed, pick-up type impression copings are secured tightly in position, linked with pattern resin, and an elastic impression material is used to modify the impression. When the impression material has polymerized, the screws securing the copings to the implant fixture are loosened and the impression is removed. Fixture analogs are then attached to the impression copings imbedded in the impression, and the impression is boxed and the master cast prepared in the usual manner.

Record bases are now fabricated. Healing abutments of the same length and diameter as those used in the patient are attached to the implant analogs and a record base is fabricated with autopolymerizing acrylic resin. The record base should positively engage these healing abutments as well as the lateral wall of the skin-lined maxillary defect. This technique will maximize

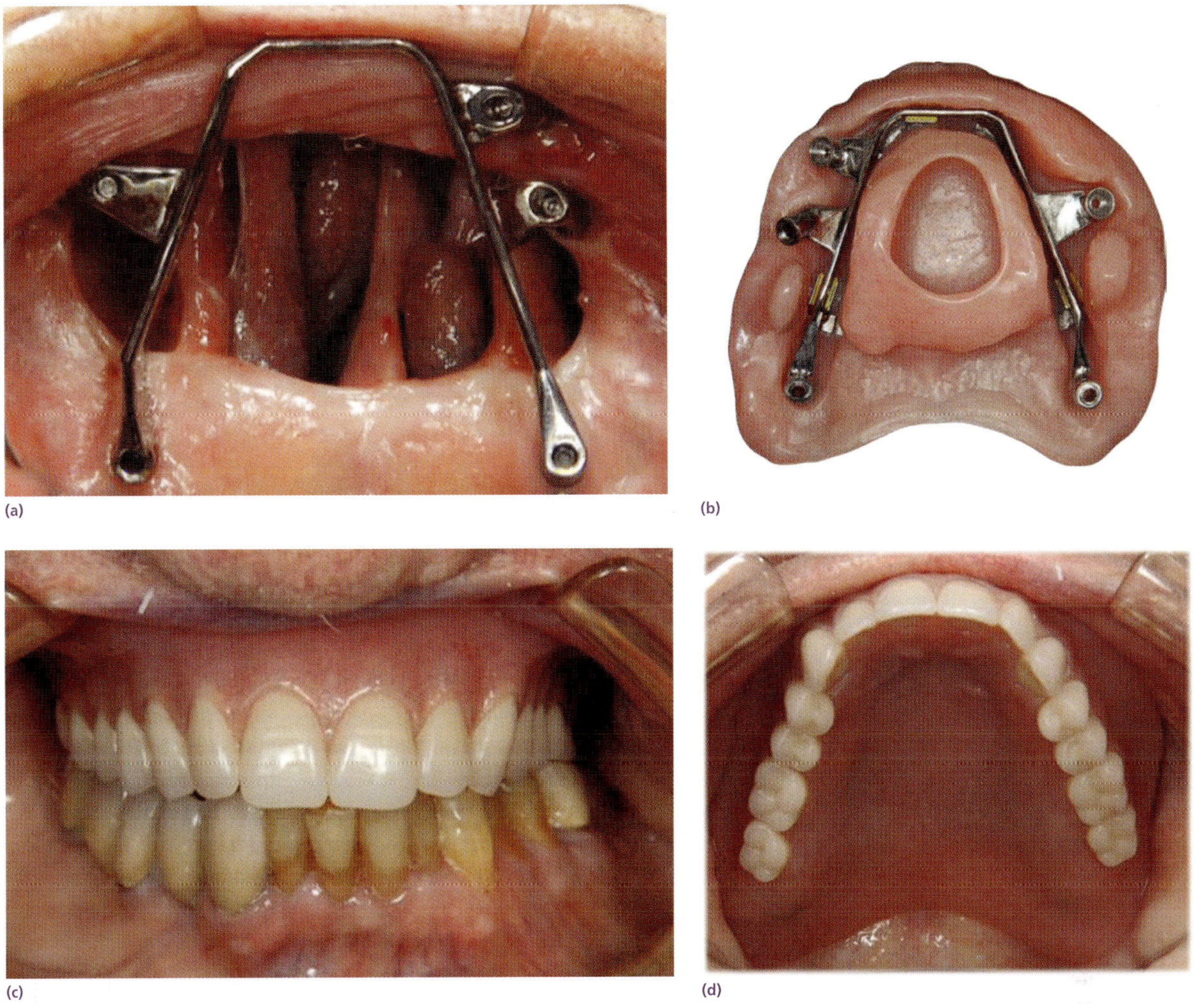

Figure 21.5 (a) A total palectomy defect restored with combination of tuberosity/pterygoid implants and zygomatic implants. (b) Obturator bar with implant connecting bar. (c, d) Prosthesis in place.

the stability and retention of the record base used to make maxillo-mandibular registrations. A face bow transfer record is obtained and transferred to an articulator that will accept the large maxillary cast.[1] The centric relation record is secured and the opposing mandibular cast is mounted on the articulator.

The anterior teeth are selected and arranged using established criteria and the posterior teeth are selected and arranged according to neutro-centric occlusal concepts. The waxed trial dentures are tried in the mouth, and the centric relation record and occlusal vertical dimension are verified. The anterior teeth are evaluated for acceptable speech and esthetics. The trial dentures are repositioned on the articulator and a silicone template is fabricated with the maxillary teeth incorporated within it. Detailed descriptions of these procedures can be found elsewhere.[1]

Design of the implant connecting bar and fabrication of the prostheses

The authors prefer implant-assisted implant connecting bar designs for this group of patients. In such designs the primary support is derived from the residual denture-bearing surfaces and key areas of the defect. The implants are used to facilitate stability and retention of the large obturator prosthesis. The authors prefer to unite the implants with a rigid, precision-fitted implant connecting bar with retentive elements attached to the bar. The potentially most damaging forces on implants will result from occlusal loading and so, ideally, the bar-attachment apparatus should be designed to direct most occlusal forces along the long axis of the implant fixtures. The implant connecting bar should be designed so that posterior occlusal forces are borne by the residual alveolar ridge and maxillary tuberosity as opposed to the implants. Gravitational forces are much less of a concern and can be reduced by aggressively engaging undercuts and the lateral wall of the maxillary defect. In large defects, lateral forces secondary to lateral displacement of a large obturator prosthesis need to be taken into account.

Numerous factors complicate the design of the bar and the distribution of occlusal forces for total maxillectomy patients. For example, when the patient is subjected to a radical maxillectomy (resection of half of the hard palate), fewer implant sites are available and the anterior–posterior (AP) spread of the implants placed in the remaining edentulous premaxilla is often limited. In addition, occlusal loads produce multiple axes of rotation of the obturator prosthesis, especially when the food bolus is excised anteriorly on the side of the defect. These axes are dependent upon the position of the implants and the point of load application on the prosthesis.

Davis *et al.*,[18] developed a photo-elastic model to determine the most favorable implant connecting bar-attachment design when implants were placed in the residual premaxilla following a radical maxillectomy. A photo-elastic model was fabricated that was based on a human maxilla that had undergone a radical maxillectomy. Photo-elastic materials were used to simulate the bone around the implants and the bone along the medial and lateral aspects of the defect. Three implants were used on the nondefect side to simulate a common clinical situation and bar designs were fabricated with a gold alloy, duplicating various clinical conditions. The following designs were tested:

- implant connecting bar with Hader clips placed to the mesial of the anterior implant and distal to the posterior implant;
- implant connecting bar with ERA (APMS, Stern Gold, Attleboro, MA) attachments placed to the mesial of the anterior implant and distal to the posterior implant;
- implant connecting bar with ERA attachments placed to the mesial of the anterior implant and distal to the posterior implants, with occlusal rests between each of the implants;
- implant connecting bar with "O" ring (Attachments International, San Mateo, CA) attachments placed between the implants;
- implant connecting bar with an ERA attachment placed to the mesial of the anterior implant and a Hader clip distal to the posterior implant;
- implant connecting bar with an OSO attachment placed on the anterior and posterior implants.

The acrylic resin obturator extension base was fabricated and the loading regions selected for testing were anterior and posterior to the implants. Each loading zone had a ramp so that a force of 5.44 kg (12 lb) could be applied in both a vertical and lateral direction at each location. The photo-elastic cast was firmly fixed to the base of the stage of a straining frame. A force of 90 g was applied to the acrylic resin extension base to correspond to the weight of the obturator. Circularly polarized light was used to illuminate the cast and the results were recorded photographically. The stress patterns developed by the different designs were compared by placing them on the cast without exerting any type of external load. The resulting stresses were observed and recorded with a camera having an appropriately oriented set of polarized and quarter-waved plates affixed to the lens.

The most pertinent conclusions of the study were as follows:

1. anterior loads caused higher and more concentrated stresses around the anterior and middle implants as compared to posterior loads, since posterior loads are partially supported by the residual edentulous denture-bearing surfaces;
2. the addition of occlusal rests on the bars between the implants increased the stability of the prostheses and alleviated the stresses around the posterior implant when a posterior force was applied;
3. the "O" ring type attachment resulted in the most favorable stress distribution as compared to the bar–clip or the bar–ERA designs. However, the "O" ring designs were not as retentive as the other attachment systems tested.

Davis and her colleagues[18] concluded that bar design is a compromise between retention and the need for stress distribution and maintenance of the bone around the implants. Based on this work and our clinical experience,[2] the authors propose the following guidelines. With the use of a resilient attachment like the ERA, which allows for a vertical compression of the prosthesis in the edentulous extension areas upon application of an occlusal load, the addition of occlusal rests improves the distribution of stresses. For example, when a load is applied to point #1, the prosthesis will rotate around the new axis AB, which passes through the distal occlusal rest (Figure 21.6). Most of the occlusal load is absorbed by the residual denture-bearing surfaces in the posterior denture extension areas, and these forces are directed more favorably along the long axis of the implants. The ERA attachments allow the prosthesis to be compressed into the bearing surfaces, but provide retention when dislodging forces are applied. The implant connecting bar provides stability for the prosthesis. The placement of rests at either end of the bar enables the prosthesis to rotate around these rests, reduces wear on the attachments, and directs more of the occlusal forces along the long axes of the implants. This design has been used with success at UCLA since the mid 1990s. These design principles are similar to those proposed by Kratochvil,[19] for class I or class II distal extension removable partial dentures using the "I" bar, mesial rest concept. The patient should be advised against applying occlusal forces posteriorly

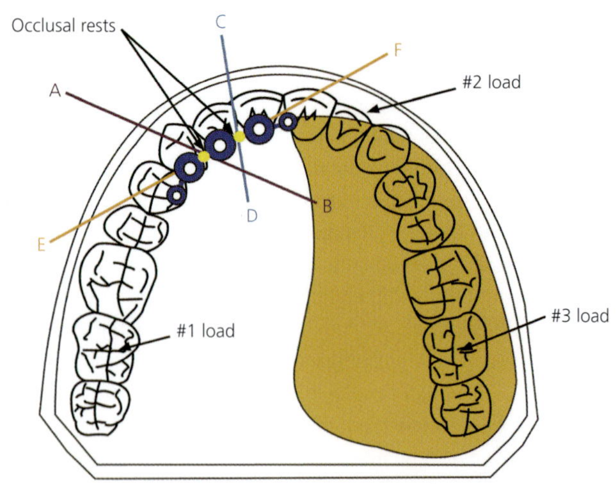

Figure 21.6 "ERA" attachments attached to each side and occlusal rests placed on top of bar. Rests on metal framework control axis of rotation and allow "ERA" attachments to function as designed. *Source:* Beumer *et al.*, 2011.[15] Reproduced with permission from Quintessence Publishing Company Inc.

on the defect side, since there is little support available to counteract these forces. Forceful occlusion on the defect side will result in rapid wear of the attachments and subsequent bone loss around the implant adjacent to the defect.

If the entire premaxilla remains, the number of implants, their distribution, and the design of retention bar follow more conventional prosthodontic guidelines. Under these circumstances we prefer that four implants be placed and suggest the design shown in Figure 21.2; see also Figure 21.9. The use of tilted implants in the posterior positions will increase the AP spread and improve biomechanics.[20–22] In this design the support is provided posteriorly by the residual denture-bearing surfaces and anteriorly by the implants. This design is particularly well suited for combination hard palate–soft palate defects. The attachments connected to the distal portion of the bar are resilient and allow for compression of the mucoperiosteum of the distal extension area engaged by the prosthesis, limiting the torquing forces applied to the implants.

Anterior maxillary defects, or large maxillary defects where only one or both maxillary tuberosities remain, are especially difficult to restore. Implants are useful in retaining these restorations but they should not be the primary means of support. Resilient type attachments are preferred, using the design principles described above (Figure 21.7). If only a single implant is available, an "O" ring type attachment is preferred, because they allow the prosthesis to rotate in multiple directions when either an occlusal load is delivered, when the prosthesis drops as a result of gravity, or when it is displaced in the horizontal plane by the facial musculature or eccentric mandibular movements (Figure 21.3).

A typical oncologic defect of a partially edentulous patient restored with implants is shown in Figure 21.8. The patient had lost most of the residual dentition following years of use of an

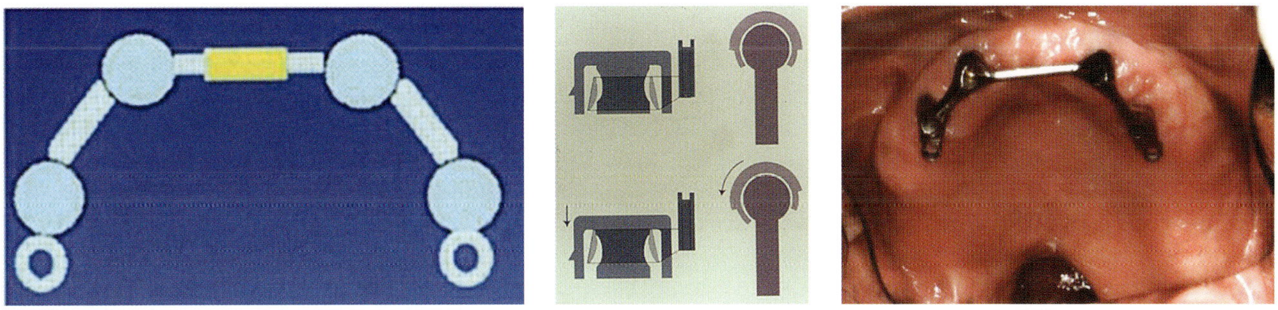

(a) (b) (c)

Figure 21.7 Suggested implant connecting bar design used to retain overdentures with soft palate obturators. (a) Note position of implants. Anterior–posterior spread should be maximized. Resilient attachments provide retention and the anterior segment of the bar provides indirect retention and support. (b) During mastication the anterior segment of the implant connecting bar serves as an axis of rotation and resilient attachments allow the posterior denture-bearing areas to support occlusal forces. *Source:* Beumer *et al.*, 2015.[23] Reproduced with permission from Quintessence Publishing Company Inc. (c) Typical patient with a soft palate defect. Anterior support is provided by the implants but support posteriorly is provided by the denture foundation areas. Implant retention ensures that the soft palate obturator extension accurately engages the residual velopharyngeal musculature, to allow the restoration of normal speech.

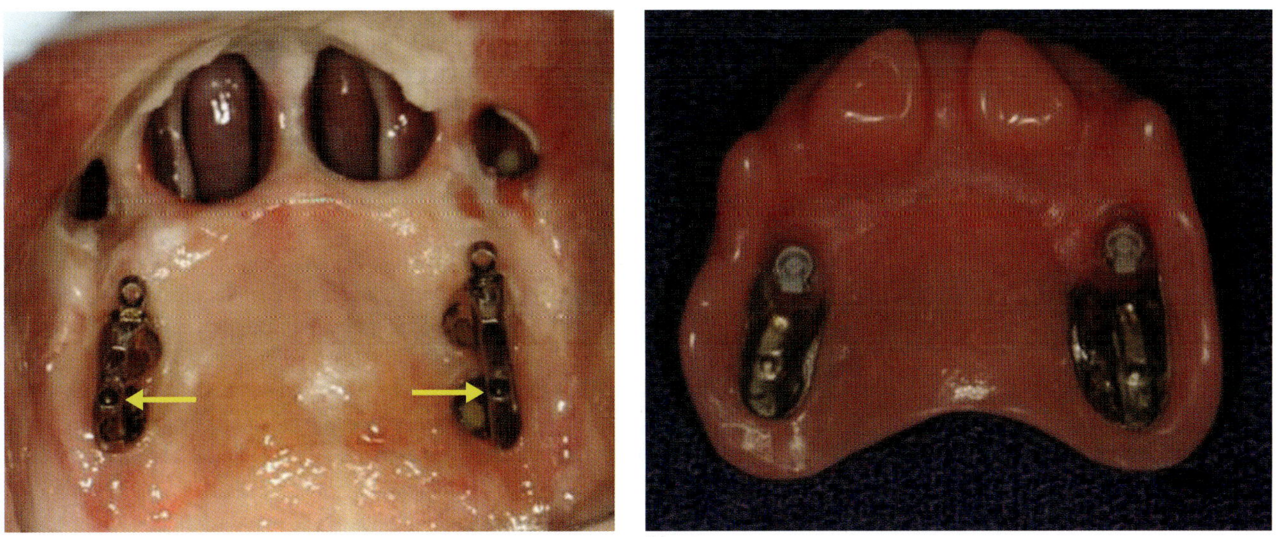

(a) (b)

Figure 21.8 (a) Implants have been placed into the posterior alveolar ridge. The posterior implants on each side engage the pterygoid plates. Note the presence of rests and the resilient attachments. (b) The definitive prosthesis.

RPD–obturator prosthesis secondary to periodontal disease. The resection included the right hard and soft palate and extended to the posterior pharyngeal wall. The implant connecting bar was designed and fabricated using conventional methods. Today, however, CAD/CAM techniques could also be employed. A detailed account of the methods used to design fabricate the implant connecting bars and the obturator prostheses can be found elsewhere.[1,23]

Lessons learned when using implants to retain large maxillary obturator prostheses

Implant connecting bar designs should be implant assisted as opposed to implant supported. The lever arms of large maxillary obturator prostheses can be excessively long and, as such, predispose to load magnification, triggering a resorptive remodeling response of the bone anchoring the implants. Given these conditions, the design of the implant connecting bar must accommodate multiple axes of rotation and direct occlusal loads along the long axis of the implants. Just as important, the ablative surgeon must create retentive, skin-lined defects for the obturator prosthesis to engage, so as to counteract the forces of gravity and provide retention and stability for the prosthesis on the defect side.

Implant-retained obturator prostheses for soft palate defects

Resection of tumors of the soft palate produces velopharyngeal insufficiency. Speech is hypernasal and the patient is unable to swallow food and liquids without nasal regurgitation. Obturator prostheses can be used to effectively obturate these defects and restore speech and swallowing. However, to do so effectively they must be securely retained and the obturator extension must be accurately positioned in the nasopharynx, so that it can properly interact with the residual velopharyngeal musculature. Retention is compromised when the residual hard palate is edentulous, because the surgical resection may compromise or extend into the posterior palatal seal area, making it difficult to obtain and/or maintain a peripheral seal.

In edentulous patients with soft palate defects, osseointegrated implants enable the design and fabrication of overdentures with retentive capacity similar to prostheses made for dentulous patients with residual dentition and a removable partial denture framework. If the soft palate defect has not resulted in compromise of the posterior palatal seal area and the residual palatal structures are favorable, two implants, placed into the premaxillary segment in the region of the canines, will be sufficient to supplement the retention, stability, and support derived from engaging the residual palatal structures. However, if the defect has compromised the posterior palatal seal area, and/or the residual palatal structures provide insufficient stability and support for the prosthesis, four or more implants should be placed. The retention provided by the implants will be enhanced if the implants are positioned to maximize AP spread. The design of the implant connecting bar and the retentive apparatus in these patients will depend upon a number of factors, such as the opposing dentition, the number and length of the implants, and the quality of the bone into which the implants were inserted, the AP spread of the implants, interocclusal space, and the size of the defect. In most patients the number and distribution of implants will require that occlusal forces be shared between the implants anteriorly and the traditional denture-bearing surfaces posteriorly, and requiring an implant-assisted design. Such a design in shown in Figure 21.9.

These implant connecting bars can be designed and fabricated by either conventional means or with CAD/CAM techniques (Figure 21.10). When the implant connecting bar is designed and fabricated with CAD/CAM techniques, and is designed to be implant assisted, soft metals such as titanium should not be used. The constant movement and rotation of such a prosthesis will rapidly wear a bar made of titanium.

Congenital defects of the maxilla

Implants are particularly valuable when restoring dental and palatal defects in patients with congenital anomalies, especially patients with incomplete repair of hard and soft palate defects associated with cleft lip and palate. Frequently, these patients present with multiple missing or malposed teeth, collapsed arch

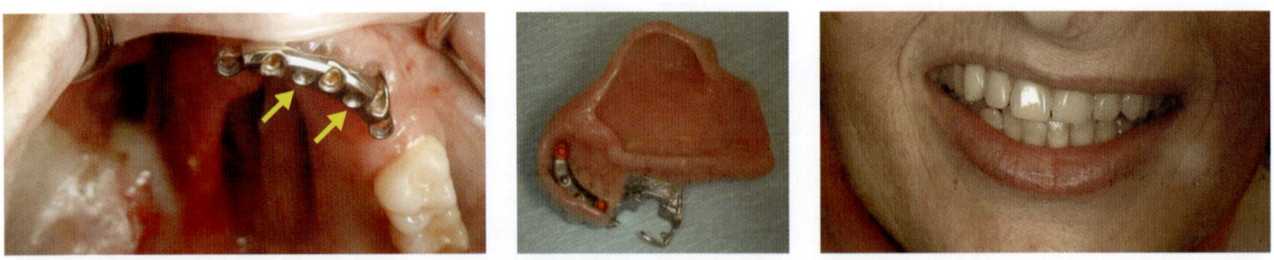

(a) (b) (c)

Figure 21.9 A typical defect restored with implants. (a) Implant connecting bar. Note the rests atop the bar between the implants. Note also that the defect extended to the posterior pharyngeal wall. Engagement of the velopharyngeal musculature will restore speech to normal. (b) Definitive prosthesis. (c) Prosthesis in position. *Source:* Beumer *et al.*, 2015.[23] Reproduced with permission from Quintessence Publishing Company Inc.

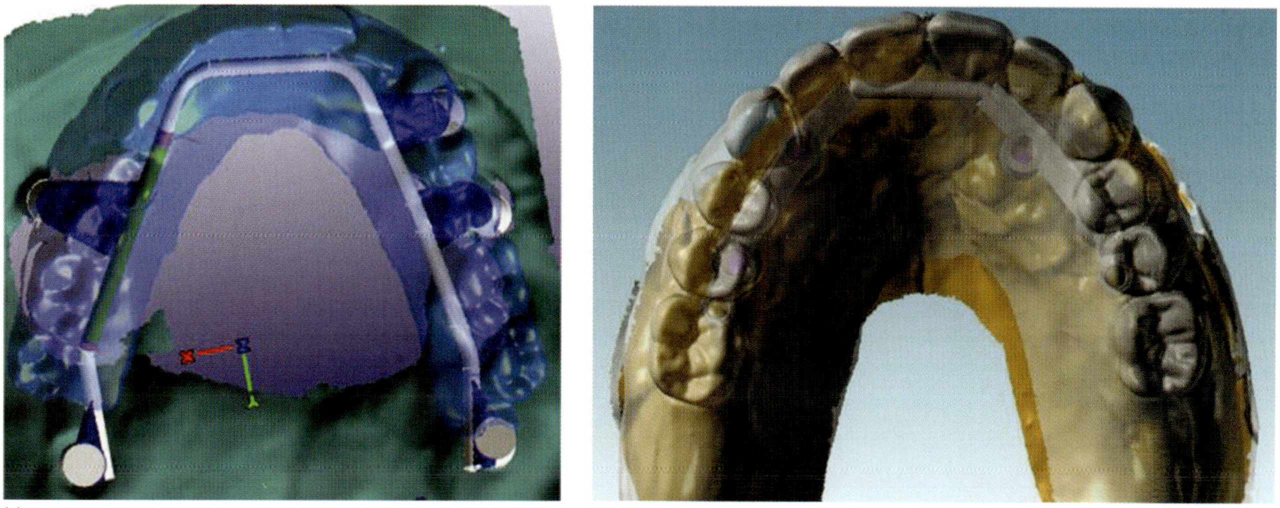

(a) (b)

Figure 21.10 These implant connecting bars were designed and fabricated with CAD/CAM programs. (a) This bar is designed to be implant supported and so was milled from titanium. (b) This bar was designed to be implant assisted and was milled from chromium–cobalt alloy.

form, oral antral fistulae, and class III jaw relations. A typical patient presenting with a partially repaired cleft palate is presented in Figure 21.11. Surveyed crowns were fabricated for the remaining maxillary molars and implants were placed anterior to these teeth in sites with suitable bone volume. Individual attachments were planned for use, so it was important that the implants be parallel to one another and their position compatible with the path of insertion of the proposed removable partial denture. They were positioned to provide anterior support for the removable overlay partial denture. To ensure parallelism, a surgical template was fashioned that permitted semi-guided implant placement, i.e. the surgical template controlled the angulation and position of the osteotomy sites but not the depth. As is the case for most individuals with partially closed clefts denied modern methods of care, the plane of occlusion and tooth positions of the teeth associated with the opposing mandibular dentition were unfavorable. These discrepancies were resolved with conventional full-veneer crowns.

Combined surgical and prosthetic rehabilitation with CAD/CAM techniques

Obturator prostheses provide excellent rehabilitation for almost all patients with maxillary or combined maxillary–soft palate defects. However, some patients will encounter lasting problems with the retention of the prosthesis or favor a surgical closure of the defect for psychological or psychosocial reasons. A computer-planned and -guided surgical reconstruction of missing soft and bony tissues, in combination with prosthetic restoration of missing teeth, may be desirable, especially in younger patients. With the advent of CAD/CAM technologies, new surgical and prosthodontic techniques are evolving, which, when properly executed in a multidisciplinary environment, provide patients with implant-supported prostheses that very effectively and predictably restore form and function for these patients.[1,24–27] However, surgical reconstruction of large maxillary defects should not be undertaken without the aid of CAD/CAM techniques. If surgical reconstructions are not properly planned and executed, irresolvable prosthodontic difficulties may be encountered due to poorly contoured, bulky tissues, lack of suitable bone volume for placement of implants, or poor positioning and alignment of implants.

In general this technique is best suited for secondary reconstruction after the patient is proven to be free of neoplastic disease. However, in selected patients, for example, those with well-defined benign tumors, a primary preplanned reconstruction can be combined with a preplanned guided tumor ablation. When a vascularized free flap is used, the condition of both the donor site and recipient site vessels needs to be carefully assessed. Vascular disease with partial occlusion of blood vessels in the donor site is considered a contraindication, as it might lead to severe vascular problems in the donor region. The status of these vessels should be verified by digital subtraction angiography. In patients who had a previous neck dissection as part of their oncologic treatment, potential recipient blood vessels must be identified and properly assessed.

The defect should be of sufficient size, because the vascularization of small free flaps with bone grafts smaller than 2 cm is not predictable. In small defects, the use of free bone grafts can be considered, particularly if sufficient, well-vascularized soft tissue is remaining or is introduced. In large defects, there is need for reasonable amounts of remaining bone at the recipient site to provide an appropriate means of fixation for the graft.

Scans are obtained from the donor site (most often the fibula) and the recipient site. The surgical reconstruction is planned based on the three-dimensional (3-D) models fabricated from these scans. Surgical guides designed to develop the osteotomy sites and the implant sites are fabricated. The implants are placed into the fibula and are allowed to osseointegrate. After a

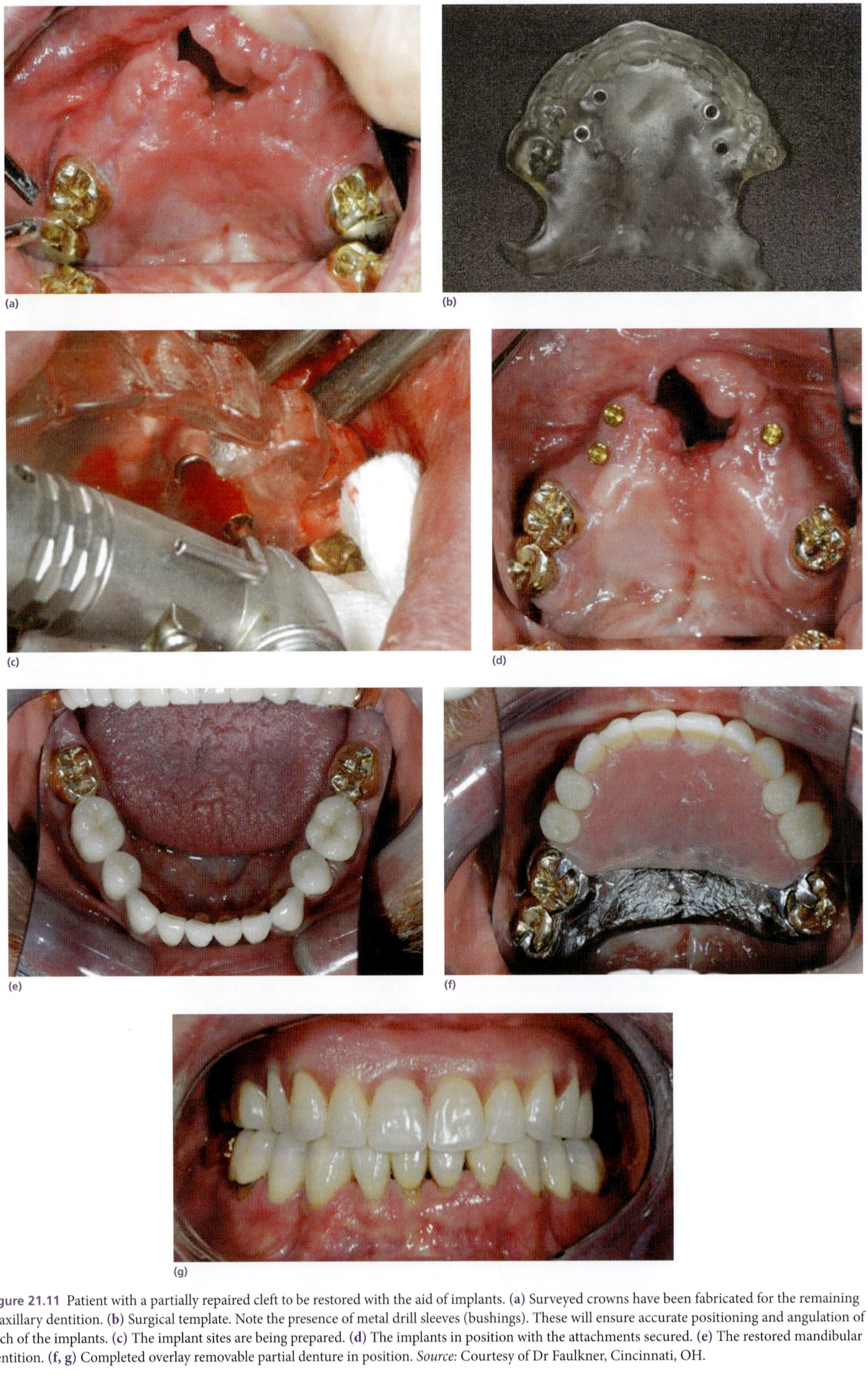

Figure 21.11 Patient with a partially repaired cleft to be restored with the aid of implants. (a) Surveyed crowns have been fabricated for the remaining maxillary dentition. (b) Surgical template. Note the presence of metal drill sleeves (bushings). These will ensure accurate positioning and angulation of each of the implants. (c) The implant sites are being prepared. (d) The implants in position with the attachments secured. (e) The restored mandibular dentition. (f, g) Completed overlay removable partial denture in position. *Source:* Courtesy of Dr Faulkner, Cincinnati, OH.

suitable period, the fibula is retrieved and osteotomized with the benefit of the surgical guide, and a prefabricated implant connecting bar or provisional prosthesis is secured to the bone flap to facilitate healing and consolidation of the graft. The graft is then secured to the recipient bone sites with mini-plates and the vascular anastomoses completed. After a suitable period of healing and soft tissue consolidation, the definitive prosthesis is fabricated.

A detailed description of the CAD/CAM methods used for work-up, the surgical templates used during surgical reconstruction and implant placement, and the fabrication of the provisional and definitive prostheses can be found elsewhere.[1]

Restoration of tongue–mandible defects with osseointegrated implants

The management of malignant tumors associated with the tongue, floor of the mouth, mandible, and adjacent structures represents a difficult challenge for the surgeon, radiation oncologist, and prosthodontist, relative to both control of the primary disease and rehabilitation following treatment. The most common intraoral sites for squamous cell carcinoma are the lateral margin of the tongue and the floor of the mouth. Both locations predispose the mandible to tumor invasion, often necessitating its resection in conjunction with resection of large portions of the tongue, the floor of the mouth, and the regional lymphatics.

Disabilities that may result from such resections are mostly due to impaired tongue function, and include impaired speech articulation, difficulty in swallowing, problems with mastication, altered mandibular movements, compromised control of salivary secretions, and cosmetic disfigurement. In the past 20 years, free tissue transfers (free flaps) and dental implants have resulted in considerable improvement in the form and function of these patients. Using these new surgical and prosthodontic methods, more patients with tongue–mandible defects can be restored in appearance and function to levels that approach their presurgical condition. However, these rehabilitative efforts are complex and require the efforts of a sophisticated, well-trained, multidisciplinary team of oncologic surgeons, maxillofacial prosthodontists, reconstructive surgeons, speech therapists, clinical psychologists, and others.

Anterior defects with mandibular continuity retained or restored

Prostheses retained and supported by osseointegrated implants placed in the anterior region of the mandible, when mandibular continuity has been retained or reconstructed, in combination with the remaining posterior teeth, enable most anterior resection patients to masticate effectively. Most of these patients retain sufficient bulk of the tongue, along with the requisite motor and sensory innervation, to permit good tongue function, but the lack of support anteriorly impairs effective incision and mastication of the food bolus. Osseointegrated implants provide this support. In patients who have undergone a marginal resection of the mandible, 8–10 mm of vertical bone is advisable before implants are considered. A similar bulk of bone is required for grafted mandibles. Before considering implants in these areas, cone-beam computed tomography (CBCT) scans are recommended to assess the 3-D bone volume of the potential implant sites.

In the marginal resection patient, the residual bone in the anterior mandible is very dense and, as a result, implant success rates are in excess of 95%. Implants placed in free grafts used to reconstruct these defects have a similar high success rate.[28] Once the graft has become consolidated and healed, free bone grafts present with a homogeneous calcification pattern, which results in an excellent bone–implant interface and implant anchorage.[29] Free flaps, particularly the fibula with its thick cortical plates, also provide excellent sites for the implants and the reports are equally favorable.[30–32]

The major challenge encountered when placing implants into the anterior mandibular resection patient, where mandibular continuity is maintained or restored, is to create thin, attached, keratinized tissues around the implants. In most instances the wound is closed primarily, and almost always requires a vestibuloplasty, with the soft tissues associated with the potential implant sites needing to be supplemented with skin or palatal grafts. The objective is to create thin, keratinized peri-implant tissues that are attached to the periosteum of the bone adjacent to the implants. When implants penetrate such tissues, oral hygiene measures are easier for the patient and the risk of peri-implant mucositis and peri-implantitis is reduced.

Defects restored with free bone grafts generally present with an excess of soft tissue overlying the graft. In most patients, a myocutaneous flap or free flap has been used to replace the soft tissues removed during the tumor extirpation. A free autogenous bone graft is usually placed at a later date and is positioned within the tissues of the soft tissue flap. Implants are placed into the bone graft 6–9 months later. Sometimes the soft tissues overlying the implants can be 10–15 mm in thickness. These tissues must be thinned and attached tissues around the implant must be created if peri-implant mucositis or peri-implantitis is to be prevented. Ideally the thickness of the tissues adjacent to the implants should not exceed 3 or 4 mm. If the tissues are not thinned sufficiently, deep peri-implant pockets will result that predispose to infection, granulation tissue formation, and hypertrophy. These soft tissue infections can spread to bone, leading to loss of bone and, ultimately, implant failure.

Of particular note is that machined titanium implants and their components (implant fixtures, healing abutments, etc.), that perforate skin that may have been used to line the bearing surface, have a tendency to trigger aggressive inflammatory tissue reactions (Figure 21.12a). However, these tissue responses can usually be eliminated by the use of polished healing abutments. Customized metal–ceramic healing abutments made

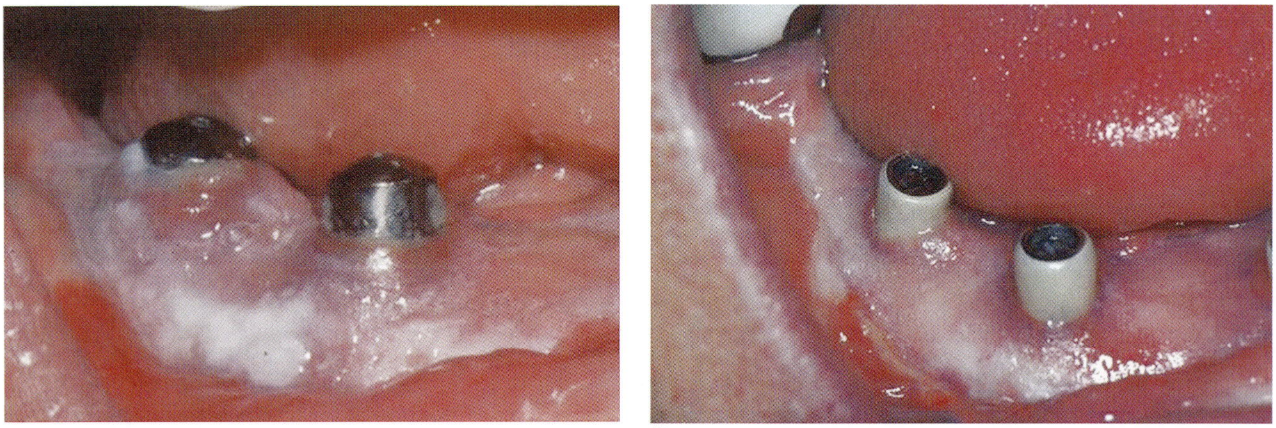

(a) (b)

Figure 21.12 **(a)** Soft tissue hypertrophy around machined-surface healing abutments following second-stage surgery. **(b)** The conventional healing abutments were replaced with metal–ceramic healing abutments made with the UCLA abutment technique. Complete healing was noted in 3 weeks.

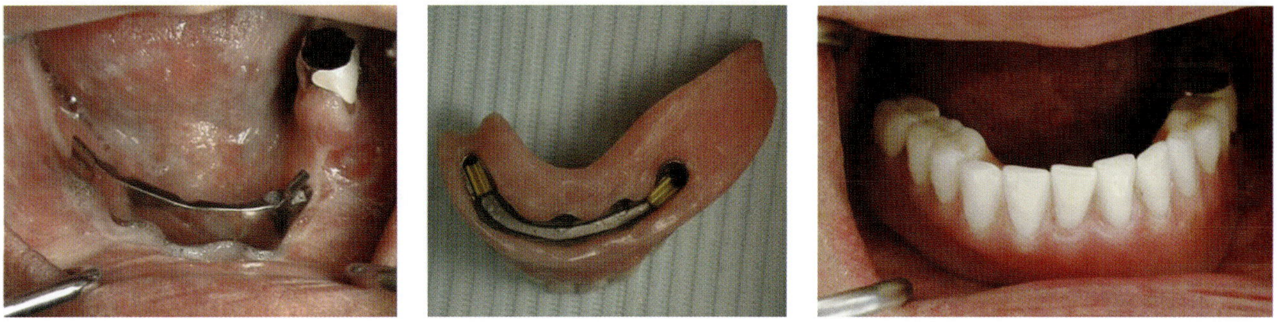

(a) (b) (c)

Figure 21.13 Anterior mandible defect restored with fibula free flap. **(a)** Implant-supported tissue bar milled to a 3° taper. The peri-implant tissues were reconstructed with free palatal grafts. **(b)** Overlay prosthesis. *Source:* Beumer *et al.*, 2011.[1] Reproduced with permission from Quintessence Publishing Company Inc. **(c)** Prosthesis in position.

from the "UCLA" abutment resolved the tissue problems in the patient shown in Figure 21.12b.

Removable overlay prostheses are preferred for restoring these defects. Support for mastication is provided by the implants anteriorly and by the residual dentition posteriorly. Denture flanges can be contoured to reposition and support the lower lip (Figure 21.13). With such designs, access for oral hygiene is easier for the patient. If an implant-supported prosthesis is preferred and the edentulous space extends into the molar region, a minimum of four or five implants must be placed. In this instance, the proper arrangement of the implants is critical. The arc of curvature of the arrangement must result in at least 1 cm AP spread. Implant-supported prostheses with less AP spread have a higher rate of implant failure and an increased number of complications associated with the prosthesis, such as screw loosening and fracture.[33] Fully guided or semi-guided implant placement is strongly recommended, utilizing a surgical template fabricated using CAD/CAM technologies.[34–36] This approach should ensure that the implants are inserted into the proper locations with proper alignment.

If a fixed restoration is planned, implants should be placed in the sites to be occupied by the individual teeth, as opposed to interproximal areas. The buccal–lingual position and angulation are also important. The authors prefer screw retention of these prostheses, and it is advised that implants should be positioned so that the screw-access channels exit through the cingulum area of anterior teeth and central fossa of the posterior teeth. Otherwise, custom substructures or custom abutments need to be fabricated and the prosthesis secured with cross-pinning screws, adding additional cost and complexity. Cement retention is discouraged in these large prostheses because of the difficulty in removing cement that inevitably becomes impacted subgingivally.[37] If a removable overlay prosthesis is planned, the buccal–lingual or labial–lingual position, angulation, and the AP spread are still of concern. Implants should be placed so that the abutments and the retentive apparatus fit within the confines of the prosthesis, allowing for proper placement of denture teeth.

Master impressions are made in the usual manner using pick-up impression copings luted together with pattern resin. We prefer this method because of its accuracy. If an overlay prosthesis is planned, the impression tray must be border molded, either during the making of the master impression or as a pick-up impression when verifying the fit of the implant connecting bar.

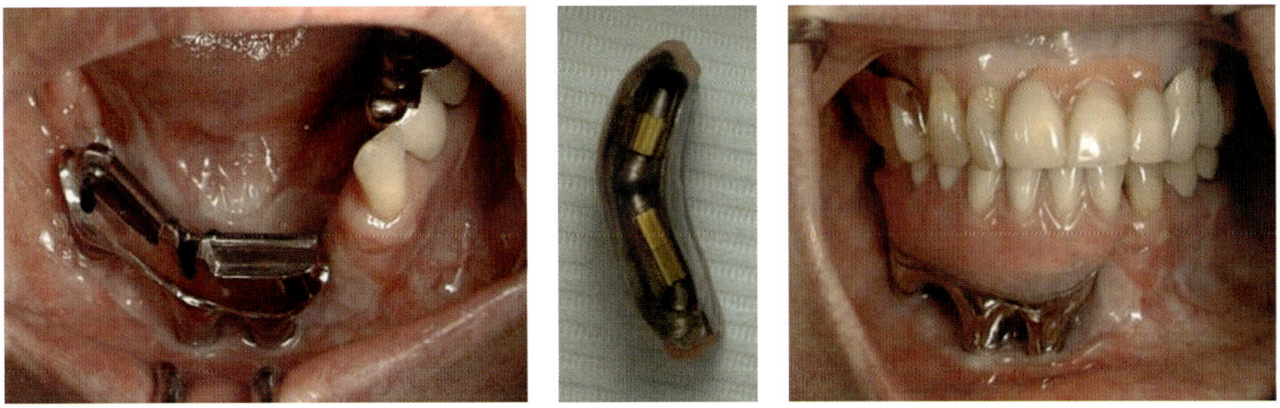

(a) (b) (c)

Figure 21.14 Lateral mandible defect reconstructed with a fibular free flap. Tongue, hypoglossal, and lingual nerves are intact on the resected side. The lack of sufficient vestibular depth and width precluded the fabrication of a denture flange. (a) Implant connecting bar milled to a 3° taper. (b) Overlay prosthesis. Clip housings were incorporated within the metal substructure. (c) Prosthesis in position. Note the hygiene access beneath the implant connecting bar. *Source:* Beumer *et al.*, 2011.[1] Reproduced with permission from Quintessence Publishing Company Inc.

Maxillo-mandibular records are made and the casts transferred to an appropriate articulator. A trial denture is then prepared. If CAD/CAM methods are to be used, the trial prosthesis is scanned and these data merged with the CBCT data of the patient. The metal framework or implant connecting bar is then designed and milled or printed in a suitable material. If a conventional method is used, a silicone template is fabricated from the trial prosthesis with the teeth imbedded. This template can be used to design any type of metal framework, whether the metal framework is for a metal–ceramic prosthesis or an implant connecting bar designed to retain an overlay prosthesis. The prosthesis is then completed using conventional prosthodontic guidelines.[33]

Lateral defects with mandibular continuity restored

In these large defects, osseointegrated implants significantly improve the retention, stability, and support for the prosthesis. In partially edentulous patients, implants are most useful when the surgical ablation of the tumor has spared the lingual and hypoglossal nerves. Under these circumstances, the patient can detect and manipulate the food bolus and the implant-supported prosthesis can be used effectively for mastication. If motor and sensory innervation has been lost on the resected side, the authors recommend that a removable partial denture be used to replace the missing dentition and support the lip and corner of the mouth.

If the marginal mandibular nerve has been resected, it is advantageous to support the corner of the mouth and recontour the lip with a denture flange incorporated within a removable overlay prosthesis. The primary purpose of the prosthesis is to provide the support necessary on the defect side for mastication and, indeed, if the hypoglossal and lingual nerves are intact, the patient will be able to detect and manipulate the food bolus sufficiently well on the resected side to permit reasonable mastication. Such patients are shown in Figure 21.13 and Figure 21.14. In some patients the lack of vestibular width and depth precludes the development of a flange (Figure 21.14).

Lessons learned from the use of implants in free vascularized flaps

- *If the defect is secondary to removal of a malignant tumor from the oral cavity, immediate placement of implants into free flaps is ill advised in most patients.* Since 80% of the recurrences occur within the first year we prefer to wait at least 12 months following tumor ablation before undertaking implant placement. In addition, especially if freehand drilling is employed, it is very difficult to properly position and angulate the implants within the graft. If immediate implant placement into the flap is considered, the authors recommend the use of CAD/CAM programs for planning and the fabrication of surgical templates, so that fully guided implant surgery can be employed.
- *At second-stage surgery the tissues surrounding the implants must be thinned. Frequently free skin or palatal grafts are needed to create a zone of attached keratinized tissue around the implants.* If the submucosal resections are not properly executed and the tissues around the implants are not thinned and tacked down properly to engage the periosteum, these tissues will be mobile, the peri-implant pockets will be excessive, and the peri-implant tissues will be susceptible to inflammation, resulting in granulation tissue formation and hypertrophy.[30,38,39] Palatal grafts are preferred over skin grafts. Best results with grafting are obtained when a pre-made border-molded stent is used to immobilize and protect the grafts during the healing period.
- *Highly polished abutment surfaces will reduce the incidence of soft tissue problems around the implants.* Frequently implants in these patients exit through skin and, in the presence of plaque, the skin surrounding the implants becomes highly

inflamed (Figure 21.12). Conventional healing abutments, with their machined surfaces, retain plaque and calculus readily and should be used with caution during the healing period after second-stage surgery. The authors also recommend against the use of machined abutments in the definitive prosthesis. When implants exit through skin the authors prefer to fabricate implant connecting bars using the "UCLA" abutment technique, so that either highly polished metal or glazed porcelain will abut the tissues of the peri-implant sulcus.

- *Overlay type prostheses are preferred because they provide better support for the corner of the mouth and the lower lip.* Most of these patients lose the marginal mandibular and inferior alveolar nerves during the resection of their tumors. As a result the lip on the resected side loses its muscle tonus, becomes fibrotic, and becomes retracted. The denture flange serves to restore lip contours and lip seal, thereby facilitating the articulation of plosive speech sounds and the control of saliva (Figure 21.13).[30,38]

Lateral discontinuity defects – implant-retained resection overdentures

Complete dentures for edentulous patients with lateral discontinuity defects (so called "resection dentures") are primarily used to restore lip contours and esthetics. Mastication is difficult because of compromised denture-bearing surfaces, deviation of the mandible, angular pathway of mandibular closure, unilateral occlusal forces, abnormal jaw relationships, impaired motor and sensory innervation of remaining tissues, and, most important, compromised tongue function. These patients are required to stabilize and retain their resection complete dentures with the tongue, while at the same time using the tongue to manipulate the bolus. This maneuver is beyond the capability of almost all patients.

The placement of osseointegrated implants enables fabrication of well-retained and stable overdentures. The support derived from the implants and the residual denture-bearing surfaces, and the retention and stability provided by the implants, is more than sufficient to allow effective mastication if the patient presents with reasonable tongue function and motor and sensory innervation on the unresected side. The tongue is no longer required to control the denture, so it can now be used solely for control and manipulation of the food bolus during mastication and swallowing. Therefore, the key, as always, to the restoration of mastication is the status of tongue function following tumor resection. When portions of the tongue are resected because of tumor, all reasonable effort should be made to restore its bulk with free flaps and avoid tethering it laterally or inferiorly.

If reasonable mastication performance is the objective, there are several measures available to determine the adequacy of tongue function. One measure is speech articulation. If the patient's speech is intelligible, the prognosis for effective manipulation of the bolus with an implant-retained prosthesis is favorable. When poor speech intelligibility is evident, the prognosis for effective mastication is less predictable. Another measure is the patient's ability to raise the dorsum of the tongue above the level of the projected plane of occlusion. If the dorsum of the tongue cannot elevate at least 10 mm above the plane, mastication with the resection denture will be problematic. A more objective measurement of tongue function and coordination can be obtained with a modified barium swallow. If the results of this study reveal prolonged oral transit times with considerable retention of the contrast medium in the oral cavity, the prognosis for improved mastication is guarded.

Most patients with poor tongue function have little to gain from the use of implants. This does not necessarily preclude the use of implants in such patients, because there are other benefits to be had from a well-retained prosthesis, such as esthetics, restoration of oral competence, and so forth. However, neither the clinician nor the patient should anticipate reasonable masticatory performance with an implant-retained overdenture unless there is good tongue function.

In patients with mandibular discontinuity defects, if implants are to be placed into the mandible to retain and support an overdenture, consideration should be given to placing implants in the opposing maxilla. The unilateral occlusal forces and the increased lateral forces, generated during the chewing cycle of these patients, tend to rock and dislodge the upper denture. Xerostomia secondary to radiotherapy or chemoradiation may further compromise peripheral seal. Therefore, implants should be considered if retention and stability of a conventional maxillary denture is marginal. Two implants, placed in the canine sites, will provide the necessary retention and stability for most patients.

Although most of these patients will receive either preoperative or postoperative radiation or chemoradiation, these treatments do not preclude the use of implants. If the patient received conventional radiation therapy via opposed lateral facial or opposed mandibular fields, the mandibular symphysis and premaxilla are out of the field in most patients. If the patient is treated with IMRT (see later section, Implants in patients treated with radiation and chemoradiation) the dose to these regions generally falls below 50 Gy and, at this dosage, sufficient viability is present in the bone to permit osseointegration. An exception would be those patients with tumors arising from the anterior floor of the mouth. In these patients the dose to the potential implant sites would approach 70 Gy or more and implant placement would predispose the patient to a significant risk of osteoradionecrosis.

Treatment procedures

Implant-retained overdentures are preferred to fixed prostheses for the following reasons. First, deviation of the mandible may require that the denture teeth be positioned buccal to the ridge on the unresected side and lingual to the ridge on the resected side. This is difficult when designing a fixed, implant-retained restoration. Second, denture flanges and lip plumpers are frequently necessary to provide support and recontour the lower lip in order to restore lip seal (oral competence). In addition, a sufficient number of implant sites may not be available to provide the number and arrangement of implants necessary to support a fixed restoration. Moreover, it is far easier for the patient to conduct proper hygiene measures for implant connecting bars than for fixed implant-retained prostheses. This is an important factor, because most resection patients are elderly and may have impaired vision and/or poor manual dexterity.

In these patients the only implant sites available in the edentulous mandible are located in the symphyseal region. A minimum of two implants should be placed, but more are desirable if space allows, not so much for retention or support, but to enhance the stability of the resection overdenture. As discussed previously, resection patients demonstrate a unilateral envelope of motion confined mainly to the defect side and their mastication is limited to the nonresected side. Thus, this occlusal pattern will tend to compromise the stability of the overdenture.

Computer-guided planning and surgical protocols have been used with increasing frequency in recent years and are recommended. The precision that can be achieved with these methods represents a significant improvement over freehand surgery. However, it may not be necessary in every patient and freehand surgical placement can still be used with effectiveness by experienced surgeons. It does, however, represent a new and sophisticated treatment planning tool to ensure that implant placement is directed by the demands of the prosthesis. Furthermore, these methods are rapidly becoming more cost effective.

If only two implants are to be placed, they should be at least 20 mm apart in order to accommodate the implant connecting bar apparatus. Implants should be placed perpendicular to the occlusal plane and, if possible, within the zone of the residual attached gingiva. For many resection patients there will usually be two implant sites on the normal side and one site on the resected side. The authors favor the bar clip designs.

Such prostheses should be "implant assisted" as opposed to "implant supported". If only two implants have been placed, the authors prefer to splint the implants together with a "Hader" type implant connecting bar as opposed to the use of individual attachments. Implant connecting bars provide more stability for the prosthesis compared to most individual attachments. The bar should be designed so that it is parallel to the axis of rotation of the prosthesis when an occlusal force is applied in the posterior extension area on the normal side. With this design, the prosthesis will rotate freely around the bar, minimizing the torquing forces delivered to the implants and minimizing the wear of the "Hader" clips. If additional retention is desired an ERA attachment (Sterngold, Attleboro, MA) can be added posteriorly on the unresected side. In this design, as an occlusal force is applied, the prosthesis will rotate freely around the bar.

When the peri-implant tissues are well healed, border-molded impressions are made and centric relation records obtained. The occlusal vertical dimension is reduced and the occlusal plane is lowered in order to ease manipulation of the bolus of food by the tongue. The trial dentures are inserted, records verified, and the esthetics and lip support refined as necessary. The implant connecting bar can be fabricated either with conventional means or using CAD/CAM techniques, and the prosthesis is completed and delivered. A detailed account of these procedures can be found elsewhere.[38]

Edentulous patients with reconstructed partial glossectomy defects and the continuity of the mandible retained or restored

Patients in this category have either undergone marginal mandibulectomy retaining mandibular continuity or have had successful reconstruction following resection of a segment of the mandible. Similar to patients with discontinuity defects, the prognosis for mastication is primarily dependent on the status of tongue function. If tongue function is unfavorable it will be difficult for the patient to achieve a reasonable level of mastication. The patient shown in Figure 21.15 presented following reconstruction of the mandible with a bone graft. However, the inability to detect, control, and manipulate the food bolus has been compromised either by the lack of tongue volume or mobility. Implants can be placed and used to retain overdentures in these patients, but significant improvements in mastication efficiency should not be anticipated.

When the tongue has been reconstructed with a free flap and the motor and sensory innervation is intact on the unresected side, the prosthetic prognosis for mastication becomes favorable (Figure 21.16). Denture-bearing surface deficiencies can be addressed with skin, palatal grafts, and vestibuloplasty, and retention provided by osseointegrated implants. With a well-retained and stable denture, the patient is able to direct his/her

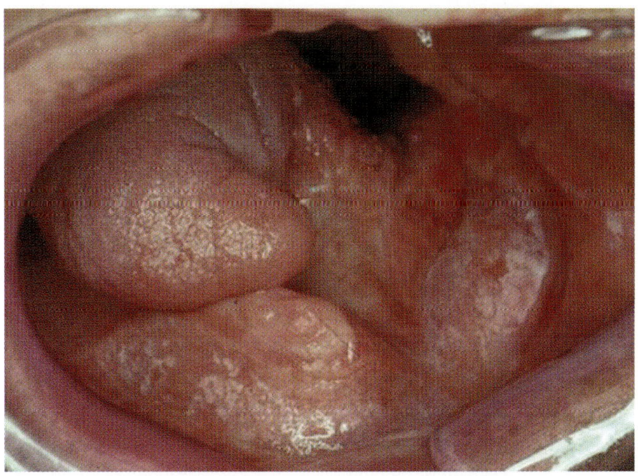

Figure 21.15 In this patient the mandible was reconstructed but not the tongue. The tongue is immobilized. Result: prognosis for mastication with complete dentures is very poor even if implants are employed. *Source:* Beumer *et al.*, 2011.[1] Reproduced with permission from Quintessence Publishing Company Inc.

attention toward manipulating the food bolus. If the opposing maxilla is edentulous and compromised by resorption, or if the clinician is unable to obtain peripheral seal because of post-radiation xerostomia, the authors consider placing implants into the premaxilla. Usually two are sufficient. In the mandible the number of implants required depends primarily on the status of the opposing maxilla. If the maxilla is edentulous, two implants are sufficient. If the opposing arch is dentate, four or more implants are recommended so that an implant-supported prosthesis can be used.

The patient shown in Figure 21.17 is characteristic of patients presenting with a partial glossectomy defect restored with a free flap where mandibular continuity has been retained. Substantial portions of the oral tongue were removed in continuity with a selective neck dissection and the tongue bulk restored with a radial forearm free flap. Following mandibulotomy the mandible was re-opposed with a reconstruction plate. Post surgery examination revealed that the bulk of the tongue was restored and its mobility was good. The mandibular bearing surface was only slightly affected by the surgery.

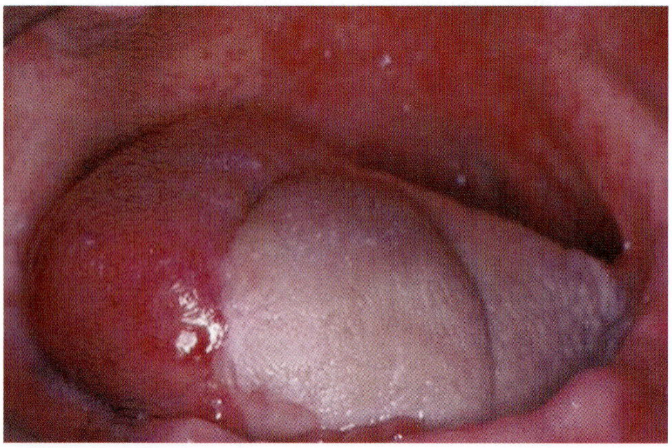

Figure 21.16 Partial glossectomy defect restored with a radial forearm flap. Portions of denture-bearing surface were resurfaced with the flap. Movement of the tongue is excellent. The prognosis for mastication is excellent, if implants are employed to retain and stabilize the mandibular denture. Mastication must be performed on the nonresected side because these flaps are nonsensate.

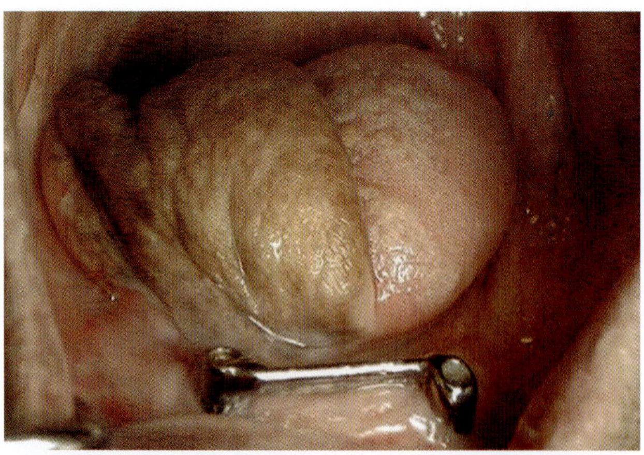

Figure 21.17 Patient with a hemi-glossectomy and reconstruction of the tongue with a free flap. Without implants, use of a mandibular complete denture would not have been possible. In this patient and the patient from Figure 21.16, the risk of additional morbidity associated with placement of implants is minimal because the dose to the implants is relatively low. *Source:* Beumer *et al.*, 2011.[1] Reproduced with permission from Quintessence Publishing Company Inc.

Sufficient bone was available for the placement of two implants in the anterior portion of both the maxilla and mandible. After a suitable period was allowed for the implants to osseointegrate the prosthodontic procedures were initiated. Implant-assisted implant connecting bars were fabricated using "Hader" bars for retention. Upon fabrication of the overdentures the occlusal vertical dimension was closed and the plane of occlusion lowered as much as feasible. The palatal contours were altered so as to idealize the interaction between the reconstructed tongue and the maxillary denture during speech and swallowing.

Implants in patients treated with radiation and chemoradiation

More than three quarters of patients with head neck tumors will be treated with radiation or chemoradiation. Radiation and chemoradiation predispose to changes in bone, skin, and mucosa, which dramatically affect the biologic processes essential to osseointegration (Figure 21.18). In normal patients, implant success requires initial implant immobilization, the formation of a fibrin clot between the surface of the implant and the osteotomy site, the activation of platelets and the release of growth factors, angiogenesis, and migration of mesenchymal stem cells to and deposition of bone on the surfaces of the implant and the osteotomy site. However these biologic processes may be compromised or completely shut down in patients exposed to high-dose radiation or chemoradiation, and, as a result, anchorage of implants in irradiated bone may be mechanical as opposed to biological. Moreover, after receiving radiation treatment, osteoclastic activity continues in some patients, reducing the mineral content of the jawbones within

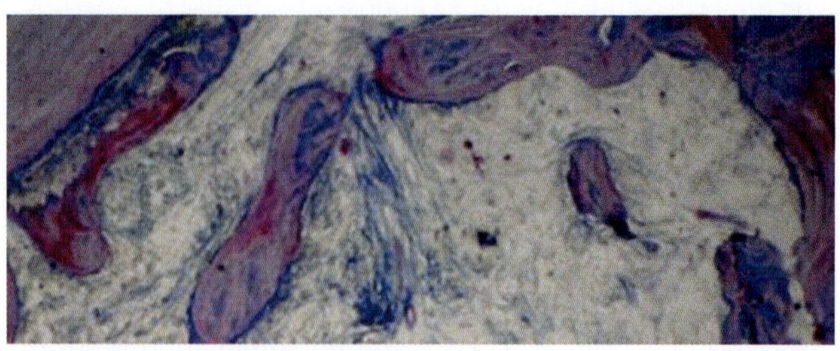

Figure 21.18 This patient received 7000 cGy to the mandible. Note the marked acelluarity, lack of vasculature, and fibrosis. Mesenchymal stem cells are lacking. Implant anchorage in such bone is achieved by mechanical means as opposed to biologic means. *Source:* Beumer *et al.*, 2015.[23] Reproduced with permission from Quintessence Publishing Company Inc.

the clinical treatment volume (the area irradiated) and reducing the thickness of the cortical layers and the volume of individual trabeculae. Such poor-quality bone makes it is more difficult to achieve initial primary implant stability[40] and the mandible is more susceptible to fracture. Moreover, long-term function of osseointegrated implants is dependent on the presence of viable bone that is capable of remodeling and turnover as the implant is subjected to stresses associated with supporting, retaining, and stabilizing prosthetic restorations. These processes are compromised or perhaps entirely lacking in bone irradiated to high dose levels (above 6500 cGy). Given these adverse affects, implants subjected to functional stresses may not be sustained indefinitely.

When implants are considered for the irradiated patient, several issues require careful consideration, including:

1 the potential benefit provided by implants;
2 the potential morbidity associated with implant placement or implant failure;
3 both short- and long-term success rates.

For example, complete denture–obturator prostheses fabricated for edentulous patients following partial palatectomy or radical maxillectomy lack the retention and stability to provide patients with significant mastication.[2] The seal between the nasal cavity and the oral cavity is imperfect, predisposing to hypernasal speech and leakage of liquids and food bolus into the nasal cavities during swallowing. The addition of implants improves the retention and stability of the prosthesis to a level where speech and swallowing are restored to normal limits in almost all patients, and, in selected patients, mastication performance may be restored to presurgical levels (Figure 21.19).[2] Unfortunately, the long-term survival rate of implants placed in edentulous palatectomy or maxillectomy patients, whose implant sites have been irradiated, is relatively low (55–65%) compared to nonirradiated patients (90–95%). However, the placement of implants in these patients is justified on the basis that the risk of osteoradionecrosis is extremely low in the maxilla and there is substantial functional benefit derived from an implant-retained maxillary obturator prosthesis in an edentulous patient.

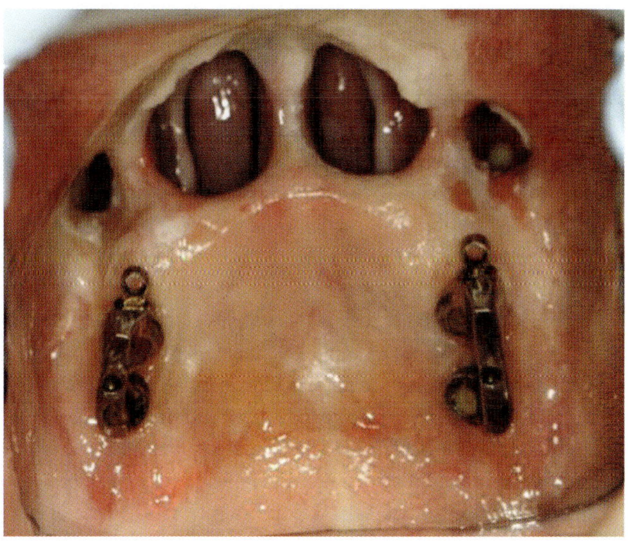

Figure 21.19 Edentulous patient with major resections for oral tumors that received postoperative radiation therapy (approximately 6000 cGy). Patient with partial palatectomy. Implants dramatically improve retention, and without appropriate retention, speech and swallowing cannot be restored to normal levels with a conventional complete denture and obturator.

The functional benefit obtained from implant placement in the irradiated edentulous mandible in patients with partial glossectomy is less clear, and depends on several factors, the most important being the status of tongue function. If the tongue and/or mandible has been resected and the mandible and the tongue have been reconstructed with a free flap, the placement of implants may significantly improve mastication even if the denture-bearing surfaces have been compromised (Figure 21.17). These patients customarily will receive a lower radiation dose than patients treated with radiation alone. The primary concern for such patients is the risk of osteoradionecrosis, and this is almost entirely dependent on the dose to the implant sites. In the mandible, when the dose to bone is 6000 cGy or below, the risk of osteoradionecrosis (ORN) is negligible. When the dose to the implant sites exceeds 6500 cGy, the risk of ORN becomes quite high.

Predictability of implants in irradiated bone

Clinical reports and animal studies indicate that the success–failure rate of osseointegrated implants in irradiated bone appears to be dependent upon the anatomical site, the dose to the site, lengths of the implants used, and the use of hyperbaric oxygen. Dosage to the potential implant sites is dependent upon the mode of radiation [conventional radiation therapy (CRT) vs. intensity-modulated radiation therapy (IMRT) vs. brachytherapy], and the clinical target volume. The use of concomitant chemotherapy during radiation (chemoradiation) increases the biologic equivalent dose by anywhere from 750–1000 cGy[41,42] and worsens the tissue effects.

Animal studies

Animal studies indicate that the wound healing potential of irradiated bone is severely compromised. In addition, the quality (density) of irradiated bone is diminished because, not only is the multicellular unit responsible for remodeling and repair of bone compromised, but bone resorption continues secondary to the presence of isolated osteoclasts. Animal experiments have shown that in irradiated bone, not only is the bone–implant contact area reduced, but also, if new bone is deposited onto the surface of the implant and in the interface zone, the quality of this bone is compromised.[43–47] Nishimura *et al.*,[48] tested the feasibility of placing implants in bone sites that had already been irradiated. They demonstrated that the quality of bone in the implant appositional zone was compromised at radiation dose levels as low as equivalent to 5200 cGy and at the highest levels of radiation (doses equivalent to 7000 cGy) there was very little if any contact or distance osteogenesis.

To summarize the animal studies, at radiation levels equivalent to tumoricidal doses (greater than 6500 cGy), little or no bone is deposited on the implant surface and the remodeling apparatus is severely compromised. Implant anchorage is essentially mechanical as opposed to biologic. At doses equivalent to those used for postoperative radiation therapy (5000–6000 cGy), a greater component of woven bone is seen in the interface and, given the reduction or absence of remodeling elements, it less likely that this immature bone will be replaced by mature lamellar bone in the usual time frame, if ever. At these doses, even if the implant becomes osseointegrated, the bone–implant contact area is decreased when compared to nonirradiated controls. This compromises the load-bearing capacity of the implant. In the event an implant does achieve osseointegration, for example, if it is placed prior to radiation, late post-radiation changes in bone (i.e., loss of blood supply, death of osteocytes, loss of the multicellular unit composed of osteoclasts and osteoblasts responsible for remodeling of bone), bone remodeling essentially ceases and eventually the bone anchorage will be degraded and the response of the implant to occlusal forces compromised.

Human data

The trends seen in human studies[4,30,43,49–60] appear to substantiate the concerns raised in the animal studies; namely, the success rates in irradiated sites are substantially less than in nonirradiated sites, the rate of implant failure increases with time, a high percentage of implants in irradiated tissues demonstrate advanced bone loss at an early stage, and the success rate diminishes as the dose increases. Even in sites with high-quality bone, such as the anterior mandible, where good initial implant anchorage can be achieved, implant failure rates increase dramatically with time.[57] The increased incidence of implant failure observed at stage I surgery indicates the difficulty in achieving initial implant anchorage, particularly in sites such as the maxilla.

The report by Granstrom[56] remains the largest series in the literature and is especially revealing. He analyzed the implant failures of 631 implants placed in 107 irradiated patients over a 25-year period. He compared the patterns of failure in this group of patients with a group of 100 nonirradiated patients with similar profiles, in which 614 implants were placed. In the irradiated group tumors associated with the orbit were most common (24), followed by the maxillary sinus (23), ear (17), skin (eight), floor of mouth (five), tonsil (four), tongue (four), maxilla (three), nasal cavity (two), palate, oropharynx, and buccal mucosa (one each). Ten additional patients presented with tumors of other sites. These patients were treated with high-energy conventional radiation therapy (CRT). Ninety-three patients received their CRT prior to surgical ablation and 14 were irradiated post tumor resection. In the study population, 528 implants were installed within the clinical target volume after radiation, 58 implants were irradiated post implant installation, and 14 others were placed into irradiated tissues but then were exposed to a second course of radiation. Doses were calculated for each implant site. Adjuvant chemotherapy was used in 29 patients and 141 implants were installed in these patients. Screw-type machined surface implants were used on all patients. Fifty-four percent (340) of the implants were placed in conjunction with hyperbaric oxygen (HBO) treatments.

One hundred forty-six implants (23%) failed in the irradiated group – 117 of 291 in the nonHBO group (40.2%) and 29 out of 340 in the HBO group (8.5%). The shortest implants demonstrated the lowest survival rates and the author suggests that this was probably due to the inability of these implants to withstand the loading forces. The use of longer "oral" type implant fixtures in craniofacial sites reduced the implant failure rate. Granstrom noted that the higher the radiation dose, the poorer the results. Particularly high losses were seen in patients who received two courses of radiotherapy – one pre implant placement and one post implant placement. He added that the more time that had elapsed after radiation therapy before implant placement, the poorer the results. The highest failure rates were seen in the frontal bone followed by the zygoma, mandible, and the nasal maxilla. Failure rates for osseointegrated implants were substantially reduced for all sites with the use of HBO except in the temporal–parietal region.

The UCLA craniofacial implant data are consistent with the pattern and distribution of failures reported by Granstrom. From 1987–1989, 92 craniofacial type machined-surface implants either 3 or 4 mm in length were placed in 30 patients to retain facial prostheses.[50] Sixty-nine were placed in nonirradiated bone sites and 23 were placed in irradiated tissues. After 1 year of follow-up, the success rates were about the same for both the irradiated and nonirradiated groups: 85–90%. In a subsequent publication, Roumanas *et al.*[55] reported the outcomes of 207 implants placed in craniofacial defects in 72 patients (follow-up 5–14 years). Of the implants placed into irradiated bone and followed for at least 5 years, only 52% were still present, as opposed to 85% at nonirradiated sites. In this report, only 27% of the implants placed in the irradiated supraorbital rim survived 5 years as compared to a 70% survival rate in the nonirradiated supraorbital rim. Doses delivered to all irradiated sites exceeded 5000 cGy.[50,55] Data reported by Parel and Tjellstrom[49] and Visser[58] suggested similar trends. Their survival rates in the irradiated sites were higher than in the UCLA report, but the follow-up periods were shorter. In an attempt to reverse these trends, in recent years clinicians have used longer length dental implants without flanges in craniofacial sites, to retain facial prostheses.[61,62] The initial data appear favorable but the long-term results of this practice have yet to be determined. Others[63] have attempted to improve implant success in craniofacial sites with adjuvant HBO.

In the maxilla, the implant failure rate in irradiated patients has been substantially higher than in normal patients.[3,4,64,65] A significantly higher failure rate has been reported at second-stage surgery compared to the nonirradiated maxilla, presumably secondary to the inability to obtain appropriate initial stabilization of the implant, but many of the failures were also seen after the implants were placed into function. Roumanas *et al.*[3] reported on the results of 102 implants placed in the irradiated maxillae of 26 patients. All patients received at least 5000 cGy to the implant sites. The implant survival rate was 63.6%. Many of the remaining implants demonstrated moderate to severe bone loss (bone loss extending to at least the level of the fourth thread) particularly those placed in the premaxillary segment. Nimi *et al.*[4] reported similar results in the irradiated maxilla. Of the 59 implants placed in the irradiated maxilla, 17 were lost at the last follow-up.

In the mandible, initial reports indicated higher short-term success rates but subsequent studies with long-term follow-up now indicate an increasing number of failures as a function of time,[57] a pattern seen previously in the craniofacial and maxilla sites. High short-term success rates can be attributed to better initial implant anchorage and stabilization achieved in the anterior mandible, while the large number of long-term failures is suggestive of mechanical anchorage.

Esser and Wagner[53] reported on their experience with 58 irradiated patients. These patients underwent surgical resections of their oral tumors and received 6000 cGy postoperatively with CRT with conventional fractionation with opposed mandibular fields. The mandibular body and symphysis were in the radiation field. Of the 221 implants placed, 35 were lost, 18 before loading and 17 after loading. The overall success rate was 84.2%, but the follow up period was short – only 18 months.

Yerit *et al.*[57] reported results of 316 implants placed in 71 patients. All patients were treated with chemotherapy (mitmycin C and 5-fluorouracil) up front, followed by CRT. These patients received 200 cGy per fraction and 25 fractions for a total of 5000 cGy. Following radiation, the local tumor site was surgically removed in combination with a neck dissection. The site was immediately reconstructed as needed with local flaps or free vascularized flaps. Free vascularized flaps from the iliac crest, radial forearm, and jejeunum were used, depending on whether the defect was soft tissue or combined bone and soft tissue. Most patients presented initially with T2–T4 squamous cell carcinomas. The implants were placed at various intervals (0.34–6.35 years) following surgery. Based on a careful review of the radiation treatment records in these patients, implants were identified as positioned in the irradiated residual mandible, the nonirradiated residual mandible, or in grafted sites. Implant success was defined by the absence of implant mobility and bone loss less than one-third of the length of the implant. The survival rate of the 154 implants placed in the irradiated residual mandibular sites was 93% at 1 year, 90% at 2 years, 84% at 5 years, and 72% at 8 years follow-up. The survival rates for the 84 implants placed in the nonirradiated residual mandibular sites were 99% at 1 year, 99% at 2 years, 99% at 5 years, and 95% at 8 years follow-up. The survival rate for 78 implants placed in grafted mandibular sites was 96% at 1 year, 96% at 2 years, 96% at 5 years, and 54% at 8 years. In his study Granstrom,[56] reported that only 63% of 15 implants placed into in irradiated mandibles survived.

What phenomenon is responsible for the differences in success between the different sites, or given sufficient follow-up time will the success rates be relatively equal? For example, why is the success rate of implants placed in the irradiated mandible higher than in the irradiated maxilla, given the fact that the better blood supply of the maxilla is not as impaired after radiation compared to the mandible? The authors believe that in heavily irradiated sites, implant anchorage is primarily mechanical as opposed to biologic. Osseointegration in the usual sense probably does not occur because the mesenchymal stem cells are either absent or substantially reduced in number and those still present are nonfunctional. The high initial success rate in the mandible can be attributed to the better initial implant anchorage achieved in the mandible as compared to the maxilla.

The use of hyperbaric oxygen

Some clinicians[29,63,66] have attempted to improve the viability of periosteum and bone with adjuvant HBO. HBO promotes angiogenesis in irradiated tissues. Expression of vascular endothelial growth factor (VEGF) is suppressed in irradiated tissues but this suppression can be reversed by HBO.[67,68] In addition, HBO has been shown to interact with other growth factors to stimulate bone growth and bone turnover.[63] Granstrom *et al.*[52] treated 13 patients with HBO who had previously been irradiated. Each patient received 20 treatments, implant surgery was performed, followed by 10 more hyperbaric treatments. Only one implant fixture was lost (2.0% of the total). Marx[29] reported similar results in a large series of patients who had implants placed in irradiated mandibles. In his most recent report, Granstrom[63] noted that 117 implants failed out of 291 placed in irradiated sites without HBO (40.2%), and 29 implants failed out of 340 implants placed in the HBO group (8.5%).

The use of adjuvant HBO remains controversial, so in 2006 the *Journal of Oral Maxillofacial Surgery* invited Professor Gosta Granstrom, of Goteburg University (pro) and Professor Bruce Donoff of the Harvard School of Dental Medicine (con) to debate the issue. Dr. Donoff expressed concern regarding the lack of randomized clinical trials but did admit "Evidence supports enhanced long term survival in all sites." He quickly added "but the clinician must weigh the availability, complications and added cost in the decision making process." He also questioned the necessity of using HBO when the dose to the implant sites was less than 5000 cGy.[69] The critical question is not whether adjuvant HBO is useful, it is rather whether HBO is necessary for any individual patient. Unfortunately today it is not possible to answer this question when considering HBO for individual patients. Reliable biomarkers that provide insights into the vitality and wound-healing capabilities of the potential implant bone sites are presently lacking, but are needed if this question is to be resolved. Hopefully they will become available in the near future.

The question of whether to use adjunctive HBO may become moot in the future. New methods are now evolving which hold the promise of improving the vitality of irradiated tissues.

The protocol proposed by Delanian *et al.*[70] and Lyons and Ghazali,[71] employing pentoxifylline and tocopherol (vitamin E), is now being used successfully in the treatment of osteoradionecrosis. Pentoxifylline is a vasodilator that facilitates blood flow by decreasing platelet aggregation and thrombus formation, and inhibits fibrosis. Tocophorol is a free radical scavenger. This drug combination has yet to be employed in irradiated patients scheduled for implant placement, but its use would appear to be potentially beneficial.

In summary, it is clear from the current data that osseointegration is impaired in bone that has received doses in excess of 5000 cGy and perhaps even at doses as low as 3000 cGy. Success rates, based on clinical reports, are reduced as compared to nonirradiated sites, particularly the maxilla and the orbit.[3,4,30,45,54,56,64,65,72–74] The success rates are lower than in normal individuals, even in the maxilla with its excellent blood supply. The results in the maxilla are not surprising, in view of the fact that implant anchorage in irradiated bone is primarily mechanical as opposed to biologic. In addition, preliminary animal studies referred to previously appear to indicate that the bone–implant interface may be significantly compromised, making the implant less able to tolerate functional loads. HBO appears to help revitalize the bone, leading to improved success rates.[63]

Risk of osteoradionecrosis

There are few reported cases of osteoradionecrosis secondary to osseointegrated implants. Esser and Wagner[53] noted two patients who developed osteoradionecrosis in the mandible out of 60 patients (3.4%). All patients received postoperative radiation after surgical resection of oral tumors. They were all treated with opposed mandibular fields to 6000 cGy. Granstrom[75] reported 10 cases of osteoradionecrosis out of 116 (8.6%) patients who received osseointegrated implants. In these studies, osteoradionecrosis was defined as exposed bone in the radiation clinical target volume of 6 months' duration or more. Doses ranged from 2300–14500 cGy (mean dose 7900 Gy) and necrosis occurred at a variety of sites (mandible, supraorbital rim, mastoid, frontal bone). Some of the patients developing bone necrosis had received a course of hyperbaric oxygen before and after implant placement.

Risk of osteoradionecrosis in the mandible secondary to implant surgery is probably best determined by an analysis of the bone necrosis rate seen following post-radiation extractions.[29,76,77] Based on this data it should be relatively safe to place implants in irradiated mandibular sites if the dose is less than 5500 cGy. The risk would be significant greater for doses above 6500 cGy. In such patients, if implants are desirable, we recommend a course of HBO as described by Granstrom.[56,66] In patients with doses to bone sites between 5500 and 6500 cGy, individual patient factors, such as the dose per fraction, a previous radical neck dissection, and so forth, may be important cofactors to consider when assessing the risk. It should be noted that most patients treated with CRT do not receive radiation to the symphyseal region, and patients treated with IMRT receive relatively low doses to the symphysis of the mandible and the premaxilla. Therefore, implants can be placed with a high degree of predictability in these regions in many irradiated patients.

In the maxilla, the risk of bone necrosis is probably negligible even at high dose levels. The use of HBO can be justified only on the basis of improving success rates.[56,66] An exception would be those patients treated with high doses as a part of a chemoradiation protocol. Under these circumstances the biological equivalent dose approaches 8000 cGy.

Recommendations – patient selection and treatment

Edentulous mandible

There are several issues to consider, the most important being the risk of osteoradionecrosis. The short- and long-term success rates, the potential life span of the patient, the feasibility of HBO treatment, and the potential benefit for the patient must also be considered. The risk of osteoradionecrosis is primarily dependent upon dose to the implant sites, although individual patient factors, such as a history of a radical neck dissection or continuation of a heavy tobacco habit, may have an impact. In addition, concomitant chemotherapy accentuates the tissue effects[41,42] and needs to be taken into account. When considering dose, for the purposes of this discussion, the levels cited refer to doses delivered with conventional fractionation (200 cGy fractions, five fractions per week). When considering patients treated with hyper-fractionation or accelerated fractionation, formulae that take into consideration dose per fraction, number of fractions, total dose, and time frame over which the therapy is delivered should be employed.[78] Doses to implant sites may be difficult to discern, particularly when the patient is irradiated with IMRT. Therefore, before proceeding with implant placement, the radiation treatment record must be carefully examined (Figure 21.20).

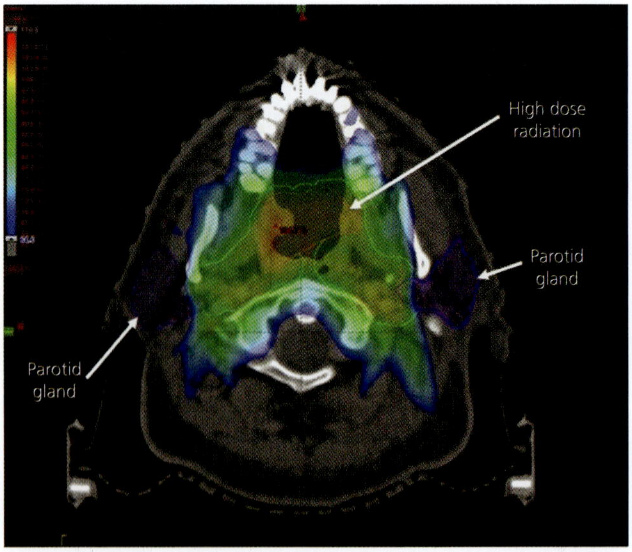

Figure 21.20 IMRT employs multiple beams in order to concentrate the dose in local areas. In this patient the anterior portion of the maxilla and mandible are spared.

Doses to the implant sites equivalent to 5500 cGy or less, imply an almost negligible risk of osteoradionecrosis unless concomitant chemotherapy is employed, whereas doses above 6500 cGy or its equivalent imply a high risk unless the patient is treated with HBO or perhaps with one of the emerging therapies being tested in the treatment of osteoradionecrosis (pentoxifylline plus tocopherol: see earlier section entitled Osteoradionecrosis). Considering the above factors, most edentulous patients will be good candidates and have much to gain from implant therapy, particularly if the patient has had a surgical procedure that compromises the denture-bearing surfaces or that negatively affects the patient's ability to control the mandibular denture with the tongue and cheeks. If the patient was treated with conventional radiation therapy (CRT), in most patients the symphysis would have been out of the field. The exception is for tumors of the anterior floor of the mouth. In these patients, the dose to the symphysis usually matches the tumor dose and will almost always exceed 65 Gy or its equivalent. If the patient is treated with IMRT, the symphyseal region will almost always be irradiated, regardless of the site of the tumor but usually the doses to the potential implant sites are less than 5500 cGy. However, there usually will be hot spots where the dose exceeds 6500 cGy, but the volume of these local areas of high dose is usually quite small.

Tumor prognosis is an important factor. Most recurrences take place within the first year and so it advisable to wait for this period to elapse before considering implants. Patients that are tumor free after this period are expected to survive an average of 10 years, so, if implants are expected to have a positive impact on function and the patient's quality of life, they should be considered.

Short-term success rates are quite favorable but long-term rates are less than first predicted.[56,57] However, HBO will improve long-term success rates.[56,66] Therefore, when developing a plan of implant treatment, implant loss rates and factors associated with implant failures in the irradiated mandible need to be taken into account. The prosthodontic treatment should be tailored to anticipate these failures and to reduce the impact of the factors leading to implant failure (fixed vs. removable, splinting vs. nonsplinting, number and lengths of implants, implant-assisted vs. implant-supported designs). The authors prefer the placement of four implants in the symphyseal region and the fabrication of an overdenture retained with an implant-assisted connecting bar. With this design all four implants are splinted together with the bar. There should be sufficient room between the two anterior implants for a "Hader" bar segment that will receive two clips. "ERA" attachments are incorporated distally. With this design when posterior occlusal forces are applied to the posterior teeth of the overdenture during mastication, the "Hader" segment acts as the axis of rotation and the "ERA" attachments, being resilient, permit the posterior forces to be absorbed by the primary mandibular support areas (retromolar pad and the buccal shelf). Strain distribution upon loading is advantageous in splinting implants.[79] As a result the occlusal forces borne by each implant are minimized, which should reduce the risk of implant overload and implant loss.

Edentulous maxilla

All edentulous patients with maxillectomy or palatectomy defects fitted with obturator prostheses derive significant benefit from implant retention, and the authors recommend their use even though the success rates are suboptimal in irradiated sites. The risk of osteoradionecrosis is negligible. Success rates depend on radiation dose and the quantity and quality of bone associated with the implant site. When implant sites are exposed to doses above 5000 cGy, initial implant anchorage is especially critical because it is highly unlikely that significant amounts of bone will be deposited on the surface of the implant or within the osteotomy site following implant placement and, as a result, anchorage is probably mechanical as opposed to biologic.

Some implant failures in the irradiated maxilla are the result of the difficulty in achieving initial implant anchorage at first-stage surgery, while others occur after loading. Therefore, when designing the implant connecting bar and selecting the attachments used for retention, the clinician should consider the altered biomechanics imposed by compromised implant anchorage. Implants should be splinted together with implant connecting bars and designs should be implant assisted as opposed to implant supported. The primary purpose of the bar should be retention. The defect and the residual denture foundation area should be employed to provide the necessary support and stability for the complete denture–obturator prosthesis. Because of the relatively high rates of failure, the implants, the implant connecting bar, and overdenture should be designed so that, in the event of selected implant failures, the bar and the prosthesis can be modified and continue to function. Success rates will be improved by careful preparation of the osteotomy site, by using the longest lengths possible given the vertical size of the implant bone site, and by obtaining *bicortical* stabilization during implant surgery. Success rates probably will be improved with the use of adjuvant HBO treatments.[56,66] Augmenting heavily irradiated maxillary sites with autogenous bone grafts has not been predictable.

Timing of implant surgery in relationship to radiation treatment

It has become increasingly clear that bone irradiated to high doses does not recover with time and, indeed, the opposite is most likely, namely that with time irradiated bone becomes more fibrotic and less vascular, with few if any mesenchymal stem cells surviving. Granstrom[56] has reported that failure rates increase as a function of the time elapsed after radiotherapy.

Irradiation of existing implants

Irradiation of titanium implants already in place produces backscatter[80] and, as a result, the tissues on the radiation source side of the implants receive a higher dose than the other tissues in the field. The dose is increased about 11–15% in the zone 1 mm from the implant surface.[81] The increase in dose locally may subject these tissues to ulceration, exposure of the underlying bone, and loss of the implants.

Of additional concern is the backscatter created by noble metals, because alloys of these metals are frequently used to fabricate implant connecting bars and implant-retained fixed prostheses. These restorations may extend subgingivally and attach directly to the implant fixture. In these cases the dose enhancement secondary to backscatter may approach 80%.[82] Because of backscatter and the increased numbers of patients presenting with implants at the time of tumor diagnosis, clinicians question if osseointegrated implants should be removed in patients about to be irradiated for head and neck tumors. Surgical removal prior to radiation has been discouraged by most knowledgeable clinicians because of the significant trauma resulting from the trephination procedure required to remove an osseointegrated implant bonded to bone. Granstrom *et al.*[83] addressed these issues in his report of 11 patients with 33 existing titanium implants who were scheduled to be irradiated. Dosages ranged from 5000–6600 cGy. Based on their findings, Granstrom *et al.*[52] recommended that all abutments and superstructures be removed prior to radiation, and skin and/or mucosa should be closed over the implant fixtures. They suggested that radiation therapy begin when healing is complete.

When considering intraoral implant-retained prosthesis, the authors initially followed the Granstrom protocol and surgically buried the implants beneath the mucosa prior to radiation. However, primary closure may be difficult to accomplish in these situations and frequently there is significant tension at the suture line. Often, the wound dehisces and the implant fixtures, with their cover screws, become exposed. As a result the protocol employed at UCLA is to remove the restoration and attach titanium healing abutments to the implant fixtures prior to initiation of radiation therapy.

Following completion of radiation, the abutments and/or superstructure (ie. prosthesis) in most instances may be reattached, but in the mandible this decision is based on a number of factors, including the dose to the implant sites, the type of prosthesis and its hygiene access, and patient compliance. The functional benefits derived from the implant prosthesis and the wishes of the patient should also be considered. The critical issue to be considered is the risk of post-radiation peri-implant tissue infections in the mandible that in turn could lead to osteoradionecrosis. There are no data to guide the clinician in this matter, and at UCLA individual patient factors drive the decision. For example, we would seriously consider permanently removing a unilateral implant-supported fixed partial denture in the posterior quadrant of the mandible, when oral hygiene is poor, the implants or abutments exit unattached, there is poorly keratinized mobile mucosa, the dose to the region is above the equivalent of 6500 cGy, and particularly if chemoradiation was employed. Such decisions are difficult and must be made following a thorough discussion with the patient of the risks and benefits of retaining the implant-retained and/or -supported prosthesis.

References

1. Beumer J, Marunick M, Garrett N, *et al.* Rehabilitation of maxillary defects. In: Beumer J, Marunick M, Esposito S (eds). *Maxillofacial Rehabilitation: Prosthodontic and Surgical Management of Cancer-Related, Acquired, and Congenital Defects of the Head and Neck.* Quintessence Publishing Co: Chicago, IL 2011; 155–212.
2. Garrett N. Outcomes of maxillectomies with conventional and implant restorations. Presented at International Congress on Maxillofacial Rehabilitation Bangkok, Thailand, September 24–27, 2008.
3. Roumanas E, Nishimura R, Davis B, *et al.* Clinical evaluation of implants retaining edentulous maxillary obturator prostheses. *J Prosth Dent* 1997; **77**: 184–190.
4. Nimi A, Ueda M, Kaneda T. Maxillary obturator supported by osseointegrated implants placed in irradiated tissues: report of cases. *J Oral Maxillofac Surg* 1993; **51**: 804–809.
5. Nimi A, Ueda M, Kaneda T. Maxillary obturator supported by osseointegrated implants placed in irradiated tissues: A preliminary report. *Int J Oral Maxillofac Implants* 1998; **13**: 407.
6. Howshaw SJ, Brunski JB, Cochran GV. Mechanical overloading of Branemark implants affects interfacial bone modeling and remodeling. *J Oral Surg* 1994; **9**: 345–360.
7. Stanford CM, Brand RA. Toward an understanding of implant occlusion and strain adaptive bone modeling and remodeling. *J Prosthet Dent* 1999; **81**: 553–561.
8. Brunski JB, Puleo DA, Nance A. Biomaterials and biomechanics of osseointegrated implants: current status and future developments. *Int J Oral Maxillofac Implants* 2000; **15**: 15–46.
9. Miyata T, Kobayashi Y, Araki T, *et al.* The influence of controlled occlusal overload on peri-implant tissue: a histologic study in monkeys. *Int J Oral Maxillofac Implants* 1998; **13**: 677–683.
10. Miyata T, Kobayashi Y, Araki T, *et al.* The influence of controlled occlusal overload on peri-implant tissue: Part 3: a histologic study in monkeys. *Int J Oral Maxillofac Implants* 2000; **15**: 425–431.
11. Miyata T, Kobayashi Y, Araki T, *et al.* The influence of controlled occlusal overload on peri-implant tissue: Part 4: a histologic study in monkeys. *Int J Oral Maxillofac Implants* 2002; **17**: 384–390.
12. Myamoto Y, Koretake K, Hirata M, *et al.* Influence of static overload on the bony interface around implants in dogs. *Int J Prosthodont* 2008; **21**: 437–444.
13. Nagasawa M, Takano R, Maeda T, *et al.* Observation of the bone surrounding an overloaded implant in a novel rat model. *Int J Oral Maxillofac Implants* 2013; **28**: 109–116.
14. Jensen OT, Shulman LB, Block MS, *et al.* Report of the sinus consensus conference of 1996. *Int J Oral Maxillfac Implants* 1996; **13**(Suppl): 11–45.
15. Aghaloo T, Moy PK. Which hard tissue augmentation techniques are the most successful in furnishing bony support for implant placement. *Int J Oral Maxillofacial Implants* 2007; **22**(suppl): 49–73.
16. Schmidt B, Pogrel M, Young C, *et al.* Reconstruction of extensive maxillary defects using zygomaticus implants. *J Oral Maxillofac Surg* 2004; **62**: 82–89.
17. Landis C, Paffrath C, Koehler C, *et al.* Zygoma implant for midfacial prosthetic rehabilitation using telescopes: 9 year followup. *Int J Prosth* 2009; **22**: 20–32.
18. Davis B, Roumanas E, Hong S, *et al.* Stress distributions of implants used for retention of maxillary obturators. in: Zlotolow I, Esposit S, Beumer, J (eds). Proceedings 1st International Congress on Maxillofacial Prosthetics, 1995: 204–208.

19. Kratochvil FJ. Influence of occlusal rest position and clasp design on movement of abutment teeth. *J Prosthet Dent* 1063; **13**: 114–124.
20. Celletti R, Pameijer CH, Bracchett G, *et al.* Histologic evaluation of osseointegrated implants restored in nonaxial functional occlusion with pre-angled abutments. *Int J Periodontics Restorative Dent* 1995; **15**: 562–573.
21. Zampelis A, Rangert B, Heijl L. Tilting of splinted implants for improved prosthodontic support: a two dimensional finite element analysis. *J Prosthet Dent* 2007; **97**(Suppl): 35–43.
22. Bevilacqua M, Tealdo T, Menini M, *et al.* The influence of cantilever length and implant angulation on stress distribution for maxillary implant-supported fixed prostheses. *J Prosthet Dent* 2011; **105**: 5–13.
23. Beumer J, Faulkner R, Lyons K, *et al.* Edentulous maxilla-overdenture prostheses. In: Beumer J, Faulkner R, Shah K, Moy P (eds). *Fundamentals of Implant Dentistry: Prosthodontic Principles.* Quintessence Publishing Co: Chicago, IL 2015; 115–149.
24. Rohner D, Kunz C, Bucher P, *et al.* New technique for reconstruction of jaw defects with a prelaminated fibula flap and dental implants. *Mund Kiefer Gesichtschir* 2000; **4**: 365.
25. Rohner D, Jacquiry C, Kunz, C, *et al.* Maxillofacial reconstruction with prefabricated osseous free flaps: A 3-year experience with 24 patients. *Plast Reconstruct Surg* 2003; **112**: 748.
26. Rohner D, Bucher P, Hammer B. Prefabricated fibular flaps for reconstruction of defects of the maxillofacial skeleton: planning, technique, and long-term experience. *Int J Oral Maxillofac Surg* 2013; **28**: 221–229.
27. Jacquiry C, Rohner D, Kunz, C, *et al.* Reconstruction of maxillary and mandibular defects using prefabricated microvascular fibular grafts and osseointegrated dental implants – a prospective study. *Clin Oral Impl Res* 2004; **15**: 598–606.
28. Keller, E.E. Mandibular discontinuity reconstruction with composite grafts: free autogenous iliac bone, titanium mesh trays, and titanium endosseous implants. *Oral Maxillofac Surg Clin N Amer* 1991; **3**: 877.
29. Marx R. Preprosthetic surgery in a radiated cancer patient (Abstract #61). In: Proceedings of the Fifth International Congress on Preprosthetic Surgery 15–18 Apr 1993, Vienna: 75.
30. Roumanas ED, Markowitz BL, Lorant JA, *et al.* Reconstructed mandibular defects: fibula free flaps and osseointegrated implants. *Plast Reconstr Surg* 1997; **99**: 356–365.
31. Garrett N, Roumanas ED, Blackwell KE, *et al.* Efficacy of conventional and implant-supported mandibular resection prostheses: study overview and treatment outcomes. *J Prosthet Dent* 2006; **96**: 13–24.
32. Salinas TJ, Desa VP, Katsnelson A, *et al.* Clinical evaluation of implants in radiated fibula flaps. *J Oral Maxillofac Surg* 2010; **68**: 524–529.
33. Beumer J, Faulkner R, Lyons K, *et al.* Restoration of edentulous mandibles with fixed prostheses. In: Beumer J, Faulkner R, Shah K, Moy P (eds). *Fundamentals of Implant Dentistry: Prosthodontic Principles.* Quintessence Publishing Co: Chicago, IL 2015; 75–113.
34. Verstreken K, Van Cleynenbreugel J, Marchal G, *et al.* Computer-assisted planning of oral implant surgery. An approach using virtual reality. *Stud Health Technol Inform* 1996; **29**: 423–434.
35. Van SteenbergheD, Glauser R, Blomback U, *et al.* A computed tomographic scan-derived customized surgical template and fixed prosthesis for flapless surgery and immediate loading of implants in fully edentulous maxillae: a prospective multicenter study. *Clin Implant Dent Relat Res* 2005; Suppl 1:S111–120.
36. Pozzi A, Moy P, Beumer J, *et al.* Computer guided planning and surgery. In: Moy P, Palacci P, Pozzi A, Beumer J (eds). *Fundamentals of Implant Dentistry: Surgical Principles.* Quintessence Publishing Co: Chicago, IL 2016 (in press).
37. Linkevicius T, Vindasiute E, Puisys A, *et al.* The influence of the cementation margin position on the amount of undetected cement. A prospective clinical study. *Clin Oral Implants Res* 2013; **24**: 71–76.
38. Beumer J, Marunick M, Garrett N, *et al.* Rehabilitation of tongue mandible defects. In: Beumer J, Marunick M, Esposito S (eds). *Maxillofacial Rehabilitation: Prosthodontic and Surgical Management of Cancer-Related, Acquired, and Congenital Defects of the Head and Neck.* Quintessence Publishing Co: Chicago, IL 2011; 61–154.
39. Dhima M, Rieck KL, Arce K, *et al.* Development of stable peri-implant soft tissue and mentolabial sulcus depth with an implant-retained soft tissue conformer after osteocutaneous flap reconstruction. *Int J Prosthodont* 2013; **26**: 265–267.
40. Karayazgan-Sarcoglu B, Atay A, Zulfikar H, *et al.* Assessment of implant stability on patients with and without radiotherapy using resonance frequency analysis. *J Oral Implantol* 2015; **41**(4): 30–35.
41. Kasibhatla M, Kirkpatrick J, Brizel D. How much radiation is chemotherapy worth in advanced head and neck cancer. *Int J Radiat Oncol Biol Phys* 2007; **68**: 1491–1495.
42. Fowler JF. Corrections to Kasibhatla *et al.* How much radiation is the chemotherapy worth in advanced head and neck cancer. *Int J Radiat Oncol Biol Phys* 2008; **71**: 326–329.
43. Jacobsson M, Tjellstrom A, Thomson P, *et al.* Integration of titanium implants in irradiated bone. Histologic and clinical study. *Ann Otol Rhinol Laryngol* 1988; **97**: 337–340.
44. Hum S, Larsen P. The effect of radiation at the titanium/bone interface. In: Laney W, Tolman D (eds). *Tissue Integration in Oral, Orthopedic and Maxillofacial Reconstruction.* Quintessence Publishing Co: Chicago, IL 1990; 234–239.
45. Nishimura R. Implants in irradiated tissues. In: Beumer J, Curtis T, Marunick M (eds). *Maxillofacial Rehabilitation: Prosthodontic and Surgical Considerations.* Ishiyaku EuroAmerica: St Louis, Tokyo 1996; 103–106.
46. Asikainen P, Kotilianinen R, Vuillemin, *et al.* Osseointegration of dental implants in radiated mandibles: An experimental study with beagle dogs. *J Oral Implant* 1993; **17**: 48–54.
47. Weinlander M, Beumer J, Kenney B, *et al.* Histomorphometric and fluorescence microscopic evaluation of interfacial bone healing around 3 different dental implants before and after radiation therapy. *Int J Oral Maxillofac Implants* 2006; **21**: 212–224.
48. Nishimura R, Roumanas E, Sugai T, *et al.* Nasal defects and osseointegrated implants: UCLA experience. *J Prosthet Dent* 1996; **76**: 597–602.
49. Parel S, Tjellstrom A. The United States and Swedish experience with osseointegration and facial prostheses. *Int J Oral Maxilllofac Implants* 1991; **6**: 75–79.
50. Roumanas E, Nishimura, R, Beumer J. Craniofacial defects and osseointegrated implants: Six year follow-up report on the success rates of craniofacial implants at UCLA. *Int J Oral Maxillofac Implants* 1994; **9**: 579–585.
51. Granstrom G, Jacobsson M, Tjellstrom A. Titanium implants in irradiated tissue: benefits from hyperbaric oxygen. *Int J Oral Maxillofac Implants* 1992; 7: 15–25.

52. Granstrom G, Bergstrom K, Tjellstrom A. A detailed analysis of fixture losses in irradiated tissue. *Int J Oral and Maxillofac Implant* 1994; **9**: 653–662.
53. Esser E, Wagner W. Dental implants following radical oral cancer surgery and adjuvant radiotherapy. *Int J Maxillofac Implants* 1997; **12**: 552–557.
54. Visch L, van Waas M, Schmitz P, *et al.* A clinical evaluation of implants in irradiated oral cancer patients. *J Dent Res* 2002; **81**: 856–859.
55. Roumanas E, Freymiller E, Chang T, *et al.* Implant retained prostheses for facial defects: An up to 14 year followup report on the survival rates of implants at UCLA. *Int J Prosth* 2002; **15**: 325–332.
56. Granstrom G. Osseointegration in irradiated cancer patients: an analysis with respect to implant failures. *J Oral Maxillofac Surg* 2005; **63**: 579–585.
57. Yerit K, Posch M, Seemann S, *et al.* Implant survival in mandibles or irradiated oral cancer patients. *Clin Oral Impl Res* 2006; **17**: 337–344.
58. Visser A. Aftercare of implant-retained facial prostheses. Presented at: Maxillofacial Rehabilitation – New technologies improve quality of life? Groningen, Netherlands 8–10 Feb 2007.
59. Chamrone L, Mandia J Jr, Shibli JA, *et al.* Dental implants installed in irradiated jaws: a systematic review. *J Dent Res* 2013; **92**(12 Suppl): 119S–130S.
60. Dholam KP, Pusalkar HA, Yadav PS, *et al.* Implant-retained dental rehabilitation in head and neck cancer patients: an assessment of success and failure. *Implant Dent* 2013; **22**: 604–609.
61. Flood T, Downie I, Ethunandan M. Prosthetic reconstruction after rhinectomy-evolution of bone anchored epistheses and adjunctive surgical techniques in nasal reconstruction from one unit. Presented at: The 2nd International Symposium. Bone Conduction Hearing – Craniofacial Osseointegration. Gothenberg, Sweden 11–13 Jun, 2009.
62. Proops D, Worrollo S, Jeynes P, *et al.* Head and neck reconstruction in adults – the Birmingham experience. Presented at: The 2nd International Symposium. Bone Conduction Hearing – Craniofacial Osseointegration. Gothenberg, Sweden 11–13 Jun, 2009.
63. Granstrom G. Pathophysiologic basis for HBO in the treatment of healing disorders in radio-injured tissues. In: Marroni A, Mathieu D, Wattel F (eds). *The ECHM Collection* vol **2**. Flagstaff, AZ: Best Publishing, 2005.
64. Sammartino G, Marenzi G, Cioffi I, *et al.* Implant therapy in irradiated patients. *J Craniofac Surg* 2011; **22**: 443–445.
65. Carr AB. Implant location and radiotherapy are the only factors linked to 2-year implant failure. *J Evid Based Dent Pract* 2012; **12**(3 Suppl): 217–219.
66. Granstrom G. Placement of dental implants in irradiated bone: The case for using hyperbaric oxygen. *J Oral Maxillofac Surg* 2006; **64**: 812–818.
67. Dudziak M, Saadeh P, Mehara B, *et al.* The effect of ionizing radiation on osteoblast-like cells in vitro. *Plast Reconstr Surg* 2000; **106**: 1049–1061.
68. Fok T, Ahmed J, Peel S, *et al.* Hyperbaric oxygen results in increased vascular endothelial growth factor (VEGF) protein expression in rabbit calvarial critical sized defects. *Oral Surg Oral Med Oral Path Oral Radiol Endo* 2008; **105**: 417.
69. Donoff RB. Treatment of the irradiated patient with dental implants: the case against hyperbaric oxygen treatment. *J Oral Maxillofac Surg* 2006; **64**: 819–822.
70. Delanian S, Depondt J, Lefaix J. Major healing of refractory mandible osteoradionecrosis after treatment combining pentoxifylline and tocopherol: a phase II trial. *Head and Neck* 2005; **27**: 114–123.
71. Lyons A and Ghazali N. Osteoradionecrosis of the jaws: current understanding of its pathophysiology and treatment. *Brit J Oral Maxillofac Surg* 2008; **46**: 653.
72. Nishimura R, Roumanas E, Shimizu K. Implants in irradiated bone. In: Proceedings of the First International Congress on Maxillofacial Prosthetics. 27-30 Apr 1994, Indian Wells, CA. New York: Memorial Sloane-Kettering Cancer Center, 1995: 199–203.
73. Nishimura R, Roumanas, E, Sugai T, *et al.* Orbital defects and osseointegrated implants: UCLA experience. *J Prosthet Dent* 1998; **79**: 304–309.
74. Nishimura R, Roumanas E, Sugai T, *et al.* Auricular prostheses and osseointegrated implants: UCLA experience. *J Prosthet Dent* 1995; **73**: 553–558.
75. Granstrom G. Implants in irradiated patients. Presented at: The 2nd International Symposium. Bone Conduction Hearing – Craniofacial Osseointegration. Gothenberg, Sweden 11–13 Jun, 2009.
76. Morrish RB Jr, Chan E, Silverman S, *et al.* Osteoradionecrosis in patients irradiated for head and neck carcinoma. *Cancer* 1981; **47**: 1980–1983.
77. Beumer J, Harrison R, Sanders B, *et al.* Postradiation dental extractions: a review of the literature and a report of 72 episodes. *Head and Neck Surg* 1983; **6**: 581–586.
78. Kirk J, Gray WM, Watson ER. Cumulative radiation effect. I. Fractionated treatment regimes. *Clin Radiol* 1971; **22**: 145–155.
79. Yilmaz B, Seidt JD, McGlumphy EA, *et al.* Comparison of strains for splinted and nonsplinted screw-retained prostheses on short implants. *Int J Oral Maxillofac Implants* 2011; **26**(6): 1176–1182.
80. Friedrich RE, Todorovic M, Helland M, *et al.* Scattering effects of irradiation on surroundings calculated for a small dental implant. *Anticancer Res* 2012; **32**: 2043–2046.
81. Schwartz HC, Wollin M, Leake D, *et al.* Interface radiation dosimetry in mandibular reconstruction. *Arch Otolaryngol* 1979; **105**; 293–295.
82. Scrimger JW. Backscatter from high atomic number materials in highenergy photon beams. *Radiology* 1977; **124**: 815–817.
83. Granstrom G, Tjellstrom A, Albrektsson T. Post implant irradiation of osseointegrated implants. In: Zlotolow I, Esposito S, Beumer J (eds). Proceedings of the First International Congress on Maxillofacial Prosthetics 1995: 292–296.

CHAPTER 22

Implant-Retained Restoration of the Craniofacial Patient

Robert Ferguson Wright, Glenn E. Minsley, and Sun-Yung Bak
University of North Carolina, Chapel Hill School of Dentistry, Chapel Hill, North Carolina, USA

Facial defects from trauma, disease, or congenital abnormality have devastating psychosocial and functional effects on the patient. Missing anatomical portions of the maxillofacial and oral environment significantly affect esthetics, which makes it difficult for the patient to experience normal social interactions with family and friends. Surgical rehabilitation has been one of the options for restoring facial defects. However, sometimes "the treatment was worse than the cure," resulting in facial disfigurement and oral dysfunction.[1] Surgery is often limited by the availability of tissues and compromise of the tissue vascularity from previous radiation. Also, it may be advantageous to have exposure of facial defects so that oncologists can visually evaluate the surgical site for future recurrence.

Restoration of facial defects with facial prostheses has aided patients to experience less psychological trauma, as well as display a more normal esthetic appearance. The traditional means of retention of facial prostheses prior to craniofacial implants were through mechanical intrinsic undercuts and extrinsic adhesives.[2] Often, mechanical retention was not adequate with the intrinsic undercuts, and patients experienced more embarrassment and psychosocial trauma when the prosthesis failed to adhere due to mobility of the adjacent tissues and failure of the adhesive itself. The adhesives used to hold the prosthesis in place damaged the prosthesis during maintenance, reducing the durability of the prosthesis and, often, it was difficult for the patient to place the prosthesis in the proper position every time.[3] In addition, the adhesives were difficult to clean from the margins of the prosthesis and dermatitis was a common complication.[4]

In 1977, Per-Ingvar Branemark and his colleagues placed the first craniofacial implant to retain a hearing aid. Craniofacial implants are extraoral endosseous implants inserted in the mastoid, orbital, and nasal regions, excluding the upper and lower jaws, which are parts of the craniofacial skeleton.[5] The length of the implant is short since the thickness of the temporal bone is usually 4 mm. Craniofacial implants are 3–4 mm in length with a flange in the coronal aspect to provide primary stability and to prevent risk of penetration through thin bones, injuring other organs.[6] Craniofacial implants enable the patients to position the facial prosthesis accurately in the same position every time the patients wear the prosthesis. Implants also extend the life of the prosthesis by not needing application of adhesives and solvents, which damage the prosthesis. In addition, they provide reliable retention to facial prostheses.[7,8,9]

The definition of "success rates" of implants is not uniform throughout the craniofacial area.[10] "Implant success rate" and "implant survival rate" are not defined in the glossary of prosthodontic terms. Various authors have defined success and survival in different ways. Esposito *et al.*[11] states that, for an implant to be successful, criteria such as function (ability to chew), tissue physiology (presence and maintenance of osseointegration, absence of pain and other pathological processes), and user satisfaction (esthetics and absence of discomfort) must be fulfilled. Otherwise, the implants are "surviving", where implants are still in function but criteria for "success" or "failure" have not been met. Abu-Serriah *et al.*[12] agrees that "surviving implants are those that are still in function, but which have not been tested against certain criteria of success." Abu-Serriah questions whether success should be defined as a firm implant without clinical complications, such as poor tissue response, or if it should be defined as implants in functional service. In a 2008 clinical study of auricular prostheses, Wright *et al.*[13] developed criteria of success. A systematic evaluation of the success of the implant prosthesis was developed. Criteria were established to organize reversible and irreversible factors with regard to both the integration of implants and qualities of the implant-retained facial prostheses (Table 22.1). Implant factors examined included position, integration, and skin reactions. Prosthetic considerations included marginal fit, stability and function, symmetry/position, texture, color stability, and patient acceptance. Irreversible factors were those factors that could not be corrected, and therefore any one factor or problem would indicate a failure. Reversible factors required reassessment, analysis, and correction (Table 22.2).

Evidence-based Implant Treatment Planning and Clinical Protocols, First Edition. Edited by Steven J. Sadowsky.

Companion website: www.wiley.com/go/sadowsky/implant

Table 22.1 Criteria for success (Pt, patient; QoL, quality of life; Rxn, reaction). Source: Wright 2008.[13] Reproduced with permission of John Wiley & Sons.

	Implant	Prosthesis
Reversible factors	Position (corrections angulated abutments, use of magnets instead of clips and bars)	Margins/marginal accuracy
	Peri-abutment skin Rxn: grades 0, 1, 2, and 3	Color stability (extrinsic) Stability/functionality Prosthesis, mobility Symmetry/position Pt acceptance/QOL
Irreversible factors	Integration vs. mobility/pathology	Color stability (intrinsic)
	Position (cannot be corrected without compromising esthetics or functionality of prosthesis)	Contour/form
	Peri-abutment skin Rxn; grade IV	Pt acceptance/QOL

Table 22.2 Catergories I–V (Pt, patient; Rxn, reaction). Source: Wright 2008.[13] Reproduced with permission of John Wiley & Sons.

	Implant	CATEGORY				
		I	II	III	IV	V
Reversible	Position *(corrects: via angulated abutments, use of magnets instead of clips and bars)*					
	Peri-abutment skin Rxn: grade 0					
	Peri-abutment skin Rxn: grade 1					
	Peri-abutment skin Rxn: grade 2					
	Peri-abutment skin Rxn: grade 3					
	Prosthesis					
	Margins/marginal accuracy					
	Color stability (extrinsic)					
	Stability/functionality					
	Prosthesis mobility					
	Symmetry position					
	Pt acceptance/quality of life					
Irreversible	**Implant**					
	Position *(cannot be corrected without compromising esthetics or functionality of prosthesis)*					
	Integration vs. mobility/pathology					
	Peri-abutment skin Rxn: grade 4					
	Prosthesis					
	Color stability (intrinsic)					
	Contour/form					
	Pt acceptance/quality of life					

Category I: ideal outcome Soft tissue and hard tissue condition healthy. Implants integrated, and prosthesis is esthetic and accepted by patient Grade 0 Holgers possible.
Category II: Minimal to no bone resorption and/or reversible soft tissue reaction up to grade 1 Holgers Prosthesis esthetically acceptable or may require minimal modification. Positioning or angulation of implants is not ideal but can be corrected.
Category III: soft tissue reaction requires prosthesis design or fabrication changes, and/or minor surgical intervention. Prosthesis requires moderate esthetic medification. Peri-abutment skin reaction up to grade 2 Holgers. Requires correction that is difficult, but possible to achieve.
Category IV: prosthesis with reservation can be used, but retention or esthetics is compromised. Result is substandard. Prosthesis should be refabricated. Peri-abutment skin reaction up to grade 3 Holgers.
Category V: prosthesis cannot be retained by implants due to lack of osseointegration or positioning that cannot be corrected. Peri-abutment skin reaction up to grade 4 Holgers. All irreversible factors qualify Patient refuses to wear prosthesis.
Note: the most complex factor determines the overall classification for the case.

Earlier papers write about success rates,[12,14,15] while later papers discuss survival rates.[16,17] The survival rate is dependent on the time of follow-up of the patient.[17] The longer the time elapsed to evaluate the patient, the higher the failure rate.[18] Therefore, the longer the follow-up period, the shorter the survival rate. The survival rate of implants at 12 months at 100% is not necessarily indicative of success. Although there is discrepancy in the definition of rate of success or survival of implants, there is an agreement that the highest survival rate is among the auricular implants. There is a correlation between anatomical location of placement of craniofacial implants and clinical success.[10,13] The highest success rate is found in the mastoid region and clinical study of 16 patients with implant-retained auricular prostheses revealed a 100% success rate and the average follow-up was 45 months.[13]

Roumanas *et al.*[16] did a retrospective multicenter study of survival rates of osseointegrated implants used to retain orbital, nasal, and auricular prostheses in a 14-year span. Out of 182 implants uncovered, 35 failed to integrate. The survival rate for all exposed implants was 80%. Auricular implants had a survival rate of 95–100%, while orbital implants had the lowest survival rate at 53%. Nasal implants had a 6-year survival rate of 87%. A study done by Nishimura *et al.* for a 7-year span (1987–1994) at UCLA found that there was 100% success rate of auricular implants, 71.4% for nasal implants, and 37.5% success rate of orbital implants.[19,20,21] Wolfaardt's *et al.*'s[15] retrospective study of a survey of centers in Canada with a follow-up period of 12–48 months found that the survival rates were 98.9% in the mastoid region and 96.6% in the orbital region. This relatively high survival rate for the orbit in the Canadian study may be explained by there being a relatively small number of patients compared to those receiving mastoid implants. In addition, the high survival rate could also be due to complex variables, such as a cohort of patients with good bone quality in the orbit. Other studies with 2 years or less of follow-up time found higher survival rates of craniofacial implants. Scolozzi *et al.*[22] reported implant survival in the mastoid region over 95%, nasal region 71–81%, and orbital region 35–91%. Wright *et al.*[13] reported 100% survival rate in the mastoid region.

The auricular area has dense cortical bone, which provides good primary stability and vasculature for maintenance of the bone–implant interface.[19] There is quite a disparity in the survival rate of implants depending on the anatomical location of the placement of implants in nasal defects. In implants restoring nasal prostheses, there is a lower success rate in the glabella compared to the anterior nasal floor. In their study, Nishimura *et al.* found 0% success rate in the glabella versus 88.1% success rate in the anterior nasal floor. The bone in the glabella site is dense, but the vascularity is poor with little marrow space, which may preclude remodeling necessary for osseointegration.[10,20] In orbital defects, due to the curvature of the orbital rim, a large amount of bone needs to be removed in order to countersink the flange of the implant, which may create excessive thermal damage, compromising blood supply to the periosteum and causing bone necrosis.[10] There is increased failure rate as more time passes, which is probably a result of the poor remodeling capacity of the bone–implant interface, lack of stabilizing bone volume in the frontal sinus, or decrease in vascular perfusion in these sites.[10]

Patients with facial defects from surgical treatment of disease often undergo radiotherapy. The effect of radiotherapy on tissues is very controversial. With radiation, some studies report progressive vascular damage while other studies find the vascular environment intact in high-dose irradiation. Some believe that there is a period of time when there is actually growth of vascularity immediately after the radiation. Some experimental animal studies show an improved bone-healing capacity 1 year after irradiation, and thus a long healing time has been recommended by some before implant placement.[11] However, fibrosis and loss of vasculature has been observed to begin 6 months after irradiation in a human study, which appears to worsen over time. Thus, the recommendation by others has been to place implants within 6 months after irradiation.[11]

Even with conflicting reports of the effect of radiation on the vascular system in the irradiation area, there is agreement that there is a higher rate of loss of implants in irradiated sites compared to nonirradiated sites. Roumanas *et al.*[14] found that the success rate of craniofacial implants for irradiated patients was 68.4% compared to 85.3% for nonirradiated patients. A stuby by Tolman *et al.*[23] found the success rate to be 85% for irradiated patient versus 97% for nonirradiated patients. In a Swedish study, the success rate of craniofacial implants was 98.4% in nonirradiated sites compared to 57.9% in irradiated sites.[24] Although the survival rates of implants are lower for patients receiving radiotherapy, radiotherapy is not a contraindication to placement of craniofacial implants.[25] The factors that impact clinical success are the dose and fractionation of the radiation, and the anatomical site of placement of the implants.[26]

For radiation doses below 48 Gy, complications are rarely seen, whereas for doses above 64 Gy, there are many complications.[11] Asikainen *et al.*[27] did a study with mandibles of beagle dogs and found that there was a loss of all implants placed in mandibles irradiated with 60 Gy, few lost implants in mandibles irradiated with 50 Gy, and no loss of implants placed in mandi bles irradiated with 40 Gy. In a meta-analysis by Esposito *et al.*,[11] there was a 2.6% loss of implants placed in jaws irradiated with less than 55 Gy while there was 10.1% loss of implants in jaws irradiated with 55 Gy or greater. The failure rate was 22.9% in the maxilla compared to 6.9% in the mandible in jaws irradiated with 55 Gy or greater. A review by Colella *et al.*[28] noted no implant failures in patients who received less than 45 Gy.

In the irradiated temporal bone, auricular implants had 100% survival in studies by Parel *et al.*[29] and Tolman *et al.*,[30] while Granstrom *et al.*[31] noted failures of 9% within a 5-year follow-up period. In a Swedish study, in the orbital sites, the success rate in the irradiated sites was 57% in a 5-year span and 45.5% in a 12-year span.[24] With high doses of radiotherapy, success in the irradiated orbital sites ranges from 33% to 57%, possibly due to cellular and vascular changes in the irradiated bone. In nasal defects, there are too few studies to make any conclusive statements. Beumer *et al.*[32] concluded from his retrospective analysis that osseointegration was impaired in bone for radiation doses in excess of 55 Gy and recommended hyperbaric oxygen therapy (HBO) to avoid risk of osteoradionecrosis if implant therapy was necessary.

HBO is a form of treatment where the patient is placed is a chamber with increased atmospheric pressure of oxygen. HBO therapy increases oxygen levels in the tissues, which increases capillary growth. It causes neovascularization, which causes epithelialization of soft tissue wounds.[33] Adjunctive HBO therapy did not increase survival rate in the mandible, but appears to increase the survival rate in the maxilla as noted by Niimi *et al.*[34,35] Also, Esposito *et al.*[11] compiled a meta-analysis and found that the implants placed in the irradiated maxilla with HBO had a 17.6% failure rate compared to a 31.7% failure rate without HBO. In the mandible, the failure rate was similar, at 4.3% with HBO and 5% without HBO.[11]

HBO may be beneficial as adjunctive treatment in irradiated tissue since it may decrease soft tissue complications and accelerate the healing process. Larsen *et al.*[36] studied the placement of implants in the tibia of rabbits. There was 54% wound dehiscence in radiated tibias compared with 15% in nonirradiated tibias in rabbits not receiving HBO. In rabbits receiving HBO, there was 7% dehiscence in both the irradiated and nonirradiated tibias. In the animal model, the histomorphometric analysis illustrated that there was a significant improvement of integration between the implant and bone in HBO-treated tibias for both irradiated and nonirradiated rabbits. With 16 weeks of healing, which is equivalent to 1 year, there was a greater percentage of integration than at 12 weeks. However, it is difficult to apply this animal model to humans. Granstrom *et al.*'s[26] randomized study of patients in Gothenburg given HBO and patients not given HBO as control found that implant failure in patients given HBO was 2.6%, compared to 58% in patients without HBO in the maxilla and orbit. However, the studies of craniofacial implants placed in irradiated sites with and without HBO are too few in number, and the parameters of each study are so different in terms of length of the study and the amount of radiation delivered, that it is difficult to make any conclusive remarks.

Craniofacial implants must be carefully considered with appropriate presurgical planning. Patients must be aware of the failure rate and that prosthesis retention, esthetics, and the psychosocial benefits often outweigh the risks. With increase in time, there is decrease in survival rate of craniofacial implants, especially with radiotherapy where the side effects of avascularity and fibrosis increase with time. The use of craniofacial implants in maxillofacial prosthetics has certainly had a revolutionary impact on the treatment and rehabilitation of our patients when compared to the adhesive-retained prostheses. The quality-of-life issues and advantages are numerous for bone-anchored facial prosthetics.

Surgical phase

Presurgical planning

Presurgical planning for the placement of craniofacial implants begins with a diagnostic evaluation. The evaluation includes clinical examination of the defect site, as well as radiographic and/or stereolithographic model examination, to determine if there is sufficient bone thickness to accommodate placement of the craniofacial implants.[37] As part of the diagnostic examination, a moulage should be made of the defect site. A diagnostic mock-up of the final prosthesis should be performed to determine appropriate positioning of the craniofacial implants. A radiographic template is fabricated from the diagnostic mock-up (Figure 22.1). The template is used to assist in assessing whether there is appropriate bone thickness for the planned craniofacial implants. The implants should be positioned in areas of the prosthesis that are of appropriate thickness to accept the abutment height and corresponding attachment components while maintaining the esthetics of the prosthesis. The average combined height for an abutment with a corresponding attachment could be in the range of 4–5 mm. Therefore, for example, in an auricular prosthesis, the implants should be positioned beneath the helical portion of the prosthesis, where the restorative material would be several millimeters greater than the 4–5 mm height range. This would adequately conceal the abutments and attachment system to provide proper esthetics for the prosthesis. Radiopaque markers are positioned within the diagnostic template where the craniofacial implants are to be placed and secured with an acceptable luting medium (Figure 22.2). The surgeon may want to select multiple sites for craniofacial implant placement, rather than a limited number, in case some sites reveal inadequate bone thickness on radiographic analysis. This could prevent any repeat of radiographic scanning with unnecessary exposure of the patient to radiation.

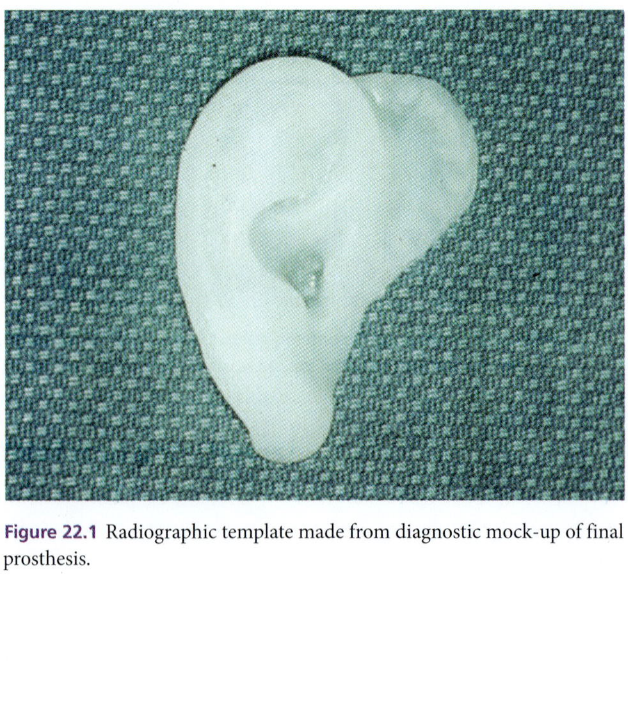

Figure 22.1 Radiographic template made from diagnostic mock-up of final prosthesis.

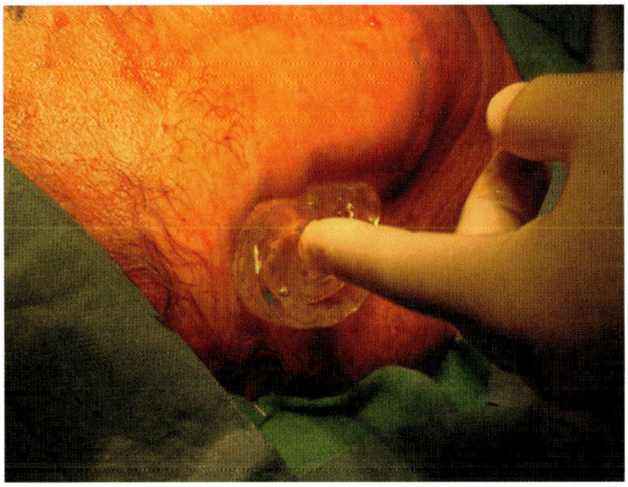

Figure 22.2 Radiographic template in position on patient's face. Radiographic markers (in this case, spherical lead shot seen as round gray balls) are embedded in the template in selected potential locations for craniofacial implant placement.

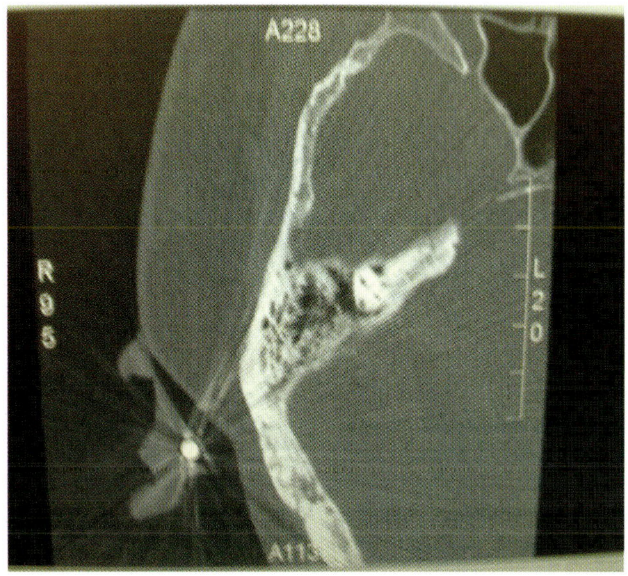

Figure 22.3 CT radiograph showing radiographic marker and associated thickness of bone adjacent to marker.

The patient is scheduled for computed tomography (CT) scan radiography of the defect site. At the time of the CT scan appointment, the radiographic template is positioned and secured within the defect and CT radiographs are made of the site. Examination of the radiographic sections will reveal the selected, proposed implant sites corresponding to the markers (Figure 22.3). The thickness of the bone can be measured to determine if adequate thickness exists for implant placement. Stereolithographic models can be employed to assist in this determination. A minimum of 3 mm of bone thickness is necessary to accept most craniofacial implants. However, it has been reported that endosseous dental implants can be substituted or combined with craniofacial implants in craniofacial regions where there is sufficient bone thickness to accept the minimum length standard endosseous dental implant.[37,38] Appropriate sites for craniofacial implant placement are selected and noted on the template. The radiographic template can then be converted into a surgical template by removing the specific markers in the selected sites and drilling holes through the template to provide initial marking of the defect tissues for surgical implant placement.

The literature reports recommended number of implants to be placed according to site.[37] This is supported by data on success of osseointegration of craniofacial implants in each site as well as the size and weight of the prosthesis. When possible, the implants should be spread far enough apart to distribute the weight of the prosthesis proportionately. Two craniofacial implants are recommended for an auricular prosthesis. Branemark and his colleagues[39] recommended positioning the two craniofacial implants based on number positions of a clock. Originally, for an auricular prosthesis on the right side of the head, the craniofacial implants would be placed at the 9 o'clock and 11 o'clock positions. For an auricular prosthesis on the left side of the head, it was suggested to place the craniofacial implants in the 1 o'clock and 3 o'clock positions. Later, the group revised the positions, moving the lower implant position to 8 o'clock for the right side and to 4 o'clock for the left side.[40] Two to three implants can be used to retain a nasal prosthesis. The usual sites for craniofacial implants are the floor of the nose and the frontal bone. Three or more craniofacial implants are recommended for an orbital prosthesis, as the literature reported that the orbit has the lowest percentage of success of osseointegration.[37] The main areas for craniofacial implant placement in the orbit are usually in the lateral wall and supraorbital rim regions of the orbit.

The craniofacial implant abutments should protrude through keratinized skin rather than nonkeratinized mucosa. The surgical placement of a split-thickness skin graft may be necessary in the site where placement of the craniofacial implants would have the abutments protruding through mucosa.

Surgery

Surgical placement of the craniofacial implants should be performed in an operating room environment. The patient is anesthetized with general anesthesia or through conscious sedation. The patient is draped appropriately and the surgical site is isolated and prepared with a disinfecting solution such as betadine. The sterilized surgical template is positioned within the defect site. The holes designating the selected positions for the craniofacial implants are located in the surgical template. The skin and underlying bone are marked by inserting either a marker or a needle, coated with a dye or ink, through the holes in the template. If a marker is used to mark the skin, then a needle, coated with a dye or ink, should be used to pierce the skin until it contacts the underlying bone to leave a tattoo mark on the bone (Figure 22.4).

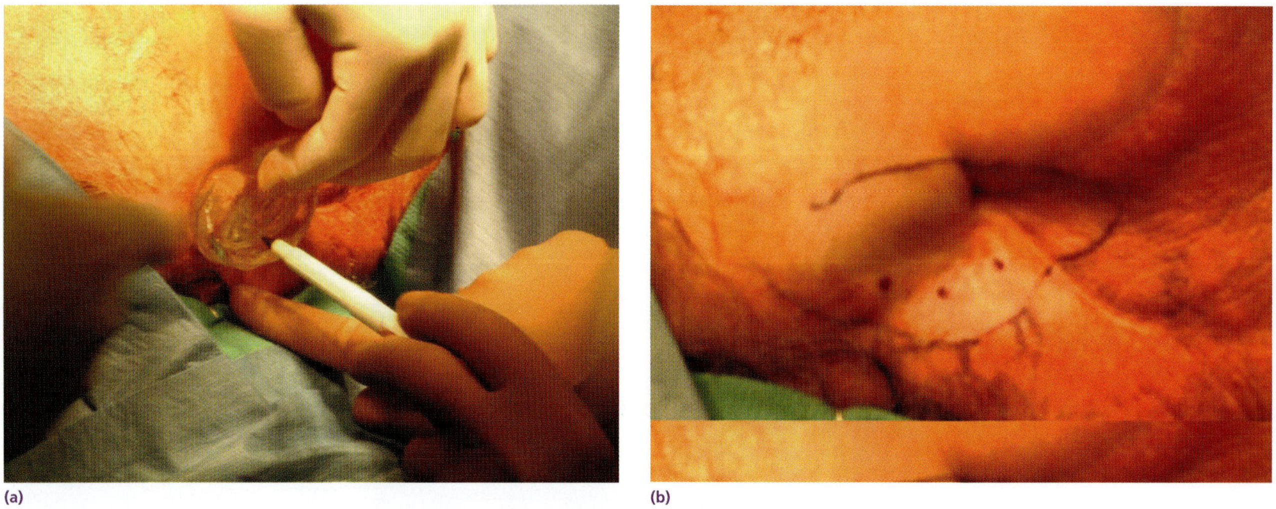

Figure 22.4 **(a)** Selected sites for craniofacial implants are marked with indelible dye or ink using a marker that penetrates holes drilled in template at the selected sites. **(b)** Marked sites for craniofacial implant placement. A needle coated with a dye or ink can then be passed through the skin at the indicated sites to tattoo the underlying bone. The curved line indicates the posterior border of the template for this case.

The surgical protocol, developed by Branemark, has been the hallmark of surgical placement of craniofacial implants.[40] The original protocol is a two-phase surgical procedure. The first surgical phase is the surgical placement of the craniofacial implants. Once the craniofacial implants are surgically implanted into the facial bone, the implants are covered by the overlying subcutaneous tissues and skin and osseointegration is allowed to proceed over a 3–4-month period. No loading of the implants occurs during this time. Following this period, a second surgical procedure is performed to uncover the craniofacial implants. The final abutments are secured to the implants. The underlying subcutaneous tissues from the raised soft tissue flap are dissected and removed leaving a thin skin flap. Perforations are made through this skin flap in the areas where the abutments are to protrude through the flap. The skin flap is repositioned and sutured in place. Healing caps are secured to the abutments. A packing is placed over the skin flap and abutments to maintain pressure against the flap. This is to prevent hematoma formation and maintain contact of the skin with the underlying bone to allow for proper attachment during the healing period; this is usually 2–3 weeks. Prosthetic treatment can be initiated following this period.

There have been several changes in the design of the craniofacial implants over the years that have resulted in changes in the surgical protocol. The original Branemark craniofacial implants, which were threaded in design, required the use of a tap to create threads in the bone socket that was created for each implant. The implants were inserted by slowly screwing the implant into the tapped bone socket. Today, the new generation of the Branemark craniofacial implant, now marketed by Cochlear Corporation (Englewood, CO) under the name of Vistafix, are self-tapping implants that do not require the creation of a pre-tapped bone socket. This is true for some other craniofacial implant systems, such as the ITI craniofacial implant system marketed by the Straumann Corporation (Basel, Switzerland).[41]

The original Branemark craniofacial implants had a perforated metal collar around the head of the implant that overlaid onto the outer cortex of the bone to prevent potential iatrogenic damage to vital structures due to overseating of the implant. In addition, the head of the implant was an external hexagonal design. The newer generation of implants include craniofacial implants without the extended metal collar as well as an internal mortise design to the head of the implant.

Healing abutments have replaced the use of having to select a final abutment of appropriate length at the time of second-stage surgery. This allows the restorative dentist or anaplastologist to carefully measure the thickness of the final skin flap and select a final abutment of correct length, following complete healing of the skin, rather than having to guess at the time of the second-stage surgery.

In addition, the protocol has changed to allow for one-stage surgical procedures.[41] According to the Cochlear Corporation (Englewood, CO), in their *Treatment and Surgery Guide* manual for their Vistafix system, this protocol can be considered only for auricular prostheses when there is bone thickness greater than 3 mm with good quality to the bone.[42]

For the first stage of the standard two-stage surgical approach, an incision is made remote to the designated areas for placement of the craniofacial implants. A full-thickness flap is elevated to expose the underlying bone (Figure 22.5). The markings, previously tattooed with a needle coated with a dye or marker, are located on the cortex of the bone. Pilot drills of the appropriate depth, previously determined by the CT scans, are used to create the initial holes in the bone at the designated implant sites (Figure 22.6). Canon drills are then used to enlarge the sockets to the appropriate diameter and depth for the corresponding craniofacial implants. If the implant has a flange at the head, the

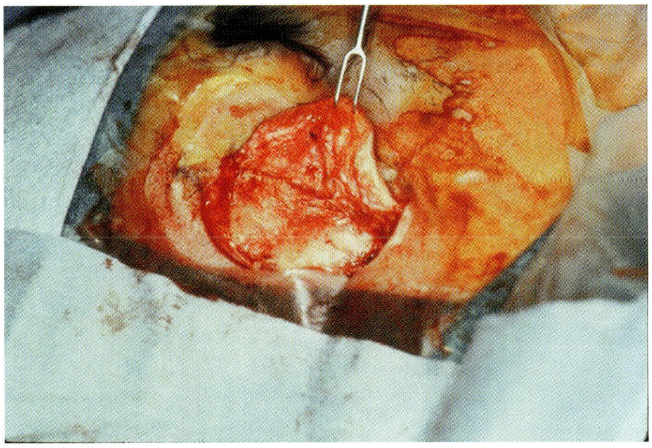

Figure 22.5 Elevation of full-thickness flap.

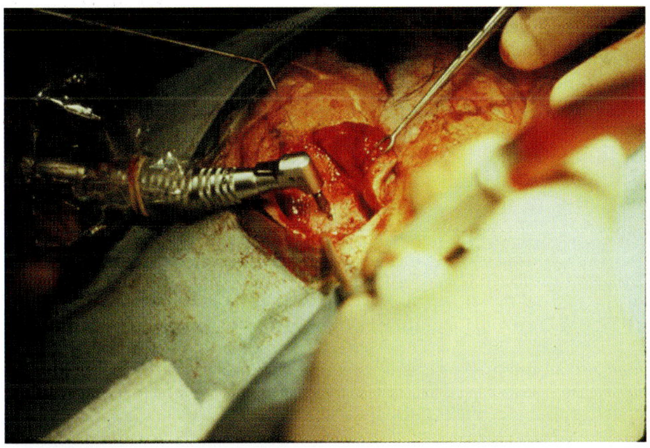

Figure 22.6 Pilot holes for craniofacial implant sockets are created with a pilot drill. Note that the pilot drill shaft has a narrow portion followed by a wider section. The wider section is at a selected distance from the drill bit (such as 3 mm or 4 mm) to define the specific depth of the pilot hole in accordance to the previously selected length of craniofacial implant for placement.

drill is designed with a countersinking part to create a countersunk perimeter around the implant socket to accommodate the flange when the implant is inserted into the prepared socket (Figure 22.7). Each craniofacial implant is slowly screwed into position until fully seated in the prepared socket (Figure 22.8). Cover screws are inserted into each implant (Figure 22.9). The full-thickness flap is repositioned and sutured into place (Figure 22.10). A surgical dressing is applied to secure the flap against the bone to insure attachment to the bone and to prevent hematoma formation beneath the flap (Figure 22.11). A period of 3–4 months is allowed for osseointegration of the implants.

The second-stage surgery is performed following the 3–4-month healing period. A repeat incision is made to elevate the full-thickness flap to expose the underlying implants (Figure 22.12). Any overgrowth of bone over the head of the implant and cover screw is carefully removed without damaging the implant. The cover screws are removed from the implants. The implants should be tested to assure stability and rigidity as

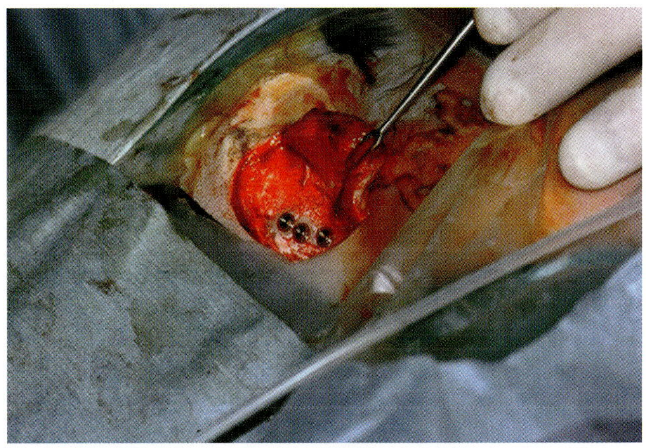

Figure 22.8 Craniofacial implants in position in respective sockets.

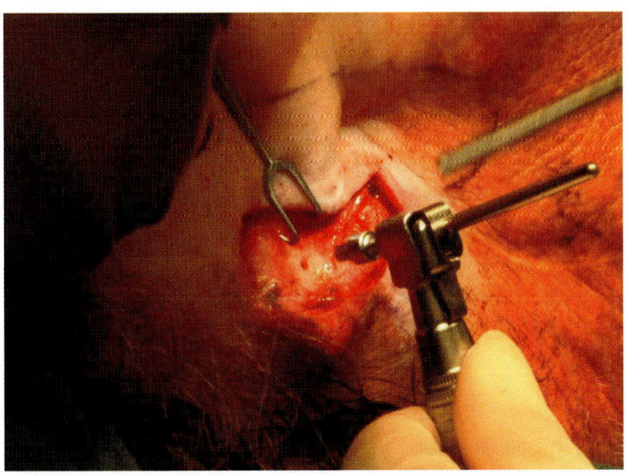

(a)

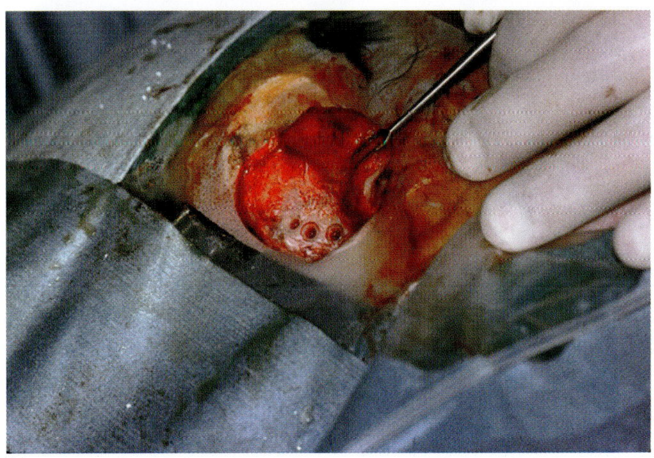

(b)

Figure 22.7 (a) Canon drill used to increase diameter of craniofacial implant socket to previously selected depth. If the craniofacial implant has a flanged head, the canon drill will also create the countersink surface to accommodate the flange. (b) Prepared craniofacial implant sockets with countersunk surfaces to accommodate flanges of the implants.

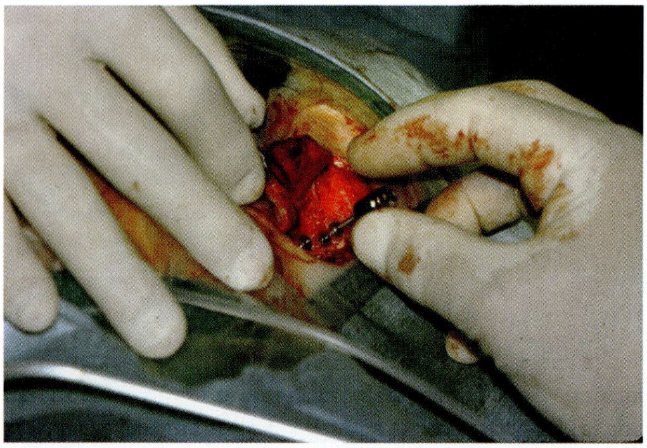

Figure 22.9 Cover screws are secured onto the craniofacial implants.

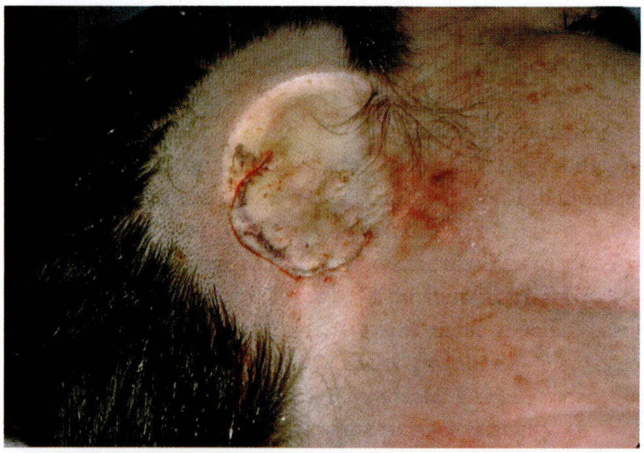

Figure 22.10 The full-thickness flap is sutured into its original position.

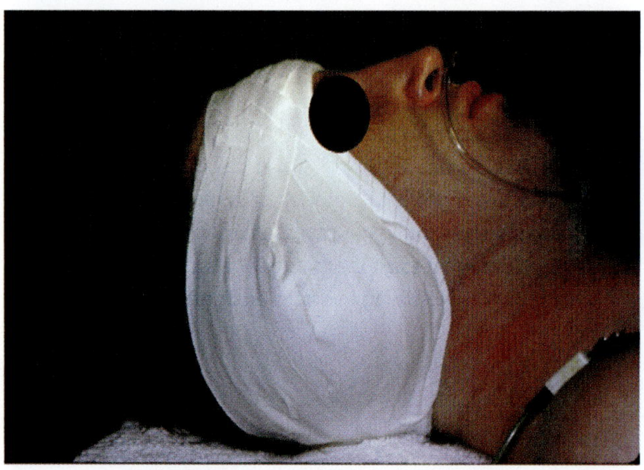

Figure 22.11 Surgical dressing is applied to maintain adaptation of the flap to the underlying bone for good attachment during the healing phase and to minimize hematoma formation.

an indication of successful osseointegration. Any mobile implant should be deemed a failure and removed at this time.

The full-thickness flap is debulked of as much subcutaneous tissue as possible to create a thin skin flap (Figure 22.13). The flap is repositioned in place and perforations through the flap over the craniofacial implants are made with a punch (Figure 22.14). Either the actual abutments or healing abutments are then attached to the implants (Figure 22.15). The abutments should be of adequate length to extend transcutaneously at least 1 mm above the skin flap (Figure 22.16). The skin flap is sutured into position. If the final abutments are used, healing caps are secured onto the abutments. Another surgical dressing is applied to maintain adaptation of the flap to the underlying bone for good attachment during the healing phase (Figure 22.17). A period of 3–4 weeks is allowed to elapse for healing of the flap before initiation of prosthetic treatment.

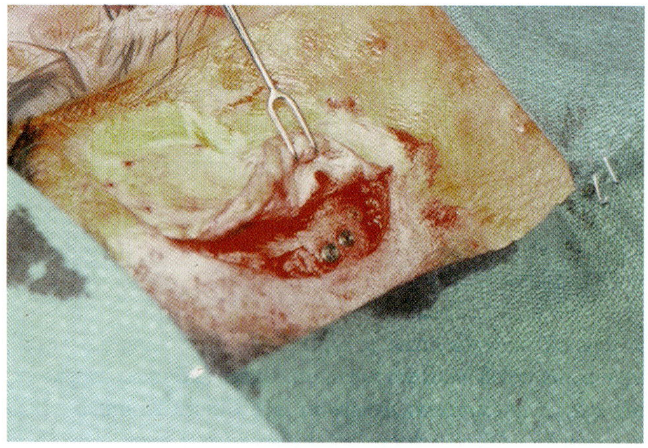

Figure 22.12 Full-thickness flap is raised again during second-stage surgery. The incision is made through the original incision site.

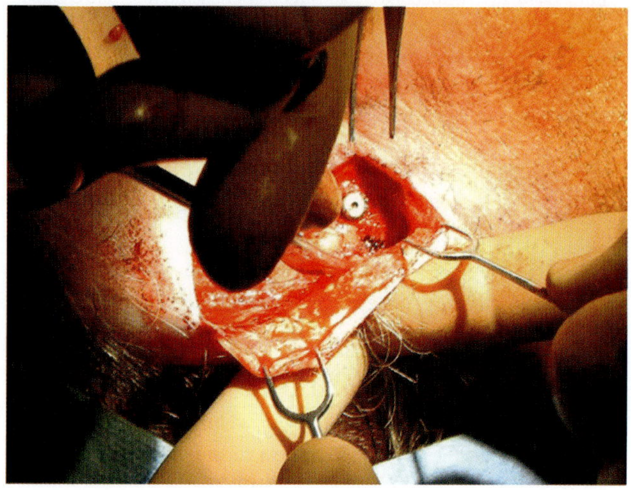

Figure 22.13 Debulking of the full-thickness flap.

Nasal prostheses

The most common sites for placement of craniofacial implants for a nasal prosthesis are the floor of the nose and the glabella region (Figure 22.18). While the literature reports good success

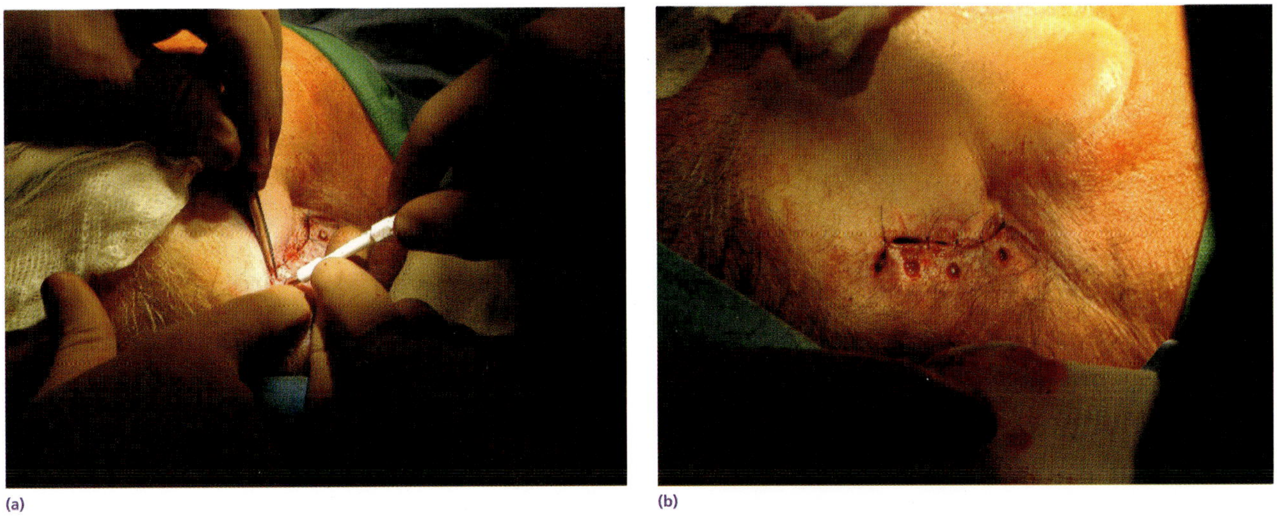

Figure 22.14 (a) The debulked flap is repositioned and holes are created through the flap over the underlying craniofacial implants using a surgical punch. (b) Punch holes through flap, exposing the underlying respective craniofacial implants.

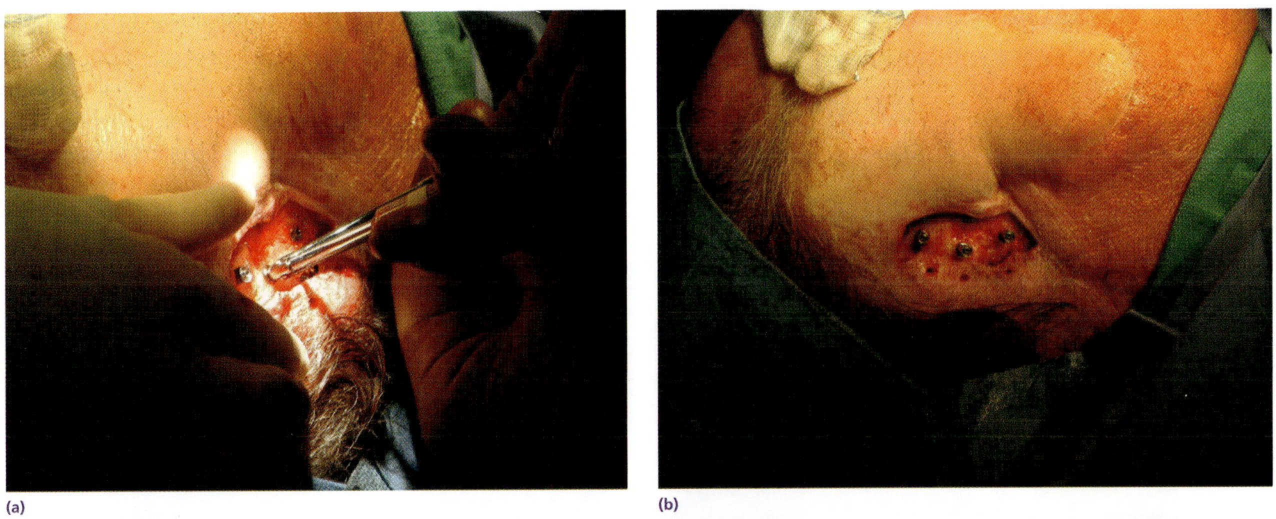

Figure 22.15 (a) Final abutments being secured to the craniofacial implants. (b) Final abutments secured to their respective craniofacial implants.

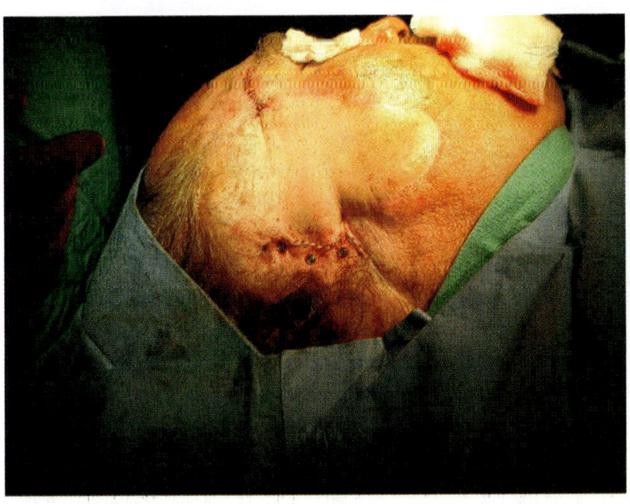

Figure 22.16 Skin flap repositioned and sutured in place. Note that the abutments protrude at least 1 mm through the skin.

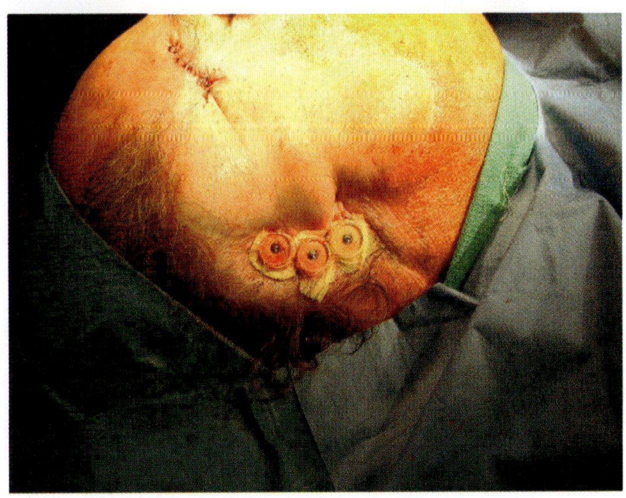

Figure 22.17 Healing caps and surgical dressing applied around the abutments and skin flap. In addition, a surgical packing will be placed to maintain light pressure against the flap to maintain position of the flap and prevent hematoma formation.

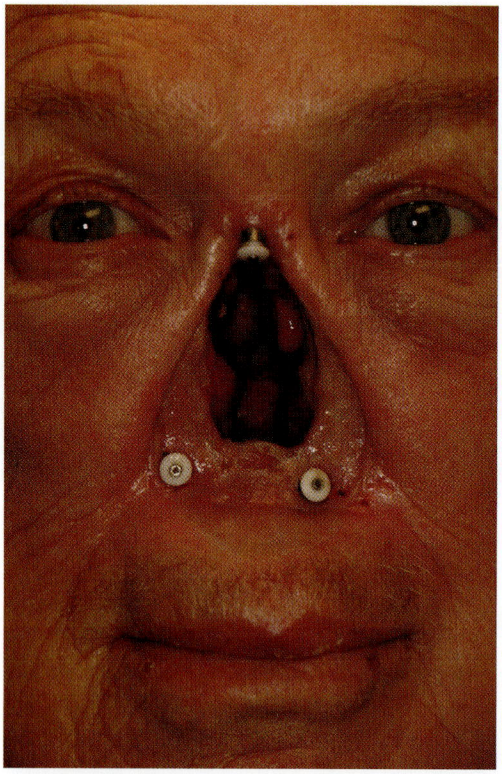

Figure 22.18 Craniofacial implants placed in floor of nose and in glabella region.

in osseointegration of craniofacial implants in the floor of the nose, there are unfavorable, albeit variable results, regarding success of osseointegration in the glabella region as has been alluded to in an earlier section.[16,20,43] Roumanas *et al.*[16] reported an overall 25% survival rate for craniofacial implants, ranging from 3–5 mm, in the glabella region. No time period before failure was reported in the article. Karakoca *et al.*[43] reported a survival period of 30–33 months for two glabella-placed craniofacial implants in their study. Based on these studies, it is recommended that the glabella region should be used as a secondary, alternate site, rather than a primary site for craniofacial implant placement in the nasal cavity.[16,43] A radiographic template with radiopaque markers can be used to identify sites of sufficient bone thickness for placement of the implants such that the abutments and subsequent retentive components will not interfere with the esthetics of the prosthesis (Figure 22.19). CT radiographic scans with the template in position are made to ascertain appropriate sites of bone thickness (Figure 22.20). In addition, the use of three-dimensional (3-D) computer-generated images or a stereolithographic generated model of the region can be helpful in making the final determination of appropriate implant sites (Figure 22.21).

Once the sites have been determined, the radiographic template can be converted into a surgical template to guide the surgeon in the location and surgical placement of the craniofacial implants (Figure 22.22). After an appropriate time period to

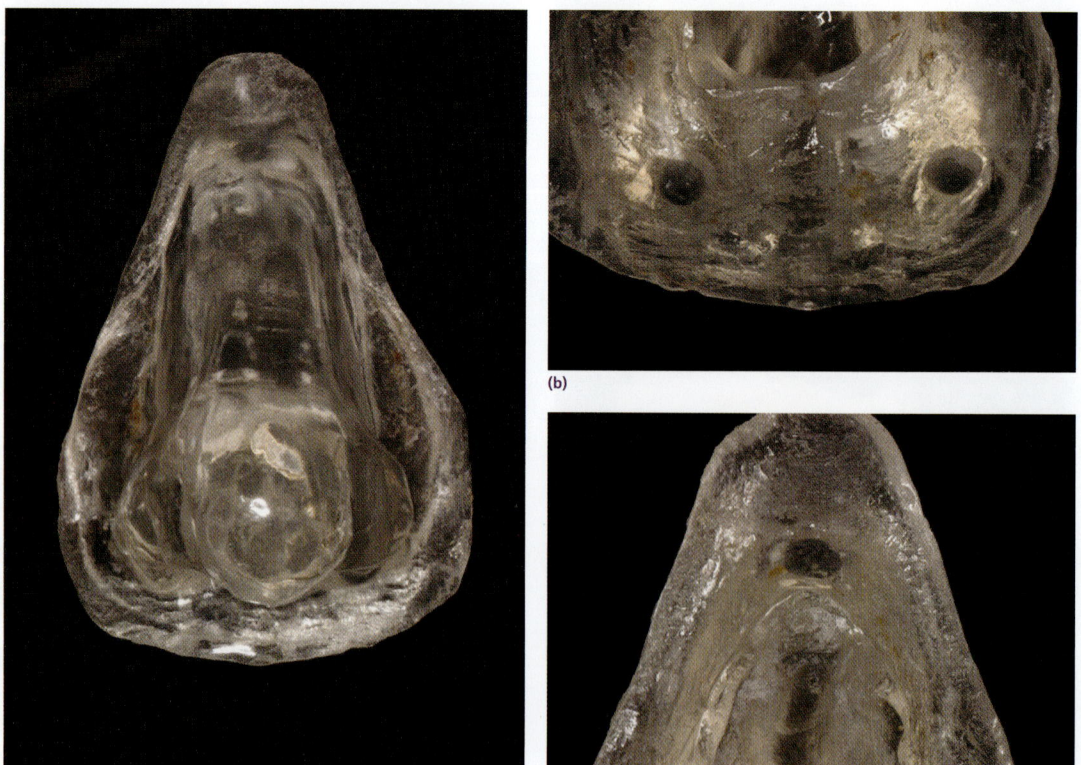

(a) (b) (c)

Figure 22.19 (a) Radiographic template. (b, c) Spherical lead shots, used as radiographic markers, embedded in template in potential locations for craniofacial implant placement.

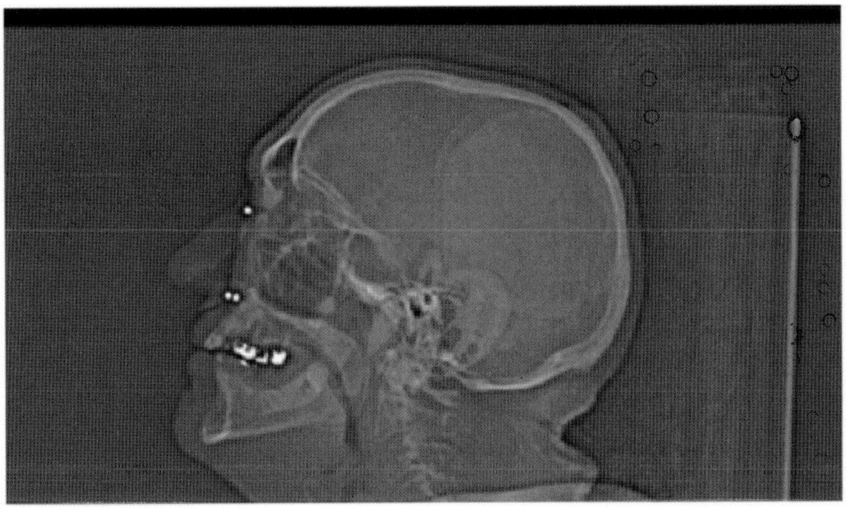

Figure 22.20 CT radiograph with radiographic template in position showing markers and thickness of adjacent bone.

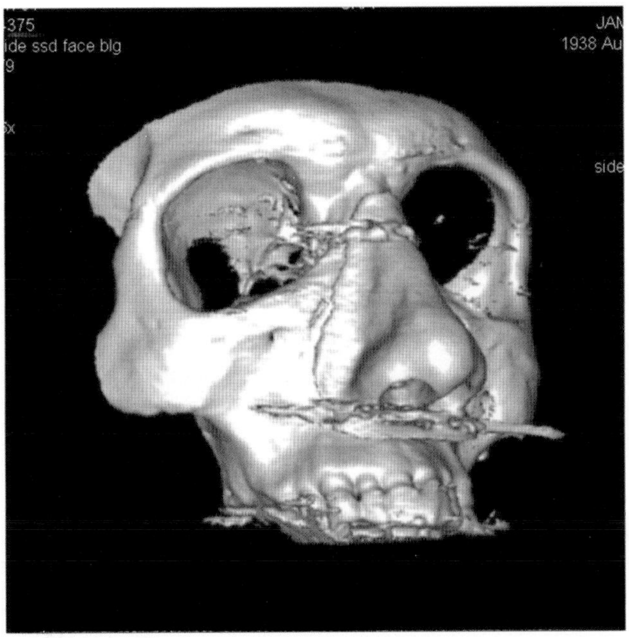

Figure 22.21 Three-dimensional computer-generated image of template and patient's skull.

allow for osseointegration of the craniofacial implants, the definitive abutments can be attached to the implants. An attachment system can be designed to retain the nasal prosthesis. In many cases, this may be a framework, attached to the abutments, which employs a clip–bar retentive mechanism or incorporation of magnets for retention with the nasal prosthesis. Other retentive designs are the use of solitary abutments incorporating attachments such as magnets.

If a framework is to be used as part of the retentive mechanism, a moulage of the nasal defect and surrounding facial regions is made. Impression copings are attached to the abutments prior to making of the moulage. The copings can be splinted together to form a stable unit that will be incorporated in the moulage (Figure 22.23). The moulage is then made of the region (Figure 22.24). Abutment analogs are attached to the impression copings and the moulage is poured with dental stone to produce the master cast.

The framework can be fabricated through a conventional method of casting in a metal alloy from a wax pattern, or soldering prefabricated metal bars to metal alloy copings. More recently, computer-assisted design/computer-assisted milled (CAD/CAM) technology is being employed in the fabrication of such frameworks (Figure 22.25). The framework should be attached to the abutments in the defect on the patient and evaluated to insure that it fits passively.

A superstructure can then be fabricated to fit over the framework. This is usually made in acrylic resin or similar material. The superstructure will incorporate the reciprocal retentive components that will join to those in the framework to provide retention for the prosthesis (Figure 22.26). The superstructure can be made hollow to allow for patency of the nasal airway in the prosthesis. This superstructure eventually becomes incorporated into the final prosthesis.

The contours for the nasal prosthesis are created in wax or in clay over the superstructure. The entire pattern is positioned on the patient's face to evaluate for accuracy of fit, anatomic detail, and marginal integrity with the adjacent skin. Further refinements are made until the final results are achieved in the pattern (Figure 22.27). The pattern, along with the master cast, are invested and the wax or clay is thoroughly removed from the mould. A material, such as silicone, is used for the outer overlay of the prosthesis. Color is incorporated intrinsically into the silicone using artist oils and/or dry earth pigments to create the intrinsic skin tones. The silicone is packed, under pressure, in the mold and processed to a complete curing of the material. The final prosthesis is then removed from the mold. The prosthesis is positioned on the patient. Margins are trimmed

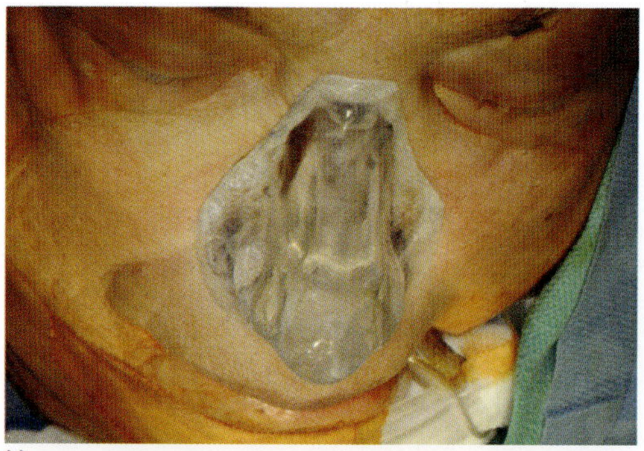

(a)

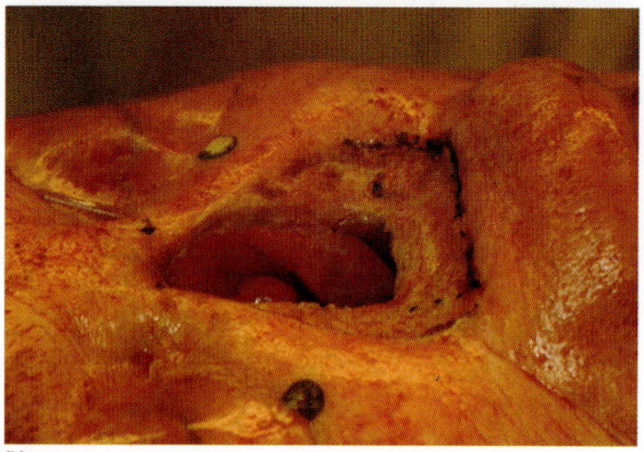

(b)

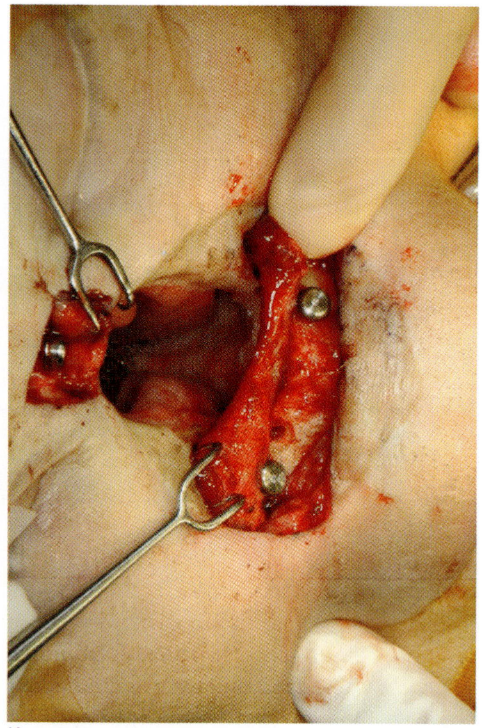

(c)

Figure 22.22 **(a)** Radiographic template converted to surgical template where holes were drilled through template in areas of radiographic markers. The surgical template is positioned on patient's face and a marker with indelible dye or ink is passed through the holes in the template to mark the positions of the craniofacial implants on the patient's skin. **(b)** Markings indicating the positions for the craniofacial implants in the floor of the nose and glabella regions. A needle coated with a dye or ink can be passed through the skin at these markings to tattoo the underlying bone. **(c)** Craniofacial implants placed in previously marked sites.

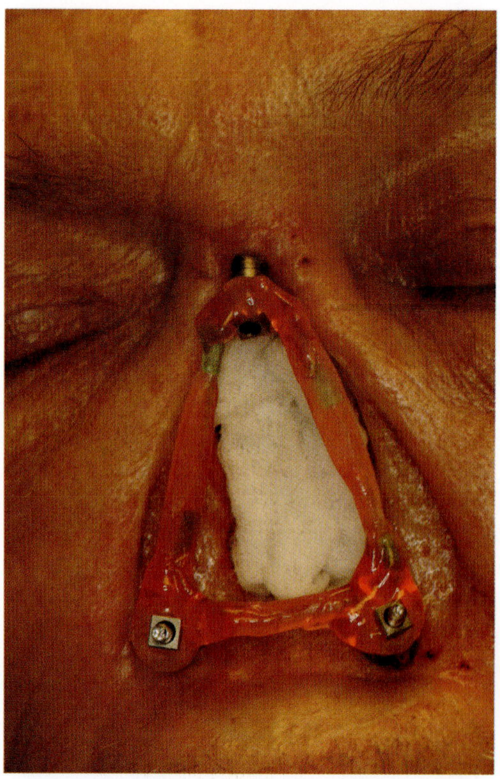

Figure 22.23 Splinted impression copings attached to craniofacial implant abutments.

accordingly for proper marginal adaptation. Extrinsic coloration is performed to create the final surface characteristics on the prosthesis that match and blend with the adjacent skin of the patient's face (Figure 22.28).

Implant-retained auricular prostheses

Patients with developmental and acquired defects of the auricle can elect to have no treatment, autogenous surgical reconstruction, or prosthetic reconstruction. Since 1986, carefully selected patients in North America have had the treatment option of the placement of craniofacial implants in the mastoid process in order to retain a prosthesis by the use of magnets or clips.

The presurgical planning must include appropriate CT radiographic imaging of the mastoid process. In addition, the presurgical planning includes a diagnostic waxing of the auricle that is converted to clear methyl methacrylate resin to be utilized as a surgical template. The templates are prepared in a manner to allow skin markings through holes where the implants will ideally be placed. A wider area can also be marked for alternative implant placement should a mastoid air cell be encountered at the time of surgery. The surgical procedure includes a full-thickness skin flap and marking of the planned implant sites with methylene blue using needle injection. Tissue remnants, skin tags, or scar tissue should be removed. Care should be

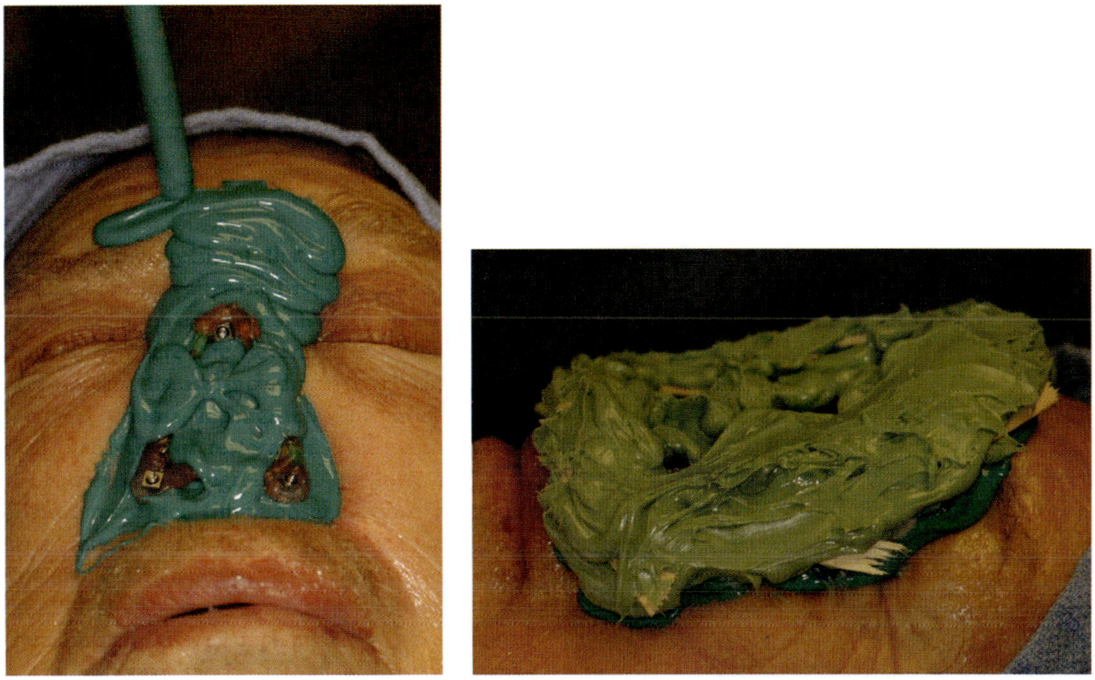

(a) (b)

Figure 22.24 (a, b) Moulage made using low-viscosity vinylpolysiloxane impression material supported by high-viscosity vinylpolysiloxane impression material with pieces of tongue blades embedded within the high-viscosity material to assist in providing a rigid "tray" to support the low-viscosity impression material.

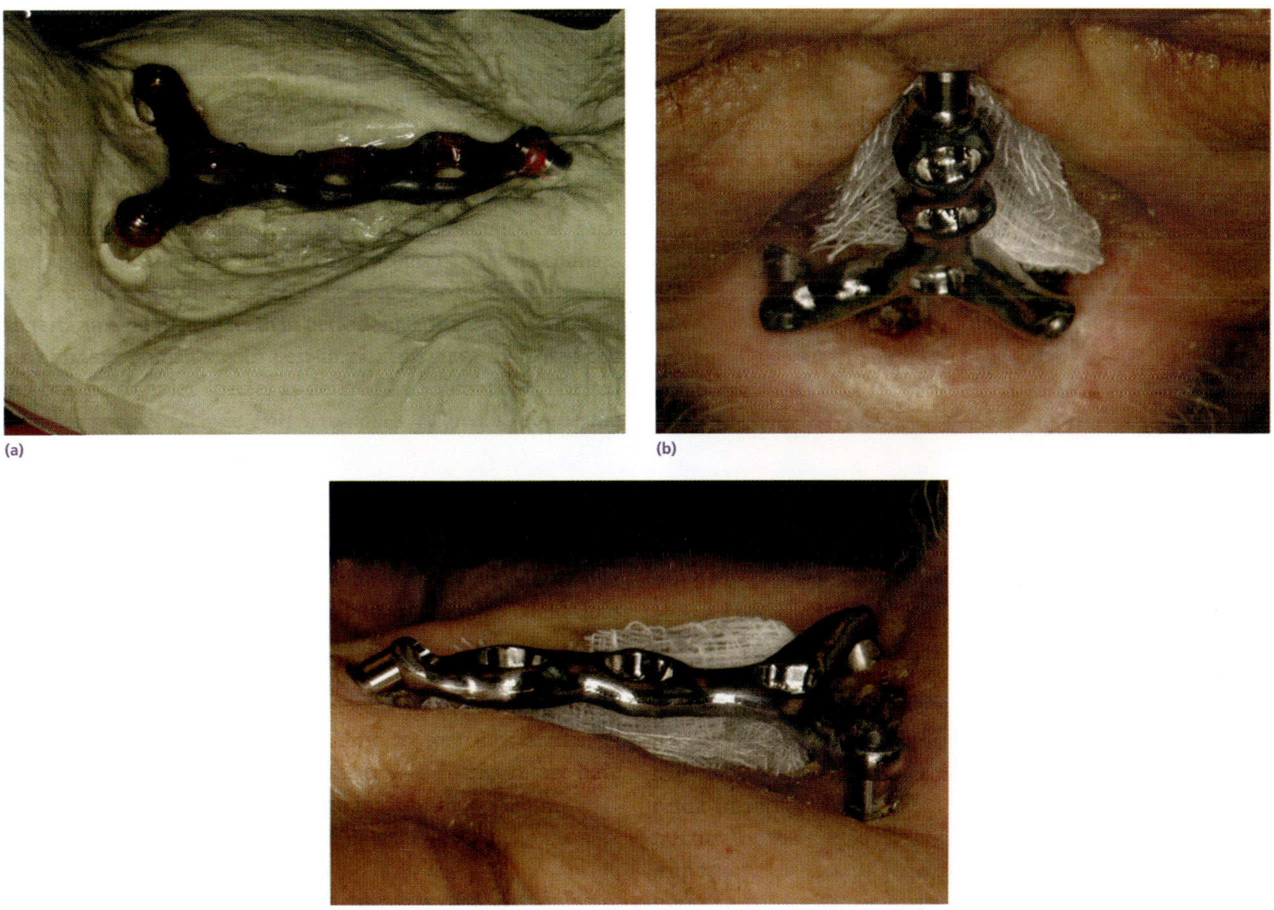

(a) (b) (c)

Figure 22.25 (a) Master cast with incorporated abutment analogs with a pattern for framework made from acrylic resin and wax. Framework will incorporate three cobalt–samarium magnets to provide retention of the nasal prosthesis to the CAD/CAM titanium alloy framework. (b) CAD/CAM titanium alloy framework made via copy mill process of framework pattern. (c) Sagittal view of CAD/CAM titanium alloy framework.

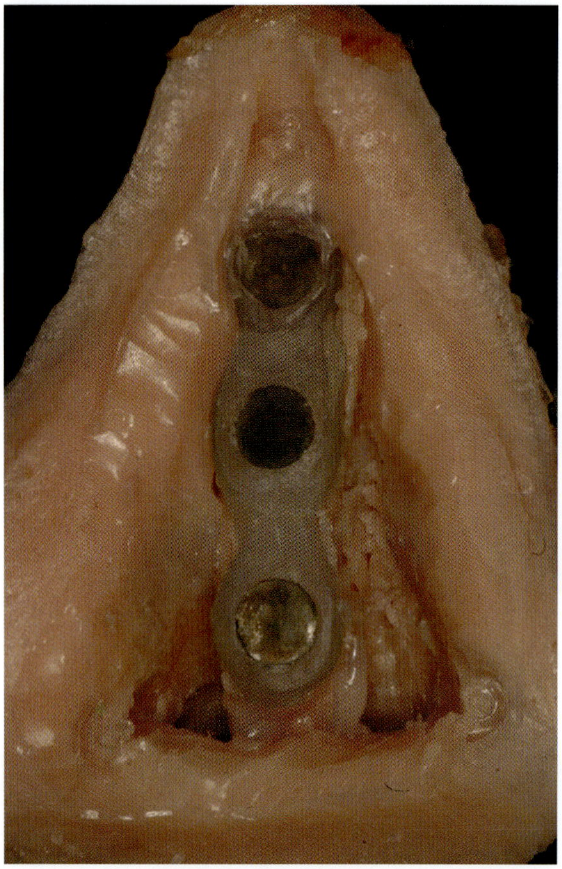

Figure 22.26 Acrylic resin superstructure framework, housing a matching set of cobalt–samarium magnets, embedded within the final prosthesis.

taken to thin the skin and subcutaneous tissue to 2 mm or less. When bone quality is very good, a one-stage procedure can be utilized. The normal healing time for the mastoid process is 3–4 months when the bone quality is good and in the absence of irradiation of the bone. The healing time for irradiated patients or patients with poor bone quality is a minimum of 6 months.

A 36-year-old patient with congenital atresia of the right auricle had numerous unsuccessful plastic and surgical reconstructive attempts (Figure 22.29). The patient was referred to the University of North Carolina and elected to have an implant-retained auricular prosthesis. A surgical template was utilized for guided surgical placement of the two craniofacial implants (Figure 22.30). The bar consisted of two magnets and a clip for the retention of the auricular prosthesis (Figure 22.31). The final silicone prosthesis was cast and custom stained (Figure 22.32). The prosthesis contained a superstructure with magnet keepers and a single clip for retention (Factor II Inc. Lakeside, AZ).

A 76-year-old patient lost his left auricle from recurrent basal cell carcinoma. The surgical procedure included excision of the left auricle, left parotidectomy, and partial reconstruction using a deltopectoral flap. The patient was treated postoperatively with radiation therapy. In anticipation of the planned craniofacial implants, a radiation shield was fabricated to protect the implant sites and allow delivery of the radiation to the tumor site.[44] Three implants were placed 4 months after radiation utilizing a surgical template (Figure 22.33). Three months' healing time was allowed before loading. The Magnacap magnet system was utilized (Technovent Ltd, Leeds, UK). Magnet keepers were

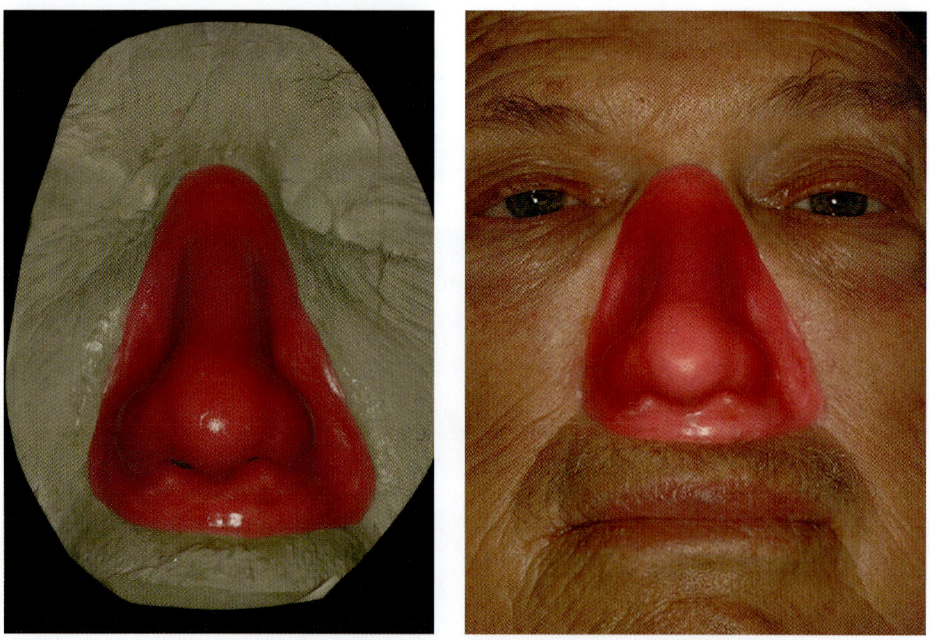

(a) (b)

Figure 22.27 (a) Final wax pattern for nasal prosthesis on master cast. The wax pattern incorporates the acrylic resin superstructure framework. (b) Final wax pattern positioned on patient's face to check for accuracy of contours and marginal integrity.

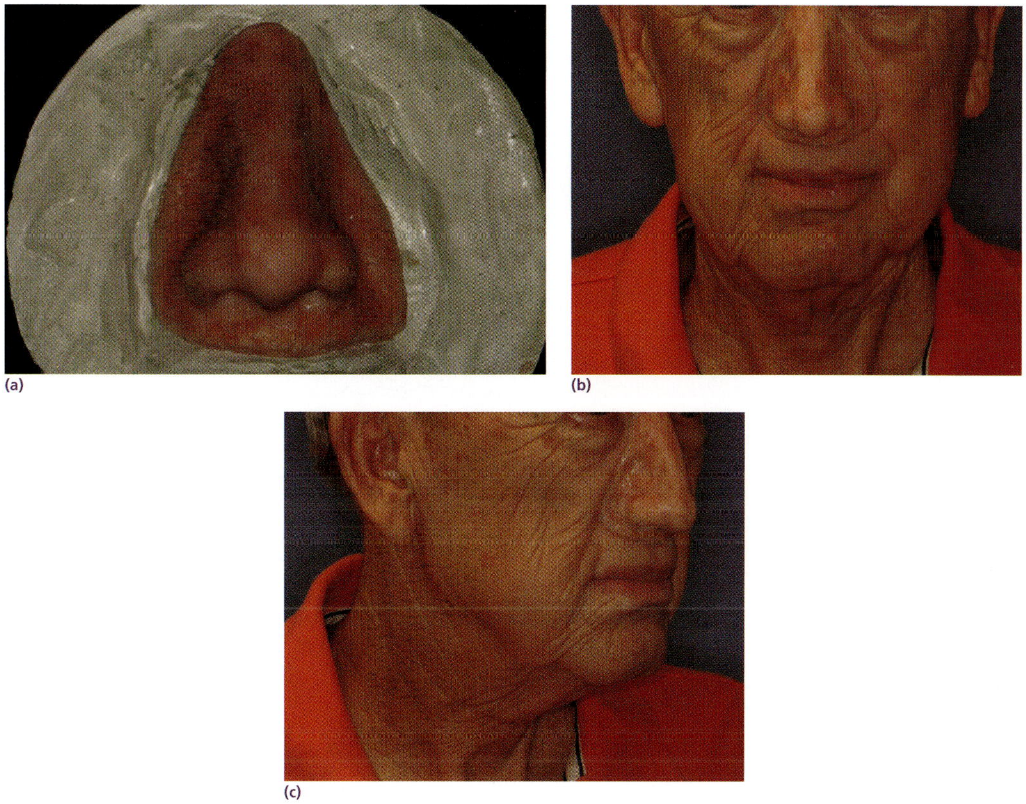

Figure 22.28 (a) Final nasal prosthesis on master cast. (b) Full face view of final nasal prosthesis positioned on patient's face. (c) Three-quarter view of final nasal prosthesis positioned on patient's face.

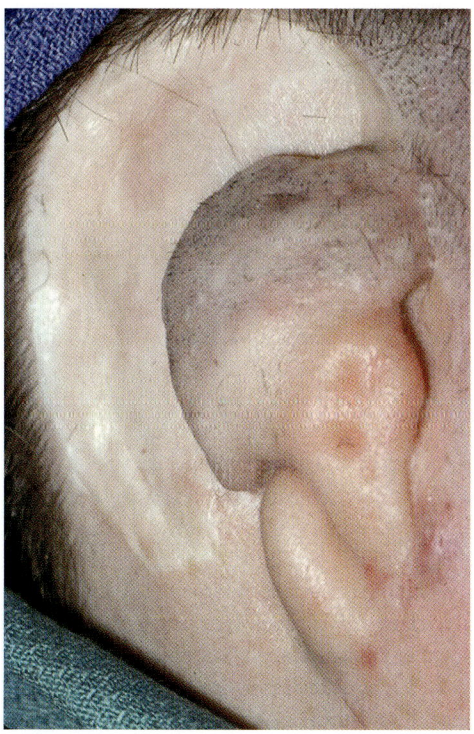

Figure 22.29 Patient with a history of congenital atresia and numerous plastic surgical reconstructions. Presurgical planning includes removal of tissue tags and thinning of the skin and subcutaneous tissue to 2 mm or less.

oriented and connected using autopolymerizing acrylic resin (Figures 22.34 and 22.35). The prosthesis was intrinsically colored and processed in silicone (A2186; Factor II Inc., Lakeside, AZ) (Figure 22.36).[44]

Implant-retained orbital prostheses

Surgical reconstruction for orbital resections is a challenge. Soft tissue flaps to close the orbital contents are not esthetic. Therefore the use of craniofacial implants to retain an orbital prosthesis is a good treatment option if patients are aware that the survival rate of orbital implants is less than that for implants in the mastoid process used to retain auricular prostheses.[15]

The presurgical planning must include a prosthodontist as part of the team since the implants must be carefully planned to be within the confines of the prosthesis and the retentive components and implants must not limit the esthetics of the final facial prosthesis. The presurgical planning should also include a CT radiographic image of the orbit, a diagnostic waxing, and a surgical template (Figure 22.37). The frontal sinus can be the limiting factor for placement of implants in the 1 and 2 o'clock positions for the right orbit and at the 10 and 11 o'clock positions for the left orbit. The supraorbital rim is the most common site for orbital implant placement.

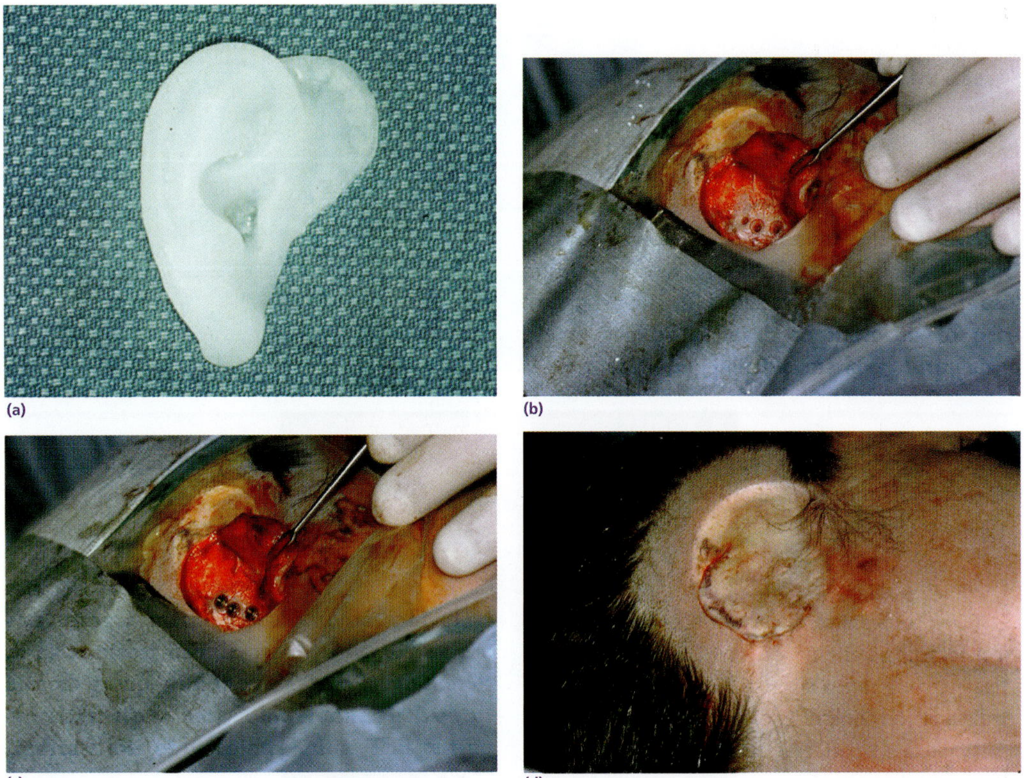

(a) (b) (c) (d)

Figure 22.30 **(a)** Surgical template. **(b)** Three implants placed with countersinking. **(c)** Abutments connected to implants. **(d)** Surgical closure.

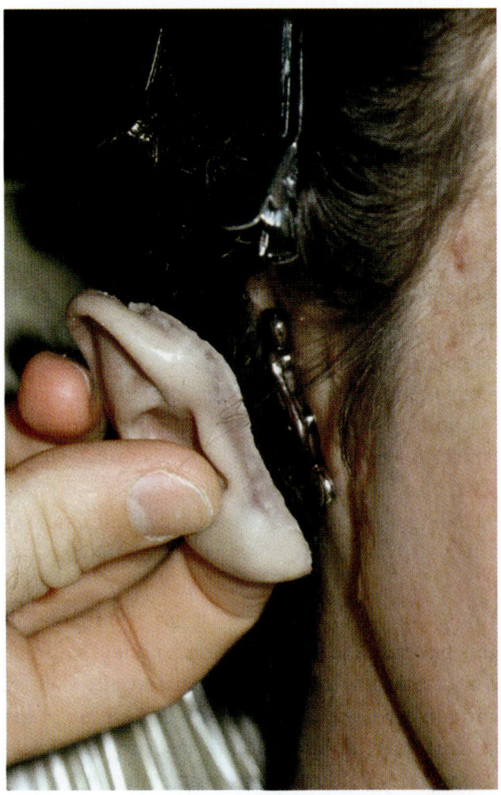

Figure 22.31 Bar framework consists of three magnets and two bar segments with keepers in the superstructure.

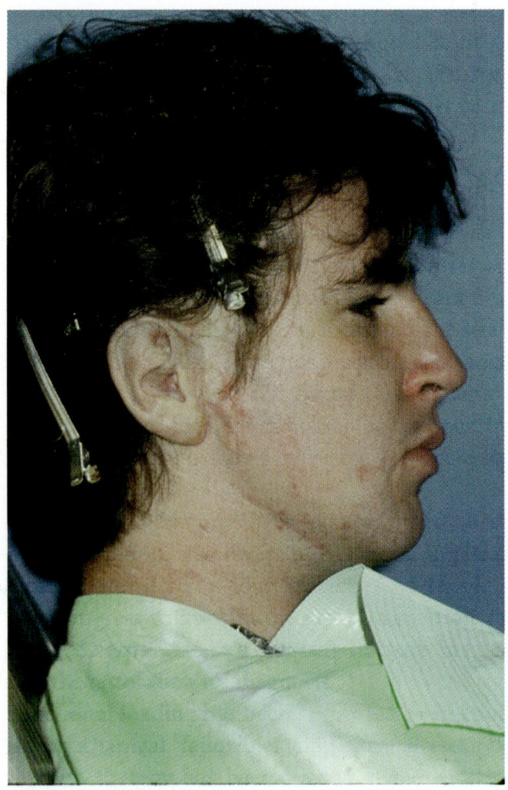

Figure 22.32 Final auricular prosthesis cast, custom stained, and engaged onto implant framework.

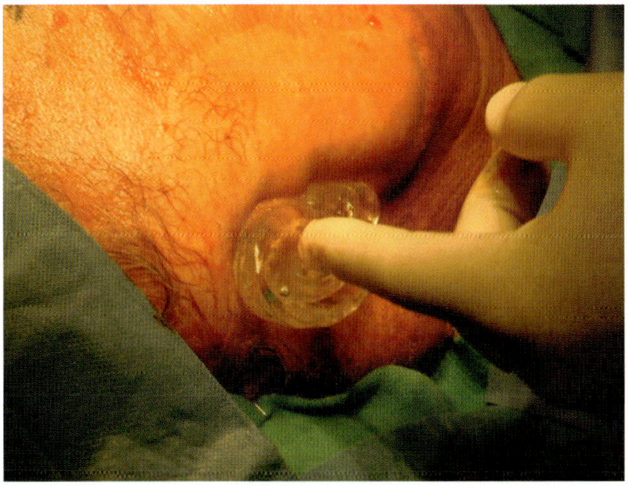

Figure 22.33 Surgical guide oriented on face.

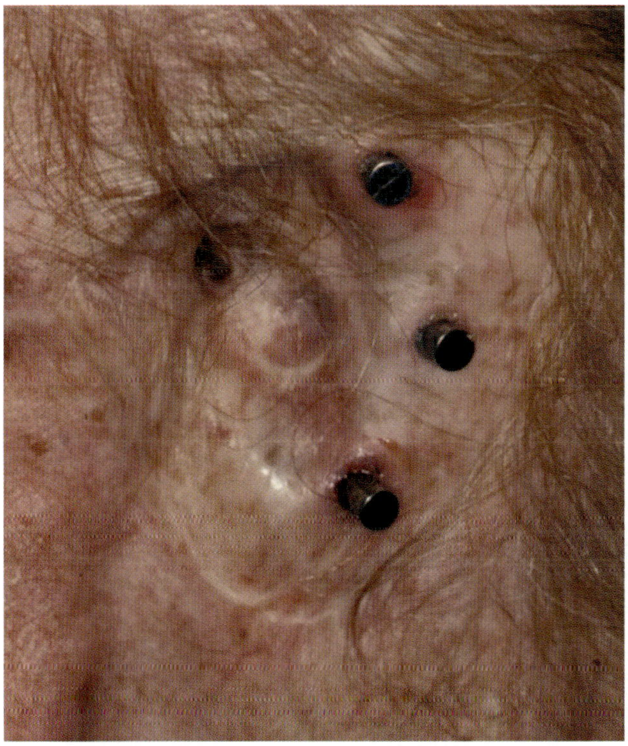

Figure 22.34 Implant healing abutments in place after 3 months of healing.

Surgical exoneration due to cancer is the most common cause of the loss of the orbital contents (Figure 22.38). In the patient in Figure 22.38, three craniofacial implants were placed in the supra- and infraorbital rims and a bar was cast to hold three magnets for retention. The orbital prosthesis has a clear acrylic magnet keeper (substructure) embedded in the intaglio surface to engage the three magnets on the framework for retention (Figure 22.39). The prosthesis provides the patient with a very

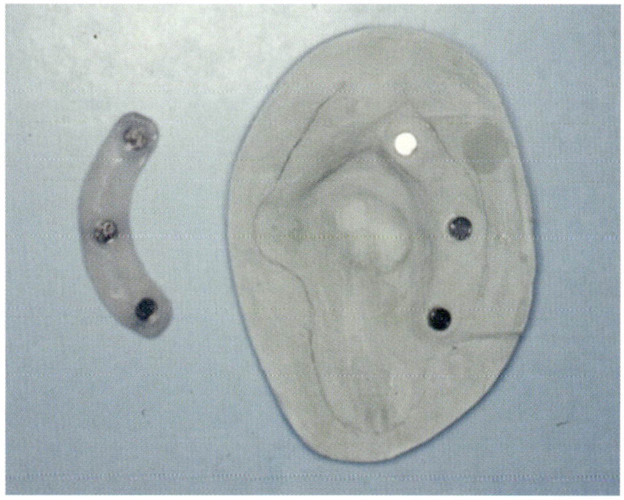

Figure 22.35 Magnet keepers oriented with autopolymerizing acrylic resin on master cast.

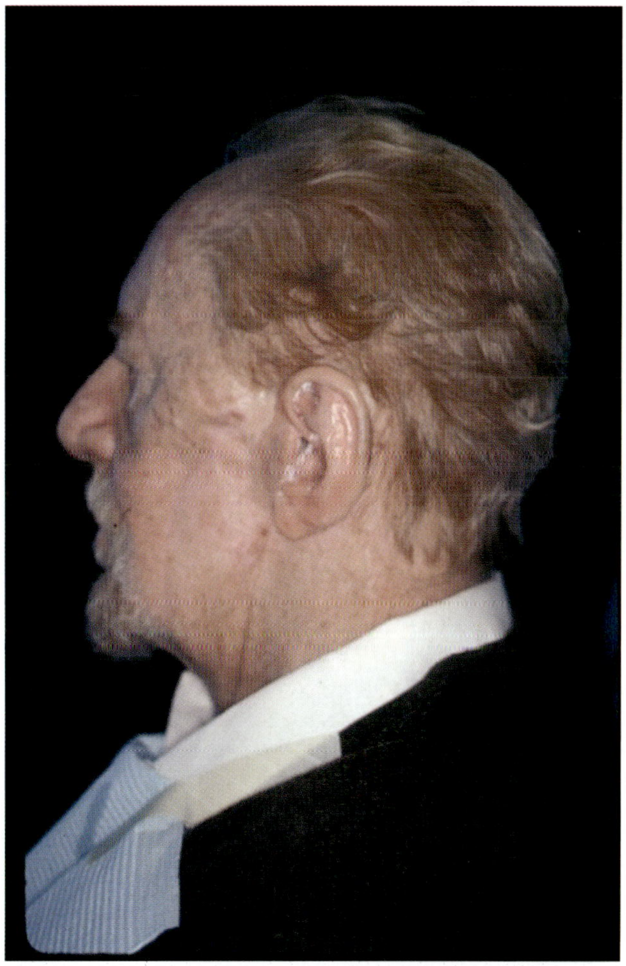

Figure 22.36 The auricular magnet-retained prosthesis after custom staining. *Source:* Hatfielt *et al.*, 2001.[44] Reproduced with permission from Elsevier.

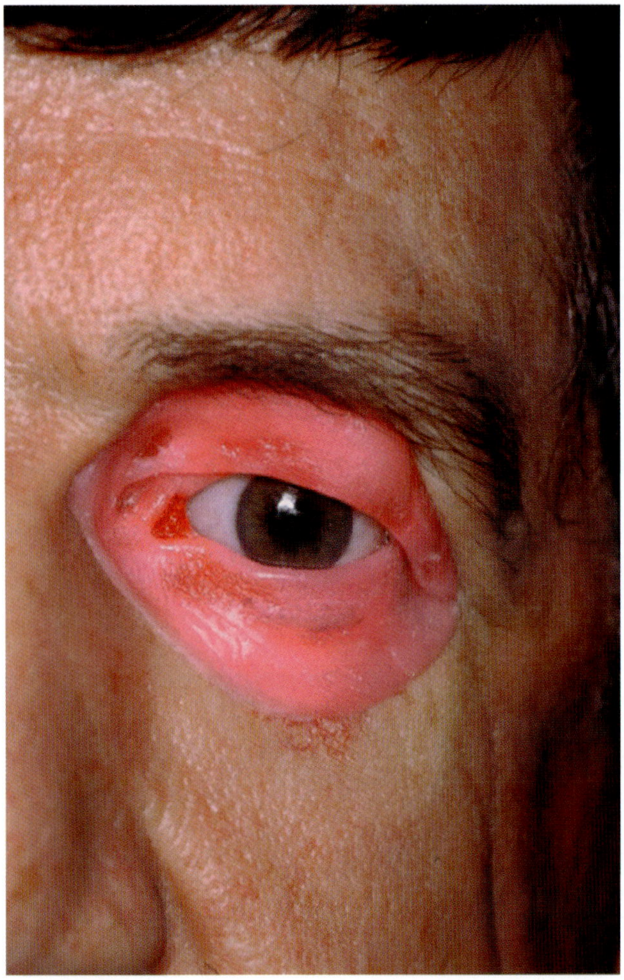

Figure 22.37 Diagnostic waxing for presurgical planning.

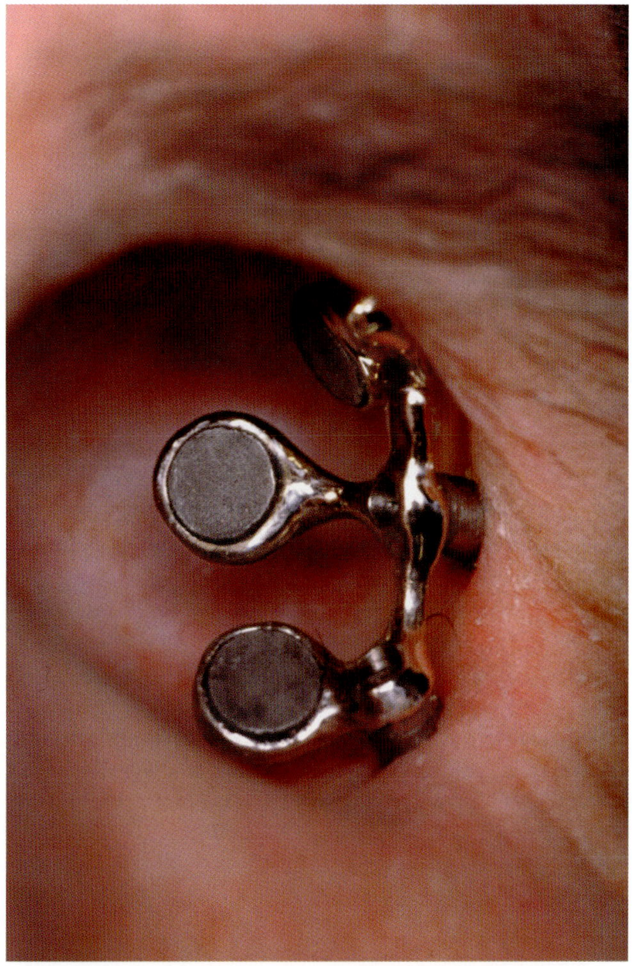

Figure 22.38 Three implants placed in the supraorbital rim and infraorbital rim with a cast bar containing three magnets for retention.

esthetic restoration of the orbit (Figure 22.40). The custom ocular prosthesis is contained within the orbital prosthesis.

A large orbital resection was necessary due to a malignancy (Figure 22.41). The patient was treated with the placement of standard intraoral implants (IMZ). A bar was cast in two sections with a nonrigid connector due to the divergent paths of insertion (Figure 22.42). The bar was cast to hold three magnets for retention (Figure 22.43). A custom ocular prosthesis was fabricated to match the patients left eye. The ocular prosthesis was positioned using this calibrated measuring device (Figure 22.44). The magnet keeper (infrastructure) was housed in the intaglio surface of the orbital prosthesis (Figure 22.45). The wax trial of the orbital prosthesis was verified on the patient (Figure 22.46). The intaglio surface of the orbital prosthesis contained the infrastructure with the magnets (Figure 22.47). The final prosthesis restored the patient's orbital defect and improved this patient's quality of life (Figure 22.48). The margins of the final prosthesis are disguised by the patient's selection of eyeglasses (Figure 22.49).

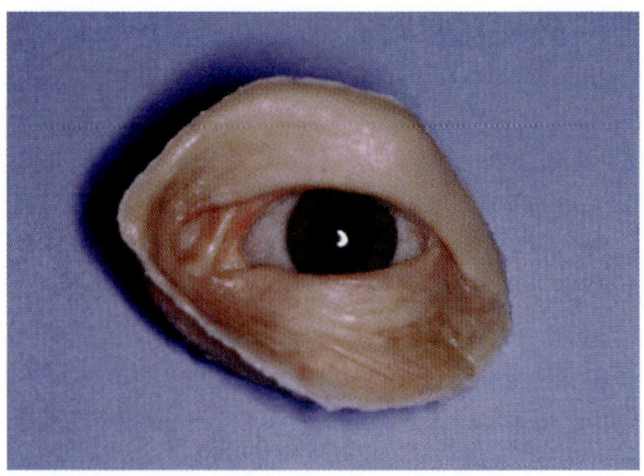

Figure 22.39 The custom orbital prosthesis which contains a custom ocular prosthesis and the substructure with the magnet keepers.

Midfacial prostheses

Midfacial defects are facial defects of the middle third of the face that have communication with the oral cavity. Midfacial defects are defined as either lateral or midline. A lateral defect would

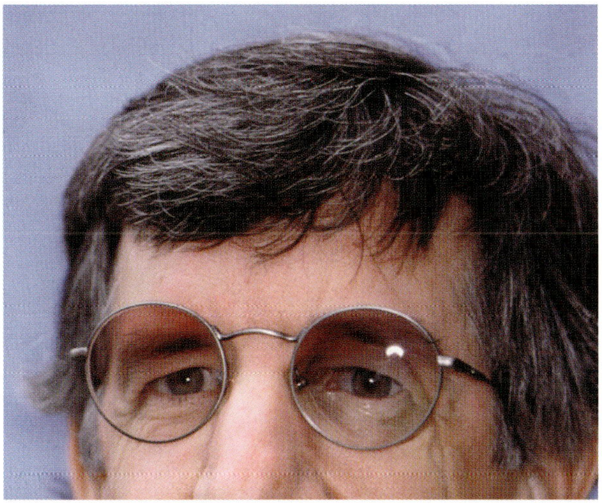

Figure 22.40 The orbital prosthesis is retained by magnets.

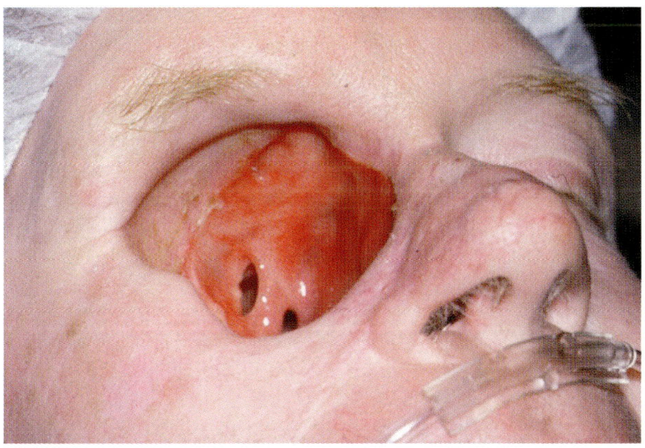

Figure 22.41 Large orbital defect due to a malignancy.

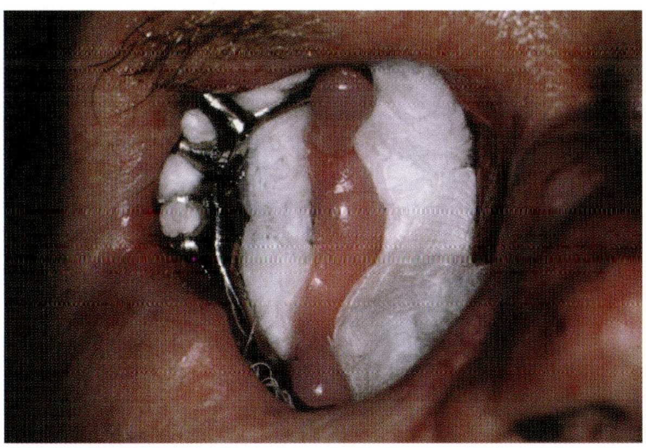

Figure 22.42 Four IMZ implants are placed to anchor a bar with magnets

extend to the cheek and have communication with the oral cavity. An example of a midline midfacial defect would be a combination nasal defect and/or upper lip defect and communication with an intraoral maxillary defect. The types of maxillofacial defects can be quite challenging due to facial defects bordering on movable tissue that limits esthetics, retention, and support.

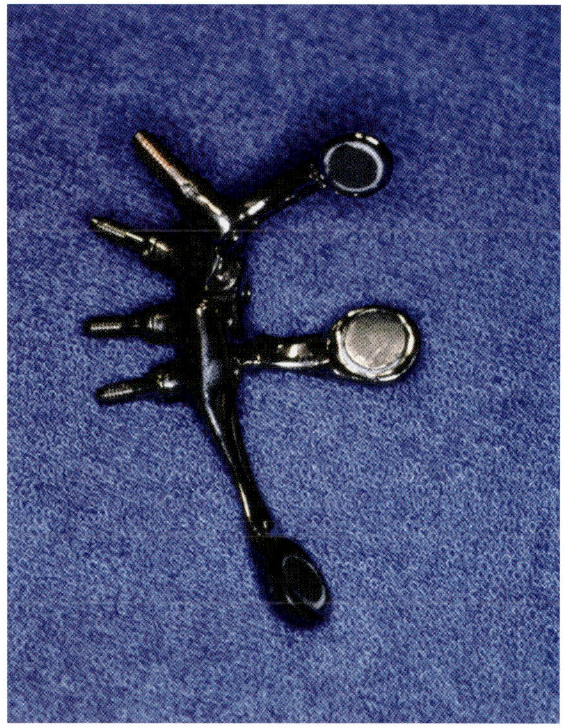

Figure 22.43 The bar has three magnets to aid in retention

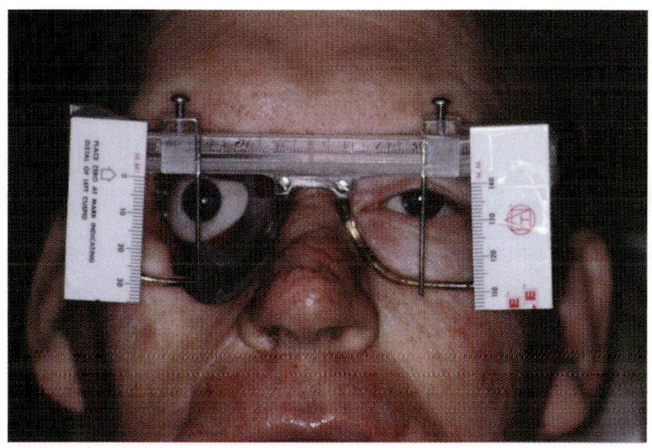

Figure 22.44 Positioning of the ocular prosthesis with a calibrated device.

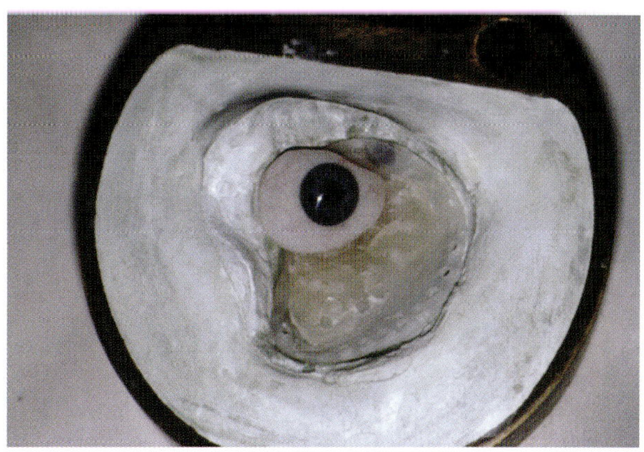

Figure 22.45 The infra-structure is the magnet keeper.

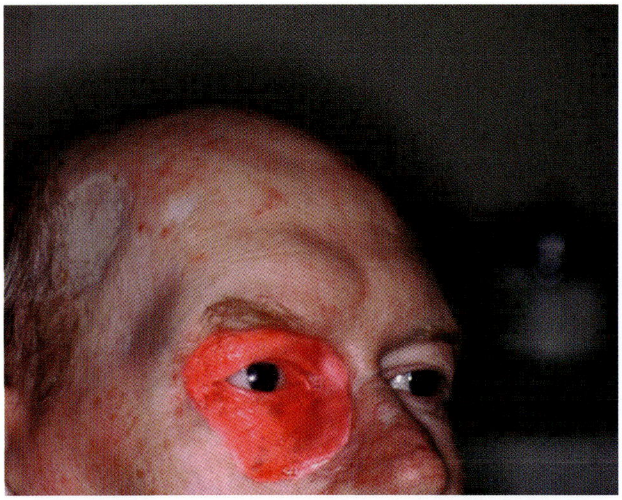

Figure 22.46 Wax trial of the orbital prosthesis.

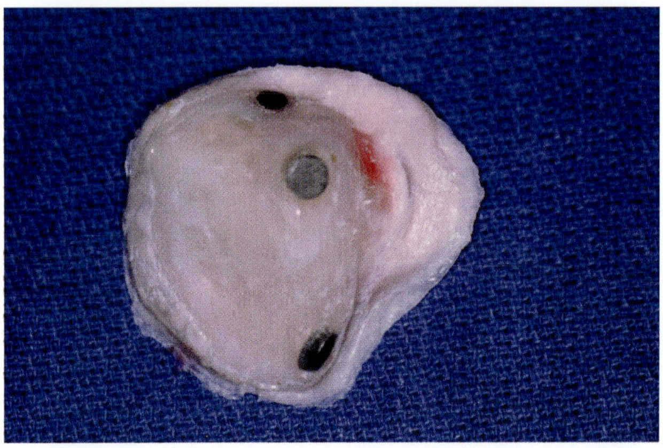

Figure 22.47 The intaglio surface of the orbital prosthesis with the magnet keeper as the substructure.

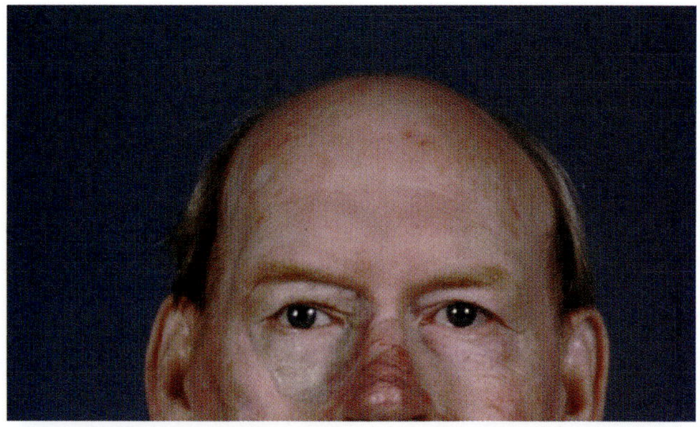

Figure 22.48 The orbital prosthesis is retained by magnets.

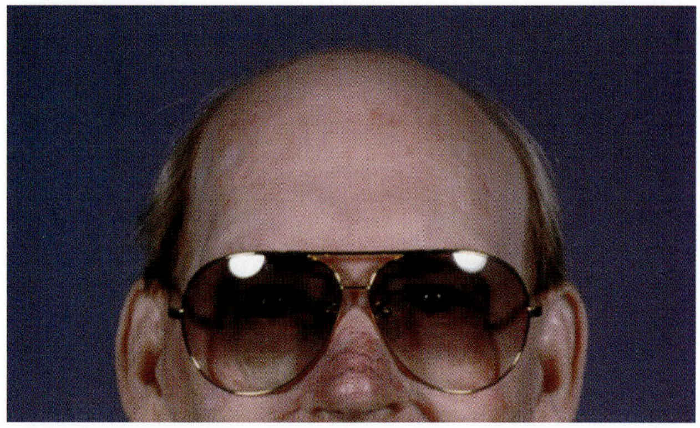

Figure 22.49 Eye glasses disguise the margins of the prosthesis.

These midfacial defects are complicated, since any intraoral prosthesis movement will be transmitted to the extraoral prosthesis (Figure 22.50). In 1975, the patient was diagnosed with advanced squamous cell carcinoma at the age of 42. The ablative surgery included a total rhinectomy, bilateral maxillectomies, and bilateral neck dissections. His midfacial defect extended to his left and right cheeks. His ablative surgery was followed by a full course of external-beam radiation. The patient wore a poorly retained maxillary obturator and facial prosthesis held on with two straps fastened around his head.

Presurgical implant planning was coordinated with the Department of Oral and Maxillofacial Surgery at Bronx V.A. Medical Center affiliated with Columbia University College of Dental Medicine. The presurgical planning included radiographic imaging of the craniofacial area. The patient was 63 years old when he received two 7 mm Branemark implants (Nobelpharma USA, Chicago) into the frontal bone and right zygoma and a 10 mm Branemark implant into the left zygoma. The implants were placed in two stages and 6 months' healing time was allowed since the patient had received radiotherapy. At stage two, 8.5 mm standard abutments were added to the implants. Three weeks' healing time was allowed after stage 2 uncovering before square impression abutments were attached and picked-up utilizing a custom tray and two-stage impression technique. The framework was cast in palladium–gold alloy (Legacy, J.F. Jelenko and Co., Armonk, NY) (Figure 22.51). The obturator was fabricated utilizing standard impression techniques and the vertical maxillomandibular relationships were established by the use of esthetics phonetics, and swallowing. A trial arrangement was performed to verify the esthetics and centric relation. The palladium–gold framework had four regions designed to engage retentive Dolder clips on the obturator (Figure 22.52). The silicone prosthesis was retained by a castable O-ring attachment system (Implant Innovations Inc., West Palm Beach, FL). The pattern was waxed and cast onto the gold alloy framework. The three patrix attachments were at the terminal ends of the framework. The matrix O-ring attachments were oriented to the intaglio surface of the facial prosthesis by mesh and acrylic resin. Three magnets (Shiner SR, Preat Corp., San Mateo, CA) were attached to the nasal region of the obturator and oriented to three magnets on the intaglio surface of the facial prosthesis (Figure 22.53). The patient was able to place and remove the

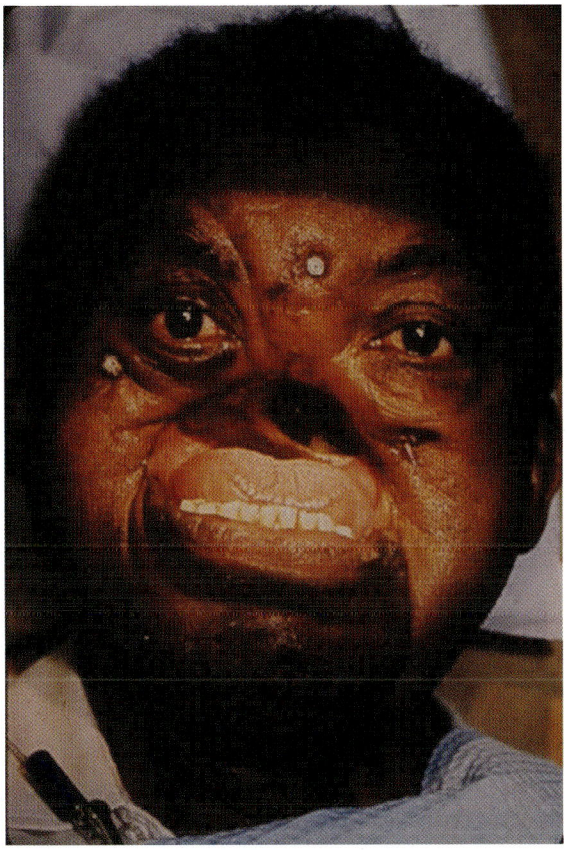

Figure 22.50 Two implants placed in the zygoma and one in the frontal bone. *Source:* Evans *et al.*, 1996.[45] Reproduced with permission from Elsevier.

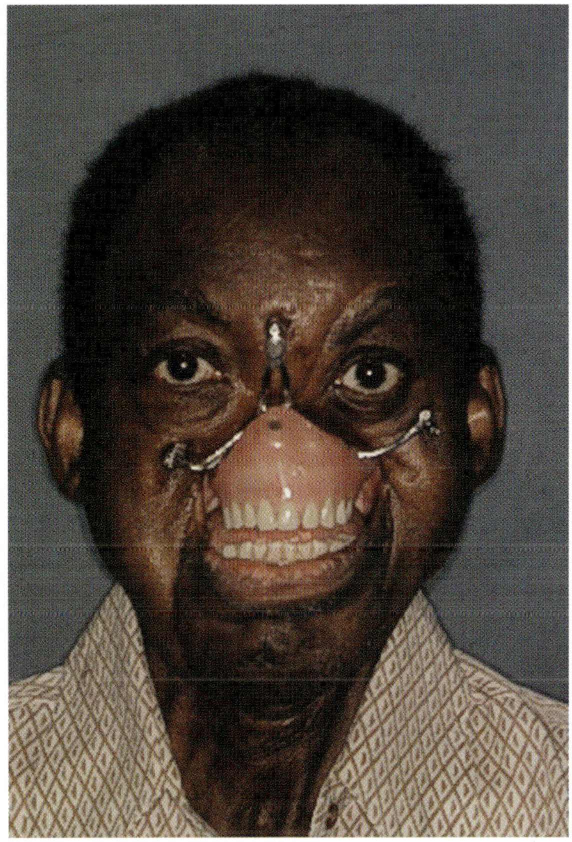

Figure 22.52 The obturator is retained by four Dolder clips. *Source:* Evans *et al.*, 1996.[45] Reproduced with permission from Elsevier.

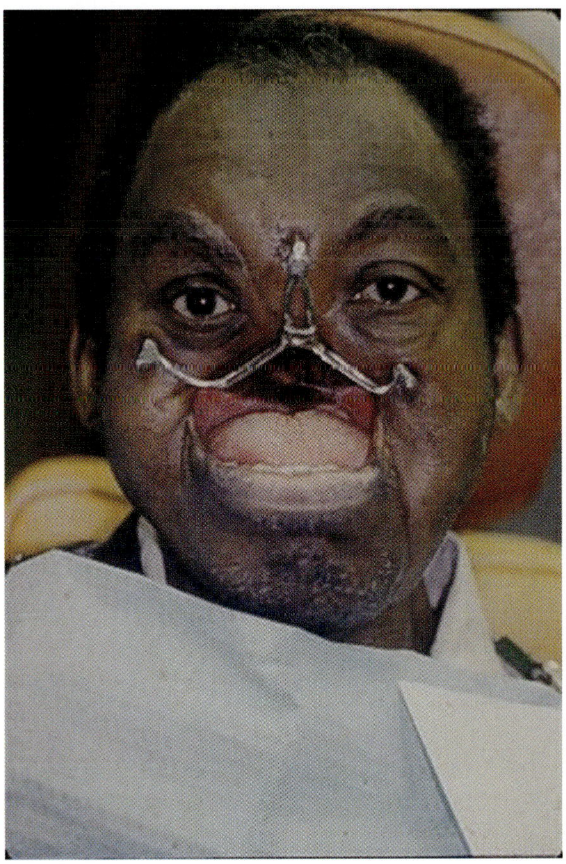

Figure 22.51 The framework is cast in a gold–palladium allow. There are three O-ring attachments. *Source:* Evans *et al.*, 1996.[45] Reproduced with permission from Elsevier.

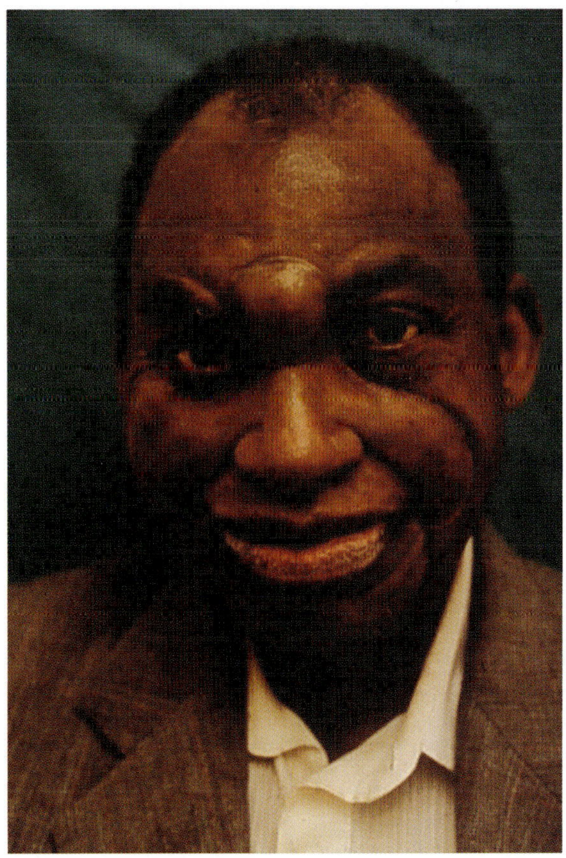

Figure 22.53 The facial prosthesis snaps onto the O-rings and engages the three magnets in the obturator in the nasal area. *Source:* Evans *et al.*, 1996.[45] Reproduced with permission from Elsevier.

facial prosthesis. The use of craniofacial implants improved this patient's quality of life and it should be noted that he sang in his church choir.[45]

Related advances in technology for cranionfacial implant-retained restorations

Computer-guided implant placement had its beginnings in intraoral prosthodontics. However, the same concept has been demonstrated in extraoral prosthetics. Van der Meer *et al.*[46] described digital presurgical planning of the implant placement and the achievement of a satisfactory surgical and prosthodontic result. The use of rapid prototyping (RP), stereolithography (STL), and modeling have allowed for digital design of maxillofacial prostheses. From imaging techniques like CT and magnetic resonance imaging (MRI), hard and soft tissues can be captured and the information converted using software into a RP or STL model. When indicated, mirror imaging of the unaffected side can be utilized to assist in the reconstruction of the craniofacial defect. Digital files of noses and other facial structures could be helpful in creating prostheses when native tissues are lost due to trauma.

Traditional moulage techniques have the disadvantage of distortion and inaccuracy. CT and MRI for sterolithography have the disadvantage of not capturing soft tissue detail. Recent advances in the area of craniofacial prostheses have been reported by the US Naval Postgraduate Dental School in Bethesda where digital capture of the facial structures with photogrammetry techniques has been succesful. Image capture, using 3dMDface™ Imaging, is fast and captures tissues in their natural state. The 3-D image capture has been utilized in the fabrication of a facial prosthesis by taking the photo data and storing it in a format to fabricate rapid prototype models. The files are exported as a virtual reality modeling language file (VRML). The VRML files are imported to create both a STL and 3-D printed RP model. The RP models can be duplicated and the duplication poured in type 4 stone for prosthesis fabrication.[47,48] Advances in digital technology are having a remarkable impact in the specialty of prosthodontics by providing patients with high-quality implant-retained prostheses.

Summary

There are numerous advantages of implant-retained craniofacial prostheses over the conventional adhesive-retained prostheses. The use of implants to restore facial defects caused by trauma, disease, or congenital abnormality has had a profound impact and revolutionized the subspecialty of maxillofacial prosthetics. A review of the classic literature provides the understanding of how craniofacial implant-retained restorations developed and came to North America in the mid 1980s. The classic and current literature provides a discussion of challenges with implant-retained prostheses, such as bone quality, irradiation versus no radiotherapy, dosage of radiation, survival rate due to site of implant placement, anatomic limitations, soft tissue complications, and prosthetic limitations due to improper implant placement. Presurgical planning for the craniofacial implant-retained prosthesis is critical, just as appropriate presurgical planning is required for all dental implants. The surgical placement of craniofacial implants has been reviewed. Important prosthodontic principals for nasal, auricular, orbital, and midfacial prostheses has been provided. Emerging technology in the area of presurgical planning, digital capture of the facial defect and design of the definitive craniofacial prosthesis continues to change the traditional practice of maxillofacial prosthetics. The advances of implant-retained craniofacial prostheses and emerging technology have had an impact on these patients' quality of life.

Postscript

A few months after Dr. Robert Ferguson Wright, lead author, submitted this chapter, he died suddenly at his home in Chapel Hill, North Carolina. He was a valued friend as well as a gifted educator and clinician. His penchant was a devotion to life-long learning while generously contributing to the scientific community. After completing his DDS degree at the University of Memphis, he continued his postgraduate education in prosthodontics at LSU Health Sciences Center and a maxillofacial prosthetics residency at Memorial Sloan Kettering Cancer Center. He held academic positions at Columbia University, Harvard University, and, most recently, at University of North Carolina. Robert was an active participant in the American College of Prosthodontics, the Academy of Prosthodontics, the Greater New York Academy of Prosthodontics, and the American Society of Dental Educators. He possessed an exceptional balance between his head and his heart and was a role model for his students and colleagues. I am most grateful that his scholarly work is featured in this chapter serving as a testament to his craft.

Steven J. Sadowsky

References

1. Beumer J III, Marunick MT, Esposito SJ. *Maxillofacial Rehabilitation*, 3rd edn. Hanover Park, IL: Quintessence Publishing 2011.
2. Del Valle V, Wolfaardt J, Tan H. Mechanical evaluation of craniofacial osseointegration retention Systems. *Int J Oral Maxillofac Implants* 1995; **10**(4): 491–498.
3. Parel SM, Branemark PI, Tjellstrom A, *et al.* Osseointegration in maxillofacial prosthetics. Part II: extraoral applications. *J Prosthet Dent* 1986; **55**(5): 600–606.
4. Schweiger JW, Wright RF. Maxillofacial prosthetic rehabilitation. In: Meyers EN (ed). *Cancer of the Head and Neck*. New York: Churchill Livingstone 1989.

5. Abu-Serriah MM, McGowan DA, Moos KF, *et al.* Extra-oral endosseous craniofacial implants: current status and future developments. *Int J Oral Maxillofac Surg* 2003; **32**(5): 452–458.
6. Tjellstrom A, Tonchev E, Lindstrom J, *et al.* Five years experience with bone-anchored auricular prostheses. *Otolaryngol Head Neck Surg* 1985; **93**(3): 366–372.
7. Wazen JJ, Wright RF, Hatfield RB, *et al.* Auricular rehabilitation with bone-anchored titanium implants. *Laryngo* 1999; **109**: 523–527.
8. Evans JH, Schweiger JW, Wright RF. Craniofacial osseointegration of a large midfacial bone-anchored combination maxillofacial prosthesis: a clinical report. *J Prosthet Dent* 1996; **75**(5): 483–486.
9. Fee Willard. *Head and Neck Cancer.* Philadelphia, PA: B.C. Decker 1990.
10. Cheng, AC, Leong E, Khin NT, *et al.* Osseointegrated implants in craniofacial application: current status. *Singapore Dent J* 2007; **29**(1): 8–18.
11. Esposito M, Hirsch J, Lekholm U, *et al.* Biological factors contributing to failures of osseointegrated oral implants. (I). Success criteria and epidemiology. *Eur J Oral Sci* 1998; **106**(1): 721–764.
12. Abu-Serriah MM, McGowan DA, Moos KF, *et al.* Outcome of extra-oral craniofacial endosseous implants. *Br J Oral Maxillofac Surg* 2001; **39**(5): 269–275.
13. Wright RF, Zemnick C, Wazen JJ, *et al.* Osseointegrated implants and auricular defects: retrospective case series study. *J Prosthodont* 2008; **17**(6): 468–475.
14. Roumanas E, Nishimura R, Beumer III J, *et al.* Craniofacial defects and osseointegrated implants: six year follow-up report on the success rates of craniofacial implants at UCLA. *Int J Oral Maxillofac Implants* 1994; **9**: 579–585.
15. Wolfaardt JF, Wilkes GH, Parel SM, *et al.* Craniofacial osseointegration: the Canadian experience. *Int J Oral Maxillofac Implants* 1993; **8**(2): 197–204.
16. Roumanas ED, Freymiller EG, Chang TL, *et al.* Implant-retained prostheses for facial defects: an up to 14-year follow-up report on the survival rates of implants at UCLA. *Int J Prosthodont* 2002; **15**(4): 325–332.
17. Toljanic JA, Eckert SE, Roumanas E, *et al.* Osseointegrated craniofacial implants in the rehabilitation of orbital defects: an update of a retrospective experience in the United States. *J Prosthet Dent* 2005; **94**(2): 177–182.
18. Granstrom G. Osseointegration in irradiated cancer patients: an analysis with respect to implant failures. *J Oral Maxillofac Surg* 2005; **63**(5): 579–585.
19. Nishimura RD, Roumanas E, Sugai T, *et al.* Auricular prostheses and osseointegrated implants: UCLA experience. *J Prosthet Dent* 1995; **73**(6): 553–558.
20. Nishimura RD, Roumanas E, Moy PK, *et al.* Nasal defects and osseointegrated implants: UCLA experience. *J Prosthet Dent* 1996: **76**(6): 597–602.
21. Nishimura RD, Roumanas E, Moy PK, *et al.* Osseointegrated implants and orbital defects: UCLA experience. *J Prosthet Dent* 1998; **79**(3): 304–309.
22. Scolozzi P, Jaques P. Treatment of midfacial defects using prostheses supported by ITI dental implants. *Plast Reconstr Surg* 2004; **114**(6): 1395–1404.
23. Tolman DE, Taylor PF. Bone-anchored craniofacial prosthesis study: irradiated patients. *Int J Oral Maxillofac Implants* 1996: **11**(5): 612–619.
24. Parel S. Tjellstrom A. The United States and Swedish experience with osseointegration and facial prostheses. *Int J Oral Maxillofac Implants* 1991; **6**(1): 75–79.
25. Schoen, PJ, Raghoebar GM, Van Oort RP, *et al.* Treatment outcome of bone-anchored craniofacial prostheses after tumor surgery. *Cancer* 2001; **92**(12): 3045–3050.
26. Granstrom G. Radiotherapy, osseointegration and hyperbaric oxygen therapy. *Periodontology* 2000; **33**: 145–162.
27. Asikainen P, Klementti E, Kotilaninen R, *et al.* Osseointegration of dental implants in bone irradiated with 40,50, or 60 Gy doses. An experimental study with beagle dogs. *Clin Oral Implants Res* 1998; **9**: 20–25.
28. Colella G, Cannavale R, Pentenero M, *et al.* Oral implants in radiated patients: a systematic review. *Int J Oral Maxillofac Implants* 2007; **22**(4): 616–622.
29. Parel SM, Tjellstrom A. The United States and Swedish experience with osseointegration and facial prostheses. *Int J Oral Maxillofac Implants* 1991; **6**(1): 75–79.
30. Tolman DE, Taylor PF. Bone-anchored craniofacial prosthesis study: irradiated patients. *Int J Oral Maxillofac Implants* 1996: **11**(5): 612–619.
31. Granstrom G, Tjellstrom A, Branemark PI, *et al.* Bone-anchored reconstruction of the irradiated head and neck cancer patient. *Otolaryngol Head Neck Surg* 1993: **108**(4): 334–343.
32. Beumer III J, Roumanans E, Nishimura RD. Advances in osseointegrated implants for dental and facial rehabilitation following major head and neck surgery. *Seminars in Surgical Oncol* 1995; **11**(3): 200–207.
33. Kindwall EP, Gottlieb LJ, Larson DL. Hyperbaric oxygen therapy in plastic surgery: a review article. *Plastic and Reconstruc Surg* 1991; **88**(5): 898–908.
34. Niimi A, Fujimoto T, Nosaka Y, *et al.* A Japanese multi-center study of osseointegrated implants placed in irradiated tissues: a preliminary report. *Int J Oral Maxillofac Implants* 1997: **12**(2): 259–264.
35. Niimi A, Ueda M, Keller EE, *et al.* Experience with osseointegrated implants placed in irradiated tissues in Japan and the United States. *Int J Oral Maxillofac Implants* 1998: **13**(3): 407–411.
36. Larsen PE, Stronczek MJ, Beck FM, *et al.* Osteointegration of implants in radiated bone with and without adjunctive hyperbaric oxygen. *J Oral Maxillofac Surg* 1993; **51**(3): 280–287.
37. Beumer III J, Ma T, Marunick M, *et al.* Restoration of facial defects etiology, disability and rehabilitation. In: Beumer III J, Curtis TA, Marunick MT (eds). *Maxillofacial Rehabilitation: Prosthodontic and Surgical Considerations.* St. Louis: Ishiyaku EuroAmerica 1996.
38. Kovacs AF, Wagner M. Orbital prostheses anchored by dental implants. *Rev Med Hosp Gen Mex* 1999; **62**(1): 22–25.
39. Tjellstrom A. Osseointegrated systems and their applications in the head and neck. *Adv Otolaryngol Head Neck Surg* 1989; **3**: 39–70.
40. Tjellstrom A. Osseointegrated implants for replacement of absent or defective ears. *Clinics in Plastic Surgery* 1990; **17**(2): 355–366.
41. Federspil PA. Implant-retained craniofacial prostheses for facial defects. *GMS Curr Top Otorhinolaryngol Head Neck Surg* 2009; **8**: Doc03.
42. Cochlear Vistafix. *Treatment and Surgery Guide* [manual]. Englewood CO: Cochlear Americas 2012.
43. Karakoca S, Aydin C, Yilmaz H, *et al.* Survival rates and periimplant soft tissue evaluation of extraoral implants over a mean follow-up period of three years. *J Prosthet Dent* 2008; **100**(6): 458–464.

44. Hatfield R, Frias VV, Wazen JJ, *et al.* A radiation-shielding device for craniofacial implant placement. *J Prosthet Dent* 2001; **86**(4): 348–351.
45. Evans JH, Schweiger JW, Wright RF. Craniofacial osseointegration of a large midfacial bone-anchored combination maxillofacial prosthesis: a clinical report. *J Prosthet Dent* 1996; **75**(5): 483-486.
46. Vander Meer WJ, Vissink A, Raghoebar GM, Visser A. Digitally designed surgical guides for placing extra-oral implants in the mastoid area. *Int J Oral Maxillofac Implants* 2012; **27**(3): 703–707.
47. Sabol JV, Grant GT, Liacouras P, *et al.* Digital image capture and rapid prototyping of the maxillofacial defect. *J Prosthodont* 2011; **20**(4): 310–314.
48. Grant GT, Aita-Holmes C, Liacouras P, *et al.* Digital capture, design, and manufacturing of a facial prosthesis: clinical report on a pediatric patient. *J Prosthet Dent* 2015; **114**(1): 138–141.

CHAPTER 23

Peri-Implant Diseases

Brian Kucey[1] and Elena Hernandez-Kucey[2]

[1] Private Practice in Prosthodontics, Edmonton, Alberta, Canada
[2] Private Practice in General Dentistry, Edmonton, Alberta, Canada

Introduction

Osseointegration is defined as a direct structural and functional connection between ordered, living bone, and the surface of a load-carrying implant.[1] There has been an exponential increase in the number of implants placed and the number of practitioners using dental implants. At the same time, there has been an extrapolation from full-arch treatment for the edentulous patient to single and multi-unit restorations in partially edentulous patients. Concurrently, a change from the initial model of osseointegration involving oral surgeons and prosthodontists to the entire range of providers has evolved. Among the many challenges facing implant dentistry is the goal to maintain and improve treatment outcomes, subjectively and objectively. It is inherent that in the treatment of human beings, despite all efforts, complications will arise. Identification of risk factors to reduce morbidity is paramount.

Executing an optimal plan is essential from the clinician's perspective, in order to achieve a level of outcome within current expectations. Practitioners agree that patient satisfaction is optimized when we prevent or reduce the incidence of clinical complications, particularly those which result in pain and/or implant loss (osseoseparation). Many quality-of-life (QOL) and patient reported outcome measures (PROMs) surveys have been published,[2,3] which have provided consumer insight of implant dentistry in addition to the goals of the clinician. Although the patient's perspective can be significantly different from the clinician's goals, it is our responsibility to educate the patient on the factors that enhance the treatment outcome, including appropriate and regular maintenance. Optimal health around a dental implant restoration is dependent on a balance between osseointegration and healthy peri-implant tissues (void of inflammation, bleeding, bacterial pathogens, pain, and suppuration). Peri-implant diseases are pathologic inflammatory changes that alter this healthy relationship and include reversible and irreversible soft and/or hard tissue changes originating in the marginal peri-implant sulcus, which can lead to ailing (minor complications), failing, and failed (major complications) implants. Potential risk indicators for peri-implant diseases include poor oral hygiene, smoking, history of periodontitis, diabetes, genetic traits, alcohol consumption, and implant surface.[4] The patient (systemic diseases), dental history (periodontitis), social habits (oral hygiene, smoking, drug abuse), and parafunctional habits are each influential in the changes that arise following osseointegration. Additionally, poor restoration design, residual cement, failing components, and trauma can lead to an untoward result.

This chapter provides insight into the diagnosis and treatment of the spectrum of diseases that afflict soft and hard tissues surrounding previously stable and healthy implants with the goal of helping to provide the clinician with evidence-based techniques to minimize and address complications.

Peri-implant diseases

Following confirmation that osseointegration has been achieved, the final restoration has been delivered, and the implant is in function, further remodeling occurs contingent on the patient's physiologic adaptive capacity. Unfavorable changes to the health of the soft and hard tissues surrounding the implant are defined as peri-implant diseases. Peri-implant diseases have been classified as peri implant mucositis and peri-implantitis.[5] A less common condition, apical peri implantitis, has been excluded from this discussion.

Distinction between natural tooth and implant attachment complex

Gingival tissues and osseous attachments differ between natural teeth and implants (Table 23.1). At the surface of an implant, the connective tissue fibers run parallel to the abutment, circumferentially around the implant to form a gingival cuff. They have a

Evidence-based Implant Treatment Planning and Clinical Protocols, First Edition. Edited by Steven J. Sadowsky.

Companion website: www.wiley.com/go/sadowsky/implant

Table 23.1 Natural tooth vs. implant gingival complex and attachment mechanism.

	Healthy natural tooth	Stable osseointegrated implant
Epithelial anatomy	Circular and trans-septal fibers connected to cementum	Collagen fibers parallel to implant with hemidesmosomes
Subepithelial anatomy	Fibroblasts and vessels	More collagen and less fibroblasts/vessels
Biological width	2.04 mm to base of sulcus	2.04 mm
Bone attachment	Lamina dura, periodontal ligament, cementum	Direct contact of osteoid to implant surface
Sulcus depth	0.69 mm plus proximal bone position	0.69 mm plus implant design and position effect
Gingival biotype	Thick or thin	Variable
Crevicular fluid	Plasma proteins, desquamating epithelial cells, neutrophilic granulocytes, and monocytes	Same
Inflamed gingival crevice	Bacterial toxins, endotoxins, lysosomal proteases, collagenolysis	Same
Color of gingival tissues	Coral pink, firmly bound to underlying periosteum of the alveolar bone	Same
Keratinized tissue attachment	2 mm minimum for maintaining periodontal health	Considerable disagreement exists as to how much is necessary around implants
Principal attachment mechanism	Sharpey's fibers from alveolus to cementum	Osteocytes, collagen bundles, glycoprotein layer, titanium oxide

tenuous adhesion relative to the strong attachment of connective tissue fibers on a natural tooth. This results in differences in susceptibility to bacterial invasion and pathways of healing as compared to natural teeth. Natural tooth connective tissue attachment can also limit a disease process laterally, as we observe with a cracked tooth. There is no periodontal ligament or crevicular fluid flow surrounding an osseointegrated implant. The junctional epithelium attachment surrounding an implant is dependent on desmosomes and hemidesmosomes.[6]

Optimal health around a dental implant restoration assumes successful osseointegration to bone, healthy soft tissues void of inflammation, bleeding or suppuration, and the presence of adequate keratinized tissue. Inflammatory and noninflammatory peri-implant diseases alter this healthy relationship and include reversible and nonreversible soft or hard tissue changes originating in the marginal peri-implant sulcus.

History

The Swedish National Board of Health and Welfare provided a formal assessment of osseointegrated implants in 1975.[7] The first widely sourced criteria for implant success was the US NIH (National Institute of Health) Harvard Consensus Development Conference (1978)[8] but this did not include osseointegrated implants, as only one center had reported their use (Brånemark). The first published criteria of success for osseointegrated implants was by Albrektsson *et al.*[9] which was based on Brånemark implant data. The five listed criteria lacked detail regarding the peri-implant soft tissue. One millimeter of vertical bone loss following the first year and then less than 0.2 mm of annual bone loss after the first year of service was the benchmark. A minimum of 85% (5 year) and 80% (10 year) success was proposed for the anterior mandible (zone 1). This was a significant increase in success from the NIH Conference. At the 10th anniversary Toronto Conference (1992)[10], Adell[11] reported at 15 years the annual bone loss of 0.1 mm after healing and remodeling periods.

Albrektsson and Zarb[12] updated the criteria of success and suggested that every implant in a reported study be evaluated as part of a four-grade scale (success, survival, unaccounted for, failures). The 1986 standard was applied to the posterior mandible and maxillae (zone 2). They proposed zone 1 success be increased to 85% (10 year) and 90% (5 year).

Peri-implant disease has been reported to be effectively managed with strict recall, even in patients with tobacco use and a history of periodontitis.[13] With close recare follow-ups, marginal bone loss was reported after the first year at 0.9 mm, then 0.05–0.07 mm/year.[14–16] With standard treatment follow-ups, the mean total bone loss was 0.16 mm/year.[17]

Adell[18] summarized the Brånemark experience in four points: implant survival may not be the same as implant success, osseointegration needs a long time to be established (over 12 months), care for the host tissue is paramount, and all requirements for osseointegration to occur must be maintained under control for the long term. Implant recare was also categorized as either one, two, or multiple visits per year.

The references listed above reported the outcomes of machined-surface external hex implants only. Considering the advent of moderately roughened implant surfaces, the previous criteria for implant success may no longer be acceptable. Numerous factors have been documented to influence marginal bone loss (MBL) surrounding dental implants.[19]

In addition, lack of a standardized methodology prevents systematic review of the majority of published studies. Some argue that cohort study results concerning MBL might be closer to daily implant practice reality than evidence-based randomized clinical trials (RCTs).[20]

A paradigm shift from bone only to prioritize soft tissue concerns

The criteria of success for osseointegrated implants concentrated on rates and extent of radiographic bone loss and marginalized concern with mucositis, as there were little available data regarding the peri-implant epithelium at the time. The causal relationship between oral microflora (biofilm) and peri-implant disease as a pathway of implant failure was drawn from periodontal literature. There was weak evidence that plaque accumulations cause inflammation of the peri-implant mucosa analogous to gingivitis. Bone-based research by Brånemark and colleagues left questions as to the barrier function of the junctional epithelium surrounding dental implants, particularly when it is compromised during inflammation.[21]

In spite of the fact that the data were not compelling to construct a periodontal model for peri-implant disease, similarities have been noted.[22] Given the ubiquity of peri-implant disease, there may have been a rush to judgment to explain the etiology. The prevalence of peri-implant mucositis has been reported as high as 80% of the subjects and surrounding 50% of the implants. Peri-implantitis was reported to occur in 28–56% of subjects affecting 12–43% implant sites.[23]

The term peri-implantitis describing peri-implant soft tissue inflammation with subsequent destruction of bone was published in 1965 by Levignac.[24] The terms "peri-implant mucositis" and "peri-implantitis" were introduced in 1993.[25] Although the periodontium and peri-implant tissues have significant architectural differences, the same bacterial pathogens that afflict the natural dentition seem to be related to peri-implant diseases. It has been postulated recently that marginal bone loss surrounding oral implants is, in reality, a foreign body response in contrast to a periodontitis-like disease. Albrektsson *et al.*[26] did admit that following severe marginal bone loss, a secondary bacteria-mediated infection may follow as a complication to the already established bone loss.

The term "osseoseparation" has been proposed to describe "crestal and interfacial bone–implant interface degradation."[27] There is a philosophical disagreement between the progression of peri-implant diseases and its relation to the eventual complete failure of osseointegration.

Biofilm

As early as 1978, the medical community stated that chronic infections in patients with implantable devices were caused by biofilms.[28,29] Dental plaque is a biofilm which encourages bacterial proliferation on both teeth and implants. The formation of biofilm is multi-stage, initiating with pellicle attachment to enamel and implants, followed by binding proteins, which promote the adhesion of bacteria and secretions of the extracellular polysaccharides to allow aggregation of bacterial colonies. Mature plaque behaves as a complex microorganism and changes in composition as probing depth increases.[30] If the implant surface is exposed, roughness significantly contributes to plaque build-up. The implant–abutment microgap is also a potential source of microbial contamination affecting the surrounding tissue health. The microbiota colonized in completely edentulous implant patients is different than that in partially edentulous implant patients.[31] In patients with a history of periodontal disease, the microbiota on implants is similar to that found in periodontal pockets around teeth, which may indicate a susceptibility to peri-implant disease.[32] Biofilms have strong bonds which require regular effective mechanical and chemical intervention to disrupt.

Peri-implant mucositis (PIM) and peri-implantitis (PI)

PIM presents as chronic or acute soft tissue reversible inflammatory changes (redness, swelling, bleeding on probing, increased supracrestal pocket depth) without concomitant loss of supporting bone (Figures 23.1 and 23.2). Suppuration and fistula may or may not be present. There may be mobility of the

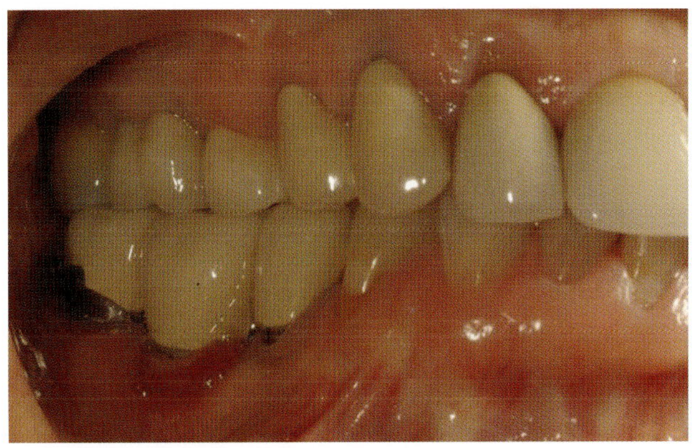

Figure 23.1 Clinical photograph of peri-implant mucositis lower right molar.

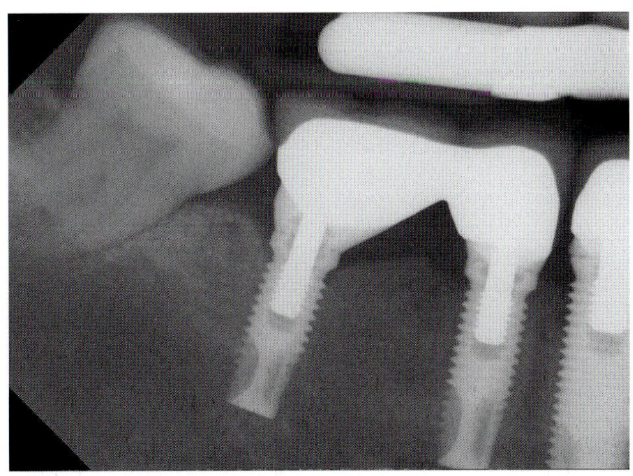

Figure 23.2 Peri-implant mucositis radiograph lower right first molar.

restoration or restorative components but this does not include mobility of the implant. Pain is limited to soft tissue.

PI has been defined as site-specific infectious disease with inflammatory changes in soft tissues and bone around a dental implant and/or its abutment in function (Figures 23.3 and 23.4).[33] Most clinicians agree that PI is a "progression" of PIM with an increase in pocket depth (subcrestal changes), bleeding on probing, presence of suppuration (exudate) with or without fistula, possible pain or discomfort, and progressive radiographically determined bone loss.[34] The definition disagreements hinge on the presence of suppuration and the percentage of bone loss around the crestal area of the implant. PI is, therefore, a progressive condition following unresolved PIM, with bony defects of increasing dimensions that ultimately could result in complete loss of osseointegration. A proposed subclassification for peri-implantitis as early, moderate, and advanced has been made.[35]

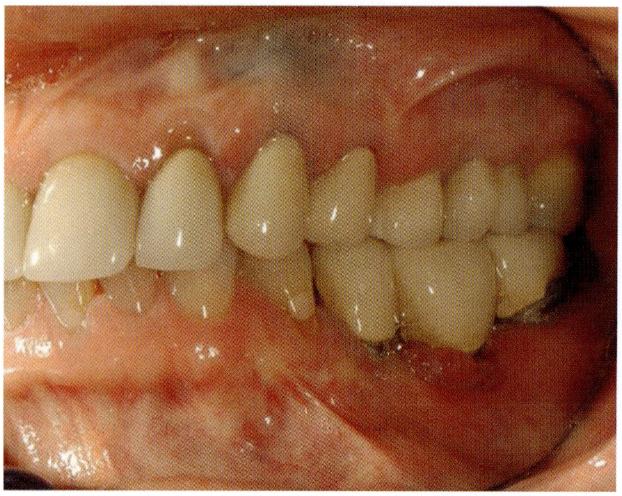

Figure 23.3 Clinical photograph of peri-implantitis in lower left first molar.

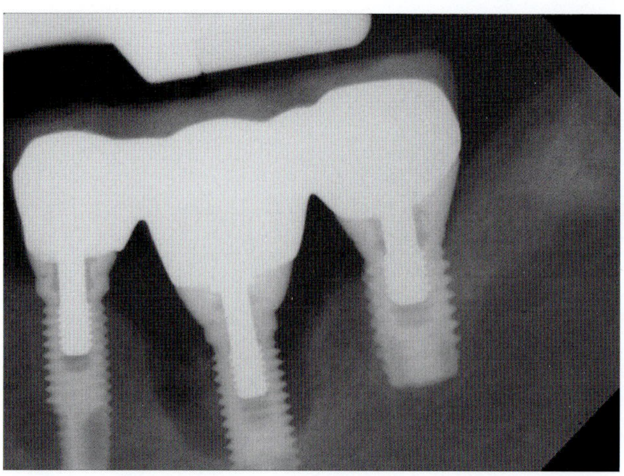

Figure 23.4 Radiograph peri-implantitis lower left molar.

Both PIM and PI are considered pathologic conditions, often initiated by bacterial insult/origin, and further complicated by trauma, such as occlusal load factors acting in concert,[36] implant surface,[37] and changes to host resistance related to systemic diseases, medications, and smoking.[38] Furthermore, food impaction or foreign object trauma (cement, floss, dental impression materials, oral hygiene aids), with or without plaque around the peri-implant sulcus, may lead to acute or chronic changes to the peri-implant soft tissue health.

Diagnosis

A baseline of data related to the original presentation of the individual implant prior to restoration, the implant restoration, soft tissue, bone levels, clinical presentation of abutment and restoration margin, emergence profile, interproximal contacts, occlusion, pre-load torque, cement type, etc. is necessary to compare findings at subsequent maintenance examinations. Diagnostic tests include accurate updated dental and medical history, evaluation of oral hygiene, probing, serial sequential radiographs, clinical photography, tissue margin changes, torque test, percussion test, bacterial assay,[39] floss/shim stock test, articulating paper/shim stock to test occlusion, and test of passive framework fit (Table 23.2). Direct visual inspection of the implant by removal of the prosthesis is recommended when other tests are inconclusive.

Radiographic signs

A sign of a peri-implantitis lesion commonly includes radiographic changes, usually "saucer-shaped" cratering or vertical changes to the crestal bone, with a normal appearance in the remaining apical portion of the implant. There may be concomitant bleeding and suppuration on probing with inflammation and hyperplasia of the peri-implant tissues. An associated symptom of pain may be related to an overlying acute infection.

A periapical radiograph 90° to the implant long axis (orthogonal) continues to be the gold standard for assessing subgingival component fit and proximal bone/implant levels. However, it does not provide information regarding bone position on the labial and lingual aspects of the implant. The original Brånemark research team advocated removal of the prostheses annually and two periapical radiographs at 90° to the long axis of the implant, with one of the radiographs with a 5° variation to account for thread pitch. Although it has been suggested that radiographic tube head angulation error within 20° will result in an acceptable radiograph for the external hex implant,[40] others have stated that analysis of interface discrepancies becomes subjective when tube angulation error exceeds 5°.[41] With the popularity of cemented restorations and numerous internal connection designs, removal of the restoration and/or abutment is not possible or recommended. A paralleling device indexed on the head of the implant and adjacent teeth by occlusal registration

Table 23.2 Diagnostic checklist for peri-implant disease.

	Healthy	Pathologic but potentially reversible	Pathologic and irreversible
Patient concerns	None	Patient awareness	Patient experiencing pain or other symptoms
Medical history update	Unchanged	Changes/unrelated	Changes affect implant
Evaluation of oral hygiene effectiveness	Good	Fair	Poor
Evaluation of tissue health: Loe & Silness Gingival index (0–3)	Mild inflammation: 0	Moderate inflammation: 1	Severe Inflammation: 2–3
Probing depth	Minimal (0–2 mm)	2–4 mm	>4–6 mm
Bleeding on probing (BOP)	None	Light to moderate	Heavy
Quantity and quality of keratinized tissue	Present and keratinized	Reduced	Reduced/absent with sequelae
Gingival recession	None	Slight recession	Advanced recession
Trauma, redness, inflammation in gingival tissues	None	Slight, reversible – asymptomatic	Severe, chronic/acute – symptomatic
Peri-implant tissue mobility	None	Mild–moderate mobility	Severe mobility
Implant restoration stability	Stable	Suspected movement	Obvious instability
Presence of food impaction	None	Occasional	Chronic
Interproximal contact	Normal	Weak	Open
Residual peri-implant cement	None	Suspected or asymptomatic	Present and symptomatic
Titanium tattoo	None	Suspected	Present
Radiographic bone changes	No change	Change within expectations	Change beyond expectations
Presence of suppuration or fistula	None	Suspected	Present/recurring
Assessment of occlusion	Normal	Heavy contacts without micromotion	Heavy contact with micromotion
Presence of pain or discomfort	None	Mild/tissue	Moderate to severe/bone
Lymphadenopathy	None	None	If present, acute emergency
Mobility of the implant	None	Suspected	Present and irreversible
Presence of pathogenic bacteria (assay)	None	Present	Present
Passivity of restoration	Passive	Early strain suspected	Non-passive, rocking or spinning of restoration, cracking of veneering materials

material and a conventional film-holding device (Rinn XCP, Dentsply Rinn, York, PA) at the time of restoration delivery has been advocated. On subsequent radiographic examinations, the paralleling device can be repositioned with the occlusal index without requiring removal of the restoration. An additional observation was, regardless of whether or not the device was applied, the clinicians in the study incorrectly identified misfit up to 30%.[42] Preservation and storage of the paralleling device is a logistical concern.

An alternative method to provide predictable radiographic tube positioning is to observe the occlusal screw access restoration for posterior units and to make slight adjustments with tube head if there is a variation from the long axis of the adjacent teeth. For anterior implants, it can be assumed that the angulation of the implant is similar to the long axis of the adjacent teeth, as the majority of these restorations will be cemented. Following the exposure of the digital intraoral radiograph, the tube head and sensor should remain in position relative to the patient for predictable angulation modification, if required. In comparison, film-based radiographs require not only additional time but increase errors with film replacement, time of developing, and operator and patient movement.

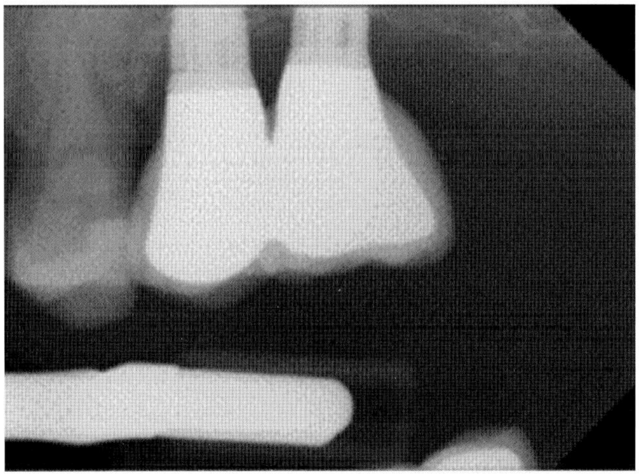

Figure 23.5 Slight abutment misfit on anterior implant with mucositis.

A fistula at implant–restoration level without suppuration may indicate a non-seated restoration, component misfit (Figure 23.5), trapped debris (compressed particulate graft) between the implant and restoration (Figure 23.6), or thin peri-implant soft tissue.

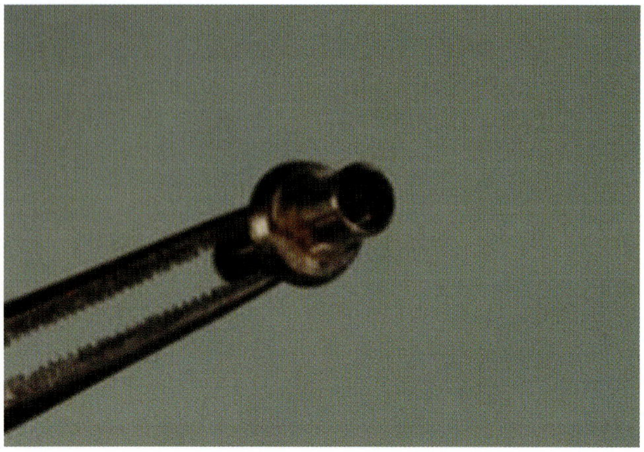

Figure 23.6 Debris identified on inferior surface of abutment.

Percussion tests

Percussion tests using a metal instrument on individual implants, such as a mirror handle, were advocated by the Brånemark research group, with the result similar to that of an ankylosed tooth (sharp sound). A lower tone pitch on an implant may indicate loss of osseointegration. This testing method requires removal of the prosthesis in a complete-arch restoration and is not quantitative or reproducible. Once the prosthesis is removed, the test will be applied either to the abutment or directly to the implant. A loose abutment screw problem needs to be eliminated prior to testing for implant stability. Percussion testing of single-tooth implant restorations or short-span implant bridges may suggest loss of pre-load torque to prosthetic and/or abutment screws and/or loss of osseointegration without removal of the restoration. This test has been refined with resonance frequency analysis (RFA) instruments (Osstell, Goteborg, Sweden) to determine an "implant stability quotient" (ISQ) which may relate to micromotion of the implant and/or components.[43,44] The challenge for single-tooth implant diagnosis is whether there is movement between the restoration and the implant (i.e. loss of abutment screw pre-load or decementation), or loss of osseointegration. The use of RFA in relationship to long-term implant component fatigue has not been established. The mirror handle test remains a simple and accessible clinical diagnostic aid in assessing osseointegration.

Bacteriological testing

Bacteriological testing/microbiological sampling has been advocated in diagnosis of periodontal diseases and dental implants. The BANA (benzoyl-DL-arginine-naphthylamide) test, DNA probes, and immunological reagents are being studied for detection of anaerobic periodontal infections[45] and may be useful in the diagnosis of peri-implant pathogens.[46,47]

Some investigations regarding the effect of interleukin-1 gene cluster (IL1A, IL1B) and the IL1RN gene on peri-implant health have shown a higher risk of peri-implant diseases in positive-risk genotype patients.[48]

Suppuration/exudate

The presence of sulcular exudate with or without a fistula has been discussed in the literature as a significant finding in the transition from peri-implant mucositis to peri-implantitis.[49] Recent reports show that crevicular fluid tests can now identify progression from health to mucositis to peri-implantitis.[50] Studies analyzing possible markers distinguishing mucositis (with ability to resolve lesion) from implantitis (impaired healing and prolonged inflammation) have suggested tissue plasminogen activators are specific to predict changes in marginal bone. Clinical presentation may include inflammation and redness, with or without discharge.

Occlusion

Use of shim stock and articulating film/paper/ribbon/tape for axial and nonaxial load analysis is a commonly utilized test for both natural teeth and implant restorations. An electronic device has been proposed for diagnosis of occlusion but has a lack of evidence to support its use. Assessment of opposing natural teeth in fremitus, testing for screw loosening, evaluating veneering materials fracture,[51] and identifying wear faceting of restorations, all may be important disclosers of overload.

At the time of implant restoration delivery, it is well accepted for the partially edentulous patient there should be no contact with the opposing dentition using shim stock. If using some type of articulating film, there should also be lighter contact on the implant restorations compared with natural teeth. The rationale for this theorem is extended from the fact that a periodontal ligament is absent in osseointegration. A debate continues as to how much occlusal relief is appropriate.

During implant recare, the occlusal contacts on restorations should be evaluated in a similar fashion. A significant finding is a change in the occlusal relief (shim stock) and the size of the contact(s) (articulating film). The proximal contacts should also be evaluated with shim stock and dental floss or tape. These findings are correlated with the radiographic findings. In cases where radiographic changes are not present, the occlusion may be left unaltered.

Occlusal overload has not been demonstrated to directly cause osseoseparation. However, it has been implicated in mechanical failure of screw-joint stability, and tensile strain, which may progress to implant fracture. On multiple implant restorations, determination of implant fracture may require removal of the restoration for diagnosis.

Parafunctional loading has been suspected as an etiological factor in mechanical failure of implants. Prescription of occlusal splint therapy has been suggested as a preventative measure in these patients.[52] However, there are no studies which clearly establish a relationship between bruxism, implant failure, and lack of occlusal splint wear. Occlusal splint wear continues to be recommended in selected bruxers based on expert opinion.[53,54]

Etiology

Although there is disagreement that all implant systems experience some bone loss after the first year post-surgically, occasionally some implants demonstrate much greater changes. Currently, there are several theories regarding causes of peri-implant disease, including bacterial infections, occlusal overload, trauma, incongruent restoration design, poor surgical placement or restoration, and host variables which can contribute to progressive bone loss, including changes in host resistance (immunosuppression or epigenetics), drug interactions (bisphosphonates, antidepressants), nutritional deficiencies, systemic diseases (diabetes), and smoking.[55] The etiology is subject to the health of the host and peri-implant tissue, implant design, presence of roughness, and excessive mechanical load. Misch summarized the etiology of the most common implant complications in his stress-based treatment plan theorem.[56]

Bacterial infections

Biologic causes of inflammatory peri-implant disease are related to the complex biofilm harboring numerous known microbes. Biofilm formation around implant surfaces occurs as early as 30 minutes after the implant is exposed to the oral cavity.[57] Osseointegration of the dental implant is influenced by surface roughness but greater surface roughness is directly linked to higher rate of biofilm formation surrounding the implant.[58] Apical migration of pathogenic bacteria with subsequent peri-implant soft tissue inflammation and progressive bone changes are thought to be more aggressive processes than sequelae of bacteria around natural teeth in periodontal disease.[59] Microflora surrounding implants with peri-implantitis have increased red and orange complex species as defined by Socransky.[60] The red complex species include *Porphyromonas gingivalis*, *Tannerella forsythia*, and *Treponema denticola,* and the orange complex species include *Fusobacterium nucleatum* and *Prevotella intermedia*. A fungal component, *Candida albicans*, has also been identified in bacterial assays and found to have increased adhesion to titanium implant surfaces.[61] Microbiota of the remaining natural teeth, particularly in the partially edentulous patient, serve as the primary source of causative pathogens and directly affect implants undergoing osseointegration.[62] Demonstrated susceptibility to periodontal disease appears to translate to increased susceptibility to peri-implantitis,[63,64] although patients under periodontal care and strict recare have been reported to have similarly high implant success.[13]

Mechanical factors

Mechanical causes of peri-implant disease include instability of the restoration, associated with loss of screw pre-load,[65–67] failure of cement retention of restoration,[68,69] failure to remove excess cement (Figures 23.7 and 23.8),[70,71] excessive contour of restoration,[72] prosthesis misfit,[73,74] and excessive depth of manufacturer implant–abutment interface,[75] hindering oral hygiene access and promoting pathogenic biofilm. Unfortunately, a lack of agreement on study design has left the profession with a conclusion that there is a lack of evidence to claim superiority for a single implant design or manufacturer. Touati[76] subdivided mechanical factors into implant related (design, surface, type of connection, and platform shifting) and prosthetic related (type of abutment connection, final abutment design, immediate provisionalization, interim abutment material and design, submergence profile, emergence profile, restoration anatomy, retention, possible excess cement, occlusion/excessive load). Lack of precision or passive fit between adjacent implant abutments can result in abutment and/or restoration loosening or fracturing, fracture of the implant, or interruption of osseointegration.[77] Impaction of foreign materials, including food particles, popcorn hulls, floss, and oral hygiene aids (brush bristles), can also cause mechanical irritation of the peri-implant tissues and this is not visible on radiographs.[78]

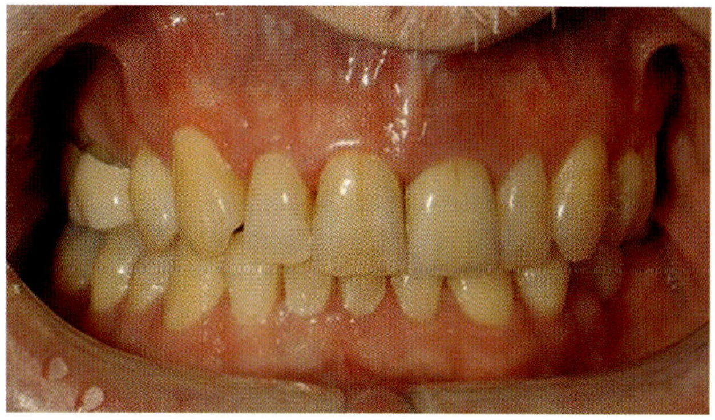

Figure 23.7 Clinical photograph of upper left central incisor implant with peri-implant mucositis due to residual cement.

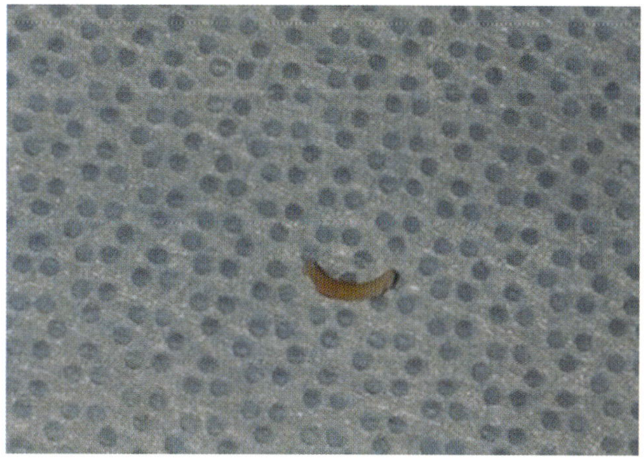

Figure 23.8 Clinical photograph of recovered residual cement fragment.

Occlusal overloading

Osseointegration changed the thinking again regarding occlusion. Several animal studies have indicated that occlusion is not a causative factor in loss of osseointegration. However, there is a lack of "shock absorption" due to the absence of a periodontal ligament around a dental implant. This means load is transmitted directly to the implant interface with the surrounding bone which, when excessive, can result in microfractures or loss of osseointegration, possibly by facilitating bacterial penetration. Crestal loads have been identified as the most concentrated, which incidentally is where initial bone change occurs. There is a wide variation of this sign of osseous change within implant designs. Lateral occlusal forces are considered more detrimental and most practitioners favor reducing lateral contacts in restoration design.

Occlusal overload is often referred to in the implant literature as a causative factor in peri-implant bone loss, or at least a cofactor along with biofilm. Occlusal overload is not listed in the Glossary of Prosthodontic Terms. However, "occlusal disharmony" is listed and occurs when contacts of opposing occlusal surfaces are not in harmony with other tooth contacts and/or the anatomic and physiologic components of the craniomandibular complex. "Occlusal trauma" has also been described as trauma to the periodontium from functional or parafunctional forces causing damage to the attachment apparatus of the periodontium by exceeding its adaptive and reparative capacities. It may be self-limiting or progressive.[79] No evidence currently exists that defines the load-bearing capability of a dental implant beyond its structural fatigue/load limits.[80] Overload was diagnosed in one study based on "the presence of parafunctional habits, radiographs, and clinical complications including screw loosening/fracture or prosthesis factor."[81] Parafunctional habits, such as bruxism, can exacerbate mechanical failure and wear,[82] but occlusal load or overload are not necessarily potential causes for late implant failure.

In the completely edentulous implant patient, occlusal overload can occur when the balance between the number of implants, their position, prosthesis design, and parameters of occlusion are not in harmony with the patients' functional loads, physiological adaptation, and habits. Occlusal overload for these patients is manifested by excessive prosthesis wear, screw loosening/fracture, and occasional implant fracture. Occlusal trauma can exacerbate existing peri-implant disease to create bone loss (angular or horizontal). Mechanical overload in the completely edentulous implant patient may result in early implant failures when osseointegration has not been established. In cases of late implant failures (after the first 18–24 months), occlusal overload is less likely to be the primary etiological factor.

In the partially edentulous implant patient, there is a wider range of the effect of occlusion depending on the stability and health of the natural dentition, the location of the implant(s) in the arch, the overall occlusal scheme, and whether a mutually protected occlusion exists prior to implant therapy. When dental implants are added to restore overall occlusal stability, the significance of occlusion is elevated. Dental providers must recognize and modify changes to the partially edentulous implant patient even more acutely than to the completely edentulous implant patient.

A debate centers on whether overloading occurs from normal forces on implants of inadequate mechanical strength, or whether the forces are abnormal on mechanically sound implant designs. Narrow-diameter implants with internal connections have been initially diagnosed as having early implantitis, only to show implant fracture subsequently. Taylor[80] has described these mechanical failures as hoop stresses from tangential stress distribution in the implant body which can be multiplied by axial loads. For external connection systems, similar mechanical failure has been reported at a level equal to the base of the abutment screw within the implant body.

Adjunctive splint therapy is recommended in patients with known bruxism parafunction habits by some practitioners, but has been refuted as effective by one paper recently.[83]

Trauma

Tissue irritation from trauma related to overzealous oral hygiene techniques, such as that seen with floss cuts,[78] toothpick use, and excessive brushing, can mimic peri-implant mucositis symptoms. Confirmation can be made by requesting the patient to demonstrate their hygiene technique. Modification of technique will usually solve the concern in a few days.

A continuous positive airway pressure machine hood can also place pressure on the maxillary anterior area peri-implant tissues and create a stomatitis from drying soft tissues. This can result in a chronic erythema around the marginal gingiva similar to that in mouth breathers.

Facial trauma involving implant restorations can result in fracturing of the veneering material, bent and/or broken screws, or damage to the implant body itself including a bent or fractured interface.[84] Soft tissue injury could also occur which may mimic peri-implant mucositis, although there may be underlying alveolar fractures which are difficult to visualize clinically or radiographically. Although there are limited publications in this area, it appears that due to the elasticity of the bone encasing the implant and osseointegration, the damage is often limited to the restoration.[85]

Growth

Incomplete growth and development of younger patients at the time of implant placement can result in future incorrect implant position compared to adjacent natural teeth, especially in the esthetic zone, due to subsequent changes in vertical facial growth affecting the dentition.[86] The best indicators of completion of growth to consider when planning implants in younger patients are referenced in the orthodontic literature. Continued skeletal changes affect implant/teeth position throughout life. The adjacent maxillary anterior natural teeth have been documented to extrude vertically and facially along with their proximal bone and soft tissues, resulting in a change in the abutment–restoration interface. This will result in an increased probing depth adjacent to the implant restoration and associated peri-implant soft tissue changes. There is no preventative solution for this concern, other than to inform patients of this possible long-term complication and make adjustments as required.

In the case of the completely edentulous implant patient, increase in residual ridge height of the body of the mandible has been documented in numerous cases directly under the cantilever portion of complete arch prostheses.[87,88] This change has been attributed to increased biting force permitted by the dental implant rehabilitation on the internal architecture of the trabeculae, followed by secondary changes to the external cortical portion of the bone (Wolff's Law). The modern explanation for this phenomenon is referred to as skeletal mechanotransduction,[89] a process through which forces or other mechanical signals are converted to biochemical signals in cellular signaling. Clinically, this apposition can severely restrict hygiene access, resulting in tissue hyperplasia and mucositis along the cantilever and surrounding the terminal implant. As a result, the design of the intaglio surface of the cantilever should permit long-term adjustment.

Restoration design

The design of implants and components continues to evolve. From single (one-piece) implants to multi-stage implants and back, a multitude of innovations and inventions has occurred. Superiority of connection interfaces and implant surfaces have been hotly contested but lack long-term evidence.

Intrusion of natural teeth splinted to implants has been mentioned in the literature and connecting natural teeth and implants is generally not recommended.[90,91] Use of individual copings and provisionally cemented restoration with nonrigid connectors may be indicated to facilitate retrievability.[92] Several authors have demonstrated short- to medium-term stability with teeth splinted to implants.[93]

Dental implants in partially edentulous patients are "immovable" objects surrounded by an ever changing dentition due to lifelong cranial growth. This phenomenon has resulted in change to the integrity of implant–tooth interproximal contacts, with resultant open contacts, food impaction (trauma), and soft tissue sequelae, such as peri-mucositis. For this reason, restoration design which allows retrievability and modification of interdental contacts is recommended, particularly for younger patients, those patients with poor occlusal stability, and posterior areas which will exhibit more total arch drift than anterior teeth.

Esthetic discoloration of circum-implant tissues

Circum-implant "titanium tattooing", resulting from mechanical failure of zirconia internal-connection implants, is a potentially serious complication, especially in the esthetic zone. Long-term studies of zirconia custom abutments have yet to appear. This complication has been linked only to internal-connection implants with zirconia abutments.[94] Alternative designs with a separate titanium interface have not demonstrated this complication to date.

Drug interactions

Although some authors have listed a significant risk for bisphosphonate-related osteonecrosis of the jaw (BRONJ), which would be manifested as chronic peri-implant mucositis, there does not appear to be a statistically significant risk for oral bisphosphonate therapy compared with intravenous bisphosphonate therapy.[95,96] A prolonged and close follow-up period has been recommended for these patients.[97]

Selective serotonin-reuptake inhibitors (SSRIs) are widely prescribed drugs in the treatment for depression, which have been reported to increase risk of bone fracture. Failure rates of SSRI patients were double that of nonSSRI patients, although small implant diameters and smoking were associated risk factors. A careful surgical treatment planning for SSRI users was recommended.[98,99]

Alcohol

The effect of alcohol on dental implant osseointegration has been reported in animal studies and indicates that a decreased bone–implant direct contact will result from excessive alcohol consumption.[100,101] Severe alcoholics have a high risk of periodontal disease which would be expected to extend to peri-implant diseases.[102] There are no published articles relating the effect of recreational or illicit drug use on dental implant treatments or peri-implant diseases. However, the clinician would be prudent to suspect other etiologies for chronic unresolved peri-implant diseases not listed in the patient's medical history.

Tobacco

A tobacco smoking habit has been implicated as a significant risk factor in peri-implant disease since the original Brånemark research was published. When comparing machined- (smooth) or rough-surface implant success, it appears that smoking is a risk factor in smooth-surface implants only.[103] Recent evidence points to an electrochemical change to the surface of the commercially pure titanium implant resulting from exposure to caffeine and nicotine, which leads to greater biofilm accumulation and increase in peri-implant disease.[104] Smokers are at higher risk for peri-implant mucositis and peri-implantitis by shaping the peri-implant microbiomes, even in states of clinical health, and supporting a pathogen-rich community which may indicate a need for personalized therapeutics.[105]

Systemic and oral conditions

Hyposalivation and xerostomia can be related to aging, but is often a drug-mediated condition.[106] A patient with three or more chronic diseases requiring drug intake is considered multi-morbid. Polypharmacy is commonly identified with xerostomia and its associated dental sequelae.

Cognitive impairment is a factor in reduced control of biofilm which can escalate to an increased risk of aspiration pneumonia in patients with dysphagia.[107] Although the natural dentition appears to be affected by rampant caries rates in patients with reduced salivary flow,[108] dental implants appear to be a successful treatment alternative for the failing dentition.[109] Autoimmune disorders, such as Sjogren's syndrome, can be challenging to manage clinically with the added difficulty of dry oral epithelium and the increased effects of biofilm.[110] However, there are scarce publications as to the long-term prognosis of implants in these patients.

The effect of aging and increased frailty is particularly significant, considering the rate at which the world population is aging. Whether the frail state exists rapidly through a sudden incident or acute disease, or through a slow and chronic pervasive change, the pathway requires intensive health maintenance over a prolonged and unpredictable period. Prosthodontic preparation for patients in the frail state should begin early and should consider access to preventative procedures and simplicity of maintenance.[111,112]

Diabetes

Diabetes has been proven to be a significant risk factor and etiology of peri-implant diseases, specifically related to impaired/atypical osseous wound healing.[113,114] Clinically, it can be expected that type I diabetics will be less predictable in their overall peri-implant health management and will require more close follow-up than type II diabetics. There is short-term evidence to indicate that well-managed type 2 diabetes patients manage peri-implant health equally to nondiabetic patients, if controlled ranges of glycemia, assessed by monitoring HbA1c levels, are maintained.[115]

Gingival biotype

Mucosal thickness and degree of keratinization in peri-implant tissues may determine susceptibility to biofilm and debris accumulation and may deter patient compliance with oral hygiene procedures due to chronic irritation.[116] Although a number of authors have recommended specific soft tissue dimension and morphology to minimize peri-implant diseases, there is no long-term evidence to support a particular philosophy.[117,118] There is emerging evidence that a thick gingival biotype, which could be pre-existing or develop through surgical augmentation as site development or in conjunction with implant placement, is favorable over a thin gingival biotype. Patients need to be informed this is a potential adjunctive requirement for long-term peri-implant tissue stability.[119,120]

Epidemiology

Peri-implant disease has been reported in numerous publications and is currently an area of interest due to the widespread increased acceptance of dental implants by the profession and the public. There continues to be disagreement in the profession as to the classification and levels of peri-implant diseases which prevents meta-analysis of the majority of the publications. For the few papers that survive meta-analysis, the indicators are that peri-implant mucositis occurs at a rate of 8–68% and peri-implantitis occurs at a rate of 1–47%.[121–125] It has been reported that patients with a history of periodontitis have almost a sixfold higher incidence in the development of peri-implantitis than those without periodontal disease.[126] The wide variations in epidemiological studies have been attributed to patient variables, clinician experience, implant hardware design, quality of prosthetic reconstruction, and conflicting definitions for the threshold of peri-implantitis. [127] Nonetheless, epidemiological reports are useful to clinicians and researchers to elevate their awareness of peri-implant diseases and ensure adequate processes are in place for diagnosis and appropriate management.

Future directions in peri-implant disease research

As technology continues to evolve, histological assay of various cytokines in peri-implant sulcular fluid is emerging as a research tool to refine the threshold for mucositis and implantitis.[128–130] Higher levels of specific cytokines appear to be linked to the inflammatory process of peri-implantitis. Inducing synthesis of other cytokines may improve the prognosis of an implant.[131] It has been suggested that histological assay should be completed prior to initiating clinical treatment.[132] Meta-analysis of peri-implant crevicular fluid studies link a definitive diagnosis of peri-implant infection to inflammatory mediators but do not discriminate between peri-implant mucositis and peri-implantitis.[133] Animal studies have demonstrated an increase in cytokine production in gingival and bone tissues when stimulated by titanium ions which may promote alveolar bone resorption.[134,135] The corrosion of implant materials is considered a dynamic interface through the healing period and is modified by oxidizing radicals created in metabolic processes.[136] The effect of long-term corrosion of titanium and titanium alloy dental implant surfaces in humans has yet to be connected to cytokine production. There remains a significant gap between reported research tools and clinical application.

Treatment

Nonsurgical treatment for PIM or PI

Following a tentative diagnosis, a decision to proceed with either nonsurgical or surgical treatment must be made. Nonsurgical treatment for peri-implant mucositis is appropriate, generally simpler, more manageable, sufficient for detoxification, and well accepted by the patient. The early detection of peri-implant diseases is essential as the treatment of peri-implantitis is not predictable, at times complex, difficult to perform, and nonsurgical therapy has proven to be ineffective.[137]

The goal of nonsurgical treatment is to control the infection and inflammation by detoxification of the implant surface, and reduction of peri implant soft tissue inflammation. The literature shows there are many different, and effective, treatment modalities to consider in detoxification of affected implant surfaces.[138] A systematic review and meta-analysis concluded that long-term maintenance care for high-risk groups is essential and informed consent for such patients must include ongoing maintenance therapy.[139]

The goal of nonsurgical management of biofilm or iatrogenic causes of peri-implant diseases is to reduce inflammation by appropriate nonsurgical mechanical debridement, using instruments that do not abrade titanium (implant plastic, resin, or carbon fiber curettes and scalers, or ultrasonic scalers with a nonmetallic tip). Adjunctive therapies include use of local or systemic antimicrobial or antibiotic agents following appropriate identification of putative pathogens, possibly with use of bacterial assay. Corrective restorative procedures to reduce sources of food impaction and recontouring of restorations to promote oral hygiene access and encourage peri-implant tissue health should be included. Debridement and disinfection of the intaglio and cameo surfaces of removable prostheses, and any mechanical attachments, must not be ignored.

The emphasis on patient homecare effectiveness around the peri-implant tissues is fundamental, irrespective of implant design and manufacturer. Improvement in plaque control is considered to be integral in the maintenance of peri-implant tissue health and in promoting reduced pocket depth. An *in vitro* study supported maintenance procedures which leave the implant neck (abutment) surface unaltered or result in reduced roughness are recommended over procedures that increase surface roughness.

Mechanical debridement

Using manual or ultrasonic instruments (with plastic coating) to clean the implant or abutment surface has a potential to affect the implant surface and/or abutment surface, therefore non-metal scalers or curettes (carbon, plastic, resin reinforced, resin-unreinforced instruments), or titanium instruments, are generally recommended. Metal curettes can alter surfaces and remove superficial material,[141] resulting in an even rougher surface.[142] Prophylaxis pastes with a rubber cup or brush to remove supragingival and shallow subgingival stains and debris should be used judiciously. There is no evidence to support or necessitate the use of nonfluoridated prophy paste, particularly in partially dentate patients. A finishing polishing agent for dental implants should include finer-grit (tin oxide or diamond polishing paste 0.5–1.0 μm) polishing pastes to decrease surface roughness. Mechanical titanium rotary bristle brushes have been introduced by various companies for implant surface decontamination. There are no published studies verifying decontamination effectiveness or the potential surface alterations of the implant/abutment.

In addition to manual instrumentation, techniques using abrasive powder propelled by compressed air to remove biofilm, as well as extrinsic stains from surfaces, have been shown to be an effective method to clean and decontaminate implant surfaces. The powder consists of sodium bicarbonate, sodium hydrocarbonate, or the amino acid glycine. The instrument mixes air, water, and the abrasive powder at pressures of 65–100 psi to result in cleaning efficiency and removal of bacterial endotoxin from 84–98% and biofilm removal up to 100% of *in vitro* studies.[143,144] Although this technique has been shown to not change the physical structure of some implant surfaces, the powder particles may adhere to the implant surface. The clinician must understand the specific surface of the implant and be cognizant of the time of exposure of the air–powder abrasive.[145] Alterations in the surfaces of machined implants may occur and residual powder particles may become embedded and be attributed to reduction of bacterial adhesion.[146,147] The use of air–powder abrasives on its own has not demonstrated complete re-osseointegration in human studies, but one monkey study achieved bone regeneration when combined with guided bone regeneration.[148] Significant bone regeneration and reduction of mucositis using air polishing for decontamination has been demonstrated in one human study involving surgical management of peri-implantitis sites, with short- to medium-term follow-up.[149] Potential adverse effects of air polishing in a nonsurgical application may include subcutaneous emphysema with inappropriate angulation of the instrument.[150,151] For this reason, air polishing cannot be recommended for decontamination in a nonsurgical approach, but may be carefully utilized in a surgical treatment modality.

Disinfection: application of topical antibacterial agents

Topical application of therapeutic agents to detoxify the implant surface is used in conjunction with mechanical debridement. Whether it is surgical or recare, a preoperative oral disinfectant rinse to decrease bacterial count is a commonly utilized protocol. As a therapy for peri-implant diseases, various antimicrobial agents have been reported, including citric acid, ethylene diamine tetraacetic acid (EDTA), cetylpyrirdium chloride (CPC), stabilized active oxygen (Ardox X), hydrogen peroxide, sodium hypochlorite (Dakin's solution), and chlorhexidine (CHX).

Citric acid demonstrated the most effectiveness at decontamination and biocompatibility and healing around a previously contaminated implant surface. However, the toxicity of citric acid should be considered, and application should be limited to the implant surface and avoid contact with surrounding bone.[152] EDTA, a neutral pH chelator used to remove smear layer prior to regenerative procedures using biomimetic materials, has shown a decrease in pocket depth when used in conjunction with titanium granules in bone-grafting treatments of peri-implantitis defects.[153] CPC 0.25% and zinc chloride ($ZnCl_2$)

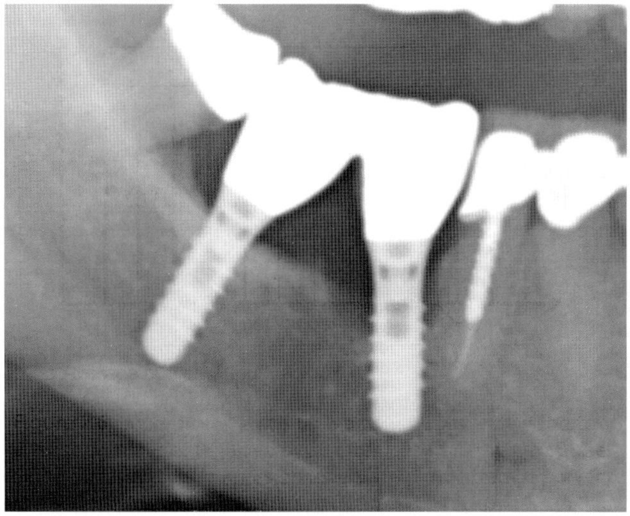

Figure 23.9 Clinical radiograph of peri-implantitis on anterior abutment.

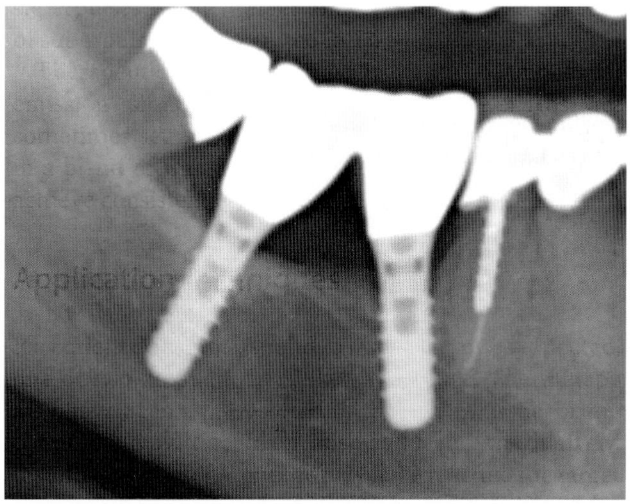

Figure 23.10 Clinical radiograph of resolved peri-implant disease 8 years after nonsurgical treatment.

2.5% were studied in commercial mouthrinses and found to be synergistic in their effect in the inhibition of bacterial growth implicated in both halitosis and peri-implant diseases.[154] Ardox X, an oxygenating agent originally used in whitening agents, has more recently been used in oxygenating mouthwash as an alternative to broad-spectrum antimicrobials.[155]

Hydrogen peroxide has been used extensively for periodontal therapy. A recent human *in vivo* pilot study concluded that all tested antiseptics reduce the total amount of microorganisms accumulating on titanium surfaces. Hydrogen peroxide 3%, 0.2% CHX, and Listerine showed significant bactericidal effect against adhering bacteria over a 12-hour period.[156] However, an animal study using 10% hydrogen peroxide and citric acid to examine re-osseointegration after decontaminating dental implants showed the hydrogen peroxide increased the levels of matrix metalloproteieinase-8 (MMP-8), resulting in poor wound healing.[157]

Sodium hypochlorite was used in wound healing in medicine prior to the discovery of antibiotics and has a broad antimicrobial activity, rapid bactericidal action, and relative nontoxicity at low concentrations. Dakin's solution (0.025% sodium hypochlorite solution) avoids tissue toxicity when used *in vivo*.[158] Subgingival irrigation with 0.1% sodium hypochlorite has been shown to cause a significantly higher and prolonged biofilm reduction as compared to water.[159] If the oral mucosa is intact, higher concentrations can be considered for decontamination but are not indicated in surgical interventions due to tissue toxicity.[160]

Chlorhexidine gluconate (CHX), the most common antiseptic used in periodontics[161] in pre- and post-surgical as well as maintenance regimes, has been studied in the nonsurgical and surgical treatment of peri-implantitis lesions.[162] There is no therapeutic benefit between 0.12% and 0.2% CHX and greater patient compliance has been demonstrated with 0.12% CHX.[163] Although CHX gel has been recommended in concentrations of 0.12–0.5%, a randomized controlled trial (RCT) did not support its efficacy over a placebo gel.[164] A common protocol for the use of CHX in peri-implant disease management is topical application to affected area b.i.d. or rinsing for 60 seconds, expectorate, no rinses or food consumption for 30 minutes b.i.d. One publication has shown benefits of combining chlorhexidine gel with an oral irrigation device.[165]

Potential side effects such as disruption of natural bacterial ecology, altered taste, and discoloration of the dentition with prolonged use of antibacterial agents should be considered and weighed against benefits of controlling peri-implant inflammation.[166] Despite isolated examples of conservative treatment resolving peri-implantitis (Figures 23.9 and 23.10), evidence suggests that mucositis can be managed with the use of mechanical/nonsurgical therapy while peri-implantitis does not respond to nonsurgical therapy and no single method can be promoted based on the current evidence.[167]

An emerging technology using ozone as a minimally invasive conservative therapy appears promising for use in management of peri-implant biofilm.[168] Oral administration of daily probiotic (*Lactobacillus reuteri prodentis*) tablets in edentulous implant patients with peri-implant mucositis showed improvement in clinical parameters and reduction in cytokine levels as compared to the placebo group. This indicates it may be an alternative therapy for the prevention and treatment of peri-implant mucositis. A larger patient study is required to positively correlate the effects of probiotics on peri-implant tissue health.[169]

Essential oils (EO) have also been considered for treatment against oral pathogens as an alternative, particularly to avoid bacterial resistance to antibiotics. These include lavender essential oil, cinnamon oil, clove oil, eucalyptus oil, peppermint oil, lemon essential oils, thyme oil, and tea tree oil (TTO).

It appears that essential oils have the potential to be developed as preventive or therapeutic agents.[170,171]

Antifungal agents, such as nystatin and fluconazole, are used in treatment of oral candida infections which may also extend to peri-implant tissues, particularly in edentulous patients. Candida infections can be notoriously difficult to control, especially in patients with poor oral hygiene or immune suppression. Recent evidence indicates that combining TTO with antifungal medications (fluconazole) is helpful to treat chronic yeast infections.[172]

Chloramine (Perisolv™, RLS Global AB, Gothenburg, Sweden), a hypochlorite solution buffered with a solution of amino acids resulting in formation of chloramines, which have an antibacterial effect, has recently been studied in treatment of peri-implantitis for nonsurgical reduction of mucosal inflammation. It has been found to be equally effective in the reduction of mucosal inflammation as conventional nonsurgical mechanical debridement up to 3 months.[173]

Mouthrinses

A review of a number of antimicrobial mouthrinses used as an auxiliary therapy in chemical peri-implant biofilm management concluded there is strong evidence that 0.12% CHX and EO have proven efficacy against oral biofilms but CHX should be prescribed with caution due to unwanted side effects. Combining a lower dose CHX (0.03%) with CPC (0.05%) was studied in a randomized, double-blind clinical trial, and found to be effective in inhibiting bacterial regrowth while reducing unpleasant subjective side effects (taste perception).[174] A clinically proven antiseptic for prevention and/or treatment of peri-implant diseases with significant efficacy without significant side effects remains elusive.

Laser disinfection of implant surfaces

Antimicrobial photodynamic therapy (aPDT) or photodisinfection is a nonsurgical, nonantibiotic therapy aimed to eliminate harmful bacteria and toxins associated with peri-implant diseases including Gram-negative pathogens.[175] Unlike thermal lasers that cut tissue, photodisinfection utilizes a cold (nonthermal) diode laser which does not produce heat or cause damage to dental materials. This treatment claims to reduce side effects associated with antibiotics, such as bacterial resistance, allergic or sensitivity reactions, opportunistic infections, or prolonged doses of medication. The aPDT has been recommended as an adjunct to conventional oral disinfection protocols.[176,177] Repeat applications (3 month intervals) with concurrent surface mechanical debridement and improved oral hygiene are recommended.[178] There is controversy as to the value of this therapy in a nonsurgical treatment, particularly if exudate has been detected. Therefore, it may be of value in treating peri-implant mucositis. It has shown some short-term clinical benefit as an adjunctive surgical treatment in the presence of pus (peri-implantitis).[179] When evaluating clinical outcomes up to 1 year post peri-implantitis treatment, it does not appear to be significantly beneficial over mechanical debridement alone and may be attributed to reduction, not elimination, of bacterial counts.[180]

Adjunctive use of diode laser in a nonsurgical approach without a photosensitizer, in addition to scaling and surface decontamination, has mixed results in the literature ranging from significant benefit[181–183] to no clinical improvements.[184] Many different lasers were examined, including neodymium-doped yttrium-aluminum-garnet (Nd:YAG), carbon dioxide (CO_2), diode, erbium/chromium-doped yttrium-scandium-gallium-garnet (Er,Cr:YSGG), and erbium-doped yttrium-aluminum-garnet (Er:YAG), in a systematic review, which stated that, due to limited sample sizes and short follow-up periods, no conclusions of laser superiority could be drawn.[185] In a different systematic review and meta-analysis of the effect of various laser wavelengths in the treatment of peri-implantitis, it was recommended that nonsurgical laser therapy may be utilized as phase 1 therapy but superiority of laser treatment compared to conventional therapy for peri-implantitis could not be identified.[186,187]

Alternative therapies

Epigenetics: enhancing host resistance with dietary phytochemicals

Until recently, the genetic predisposition of the patient was acknowledged but thought to be unalterable in the treatment of their condition. The majority of epigenetic changes are influenced by lifestyle and diets. Epigenetics studies the trait variations caused by external or environmental factors that switch genes on and off and affect how cells read genes, rather than by changes in the DNA sequence. One such example is the use of curcumin (diferuloylmethane), an extracted polyphenol (PP) from the root of turmeric; it is well known as an anti-inflammatory, anti-oxidative, and anti-lipidemic agent which modulates diseases via epigenetic regulation. It has shown ability to suppress periodontopathic bacteria in a cultured medium. The result was a suppression of *P. gingivalis* biofilm and infers curcumin has antibacterial effects and may be useful in preventing periodontal diseases.[188–190] Dietary phytochemicals as dietary supplements are emerging as a possible agent to reverse epigenetic alterations and regulate gene expression and molecular targets.

Oil pulling

It is recognized that a diminished salivary flow rate results in changes to the oral mucosa which can be a significant problem surrounding dental implants, particularly where there is a lack of attached gingiva. Whether this is due to aging, medications, chronic diseases, or radiation-induced stomatitits, the resulting plaque-induced gingivitis can be very difficult to manage. An alternative treatment to conventional oral hygiene procedures is the use of oil pulling or oil swishing therapy as a traditional Indian folk remedy. Sesame, sunflower, and coconut oils have been described but the evidence is minimal. Coconut oil is unique due to the 45–50% lauric acid content which has anti-inflammatory and antimicrobial effects. A preliminary report has shown that oil pulling using coconut oil could be an effective adjuvant procedure in decreasing plaque formation and plaque-induced gingivitis.[191] When comparing sesame oil pulling and CHX mouthwash prior to brushing, there was a significant reduction in aerobic bacteria in both groups.[192] Therefore, in patients with dry mouth syndrome who are intolerant of CHX as an antibacterial rinse, oil pulling may be considered. The current recommendation is 1 tbsp (15 ml) of coconut oil to be swished for 20 minutes and expectorated in a waste container as it will solidify and obstruct plumbing. However, there are no publications specifically using this technique for peri-implant diseases.

Antibiotic therapy

Topical antibiotics

In an effort to reduce the use of systemic antibiotics when treating local diseases such as peri-implant diseases, there is increasing interest in using topical antibiotic therapies, particularly for a nonsurgical approach to peri-implant mucositis and early peri-implantitis. Tetracycline hydrochloride paste has been used as a decontamination agent for peri-implantitis[193] but its low pH can decalcify peri-implant bone and delay the healing process.[194] The use of tetracycline as topical sustained-release micro-spherical minocycline (MSM) (Arestin, OraPharma, Valeant Pharmaceuticals North America Bridgewater, New Jersey) has been compared to topical CHX gel as an adjunct to mechanical debridement of early peri-implantitis lesions, and found to improve probing depths and bleeding scores over CHX for a 12-month period.[195,196] MSM used following mechanical debridement and 0.2% CHX gel in peri-implantitis sites greater than or equal to 5 mm followed over a 12-month period resulted in reduction in PPD and BOP and positive effects on clinical parameters.[197] A prospective randomized clinical trial compared aPDT and MSM adjunctive with mechanical debridement for initial peri-implantitis (PD 4–6 mm, BOP, MBL 0.5–2 mm) therapy. Both were equally effective in reduction of mucosal inflammation for up to 6 months but complete resolution of inflammation was not routinely achieved with either of the adjunctive therapies.[198]

Metronidazole has been advocated as a topical antibiotic therapy for peri-implant diseases. Metronidazole dental gel 25% applied in two applications 1 week apart decreased Gram-negative (60–70%) and increased Gram-positive (40–50%) bacteria to near normal levels with healing of peri-implant soft tissues.[199]

Systemic antibiotics

Systemic antibiotics have long been used prophylactically as part of the surgical protocol for the placement of dental implants. Historically they were utilized therapeutically in the management of nonosseointegrated implant complications, in conjunction with surgical drainage. For osseointegrated implant surgery, systemic antibiotics are commonly given prophylactically. Therapeutically, they have been utilized following mechanical debridement and CHX irrigation. The treatment was aimed at reducing subgingival bacterial volume and suppressing the anaerobic component, which had a beneficial effect on peri-implantitis for up to 1 year.[200] No sound scientific basis is available for the use of systemic antibiotics.[201] In a review of studies from 1992 to 2013 asking the question, "Are locally and systemically delivered antibiotics useful in the treatment of peri-implantitis?" the conclusion was the significance of adjunctive antibiotic therapy in the treatment of peri-implantitis remains debatable.[202] In an RCT comparing nonsurgical treatment of peri-implant mucositis with or without systemic Azithromax® (4 days) in patients followed for 6 months, no short-term differences were found and clinical improvements were attributed to improvements in oral hygiene. It determined a lack of evidence for the use of systemic antibiotics in the treatment of peri-implant mucositis.[203] Given the concern over the development of resistant bacteria and diminished effectiveness of current antibiotics, the use of systemic antibiotics solely or as an adjunct to mechanical therapy cannot be supported.[204]

Enamel matrix derivative

Enamel matrix derivative (EMD – Emdogain, Straumann AG, Andover, MA) is an extract of porcine fetal tooth material, and is used to biomimetically stimulate the soft and hard periodontal tissues. There are minimal published studies of the effect of EMD on peri-implant hard and soft tissues. However, EDM has been compared to MSM as an adjunctive nonsurgical treatment of peri-implant mucosal inflammation and mechanical debridement alone. There was a significant reduction in probing depth and BOP with both adjunctive groups vs. mechanical debridement solely for the duration of the 3-month study.[196] Furthermore, an EMD *in vitro* study with human gingival fibroblasts on an acid-etched titanium surface increased cell growth, spreading, and synthesis of an extracellular matrix. Although animal and human studies are required to substantiate the beneficial effects of EMD for soft tissue regeneration surrounding implants, it appears EMD may speed up the quality of soft tissue integration around dental implants.[205] EMD has been studied to investigate the proliferation and differentiation of osteoblasts grown on the titanium implant surface. This *in vitro* study also indicated that EMD may have a positive effect on implant osseointegration.[206]

Surgical therapy

Surgical therapies combine the above nonsurgical therapy with resective and/or regenerative procedures when peri-implant diseases persist (Figure 23.11). Surgical access to the affected site(s) facilitates removal of foreign bodies, removal of granulation tissue (Figures 23.12, 23.13 and 23.14), detoxification of implant surfaces with laser (Figure 23.15) or chemical agents, implantoplasty, graft (Figure 23.16) with or without

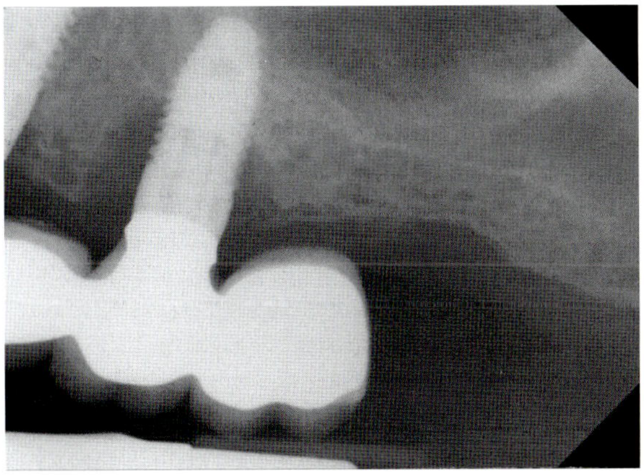

Figure 23.11 Radiograph of peri-implantitis defect.

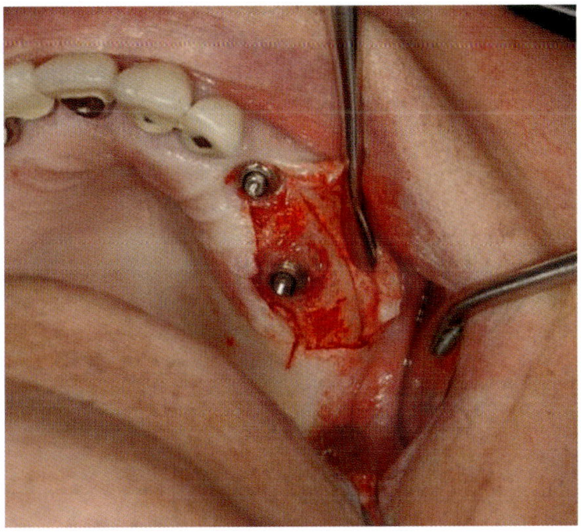

Figure 23.12 Clinical photograph of surgical exposure of peri-implantitis defect.

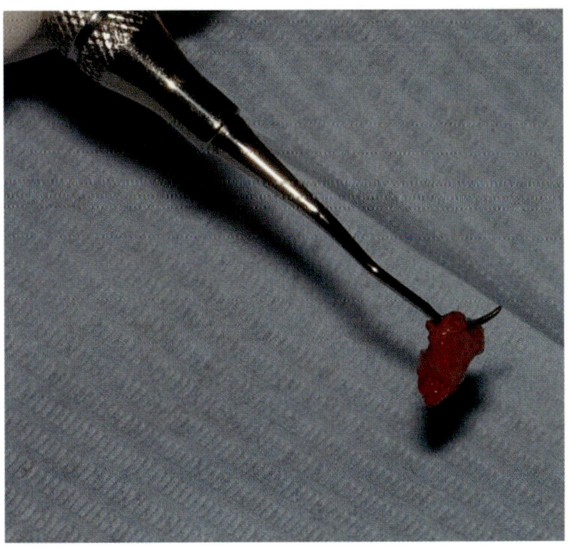

Figure 23.13 Clinical photograph of curetted granulation tissue in peri-implantitis defect.

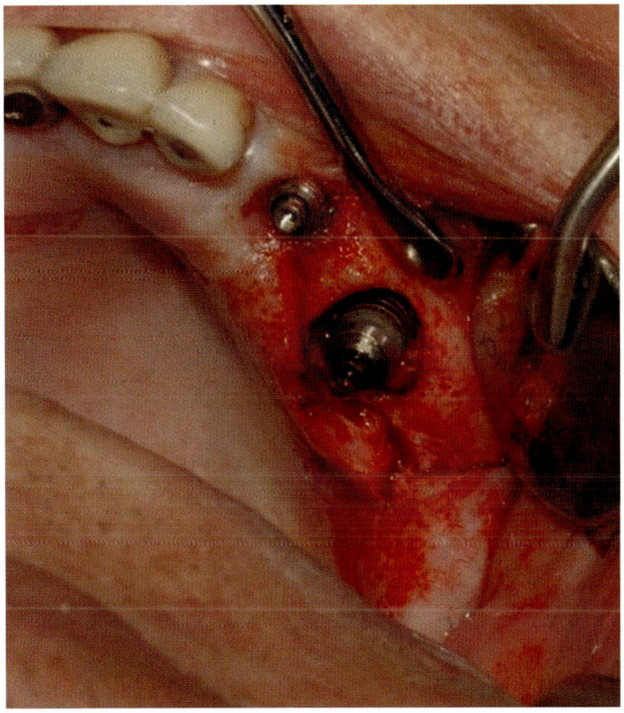

Figure 23.14 Clinical photograph of circumferential defect following debridement.

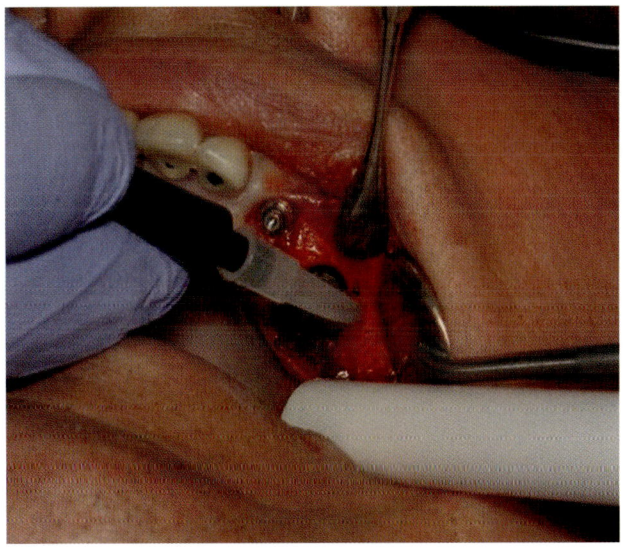

Figure 23.15 Clinical photograph of diode laser decontamination.

membrane as indicated, and is followed with postoperative systemic antibiotics and therapeutic agents. The approach taken depends on the extent and shape of the lesion as well as the esthetic compromise posed by surgical intervention. Resective surgery is used to reduce or eliminate peri-implant lesions and regenerative therapy attempts to restore hard and soft tissue contours. The cumulative interceptive supportive therapy protocol (CIST) is a guide for clinical decisions based on mucosal

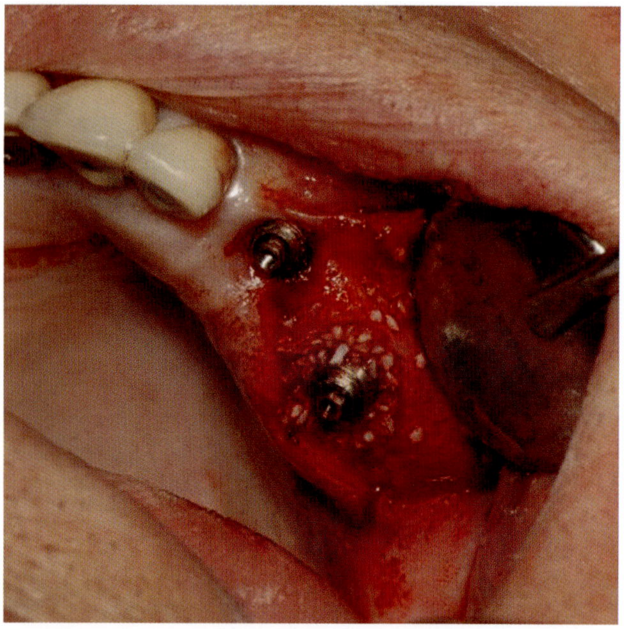

Figure 23.16 Clinical photograph of regenerative alloplastic graft placement.

condition and probing depth (PD).[207] The diagnosis is based on PD, plaque deposits, bleeding, and bone loss as determined by radiography. Treatments range from no treatment, to mechanical debridement, addition of antiseptics, systemic or local antibiotic therapy, and, ultimately, resective or regenerative surgery.

A Cochrane systematic review of different interventions for treating peri-implantitis with a 3-month to 1-year follow-up concluded there is no reliable evidence suggesting which is the most effective intervention; more complex and expensive therapies were not necessarily more beneficial than control therapies of mechanical debridement.[208]

Resective procedures

Dentistry has a long history of resective surgery for the treatment of periodontitis with a goal in reduction of BOP, probing depths, and clinical signs of inflammation. These same surgical principles can be extended to peri-implantitis to include the modification or elimination of the peri-implant osseous defect using ostectomy and osteoplasty, along with bacterial decontamination.[209] Implantoplasty (mechanical smoothing and polishing of exposed rough surfaces and/or threads) has also been recommended and shown that MBL following implantoplasty was significantly lower than after resective therapy only.[210] In addition, the implantoplasty group had significantly lower PD and BOP for more than 2 years post resective surgery.[211] Because there is an inevitable reduction in the diameter of the implant in the treated areas, implantoplasty should be avoided in narrower implants, particularly in areas of heavy occlusal loading.[212] Implant surface decontamination with 0.12% CHX + 0.05% CPC vs. a placebo solution in resective peri-implantitis surgery leads to a superior immediate suppression of anaerobic bacteria on the implant surface but not superior clinical results.[213] Another study used 2% CHX solution vs 0.12% CHX + 0.05% CPC (control group) for implant decontamination during resective surgery, with no improved outcomes.[214] A RCT studied adjunctive systemic antibiotic and local antimicrobial therapy (CHX) in surgical peri-implantitis treatment for modified-surface and nonmodified-surface implants. The authors concluded local CHX had no effect on outcomes, and systemic antibiotics had no effect on treatment success in nonmodified implants but a positive effect on modified-surface implants.[215] A 12-month prospective clinical study of 36 implants in 24 patients with moderate to advanced peri-implantitis received surgical treatment using an anti-infective surgical protocol (open flap debridement, implant decontamination, and systemic antibiotics – amoxicillin and metronidazole). They concluded an anti-infective surgical protocol was effective at 3 months with the results maintained up to 12 months.[216] As in treating periodontitis with resective surgery, postoperative recession is expected which limits this surgical technique in peri-implantitis sites to nonesthetic areas.

Regenerative procedures

The principles of guided bone regeneration (GBR) and soft tissue augmentation procedures have been applied to regenerative peri-implant surgeries. Considering the complexity, time, and expense of implant dentistry in general, complete regeneration and re-osseointegration is the ultimate goal of surgical interventions. Of course, GBR procedures for peri-implantitis treatment are complex procedures usually reported by expert experienced clinicians who are demonstrating pushing the boundaries of regenerative possibilities, rather than application to routine implant dentistry. Many decisions are required prior to and during regenerative surgical interventions, including implant explantation and future re-entry. Post-surgical management and follow-up to minimize healing complications is a common characteristic of successful case reports.

A case series report of 38 patients with 51 implant sites with peri-implantitis (BOP, PD ≥6 mm, MBL ≥4 mm) treated with regenerative treatment protocols with follow-up from 3 to 7.5 years concluded PD reduction, bone level gain, and no loss of implants.[217] Another case series of six patients with nine implants with re-entry to regenerative submerged and nonsubmerged approaches in peri-implant defects reported a mean bone fill of 91.3% with a 4.88 mm mean bone gain without additional bone-augmentation procedures.[218] There are additional recent case reports discussing surgical re-entry,[219] long-term follow-up to 17 years,[220] and combined surgical resective and regenerative therapy with concomitant soft tissue augmentation, which show improved clinical results with regenerative treatments.[221]

A retrospective longitudinal study in a periodontal private practice followed 382 implants with peri-implantitis in 150 patients. The mean follow-up time was 26 ± 20 months and the mean time between implant placement and baseline was

6.4 years. Resective surgery was done 47% and regenerative surgery with bone augmentation materials 20% of the time. Mean success rate reported was 69%. The success rate was significantly lower for individuals with the diagnosis of severe periodontitis, severe MBL, poor oral hygiene, and low compliance.[222] A more recent case report presented the results of 170 treated peri-implantitis sites in 100 patients with 2–10 years' follow-up. The treatments included most of the current therapies, including EMD, in a layered/combined regenerative approach of one to three procedures. BOP was resolved in 91% of implants, PD reduced an average of 5.1 mm, MBL gain averaged 1.77 mm, and soft tissue marginal gain averaged 0.52 mm. The authors suggested a layered/combined regenerative approach for the treatment of peri-implantitis may be recommended.[223]

Regenerative surgery utilizes autogenous, allograft, or xenograft bone replacement materials with or without resorbable (collagen) or nonresorbable (PTFE) membranes, and soft tissue augmentation materials (connective tissue, acellular dermal matrix, others). A recent addition for hard tissue replacement is porous titanium granules (PTGs).[224] A multicenter RCT was done with 63 patients, comparing open-flap debridement with or without PTGs following decontamination with titanium brushes and hydrogen peroxide. Although PTGs resulted in a significantly enhanced radiographic appearance (defect fill), an inability to discern biomaterial from osseous tissue was a limitation in determining new bone formation.[225] Implant decontamination techniques also have significant variation and the methods discussed previously in the nonsurgical approaches have also been applied to the surgical approaches to peri-implantitis treatment. Complete elimination of biofilm is difficult to achieve nonsurgically and re-osseointegration is difficult, if not impossible, to achieve without surgical access.[226]

Complete disease resolution seems to depend on initial bone loss surrounding the implant prior to surgical intervention, and implants with no signs of peri-implantitis following corrective therapy tend to remain healthy, while disease progression is observed for implants that still have residual peri-implantitis after surgical management.[227] The success of surgical peri-implant treatment is influenced by the experience of the surgical team, amount of peri-implant bone loss at baseline, smoking, probing pocket depth at baseline, and presence of plaque during follow-up. Early diagnosis of peri-implantitis and control of behavioral factors are crucial in achieving peri-implantitis treatment success.[228] Educating patients about the lack of evidence regarding success of surgical interventions, particularly in more advanced peri-implant diseases, will promote earlier intervention and encourage patient participation in homecare to further mitigate disease progression.

Occlusal therapy

Occlusal loads can be a modifying or secondary factor in peri-implant disease, particularly if the osseointegration is marginal, quality of crestal bone surrounding the implant is poor (large grafts), implant position and size violate basic planning principles, the quality of the restoration is poor (fit, design, contour), quality and quantity of surrounding soft tissues are poor, the patient exhibits inadequate biofilm control, and parafunctional habits are suspected. In other words, if conditions for osseointegration and the restoration are marginal and have several risk factors, then control of occlusion may be significant. Heavy occlusal loads in known bruxers has been linked to excessive prostheses wear and mechanical failure of implant components. Bending moments may cause component micromotion beyond the adaptive capacity of the surrounding bone and lead to screw loosening or implant fracture. Occlusion design and adjustment to minimize bending moments of implants whether single teeth, short-span bridges, or full-arch restorations is desirable.

Dental implant stability assumes occlusal stability. Occlusal instability is more the mode than the exception, particularly in the partially edentulous implant patient. Tooth migration, degenerative joint disease, missing teeth, loss of vertical dimension of occlusion, skeletal pattern, lifelong growth changes, and parafunctional habits all contribute to occlusal instability. Implant restorations delivered with meticulous attention in a stable occlusal environment may require adjustment and/or modification as circumstances change.[229] Keeping occlusal forces below the threshold of mechanical complications, while allowing continuous routine control of biofilm is the goal. The authors' experience is that maximum occlusal stability is achieved with complete-arch restorations or partially edentulous restorations when tooth position is controlled with lifelong retention. A mutually protected occlusion with long-term stability appears to favor a class I occlusion in a class I skeletal pattern.

Cross-arch stabilization with splinted screw-retained restorations and moderate cantilevers was the original design in the Brånemark studies. This design is appreciated when observing complications of restorative wear and component failure requiring retrievability. A competing design has been the use of larger numbers of implants, spaced around the arches, restored with cemented short-span bridges. Both designs have a proven long-term success and pose different risks in follow-up care.[230,231]

Cement removal

Excess cement was implicated surrounding methacrylate (Premier Implant Cement, Premier Dental Products) cement-retained implant restorations in a retrospective clinical follow-up. Signs of inflammation were present in a large proportion of implants in a short- to medium-term follow-up, which resolved following restoration removal, decontamination, and recementation with TempBond (TempBond, Kerr Sybron Dental Specialties, Orange, CA). A significant observation was that when excess cement removal was done early (<1 year) suppuration was reduced by 100%, in contrast with delayed revision (>4 years), where suppuration decreased by 88%. After recementation with zinc oxide–eugenol (ZOE) cement (TempBond), considerably fewer signs of inflammation were found.[232] ZOE has shown a strong antibacterial activity *in vitro*,[233] and its ability to dissolve in contact with oral fluids may cause less residual cement in the peri-implant sulcus, which results in fewer complications.[234] The authors recommend the use of ZOE cement as a first choice for cementing implant restorations. If additional retention is required, the surface of the abutment can be modified by air abrading, adding retentive undercuts, and utilizing the screw channel internally as a retentive element. A positive relationship between excess cement and peri-implant disease was established by a 5-year prospective clinical endoscopic study. Excess dental cement was associated with signs of peri-implant disease in 81% of the cases, which resolved in 74% of treated implants after the cement removal. There was an average of 3 years before there were clinical signs of a problem.[235] This problem is magnified with the amount of horizontal undercut from the abutment/restoration interface to the surrounding peri-implant gingival margin. The clinician should evaluate if there is residual cement (around a cement-retained restoration) present in the peri-implant tissues using direct inspection with magnification and radiographs. A radiographic angulation error of over 5° can hide a gap of 50 μm or more.[236] Custom abutments with CAD/CAM design can create an abutment profile and margin placement to significantly reduce the concern of cement removal.[237]

If the cement is accessible, it should be removed, and, if not, the restoration is removed or a flap raised to access the site. This is followed by detoxification of the surface and postoperative use of antimicrobial agents and good oral hygiene. One 5-year retrospective study of 129 implants in 77 patients concluded implants with cement remnants in patients with a history of periodontitis may be more likely to develop peri-implantitis, compared with patients without a history of periodontal infection.[238] An interesting observation in this study was regarding the influence of a transmucosal undercut in the abutment; if it was 1 mm or more in any direction, the result was more cement embedded in soft tissue, if 3 mm or more, there was more cement attached to the crown/abutment. Regardless, there appears to be cement embedded in the soft tissue as well as attached to the restoration.[74]

Platform switching has been advocated as a method to reduce MBL by redirecting the effect of the implant connection biofilm more vertically vs. horizontally.[239,240] A concern of platform switching is the creation of an additional horizontal undercut which further complicates cement removal.[241]

Various modifications of the abutment have been advocated to encourage cement intrusion into the screw access channel vs. exterior restoration margin, and potentially into the sulcus, including two 1 mm horizontal holes mid-way in the screw channel (metal abutments) and placement of a hollow cannula vertically within the screw channel (ceramic abutments).[242] A third option is the lingual lug design which can be used on both metal and ceramic abutments. The lingual lug is a laboratory fabricated abutment (male) modification, approximately 3 mm wide, 3 mm high trapezoidal shape converging with a rounded top. The restoration has a corresponding (female) mirror-image recipient. There are three benefits of this design: verification of complete seating, an anti-rotational feature, and a vent channel to direct cement extrusion coronally (Figures 23.17, 23.18 and 23.19).

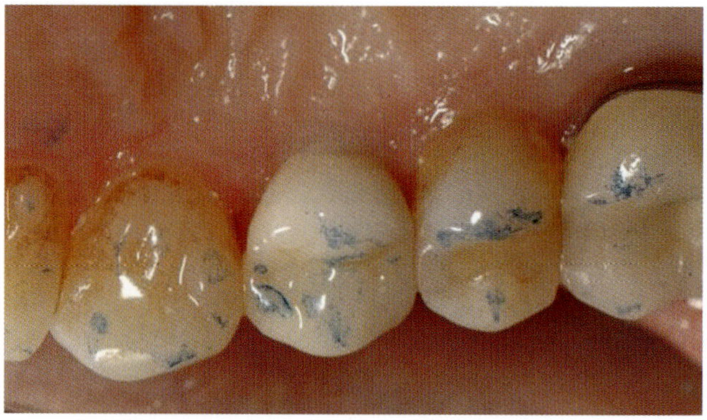

Figure 23.17 Clinical photograph of lingual lug in zirconia abutment/crown replacing the first premolar.

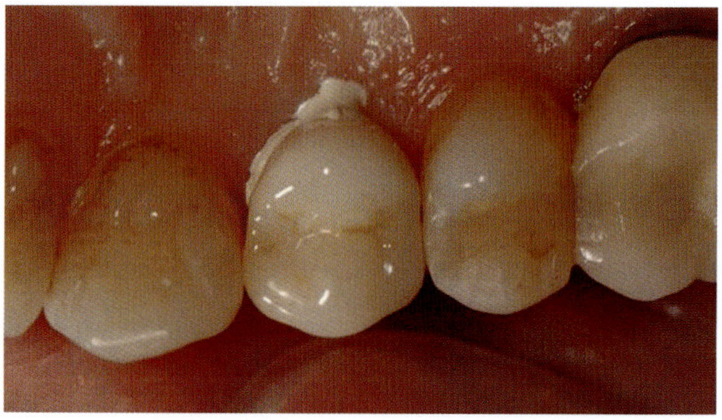

Figure 23.18 Clinical photograph of cement extrusion in lingual lug abutment/crown design.

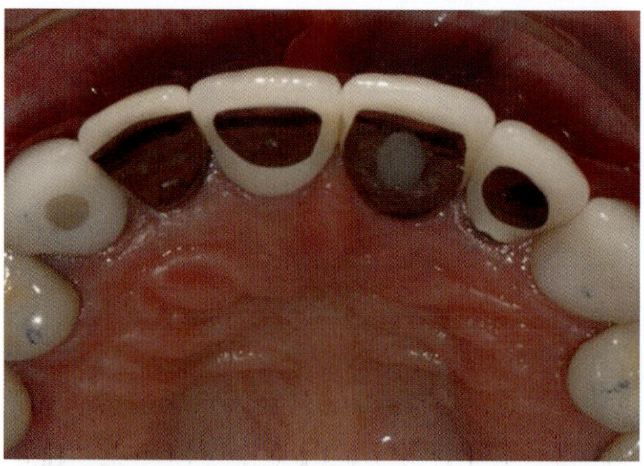

Figure 23.19 Clinical photograph of lingual lug in metal abutment/PFM crown design replacing the upper right lateral incisor verifying seating.

Whenever possible, the restoration should be removed to permit complete access to the peri-implant tissues and ensure removal of foreign body (cement) and detoxification. As this is the only method of retrievability for this type of restoration, the clinician should select an appropriate cement that permits removal of the restoration. Modified resin ionomer, polycarboxylate, glass ionomer, and resin cements are not recommended.

Confirmation of component integrity

The fit of the restoration needs to be confirmed, including checking for failing restorative components (failure of cement, loose implant abutment screws, or loose restorative screws), misfit or wear of components, or fracture of framework or connectors. Occlusal adjustment to reduce lateral or excessive occlusal forces, reducing extensive cantilever forces, and prescribing occlusal splint therapy are also recommended to mitigate stress. A systematic review spanning data from 1990–2006 suggested that abutment screw loosening occurred less than 3% in single-implant restorations, regardless of geometry of the implant–abutment connection.[243] Clinical performance of screw- versus cement-retained fixed implant-supported reconstructions was analyzed in a systematic review and concluded no statistical differences between cement- and screw-retained designs for survival or failure rates. However, screw-retained restorations exhibited fewer technical and biological complications.[244]

In a systematic review evaluating internal vs. external abutment connections, they found loosening of abutment screws was the most frequently occurring technical complication. More loose screws were reported for externally connected implant systems. Proper pre-load may decrease the incidence of such a complication.[245] A consecutive torquing protocol for prosthetic and abutment screws was recommended in a 5-year retrospective study which reported a 99.4% restorative success rate. The consecutive torquing protocol includes appointments 1 month apart to test screw pre-load until no detectable change.[246] Although manufacturers claim that titanium alloy screws have eliminated the need for consecutive torquing protocol, some clinicians continue this practice, suspecting some inter-component change over time. However, replacement intervals for screws has not been established.

Splinted restorations have been recommended for superior load sharing over nonsplinted restorations.[247] However, a compelling study using a split-mouth design in a 10-year randomized controlled trial, evaluated marginal bone level changes around adjacent splinted and nonsplinted cemented posterior maxillary implant restorations and concluded a difference in bone loss was seen between the groups but it was not clinically significant.[248] An acceptable clinical level of passivity should not cause problems to the biologic, esthetic, or functional parameters of the restoration or the patient.[249] Deep restorative interfaces that are difficult to assess for fit and passivity can create long-term problems which may simulate peri-implantitis (Figures 23.20 and 23.21).

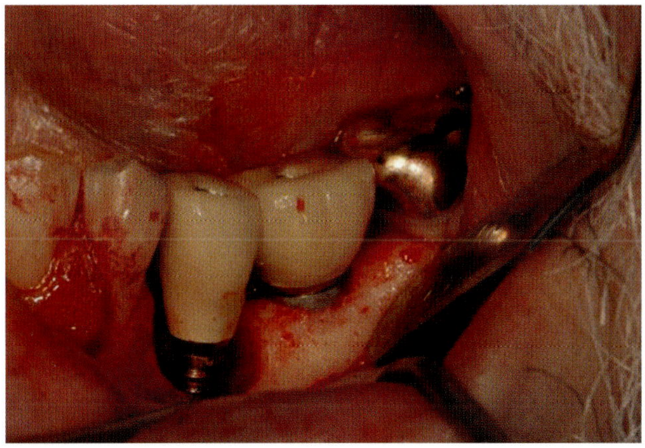

Figure 23.20 Clinical photograph of splinted screw-retained restorations with lack of restoration fit on distal implant and resulting extreme bone loss on anterior implant.

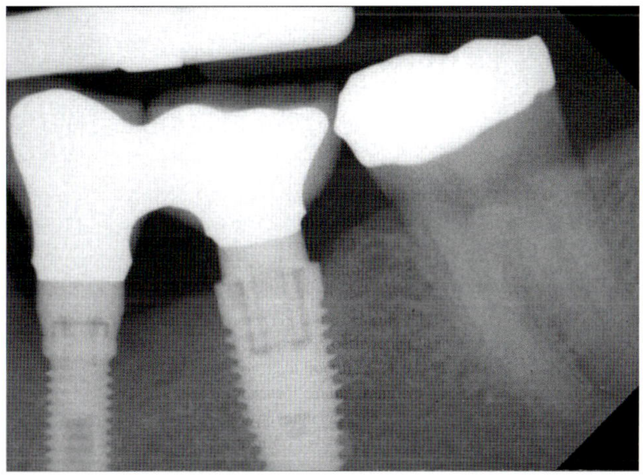

Figure 23.21 Clinical photograph of new restoration following regenerative procedure, platform switched distal abutment, and new restoration.

Explantation/implant removal

If any mobility is present with the implant, it must be removed immediately. A report of 281 patient cases selected consecutively, treated for peri implantitis, found in 51% of the patients it was not feasible to arrest progression of the disease. Smoking and smoking dose were found to be significant factors.[250] When it is determined that a nonmobile implant cannot be maintained and surgical interventions have not been markedly successful, explantation or implant removal should be considered within an appropriate interval to avoid additional bone loss.[251] An *in vitro* study investigating the effects of simulated bone loss on the implant assembly of 3.0 mm implant–abutment assemblies concluded that bone loss influenced the functional life and reliability of the implant–abutment assemblies, and that maintaining crestal bone is important in insuring biomechanical sustainability and predictable long-term function.[252]

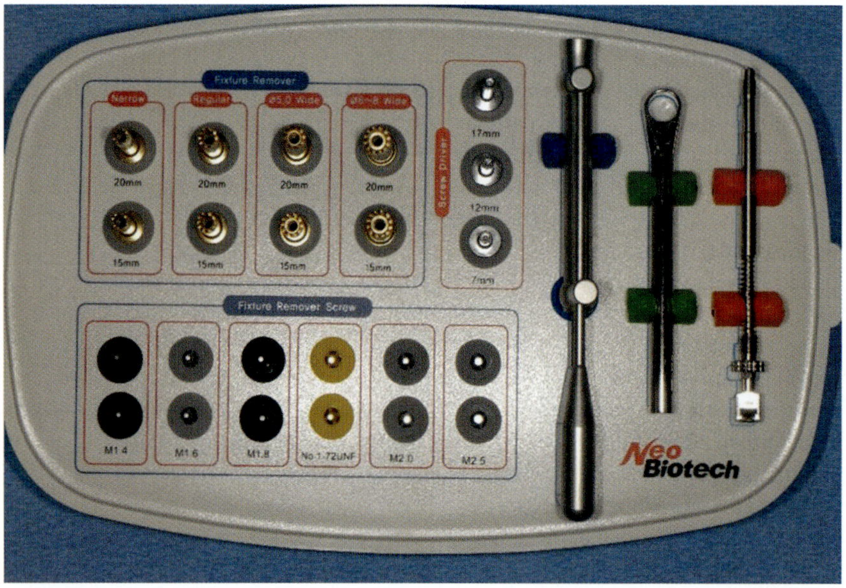

Figure 23.22 NeoBiotech Fixture Remover Kit (Biomet 3i, Palm Beach Gardens, FL).

Explantation of integrated implants may be by trephination or reverse torque or a combination of both methods. Several different manufacturers have introduced devices to apply reverse torque to a variety of implant connections and designs (Figures 23.22 and 23.23). Reverse torque can atraumatically achieve explantation by induced osseoseparation. A report of 81 patients, who received explantation of 158 nonmobile implants in the maxilla and mandible with a diagnosis of peri-implantitis or implant malposition, advocated a counter-torque technique which was successful in 88% of implant sites, and the remainder required the use of trephine burs to cut into the first 3–4 mm then counter-torque applied. The removal torque range was 146 ± 5 Ncm for the counter-torque only group, and 161 ± 13 Ncm for the trephine-assisted group. All titanium plasma-sprayed implants were removed at a significantly lower torque when compared to acid-etched, particle-blasted, and oxidized implants.[253]

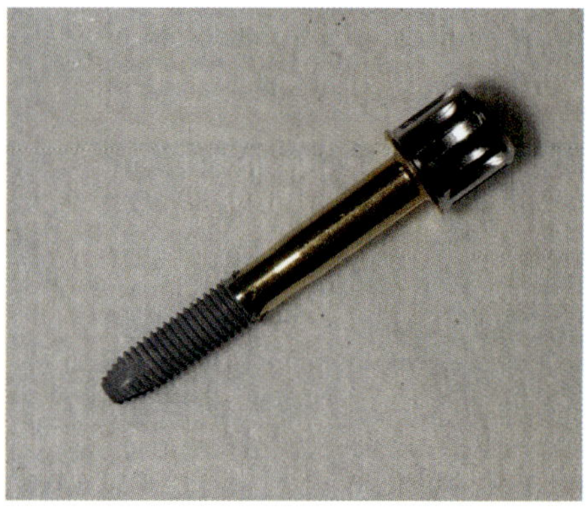

Figure 23.23 NobelSpeedy implant removed with Neobiotech Fixture Remover Kit.

Reimplantation

Reimplantation of a new implant in the same site of a previously removed implant may appear to be the most desirable option, but may be limited by osseous damage from the peri-implantitis, the explantation procedure, or both. A retrospective cohort study on 194 patients during a 6-year period showed the chances of a patient with minor bone loss in the site having reimplantation was 20 times greater than patients with severe bone loss. The conclusion stated that removal of a failing implant as soon as it is diagnosed as hopeless will improve the chances for reimplantation. Included in the patient-related reasons for avoiding reimplantation are cost (27%), fear of pain (18%), and fear of a repeated failure (16%).[254] Survival and success rates of reimplantation in previous failed implant sites ranges from 71–88%.[255–257]

In reviewing publications regarding reimplantation, the majority appear to address reimplantation in a site where initial osseointegration did not occur, in contrast to late failure implants due to peri-implant diseases. It is expected that reimplantation in the latter group is less successful if immediate reimplantation is attempted rather than using bone augmentation procedures followed by adequate healing.

Future directions

Early detection of inflammatory changes surrounding the implant is crucial in deciding when to intervene. Clinical examinations, which include pocket depth recording, detection of bleeding on probing, determining bone loss radiographically, and using our current gold standard diagnostic tools, are limited in detecting initiation of a disease state. We have discussed the role of cytokines in peri-implant crevicular fluid but the results are not firmly accepted. Circulating plasma DNA is used as a diagnostic tool routinely in medicine.[258] DNA fragment lengths of β-globin gene in gingival crevicular fluid samples have been correlated with periodontal health and disease.[259] A pilot study completed on 19 partially edentulous patients with a single posterior mandibular implant was able to demonstrate a difference of the host β-globin gene fragment lengths in peri-implant crevicular fluid (PICF) during wound healing. The authors concluded more research is needed to optimize the sampling process and correlate gene amplicon lengths with the degree of inflammation around implants.[260] In the meantime, from a clinical diagnostic perspective, the above gold standard remains.

Conclusion

Maintenance of dental implants and surrounding tissues has been shown to enhance the treatment outcome and reduce complications. The absence of preventive maintenance in individuals with pre-existing peri-implant mucositis is associated with a high incidence of peri-implantitis. Patients with a history of periodontal disease should be informed that they are more at risk for peri-implant disease. Despite the obvious need for preventive maintenance recare for implant patients, there are few available studies evaluating the long-term effect of recare programs and there is no evidence to suggest the frequency of recare intervals or to propose specific hygiene treatments. The maintenance recare visit needs to be tailored to the individual needs of the implant patient and consider systemic and past dental history (including history of periodontal disease), clinical and radiographic findings, diagnosis, and proposed interventions.

Utilizing checklists on a routine basis to provide consistent assessment of dental implant patients, and an accurate diagnosis, with appropriate therapies to promote peri-implant tissue health at the earliest opportunity, will help reduce progression of peri-implant diseases. Therefore, regular and frequent patient participation in daily prescribed maintenance and appropriate intervals of professional assessment provides the clinician an opportunity to identify subtle changes and provide intervention. The idea that implants are not "real teeth" does not mean they require less maintenance. In fact, the opposite appears to be the case, particularly in the aging population with an increased incidence of systemic inflammatory related diseases, reduced salivary flow, high stress with parafunction, and reduced dexterity and oral hygiene effectiveness. A prudent approach is to closely monitor implant and peri-implant health with a close interval of periodontal and prosthodontic maintenance.

We need to look beyond the bacterial causes of peri-implant disease and isolating the problem to the tissue or bone, understanding that the restorative considerations are equally impactful. Prosthodontic considerations and management of implant complications require a broad knowledge of components, materials, and understanding the properties of each. Which oral healthcare provider delivers the implant maintenance is one of the largest variables in the implant maintenance recare. The traditional delivery model for implant dentistry has changed significantly in the past 15 years and, like the planning of implant dentistry being restorative driven, management of peri-implant diseases also has a strong link to the restorative interface. The ability to retrieve and modify restorations for long-term peri-implant and restorative maintenance is proving to be a necessity in order to control peri-implant diseases and thereby maintain osseointegration in the long term.

There is no substitute for engaged patients, astute clinicians, and decisive evidence based protocols. "Persistent precision provides predictable prognosis" (PI Brånemark).

References

1. Brånemark P, Zarb G, Albrektsson T. *Tissue-Integrated Prostheses*. Chicago: Quintessence Publishing, Inc. 1985; 11.
2. McGrath C, Lam O, Lang N. An evidence-based review of patient-reported outcome measures in dental implant research among dentate subjects. *J Clin Periodontol* 2012; **39**(Suppl 12): 193–201.
3. Yao J, Tang H, Gao X, *et al.* Patient's expectations to dental implant: a systematic review of the literature. *Health Qual Life Outcomes* 2014; **12**: 153.
4. Heitz-Mayfield LJ. Peri-implant diseases: diagnosis and risk indicators. *J Clin Periodontol* 2008; **35**(8 Suppl): 292–304.
5. Iacono V. Committee on Research, Science and Therapy, the American Academy of Periodontology. Dental implants in periodontal therapy. *J Periodontol* 2000; **71**(12): 1934–1942.
6. Langer B, Becker W. Osseointegration and treatment planning: periodontists' perspectives. In: Albrektsson T, Zarb G (eds). *The Brånemark Osseointegrated Implant*. Chicago: Quintessence Publishing Co 1989; 127–138.
7. Brånemark P, Hansson B, Adell R, *et al. Osseointegrated Implants in the Treatment of the Edentulous Jaw. Experience from a 10-year Period*. Stockholm, Sweden: Almqvist & Wiksell 1977; 7–132.
8. Schnitman P, Schulman L. The US National Institute of Health Harvard Consensus Development Conference. Dental implants: benefit & risk. Dec 1980 NIH Publication No. 81–1531.
9. Albrektsson T, Zarb G, Worthington P, *et al.* The long-term efficacy of currently used dental implants: a review and proposed criteria for success. *Int J Oral Maxillofac Implants* 1986; **1**: 11–25.
10. Jokstad A. Osseointegration and dental implant research – contributions from the University of Toronto. *J Can Dental Assoc* 2008; **74**: 47–50.
11. Adell R, Lekholm U, Rockler B, *et al.* A 15-year study of osseointegrated implants in the treatment of the edentulous jaw. *Int J Oral Surg* 1981; **10**: 387–416.
12. Albrektsson T, Zarb G. Current interpretations of the osseointegrated response: clinical significance. *Int J Prosthodont* 1993; **6**(2): 95–105.
13. García-Bellosta S, Bravo M, Subirá C, *et al.* Retrospective study of the long-term survival of 980 implants placed in a periodontal practice. *Int J Oral Maxillofac Implants* 2010; **25**(3): 613–619.

14. Adell R, Eriksson B, Lekholm U, *et al.* Long-term follow-up study of osseointegrated implants in the treatment of totally edentulous jaws. *Int J Oral Maxillofac Implants* 1990; **5**: 347–359.
15. Lekholm U, Ericsson I, Adell R, *et al.* The condition of the soft tissues at tooth and fixture abutments supporting fixed bridges. A microbiological and histological study. *J Clin Periodontol* 1986; **13**(6): 558–562.
16. Astrand P, Ahlqvist J, Gunne J, *et al.* Implant treatment of patients with edentulous jaws: a 20-year follow-up. *Clin Implant Dent Relat Res* 2008; **10**: 207–217.
17. Pinkner S, Grondahl K, Jemt T. Marginal bone loss at implants: a retrospective, long-term follow-up of turned Brånemark System implants. *Clin Implant Dent Relat Res* 2009; **11**(1): 11–23.
18. Adell R. Nobelbiocare Gothenburg Symposium 16 April 2012. Presentation.
19. Quian J, Wennerberg A, Albrektsson T. Reasons for marginal bone loss around oral implants. *Clin Implant Dent Relat Res* 2012; **14**(6): 792–807.
20. Monje A, Hom-Lay W. Interpretation of study design on marginal bone loss in implant dentistry: evidence-based science versus clinical-based experience. *Int J Oral Maxillofac Implants* 2014; **29**(2): 279.
21. Carmichael R, Apse P, Zarb G, *et al.* Biological, microbiological, and clinical aspects of the peri-implant mucosa. In: Albrektsson T, Zarb, G (eds). *The Brånemark Osseointegrated Implant.* Chicago: Quintessence Publishing Co 1989; 39–78.
22. Mombelli A, van Ooosten M, Schurch E. The microbiota associated with successful or failing osseointegrated titanium implants. *Oral Microbiol Immunol* 1987; **2**(4): 145–151.
23. Zitzmann N, Berglundh T. Definition and prevalence of peri-implant diseases. *J Clin Periodontol* 2008; **35**(8 Suppl): 286–291.
24. Levinac J. Periimplantation osteolysis – periimplantosis – periimplantitis. *Rev Fr Odontostomatol* 1965; **12**(8): 1251–1260.
25. Lang NP. Proceedings on the 1st European Workshop on Periodontology. Karring, T (ed). Quintessence Publishing Co 1994.
26. Albrektsson T, Dahlin C, Jemt T, *et al.* Is marginal bone loss around oral implants the result of a provoked foreign body reaction? *Clin Implant Dent Relat Res* 2014; **16**(2): 155–165.
27. Koka S, Zarb G. On osseointegration: the healing adaptation principle in the context of osseosufficiency, osseoseparation, and dental implant failure. *Int J Prosthodont* 2012: **25**: 48–52.
28. Ehrlich G, Arciola C. From Koch's postulates to biofilm theory. The lesson of Bill Costerton. *Int J Artif Organs* 2012; **35**(10): 695–699.
29. Costerton J, Sterwar P, Greenberg E. Bacterial biofilms: a common cause of persistent infections. *Science* 1999; **284**(5418): 1318–1322.
30. Sangeeta D. Biofilm and dental implant: the microbial link. *J Ind Soc Periodontol* 2013; **17**(1): 5–11.
31. Kalykakis G, Nissengard, R. Clinical and microbial findings on osseointegrated implants, comparison between partially dentate and edentulous subjects. *Eur J Prosth Rest Dent* 1998; **6**: 155–159.
32. Ong C, Ivanovski S, Needleman I. Systematic review of implant outcomes in treated periodontitis subjects. *J Clin Periodontol* 2008; **35**: 438–462.
33. Lindhe J, Meyle J. Group D of European Workshop on Periodontology. Peri-implant diseases: Consensus Report of the Sixth European Workshop on Periodontology. *J Clin Periodontol* 2008; **35**(8 Suppl): 282–285.
34. Canullo L, Schlee M, Wagner W, *et al.* International Brainstorming Meeting on Etiologic and Risk Factors of Peri-implantitis, Montegrotto (Padua, Italy), August 2014. *Int J Oral Maxillofac Implants* 2015; **30**(5): 1093–1104.
35. Froum S, Rosen P. A proposed classification for peri-implantitis. *Int J Periodontics Restorative Dent* 2012; **32**(5): 532–540.
36. Naert I, Duyck J, Vandamme K. Occlusal overload and bone/implant loss. *Clin Oral Implants Res* 2012: **23**(Suppl 6): 95–107.
37. Balshe A, Assad D, Eckert S, *et al.* A retrospective study of the survival of smooth- and rough-surface dental implants. *Int J Oral Maxillofac Implants* 2009; **24**: 1113–1118.
38. Goldstep, F. Periodontal Inflammation: simplified. *Oral Health* 2013; Dec: 8–17.
39. Casado P, Otazu I, Balduino A, *et al.* Identification of periodontal pathogens in healthy peri-implant sites. *Implant Dent* 2011; **20**(3): 226–235.
40. Cameron S, Joyce A, Brousseau J, *et al.* Radiographic verification of implant abutment seating. *J Prosthet Dent* 1998; **79**: 298–303.
41. Ormaechea M, Millstein P, Hirayama H. Tube angulation effect on radiographic analysis of the implant-abutment interface. *Int J Oral Maxillofac Implants* 1999; **14**: 77–85.
42. Lin K, Wadwani C, Cheng J, *et al.* Assessing fit at the implant-abutment junction with a radiographic device that does not require access to the implant body. *J Prosth Dent* 2014; **112**(4): 817–823.
43. Manzano-Moren F, Herrera-Briones FJ, Bassam T, *et al.* Factors affecting dental implant stability measured using the Ostell Mentor Device: a systematic review. *Implant Dent* 2015; **24**(5): 565–577.
44. Van Eekeren P, Said C, Tahmaseb A, *et al.* Resonance frequency analysis of thermal acid-etched, hydrophilic implants during first 3 months of healing and osseointegration in an early-loading protocol. *Int J Oral Maxillofac Implants* 2015; **30**(4): 843–850.
45. Loesche W, Lopatin D, Giordano J, *et al.* Comparison of the Benzoil-DL-arginine-naphthylamide (BANA) test, DNA probes, and immunological reagents for ability to detect anaerobic periodontal infections due to *Porphyromonas gingivalis, Treponema denticola*, and *Bacteroides forsythus. J Clin Microbiol* 1992; **30**(2): 427–433.
46. Tang Z, Cao C, Sha Y, *et al.* Effects of non-surgical treatment modalities on peri-implantitis. *Chinese J of Stomatology* 2002; **37**(3): 173–175.
47. Albertini M, Lopez-Cerero L, O'Sullivan M, *et al.* Assessment of periodontal and opportunistic flora in patients with peri-implantitis. *Clin Oral Implants Res* 2015; **26**(8): 937–941.
48. Greenstein G, Hart T. Clinical utility of a genetic susceptibility test for severe chronic periodontitis: a critical evaluation. *J Am Dent Assoc* 2002; **133**(4): 452–459.
49. Misch C, Perel M, Wang H, *et al.* Implant success, survival, and failure: the International Congress of Oral Implantologists (ICOI) Pisa Consensus Conference. *Implant Dent* 2008; **17**(1): 5–15.
50. Hall J, Pehrson N, Ekestubbe A, *et al.* Controlled, cross-sectional exploratory study on markers for the plasminogen system and inflammation in crevicular fluid samples from healthy, mucositis and peri-implantitis sites. *Eur J Oral Implantol* 2015; **8**(2): 153–166.

51. Noda K, Arakawa H, Maekawa K, *et al.* Identification of risk factors for fracture of veneering materials and screw loosening of implant-supported fixed partial dentures partially edentulous cases. *J Oral Rehabil* 2013; **40**: 214–220.
52. Gittelson, G. Occlusion, bruxism and dental implants: Diagnosis and treatment for success. *Dent Implantol Update* 2005; **16**: 17–24.
53. Teixeira F, de Assis Claro C, Neves A, *et al.* Influence of loading and use of occlusal splint in implant-supported fixed prostheses. *J Crainiofac Surg* 2012; **23**: e477–e480.
54. Manfredini D, Bucci M, Sabattini V, *et al.* Bruxism: overview of current knowledge and suggestions for dental implants planning. *Cranio* 2011; **29**(4): 304–312.
55. Renvert S, Quirynen M. Risk indicators for peri-implantitis. A narrative review. *Clin Oral Implants Res* 2015; **26**(Suppl 11): 15–44.
56. Misch, C. Stress treatment theorem for implant dentistry. In: *Contemporary Implant Dentistry* 3rd edn. Mosby: Elsevier 2008; 68–91.
57. Furst M, Salvi G, Lang N. Bacterial colonization immediately after installation of oral titanium implants. *Clin Oral Implants Res* 2007; **18**: 501–508.
58. Teughels W, Van Assche N. Effect of material characteristics and surface topography on biofilm development. *Clin Oral Implants Res* 2006; **17**: 68–81.
59. Lindhe J, Berglundh T, Ericsson I, *et al.* Experimental breakdown of peri-implant infections. *Clin Oral implants Res* 1992; **3**: 162–168.
60. Socransky S, Haffajee A, Cugini M. Microbial complexes in subgingival plaque. *J Clin Periodontol* 1998; **25**: 134–144.
61. Blankenship J, Mitchell A. How to build a biofilm: a fungal perspective. *Curr Opin Microbiol* 2006; **19**: 342–347.
62. Ong C, Ivanovski S, Needleman I. Systematic review of implant outcomes in treated periodontitis subjects. *J Clin Periodontol* 2008; **35**: 438–462.
63. Karousis I, Fourmousis I. A comprehensive and critical review of dental implant prognosis in periodontally compromised partially edentulous patients. *Clin Oral Implant Res* 2007; **6**: 669–679.
64. Karousis I, Salvi G, Heitz-Mayfield L. Long term prognosis in patients with and without a history of chronic periodontitis: a 10 year prospective cohort study of the ITI dental implant system *Clin Oral Implants Res* 2003: **14**: 329–339.
65. Binon P. Evaluation of machining accuracy and consistency of selected implants, selected abutments, and laboratory analogs. *Int J Prosthodon* 1995; **8**: 162–178.
66. Rangert B, Jemt T, Jorneus L. Forces and moments on Brånemark implants. *Int J Oral Maxillofac Implants* 1989; **4**: 241–247.
67. Brunski J, Skalak R. Biomechanical considerations for osseointegrated fixtures. In: Worthington P, Brånemark PI (eds). *Advanced Osseointegration Surgery: Applications in the Maxillofacial Region.* Chicago: Quintessence Publishing Co 1992; 15–39.
68. Preiskel H, Tsoika P. Cement- and screw-retained implant-supported prostheses: up to 10 years of follow-up of a new design. *Int J Oral Maxillofac Implants* 2004; **19**(1): 87–91.
69. Michalakis K, Pissiotis A, Hirayama H. Cement failure loads of 4 provisional luting agents used for the cementation of implant-supported fixed partial dentures. *Int J Oral Maxillofac Implants* 2000; **15**: 545–549.
70. Burbano M, Wilson T, Valderrama P, *et al.* Characterization of cement particles found in peri-implantitis – affected human biopsy specimens. *Int J Oral Maxillofac Implants* 2015; **30**(5): 1168–1173.
71. Korsch M, Robra B, Walther W. Cement-associated signs of inflammation: retrospective analysis of the effect of excess cement on peri-implant tissue. *Int J Prosthodont* 2015: **28**(1): 11–18.
72. Sones A. Complications with osseointegrated implants. *J Prosthet Dent* 1989; **62**: 581–585
73. Jemt T, Book K. Prosthesis misfit and marginal bone loss in edentulous implant patients. *Int J Oral Maxillofac Implants* 1996; **11**: 620–625.
74. Jemt T, Rubenstein J, Carlsson L, *et al.* Measuring fit at the implant prosthodontic interface. *J Prosthet Dent* 1996; **75**: 314–325.
75. Linkevicius T, Vindasiute E, Puisys A, *et al.* The influence of the cementation margin position on the amount of undetected cement. A prospective clinical study. *Clin Oral Implants Res* 2013; **24**(1): 71–76.
76. Touati B. Major factors affecting hard and soft tissue remodeling around implants. NobelBiocare Global Symposium, June 2013. New York, NY.
77. al-Turki L, Chai J, Lautenschlager E, *et al.* Changes in prosthetic screw stability because of misfit of implant-supported prostheses. *Int J Prosthodont* 2002; **15**: 38–42.
78. Van Velzen FJ, Lang N, Schulten E, *et al.* CM Dental floss as a possible risk for the development of peri-implant disease: an observational study of 10 cases. *Clin Oral Implants Res* 2016; **27**(5): 618–621.
79. Glossary of Prosthodontic Terms, 8th edn. Academy of Prosthodontics. *J Prosthet Dent* 2005; **94**(1): 10–92.
80. Taylor T. Occlusal concepts for long-term success in implant dentistry. ACP Prosth Review Course, 2015 San Francisco, CA.
81. Han H, Kim, Han D. Multifactorial evaluation of implant failure: a 19-year retrospective study. *Int J Oral Maxillofac Implants* 2014; **29**: 303–310.
82. Chrcanovic B, Albrektsson T, Wennerberg A. Reasons for failures of oral implants. *J Oral Rehab* 2014; **41**: 443–476.
83. Zarb G. On parafunctional considerations in implant therapy. *Int J Prosthodont* 2014; **27**(3): 199.
84. Cardoso L de C, Luvizuto E, Trevisan C, *et al.* Resolution of a titanium implant fracture after a recurrent trauma. *Dent Traumatol* 2010; **26**(6): 512–515.
85. Flanagan D. External and occlusal trauma to dental implants and a case report. *Dent Traumatol* 2003; **19**(3): 160–164.
86. Daftary F, Mahallati R, Bahat O, *et al.* Lifelong craniofacial growth and the implications for osseointegrated implants. *Int J Oral Maxillofac Implants* 2013; **28**(1): 163–169.
87. Davis W, Lam P, Marshall M, *et al.* Using restorations borne totally by anterior implants to preserve the edentulous mandible. *J Am Dent Assoc* 1999; **130**(8): 1183–1189.
88. Jacobs R, Schotte A, van Steenberghe D, *et al.* Posterior jaw bone resorption in osseointegrated implant-supported overdentures. *Clin Oral Implants Res* 1992; **3**(2): 63–70.
89. Huang C, Ogawa R. Mechanotransduction in bone repair and regeneration. *FASEB J* 2010; **24**(10): 3625–3632.
90. Sheets C, Earthman J. Natural tooth intrusion and reversal in implant-assisted prostheses: evidence of and a hypothesis for the occurrence. *J Prosthet Dent* 1993; **70**: 513–520.

91. Sheets C, Earthman J. Tooth intrusion in implant-assisted prostheses. *J Prosthet Dent* 1997; **77**: 39–45.
92. Block M, Lirette D, Gardiner D, *et al.* Prospective evaluation of implants connected to teeth. *Int J Oral Maxillofac Implants* 2002; **17**(4): 473–487.
93. Pjetursson B, Bragger U, Lang N, *et al.* Comparison of survival and complication rates of tooth-supported fixed dental prostheses (FPDs) and implant-supported FDPs and single crowns (SCs). *Clin Oral Implants Res* 2007; **18**(Suppl 3): 97–113.
94. Taylor T, Klotz M, Lawton R. Titanium tattooing associated with zirconia implant abutments: a clinical report of two cases. *Int J Oral Maxillofac Implants* 2014: **29**(4): 958–960.
95. Lazarovici T, Yahalom R, Taicher S, *et al.* Bisphosphonate-related osteonecrosis of the jaw associated with dental implants. *J Oral Maxillofac Surg* 2010; **68**(4): 790–796.
96. Pazianas M, Miller P, Blumentals W, *et al.* A review of the literature on osteonecrosis of the jaw in patients with osteoporosis treated with oral bisphosphonates: prevalence, risk factors, and clinical characteristics. *Clin Ther* 2007; **29**(8): 1548–1558.
97. Grant B, Amenedo C, Freeman K, *et al.* Outcomes of placing dental implants in patients taking oral bisphosphonates: a review of 115 cases. *J Oral Maxillofac Surg* 2008; **66**(2): 223–230.
98. Koka S, Babu N, Norell A. Survival of dental implants in post-menopausal bisphosphonate users. *J Prosthodont Res*; **54**(3): 108–111.
99. Wu X, Al-Abedalia K, Rastikerdar E, *et al.* Selective serotonin reuptake inhibitors and the risk of osseointegrated implant failure: a cohort study. *J Dent Res* 2014; **93**(11): 1054–1061.
100. Clementini M, Rossetti P, Penarrocha D, *et al.* Systemic risk factors for peri-implant bone loss: a systematic review and meta-analysis. *Int J Oral Maxilllofac Surg* 2014; **43**(3): 323–334.
101. Ekfeldt A, Christiansson U, Eriksson T, *et al.* A retrospective analysis of factors associated with multiple implant failures in maxillae. *Clin Oral Implants Res* 2001: **12**(5): 462–467.
102. Hornecker E, Muuss T, Ehrenreich H, *et al.* A pilot study on the oral conditions of severely alcohol addicted persons *J Contemp Dent Pract* 2003; **4**(2): 51–59.
103. Balshe A, Assad D, Eckert S, *et al.* The effects of smoking on the survival of smooth- and rough-surface dental implants. *Int J Oral Maxillofac Implants* 2008; **23**: 1117–1122.
104. Barao V, Ricomini-Filho A, Faverani L, *et al.* The role of nicotine, cotinine, and caffeine on the electrochemical behavior and bacterial colonization to cp-Ti. *Mater Sci Eng C Mater Biol Appl* 2015; **56**: 114–124.
105. Tsiquarida A, Dabdoub S, Nagaraja H, *et al.* The influence of smoking on the peri-implant microbiome. *J Dent Res* 2015; **94**(9); 1202–1217.
106. Sugerman P, Barber M. Patient selection for endosseous dental implants: oral and systemic considerations. *Int J Oral Maxillofac Implants* 2002; **17**(2): 191–201.
107. Muller F. Prosthodontics for multimorbid and frail elders. Abstracts from the 2015 ICP Meeting's Special Session on Geriatrics in Seoul, Korea. *Int J Prosthodont* 2015; **28**(5): 466.
108. Epstein J, Beier Jensen S. Management of hyposalivation and xerostomia: criteria for treatment strategies. *Compend Contin Educ Dent* 2015; **36**(8): 600–603.
109. Muller, F. Interventions for edentate elders – what is the evidence? *Gerodontology* 2014; **31**(Suppl 1): 44–51.
110. Isidor F, Brøndum K, Hansen H. Outcome of treatment with implant-retained dental prostheses in patients with Sjögren syndrome. *Int J Oral Maxillofac Implants* 1999; **14**(5): 736–743.
111. Fitzpatrick, B. Accommodating frail patients in a prosthodontic practice. Abstracts from the 2015 ICP Meeting's Special Session on Geriatrics in Seoul, Korea. *Int J Prosthodont* 2015; **28**(5): 466.
112. Bornstein M, Cionca N, Mombelli A. Systemic conditions and treatments as risks for implant therapy. *Int J Oral Maxillofac Implants* 2009; **24**(Suppl): 12–27.
113. Gomez-Moreno G, Aguilar-Salvatierra A, Rubio Roldan J, *et al.* Peri-implant evaluation in type 2 diabetes mellitus patients: a 3-year study. *Clin Oral Implants Res* 2015; **26**(9): 1031–1035.
114. Retzepi M, Donos N. The effect of diabetes mellitus on osseous healing. *Clin Oral Implants Res* 2010; **21**(7): 673–681.
115. Daubert D, Weinstein B, Bordin S, *et al.* Prevalence and predictive factors for peri-implant disease and implant failure: a cross sectional analysis. *J Periodontol* 2015; **86**(3): 337–347.
116. Bassetti M, Kaufmann R, Salvi G. Soft tissue grafting to improve the attached mucosa at dental implants: a review of the literature and proposal of a decision tree. *Quintessence Int* 2015; **46**(6): 499–510.
117. Cox J, Zarb G. The longitudinal clinical efficacy of osseointegrated dental implants. *Int J Oral Maxillofac Implants* 1987; **2**: 91–99.
118. Rungcharassaeng K, Kan J, Yoshino S. Immediate implant placement and provisionalization with and without a connective tissue graft: an analysis of facial gingival tissue thickness. *Int J Periodontics Restorative Dent* 2012; **32**(6): 657–663.
119. Tsuda H, Rungcharassaeng K, Kan J. Peri-implant tissue response following connective tissue and bone grafting in conjunction with immediate single-tooth replacement in the esthetic zone: a case series. *Int J Oral Maxillofac Implants* 2011; **26**(2): 427–436.
120. Kan J, Rungcharassaeng K, Lozada J. Facial gingival tissue stability following immediate placement and provisionalization of maxillary anterior single implants: a 2- to 8-year follow-up. *Int J Oral Maxillofac Implants* 2011; **26**(1): 179–187.
121. Berglundh T, Persson L, Klinge B. A systematic review of the incidence of biological and technical complications in implant dentistry reported in prospective longitudinal studies of at least 5 years. *J Clin Periodontol* 2002; **29**(Suppl 3): 197–212.
122. Zitzman N, Berglundh T. Definition and prevalence of peri-implant diseases. *J Clin Periodontol* 2008; **35**(Suppl 8): 286–291.
123. Mombelli A, Muller N, Cionca N. The epidemiology of peri-implantitis. *Clin Oral Implants Res* 2012; **23**(Suppl 6): 67-76.
124. Atieh M, Alsabeeha N, Faggion C, *et al.* The frequency of peri-implant diseases: a systematic review and meta-analysis. *J Periodontol* 2013; **84**(11): 1586–1598.
125. Derks J, Tomasi C. Peri-implant health and disease. A systematic review of current epidemiology. *J Clin Periodontol* 2015; **42**(Suppl 16): S158–171.
126. Koldsland O, Scheie A, Aass A. Prevalence of peri-implantitis related to severity of the disease with different degrees of bone loss. *J Periodontol* 2010; **81**(2): 231–238.
127. Macthei, E. Treatment alternatives to negotiate peri-implantitis. *Advances in Medicine* 2014, Article ID 487903.
128. Renvert S, Widén C, Persson G. Cytokine expression in peri-implant crevicular fluid in relation to bacterial presence. *J Clin Periodontol* 2015; **42**(7): 697–702.

129. Ata-Ali J, Flichy-Fernández A, Alegre-Domingo T. Clinical, microbiological, and immunological aspects of healthy versus peri-implantitis tissue in full arch reconstruction patients: a prospective cross-sectional study. *BMC Oral Health* 2015; **15**: 43.
130. de Araújo M, Filho A, da Silva G. Evaluation of peri-implant mucosa: clinical, histopathological and immunological aspects. *Arch Oral Biol* 2014; **59**(5): 470–478.
131. Recker E, Avila-Ortiz G, Fischer C. A cross-sectional assessment of biomarker levels around implants versus natural teeth in periodontal maintenance patients. *J Periodontol* 2015; **86**(2): 264–272.
132. Faot F, Nascimento G, Bielemann A. Can peri-implant crevicular fluid assist in the diagnosis of peri-implantitis? A systematic review and meta-analysis. *J Periodontol* 2015; **86**(5): 631–645.
133. Nishimura K, Kato T, Ito T, *et al.* Influence of titanium ions on cytokine levels of murine splenocytes stimulated with periodontopathic bacterial lipopolysaccharide. *Int J Oral Maxillofac Implants* 2014; **29**(2): 472–477.
134. Wachi T, Shuto T, Shinohara Y. Release of titanium ions from an implant surface and their effect on cytokine production related to alveolar bone resorption. *Toxicology* 2015; **327**: 1–9.
135. Kasemo B, Lausmaa J. Metal selection and surface characteristics. In: Brånemark PI, Zarb G, Albrektsson T (eds). *Tissue-Integrated Prostheses*. Chicago: Quintessence Publishing Inc 1985; 107.
136. Rosen P, Clem D, Cochran D, *et al.* Peri-implant mucositis and peri-implantitis: a current understanding of their diagnoses and clinical implications. *J Periodontol* 2013; **84**(4): 440.
137. Suarez F, Monje A, Galindo-Moreno P, *et al.* Implant surface detoxification: a comprehensive review. *Implant Dent* 2013; **22**(5): 465–473.
138. Atieh M, Alsabeeha N, Faggion C, *et al.* The frequency of peri-implant diseases: a systematic review and meta-analysis. *J Periodontol* 2013; **84**(11): 1586–1598.
139. Gabay E, Levin L, Zuabi O, *et al.* Plaque score change as an indicator for peri-implant health in periodontal patients with immediately restored dental implants. *Implant Dent* 2015; **24**(3): 323–327.
140. Matarasso S, Quaremba G, Coraggio F, *et al.* Maintenance of implants: an in vitro study of titanium implant surface modifications subsequent to the application of different prophylaxis procedures. *Clin Oral Implants Res* 1996; **7**(1): 64–72.
141. Louropoulou A, Slot D, Van der Weijden F. Influence of mechanical instruments on the biocompatibility of titanium dental implants surfaces: a systematic review. *Clin Oral Implants Res* 2015; **6**(7): 841–850.
142. Schwarz F, Becker K, Renvert S. Efficacy of air polishing for the non-surgical treatment of peri-implant diseases: a systematic review. *J Clin Periodontol* 2015; **42**(10): 951–959.
143. Tastepe C, van Waas R, Liu Y, *et al.* Air powder abrasive treatment as an implant surface cleaning method: a literature review. *Int J Oral Maxillofac Implants* 2012; **27**(6): 1461–1473.
144. Mengel R, Buns C, Mengel C, *et al.* An in vitro study of the treatment of implant surfaces with different instruments. *Int J Oral Maxillofac Implants* 1998; **13**(1): 91–96.
145. Chairay J, Boulekbache H, Jean A, *et al.* Scanning electron microscopic evaluation of the effects of an air-abrasive system on dental implants: a comparative in vitro study between machined and plasma-sprayed titanium surfaces. *J Periodontol* 1997; **68**(12): 1215–1222.
146. Mouhyi J, Sennerby L, Pireaux J, *et al.* An XPS and SEM evaluation of six chemical and physical techniques for cleaning of contaminated titanium implants. *Clin Oral Implants Res* 1998; **9**(3): 185–194.
147. Duarte P, Reis A, de Freitas P, *et al.* Bacterial adhesion on smooth and rough titanium surfaces after treatment with different instruments. *J Periodontol* 2009; **80**(11): 1824–1832.
148. Schou S, Holmstrup P, Jørgensen T, *et al.* Implant surface preparation in the surgical treatment of experimental peri-implantitis with autogenous bone graft and ePTFE membrane in cynomolgus monkeys. *Clin Oral Implants Res* 2003; **14**(4): 412–422.
149. Froum S, Froum S, Rosen P. Successful management of peri-implantitis with a regenerative approach: a consecutive series of 51 treated implants with 3- to 7.5-year follow-up. *Int J Periodontics Restorative Dent* 2012; **32**(1): 11–20.
150. Finlayson R, Stevens F. Subcutaneous facial emphysema secondary to use of the Cavi-Jet. *J Periodontol* 1988; **59**(5): 315–317.
151. Bergendal T, Forsgren L, Kvint S, *et al.* The effect of an airbrasive instrument on soft and hard tissues around osseointegrated implants. A case report. *Swed Dent J* 1990; **14**(5): 219–223.
152. Ntrouka V, Hoogenkamp M, Zaura E. The effect of chemotherapeutic agents on titanium-adherent biofilms. *Clin Oral Implants Res* 2011; **22**(11): 1227–1234.
153. Wohlfahrt J, Lyngstadaas S, Rønold H, *et al.* Porous titanium granules in the surgical treatment of peri-implant osseous defects: a randomized clinical trial. *Int J Oral Maxillofac Implants* 2012; **27**(2): 401–410.
154. Kang J, Jang Y, Kim D, *et al.* Antimicrobial effectiveness of cetylpyridinium chloride and zinc chloride-containing mouthrinses on bacteria of halitosis and peri-implant disease. *Int J Oral Maxillofac Implants* 2015; **30**(6): 1341–1347.
155. Fernandez y Mostajo M, van der Reijden W, Buijs M, *et al.* Effect of an oxygenating agent on oral bacteria in vitro and on dental plaque composition in healthy young adults. *Front Cell Infect Microbiol* 2014; **4**: 95.
156. Gosau M, Hahnel S, Schwarz F, *et al.* Effect of six different peri-implantitis disinfection methods on in vivo human oral biofilm. *Clin Oral Implants Res* 2010; **21**(8): 866–872.
157. Alhag M, Renvert S, Polyzois I, *et al.* Re-osseointegration on rough implant surfaces previously coated with bacterial biofilm: an experimental study in the dog. *Clin Oral Implants Res* 2008; **19**(2): 182–187.
158. Heggers J, Sazy J, Stenberg B, *et al.* Bactericidal and wound healing properties of sodium hypochlorite solutions: the 1991 Lindberg Award. *J Burn Care Rehabil* 1991; **12**(5): 420–424.
159. Slots J. Selection of antimicrobial agents in periodontal therapy. *J Periodontol Res* 2002; **37**(5): 389–398.
160. Ferreira C, Babu J, Tipton D. Assessment of the effect of chemical agents used in dentistry on the removal of *Porphyromonas gingivalis* and *Escherichia coli* from sandblasted acid-etched titanium dental implants: an *in vitro* study. *Int J Oral Maxillofac Implants* 2015; **30**(2): 299–307.
161. Cohen D, Atlas S. Chlorhexidine gluconate in periodontal treatment. *Compend Suppl* 1994; **18**: S711–713.
162. Dennison D, Huerzeler MB, Quinones C, *et al.* Contaminated implant surfaces: an in vitro comparison of implant surface

coating and treatment modalities for decontamination. *J Periodontol* 1994; **65**(10): 942–948.
163. Rath S, Singh M. Comparative clinical and microbiological efficacy of mouthwashes containing 0.2% and 0.12% chlorhexidine. *Dent Res J (Isfahan)* 2013; **10**(3): 364–369.
164. Heitz-Mayfield L, Salvi G, Botticelli D, *et al.* Anti-infective treatment of peri-implant mucositis: a randomised controlled clinical trial. *Clin Oral Implants Res* 2011; **22**(3): 237–241.
165. Levin L, Frankenthal S, Joseph L. Water jet with adjunct chlorhexidine gel for nonsurgical treatment of peri-implantitis. *Quintessence Int* 2015; **46**(2): 133–137.
166. Ros-Llor I, Lopez-Jornet P. Cytogenetic analysis of oral mucosa cells, induced by chlorhexidine, essential oils in ethanolic solution and triclosan mouthwashes. *Environ Res* 2014; **132**: 140–145.
167. Romanos G, Weitz D. Therapy of peri-implant diseases. Where is the evidence? *J Evid Based Dent Pract* 2012; **12**(3 Suppl): 204–208.
168. Hauser-Gerspach I, Vadaszan J, Deronjic I, *et al.* Influence of gaseous ozone in peri-implantitis: bactericidal efficacy and cellular response. An *in vitro* study using titanium and zirconia. *Clin Oral Investig* 2012; **16**(4): 1049–1059.
169. Flichy-Fernández A, Ata-Ali J, Alegre-Domingo T, *et al.* The effect of orally administered probiotic Lactobacillus reuteri-containing tablets in peri-implant mucositis: a double-blind randomized controlled trial. *J Periodontal Res* 2015; **50**(6): 775–785.
170. Dagli N, Dagli R, Mahmoud R, *et al.* Essential oils, their therapeutic properties, and implication in dentistry: a review. *J Int Soc Prev Community Dent* 2015; **5**(5): 335–340.
171. Thosar N, Basak S, Bahadure R, *et al.* Antimicrobial efficacy of five essential oils against oral pathogens: an in vitro study. *Eur J Dent* 2013; **7**(Suppl 1): S71–77.
172. Mertas A, Garbusińska A, Szliszka E. The influence of tea tree oil on fluconazole activity against fluconazole-resistant *Candida albicans* strains. *Biomed Res Int* 2015; 590470.
173. Roos-Jansåker A, Almhöjd U, Jansson H. Treatment of peri-implantitis: clinical outcome of chloramine as an adjunctive to non-surgical therapy, a randomized clinical trial. *Clin Oral Implants Res* 2015 May 26; doi: 10.1111/clr.12612. [Epub ahead of print]
174. Mor-Reinoso C, Pascual A, Nart J, *et al.* Inhibition of de novo plaque growth by a new 0.03 % chlorhexidine mouth rinse formulation applying a non-brushing model: a randomized, double blind clinical trial. *Clin Oral Investig* 2015 Oct 17. [Epub ahead of print]
175. Ricardo R, Ney S, Marco A, *et al.* Comparative study between the effects of photodynamic therapy and conventional therapy on microbial reduction in ligature-induced peri-implantitis in dogs. *J Periodontol* 2005; **76**: 1275–1281.
176. Javed F, Romanos GE. Does photodynamic therapy enhance standard antibacterial therapy in dentistry? *Photomed Laser Surg* 2013; **31**(11): 512–518.
177. Periowave Photodynamic Disinfection System User Manual (Ondine Biopharma Corporation, Vancouver, BC, Canada) 2010: 8–9.
178. Haas R, Dörtbudak O, Mensdorff-Pouilly N, *et al.* Elimination of bacteria on different implant surfaces through photosensitization and soft laser. An *in vitro* study. *Clin Oral Implants Res* 1997; **8**: 249–254.
179. Dörtbudak O, Haas R, Bernhart, *et al.* Lethal photosensitization for decontamination of implant surfaces in the treatment of peri-implantitis. *Clin Oral Implants Res* 2001; **12**: 104–108.
180. Thierbach R, Eger T. Clinical outcome of a nonsurgical and surgical treatment protocol in different types of peri-implantitis: a case series. *Quintessence Int* 2013; **44**(2): 137–148.
181. Esposito M, Grusovin MG, De Angelis N. The adjunctive use of light-activated disinfection (LAD) with FotoSan is ineffective in the treatment of peri-implantitis: 1-year results from a multicentre pragmatic randomised controlled trial. *Eur J Oral Implantol* 2013; **6**(2): 109–119.
182. Mettraux G, Sculean A, Burgin W. Two-year clinical outcomes following non-surgical mechanical therapy of peri-implantitis with adjunctive diode laser application. *Clin Oral Implants Res* 2015 Sep 16. doi: 10.1111/clr.12689. [Epub ahead of print]
183. Lerario F, Roncati M, Gariffo A, *et al.* Non-surgical periodontal treatment of peri-implant diseases with the adjunctive use of diode laser: preliminary clinical study. *Lasers Med Sci* 2016: **31**(3): 1–6.
184. Arısan V, Karabuda Z, Arıcı S, *et al.* A randomized clinical trial of an adjunct diode laser application for the nonsurgical treatment of peri-implantitis. *Photomed Laser Surg* 2015; **33**(11): 547–554.
185. Natto Z, Aladmawy M, Levi P Jr, *et al.* Comparison of the efficacy of different types of lasers for the treatment of peri-implantitis: a systematic review. *Int J Oral Maxillofac Implants* 2015; **30**(2): 338–345.
186. Kotsakis G, Konstantinidis I, Karoussis I, *et al.* Systematic review and meta-analysis of the effect of various laser wavelengths in the treatment of peri-implantitis. *J Periodontol* 2014; **85**(9): 1203–1213.
187. Mailoa J, Lin G, Chan H, *et al.* Clinical outcomes of using lasers for peri-implantitis surface detoxification: a systematic review and meta-analysis. *J Periodontol* 2014; **85**(9): 1194–1202.
188. Izui S, Sekine S, Maeda K. Antibacterial activity of curcumin against periodontopathic bacteria. *J Periodontol* 2016; **87**(1): 83–90.
189. Shahzad M, Millhouse E, Culshaw S, *et al.* Selected dietary (poly) phenols inhibit periodontal pathogen growth and biofilm formation. *Food Funct* 2015; **6**(3): 719–729.
190. Boyanapalli S, Tony Kong A. "Curcumin, the King of Spices": epigenetic regulatory mechanisms in the prevention of cancer, neurological, and inflammatory diseases. *Curr Pharmacol Rep* 2015; **1**(2): 129–139.
191. Peedikayil F, Sreenivasan P, Narayanan A. Effect of coconut oil in plaque related gingivitis – a preliminary report. *Niger Med J* 2015; **56**(2): 143–147.
192. Asokan S, Emmadi P, Chamundeswari R. Effect of oil pulling on plaque induced gingivitis: a randomized, controlled, triple-blind study. *Indian J Dent Res* 2009; **20**(1): 47–51.
193. Mombelli A, Feloutzis A, Brägger U, *et al.* Treatment of peri-implantitis by local delivery of tetracycline. Clinical, microbiological and radiological results. *Clin Oral Implants Res* 2001; **12**(4): 287–294.
194. Flanagan D. Calcium hydroxide paste as a surface detoxifying agent for infected dental implants: two case reports. *J Oral Implantol* 2009; **35**(4): 204–209.
195. Renvert S, Lessem J, Dahlén G, *et al.* Topical minocycline microspheres versus topical chlorhexidine gel as an adjunct to mechanical debridement of incipient peri-implant infections: a randomized clinical trial. *J Clin Periodontol* 2006; **33**(5): 362–369.
196. Faramarzi M, Goharfar Z, Pourabbas R, *et al.* Microbiological and clinical effects of enamel matrix derivative and sustained release micro-spherical minocycline application as an adjunct to

non-surgical therapy in peri-implant mucosal inflammation. *J Korean Assoc Oral Maxilllofac Surg* 2015; **41**(4): 181–189.
197. Salvi G, Persson G, Heitz-Mayfield L. Adjunctive local antibiotic therapy in the treatment of peri-implantitis II: clinical and radiographic outcomes. *Clin Oral Implants Res* 2007; **18**(3): 281–285.
198. Schär D, Ramseier C, Eick S. Anti-infective therapy of peri-implantitis with adjunctive local drug delivery or photodynamic therapy: six-month outcomes of a prospective randomized clinical trial. *Clin Oral Implants Res* 2013; **24**(1): 104–110.
199. Stellini E, Migliorato A, Mazzoleni S. Topical treatment of peri-implantitis with metronidazole dental gel 25%. Clinical analysis and microbiological control. *Minerva Stomatol* 2000; **49**(1–2): 59–67.
200. Mombelli A, Lang N. Antimicrobial treatment of peri-implant infections. *Clin Oral Implants Res* 1992; **3**: 162–168.
201. van Winkelhoff A. Antibiotics in the treatment of peri-implantitis. *Eur J Oral Implantol* 2012; **5**(Suppl): S43–50.
202. Javed F, Alghamdi A, Ahmed A, *et al.* Clinical efficacy of antibiotics in the treatment of peri-implantitis. *Int Dent J* 2013; **63**(4): 169–176.
203. Hallström H, Persson G, Lindgren S, *et al.* Systemic antibiotics and debridement of peri-implant mucositis. A randomized clinical trial. *J Clin Periodontol* 2012; **39**(6): 574–581.
204. Rams T, Degener J, van Winkelhoff A. Antibiotic resistance in human peri-implantitis microbiota. *Clin Oral Implants Res* 2014; **25**(1): 82–90.
205. Wang Y, Zhang Y, Jing D, *et al.* Enamel matrix derivative improves gingival fibroblast cell behavior cultured on titanium surfaces. *Clin Oral Investig* 2016; **20**(4): 685–695.
206. Qu Z, Andrukhov O, Laky M, *et al.* Effect of enamel matrix derivative on proliferation and differentiation of osteoblast cells grown on the titanium implant surface. *Oral Surg Oral Med Oral Pathol Oral Radiol Endod* 2011; **111**(4): 517–522.
207. Lang N, Wilson T, Corbet E. Biological complications with dental implants: their prevention, diagnosis and treatment. *Clin Oral Implants Res* 2000; **11**(Suppl 1): 146–155.
208. Esposito M, Grusovin G, Worthington H. Treatment of peri-implantitis: what interventions are effective? A Cochrane systematic review. *Eur J Oral Implantol* 2012; **5**(Suppl): S21–41.
209. Smeets R, Henningsen A, Jung O, *et al.* Definition, etiology, prevention and treatment of peri-implantitis – a review. *Head Face Med* 2014; **10**: 34.
210. Romeo E, Lops D, Chiapasco M, *et al.* Therapy of peri-implantitis with resective surgery. A 3-year clinical trial on rough screw-shaped oral implants. Part II: radiographic outcome. *Clin Oral Implants Res* 2007; **18**(2): 179–187.
211. Romeo E, Ghisolfi M, Murgolo N, *et al.* Therapy of peri-implantitis with resective surgery. A 3-year clinical trial on rough screw-shaped oral implants. Part I: clinical outcome. *Clin Oral Implants Res* 2005; **16**(1): 9–18.
212. Chan HL, Oh WS, Ong HS, *et al.* Impact of implantoplasty on strength of the implant–abutment complex. *Int J Oral Maxillofac Implants* 2013; **28**(6): 1530–1535.
213. de Waal YC1, Raghoebar GM, Huddleston Slater J, *et al.* Implant decontamination during surgical peri-implantitis treatment: a randomized, double-blind, placebo-controlled trial. *J Clin Periodontol* 2013; **40**(2): 186–195.
214. de Waal Y, Raghoebar G, Meijer H, *et al.* Implant decontamination with 2% chlorhexidine during surgical peri-implantitis treatment: a randomized, double-blind, controlled trial. *Clin Oral Implants Res* 2015; **26**(9): 1015–1023.
215. Carcuac O, Derks J, Charalampakis G, *et al.* Adjunctive systemic and local antimicrobial therapy in the surgical treatment of peri-implantitis: a randomized controlled clinical trial. *J Dent Res* 2016; **95**(1); 50–57.
216. Heitz-Mayfield L, Salvi G, Mombelli A, *et al.* Anti-infective surgical therapy of peri-implantitis. A 12-month prospective clinical study. Implant Complication Research Group. *Clin Oral Implants Res* 2012; **23**(2): 205–210.
217. Froum S, Froum S, Rosen P. Successful management of peri-implantitis with a regenerative approach: a consecutive series of 51 treated implants with 3- to 7.5-year follow-up. *Int J Periodontics Restorative Dent* 2012; **32**(1): 11–20.
218. Parma-Benfenati S, Roncati M, Galletti P, *et al.* Peri-implantitis treatment with a regenerative approach: clinical outcomes on re-entry. *Int J Periodontics Restorative Dent* 2015; **35**(5): 625–636.
219. Schwarz F, John G, Becker J. Reentry after combined surgical resective and regenerative therapy of advanced peri-implantitis: a retrospective analysis of five cases. *Int J Periodontics Restorative Dent* 2015; **35**(5): 647–653.
220. Bassi F, Poli P, Rancitelli D, *et al.* Surgical treatment of peri-implantitis: a 17-year follow-up clinical case report. *Case Rep Dent* 2015; 574676.
221. Schwarz F, John G, Sahm N, *et al.* Combined surgical resective and regenerative therapy for advanced peri-implantitis with concomitant soft tissue volume augmentation: a case report. *Int J Periodontics Restorative Dent* 2014; **34**(4): 489–495.
222. Lagervall M, Jansson L. Treatment outcome in patients with peri-implantitis in a periodontal clinic: a retrospective study. *J Periodontol* 2013; **84**(10): 1365–1373.
223. Froum S, Froum SH, Rosen P. A regenerative approach to the successful treatment of peri-implantitis: a consecutive series of 170 implants in 100 patients with 2- to 10-year follow-up. *Int J Periodontics Restorative Dent* 2015; **35**(6): 857–863.
224. Mijiritsky E, Yatzkaier G, Mazor Z, *et al.* The use of porous titanium granules for treatment of peri-implantitis lesions: preliminary clinical and radiographic results in humans. *Br Dent J* 2013; **214**(5): E13.
225. Jepsen K, Jepsen S, Laine M, *et al.* Reconstruction of peri-implant osseous defects: a multicenter randomized trial. *J Dent Res* 2015 Oct 8. pii: 0022034515610056.
226. Valderrama P, Blansett J, Gonzalez M, *et al.* Detoxification of implant surfaces affected by peri-implant disease: an overview of non-surgical methods. *Open Dent J* 2014; **8**: 77–84.
227. Serino G, Turri A. Outcome of surgical treatment of peri-implantitis: results from a 2-year prospective clinical study in humans. *Clin Oral Implants Res* 2011; **22**(11): 1214–1220.
228. de Waal Y, Raqhoebar G, Meijer H, *et al.* Prognostic indicators for surgical peri-implantitis treatment. *Clin Oral Implants Res* 2015 Mar 29. doi: 10.1111/clr.12584. [Epub ahead of print]
229. Bergmann R. Occlusal considerations for dental implant restorations. *Compend Contin Educ Dent* 2014; **35**(7): 455–458.
230. Michalakis K, Hirayama H, Garefis P. Cement-retained versus screw-retained implant restorations: a critical review. *Int J Oral Maxillofac Implants* 2003; **18**(5): 719–728.
231. Lee A, Okayasu K, Wang H. Screw- versus cement-retained implant restorations: current concepts. *Implant Dent* 2010; **19**(1): 8–15.
232. Korsch M, Robra B, Walther W. Cement-associated signs of inflammation: retrospective analysis of the effect of excess cement on peri-implant tissue. *Int J Prosthodont* 2015; **28**(1): 11–18.

233. Boeckh C, Schumacher E, Podbielski A, et al. Antibacterial activity of restorative dental biomaterials in vitro. *Caries Res* 2002; **36**(2): 101–107.
234. Yanikoğlu N, Yeşil Duymuş Z. Evaluation of the solubility of dental cements in artificial saliva of different pH values. *Dent Mater J* 2007; **26**(1): 62–67.
235. Wilson T. The positive relationship between excess cement and peri-implant disease: a prospective clinical endoscopic study. *J Periodontol* 2009; **80**(9): 1388–1392.
236. Wadhwani C, Rapoport D, La Rosa S, *et al.* Radiographic detection and characteristic patterns of residual excess cement associated with cement-retained implant restorations: a clinical report. *J Prosthet Dent* 2012; **107**(3): 151–157.
237. Kucey B, Fraser D. The Procera abutment – the fifth generation abutment for dental implants. *J Can Dent Assoc* 2000; **66**(8): 445–449.
238. Linkevicius T, Puisys A, Vindasiute E, *et al.* Does residual cement around implant-supported restorations cause peri-implant disease? A retrospective case analysis. *Clin Oral Implants Res* 2013; **24**(11): 1179–1184.
239. Hürzeler M, Fickl S, Zuhr O, *et al.* Peri-implant bone level around implants with platform-switched abutments: preliminary data from a prospective study. *J Oral Maxillofac Surg* 2007; **65**(7 Suppl 1): 33–39.
240. Stafford G. Platform switching of implants may decrease bone loss. *Evid Based Dent* 2015; **16**(3): 84–85.
241. Vindasiute E, Puisys A, Maslova N, *et al.* Clinical factors influencing removal of the cement excess in implant-supported restorations. *Clin Implant Dent Relat Res* 2015; **17**(4): 771–778.
242. Wadhwani C, Piñeyro A, Hess T, *et al.* Effect of implant abutment modification on the extrusion of excess cement at the crown-abutment margin for cement-retained implant restorations. *Int J Oral Maxillofac Implants* 2011; **26**(6): 1241–1246.
243. Theoharidou A, Petridis H, Tzannas K, *et al.* Abutment screw loosening in single-implant restorations: a systematic review. *Int J Oral Maxillofac Implants* 2008; **23**(4): 681–690.
244. Wittneben JG, Millen C, Brägger U. Clinical performance of screw- versus cement-retained fixed implant-supported reconstructions – a systematic review. *Int J Oral Maxillofac Implants* 2014; **29**(Suppl): 84–98.
245. Gracis S, Michalakis K, Vigolo P, *et al.* Internal vs. external connections for abutments/reconstructions: a systematic review. *Clin Oral Implants Res* 2012; **23**(Suppl 6): 202–216.
246. Kucey B. Implant placement in prosthodontics practice: a five-year retrospective study. *J Prosthet Dent* 1997; **77**(2): 175.
247. Guichet D, Yoshinobu D, Caputo A. Effect of splinting and interproximal contact tightness on load transfer by implant restorations. *J Prosthet Dent* 2002; **87**(5): 528–535.
248. Vigolo P, Mutinelli S, Zaccaria M, *et al.* Clinical evaluation of marginal bone level change around multiple adjacent implants restored with splinted and nonsplinted restorations: a 10-year randomized controlled trial. *Int J Oral Maxillofac Implants* 2015; **30**(2): 411–418.
249. Monteiro D, Goiato M, Gennari Filho H, *et al.* Passivity in implant-supported prosthesis. *J Craniofac Surg* 2010; **21**(6): 2026–2029.
250. Charalampakis G, Rabe P, Leonhardt A, *et al.* A follow-up study of peri-implantitis cases after treatment. *J Clin Periodontol* 2011; **38**(9): 864–871.
251. Machtei E. What do we do after an implant fails? A review of treatment alternatives for failed implants. *Int J Periodontics Restorative Dent* 2013; **33**(4): e111–119.
252. Manzoor B, Suleiman M, Palmer R. The effects of simulated bone loss on the implant-abutment assembly and likelihood of fracture: an *in vitro* study. *Int J Oral Maxillofac Implants* 2013; **28**(3): 729–738.
253. Anitua E, Murias-Freijo A, Alkhraisat M. Conservative implant removal for the analysis of the cause, removal torque, and surface treatments of failed nonmobile dental implants. *J Oral Implantol* 2016; **42**(1): 69–77.
254. Mardinger O, Oubaid S, Manor Y. Factors affecting the decision to replace failed implants: a retrospective study. *J Periodontol* 2008; **79**(12): 2262–2266.
255. Grossmann Y, Levin L. Success and survival of single dental implants placed in sites of previously failed implants. *J Periodontol* 2007; **78**(9): 1670–1674.
256. Machtei E, Mahler D, Oettinger-Barak O, *et al.* Dental implants placed in previously failed sites: survival rate and factors affecting the outcome. *Clin Oral Implants Res* 2008; **19**(3): 259–264.
257. Alsaadi G, Quirynen M, van Steenberghe D. The importance of implant surface characteristics in the replacement of failed implants. *Int J Oral Maxillofac Implants* 2006; **21**(2): 270–274.
258. Gahan P, Swaminathan R. Circulating nucleic acids in plasma and serum. Recent developments. *Ann N Y Acad Sci* 2008; **1137**: 1–6.
259. Thaweboon B, Laohapand P, Amornchat C, *et al.* Host beta-globin gene fragments in crevicular fluid as a biomarker in periodontal health and disease. *J Periodontal Res* 2010; **45**(1): 38–44.
260. Doan T, Kriangcherdsak Y, Thaweboon S, *et al.* Evaluation of host β-Globin gene fragment lengths in peri-implant crevicular fluid during the wound healing process: a pilot study. *Int J Oral Maxillofac Implants* 2015; **30**(6): 1295–1302.

Epilogue

Shakespeare thought that a good play required no epilogue; therein lies the difference between fact and fiction. This seminal work is no play. It is devoted to facts, hard facts, with compelling evidence for each of the recommendations by the chapters' authors. Since the original osseointegration breakthroughs more than four decades back, techniques based upon folklore have been usurped by evidence-based approaches and therapeutic possibilities expanded exponentially.

Those of a certain experience can well remember the early days of what appeared to be a life-changing development, little short of a miracle. They will also remember washing implants with copious quantities of ethyl alcohol, avoiding postoperative radiographs, and treating any exposed implant surface as a surgical emergency. Early, let alone immediate, loading was to be avoided at all costs as were nonaxial forces. Treatment was confined to the edentulous mandible with osseointegration principally a surgical exercise; prosthodontic considerations were secondary. How things have changed!

Read about today's osseointegration applications in every aspect of prosthodontics, the revolution in imaging, treatment planning, and execution, together with the advent of digital technology. Our knowledge of nanotechnology, surface chemistry, and immunology extends rapidly. We venture into the maxillary sinuses, rebuild the facial skeleton, and make approaches undreamt of just a generation back. Maxillofacial prosthodontics has been revolutionized. Similarly implant site preparation and enhancement have progressed significantly. Such advances are unlikely to cease as the skill and ingenuity of new prosthodontists develop.

The Bard relied upon his unique astute observations of human behavior, a subject no clinician can afford to overlook. But we need more; the methodology we employ today must be objective and the instrumentation well proven, salient points made clear from the outset of the book.

Osseointegration is a valuable tool; it is not an icon before which all principles of prosthodontics can be sacrificed. Neither is osseointegration a complete substitute for the periodontal ligament that has taken millions of years to develop. Those who thoughtlessly overprescribe jeopardize this valuable treatment modality. So do colleagues who subscribe to the "Lived Happily Ever After" syndrome, ignoring the possibility that not all integrations succeed in the long term. Peri-implant complications can and do occur: some are predictable. All these factors are well covered in this book and deserve assiduous study.

Osseointegration represents more than an interim step before further development of regenerative medical and dental technology. It is likely to take its place side by side with regenerative science, like the internal combustion engine with its myriad of reciprocating components still providing sterling service after 150 years of development alongside the more recent turbine.

With 23 chapters authored by world-renowned experts, this text represents an unrivalled compendium of today's knowledge. For sure, techniques will be further refined, but the principles are likely to be with us for years to come.

Having read this work once, now return, dip into the chapters, and profit. Read them thoroughly and profit more. Understand the concepts and you will be a wiser clinician.

Harold Preiskel

Evidence-based Implant Treatment Planning and Clinical Protocols, First Edition. Edited by Steven J. Sadowsky.

Companion website: www.wiley.com/go/sadowsky/implant

Index

Notes: Page numbers in *italics* indicate figures and those in **bold** denote tables and boxes.

Evidence-based Implant Treatment Planning and Clinical Protocols, First Edition. Edited by Steven J. Sadowsky.

Companion website: www.wiley.com/go/sadowsky/implant